EVIDENCE-BASED PRACTICES
FOR SOCIAL WORKERS

Also available from Lyceum Books, Inc.

Advisory Editor: Thomas M. Meenaghan, *New York University*

MENTAL HEALTH IN LITERATURE, edited by Glenn Rohrer

USING EVIDENCE IN SOCIAL WORK PRACTICE: BEHAVIORAL PERSPEC-
TIVES, by Harold E. Briggs and Tina L. Rzepnicki

MODERN SOCIAL WORK THEORY: A CRITICAL INTRODUCTION, 3E, by
Malcolm Payne, foreword by Stephen C. Anderson

ENDINGS IN CLINICAL PRACTICE: EFFECTIVE CLOSURE IN DIVERSE SET-
TINGS, by Joseph Walsh

CLINICAL ASSESSMENT FOR SOCIAL WORKERS: QUALITATIVE AND QUAN-
TITATIVE METHODS, 2E, edited by Catheleen Jordan and Cynthia Franklin

A PRACTICAL GUIDE TO SOCIAL SERVICE EVALUATION, by Carl F. Brun

ADVOCACY PRACTICE FOR SOCIAL JUSTICE, by Richard Hoefer

USING STATISTICAL METHODS IN SOCIAL WORK PRACTICE WITH SPSS,
by Soleman H. Abu-Bader

ETHICS IN END-OF-LIFE DECISIONS FOR SOCIAL WORK PRACTICE, by
Ellen Csikai and Elizabeth Chaiten.

TEAMWORK IN MULTIPROFESSIONAL CARE, by Malcolm Payne, foreword
by Thomas M. Meenaghan

Evidence-Based Practices for Social Workers

An Interdisciplinary Approach

Thomas O'Hare

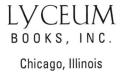

LYCEUM
BOOKS, INC.

Chicago, Illinois

Published by

Lyceum Books, Inc.
5758 S. Blackstone Ave.
Chicago, Illinois 60637
773+643-1903 (Fax)
773+643-1902 (Phone)
lyceum@lyceumbooks.com
http://www.lyceumbooks.com

Library of Congress Cataloging-in-Publication Data

O'Hare, Thomas.
    Evidence-based practices for social workers : an interdisciplinary approach /
Thomas O'Hare.
        p. cm.
    Includes bibliographical references and index.
    ISBN 0-925065-68-4
    1. Psychiatric social work. 2. Evidence-based psychiatry. I. Title.
HV689.043   2005
361.3′2—dc22

                                                            2005008943

For my loves: Peg, Matt, and Mick the One-Eared Wonder

.

CONTENTS

PREFACE

Thinking back over many years as a clinical practitioner, researcher, and social work instructor, I have had the opportunity to puzzle over a number of important and related questions: What are the causes of our clients' problems? How do we know which human behavior theories are valid? Is knowledge of risk factors useful in assessment? What is the best way to conduct an assessment? Outside of research, are scales really of any use in clinical practice? What theories explain how people change (with or without psychosocial interventions)? How do we determine which interventions are the most effective for our clients? Do effective practitioners use common methods even though they subscribe to different theories? What can the evaluation of a specific case teach us about the effectiveness of an intervention? What is the value of controlled practice research? Is the client's unique view of the problem an adequate basis for guiding practice decisions? If so, how can we make general recommendations about assessment or treatment effectiveness in order to teach, supervise, and evaluate practitioners?

Practicing clinical (direct practice) social work has become an increasingly challenging and complex enterprise. Not long ago, practitioners could comfortably embrace one or two practice theories, take their time engaging a client in treatment and working through some dilemma, and pay little heed to formal evaluation of client outcomes or treatment costs. But things have changed for most practicing social workers. Managed care, in both the private and public sectors, has become the norm, and with it, terms like *utilization review, cost effectiveness, manualized treatments*, and *best practices* have become part of the everyday practice lexicon. Clinical decisions are often heavily monitored, evaluated, and micromanaged. Many social workers are feeling a loss of control over their professional autonomy, and are having difficulty reconciling good practice with many of these administrative demands.

Within this transformed practice environment, social workers are increasingly required to use interventions supported by outcome research, and they must also evaluate the implementation of those efforts in everyday practice. However, practitioners and researchers often have widely disparate views regarding the relationship of assessment, intervention, and evaluation processes and methods. Some feel that the client's perspective should be sufficient for assessment; others see a need for practitioners to be knowledgeable about current science regarding serious psychosocial problems. Some see a need for strict application of "manualized" interventions; others dismiss the need to consult research findings at all. Some feel that evaluation of the individual case is sufficient for demonstrating practice effectiveness, yet others see a need for both individual and program evaluation methods to document positive outcomes. With full appreciation for the vagaries and complexities of daily practice as well as the need to inform and guide interventions with evidence, I have endeavored to strike a pragmatic balance in this text between flexibility and adherence to empirical guidelines in conducting routine assessment, intervention, and evaluation.

Evidence-based practice in social work is not a new theory or a new practice fad. In fact, it is not new at all. The emergence of evidence-based practice is a naturally evolving convergence of social work's pragmatic person-in-environment mission, the applied psychosocial sciences, and the growing demands for ethical, legal, and fiscal accountability. Because of its historically interdisciplinary emphasis on the interactions between psychological factors and social-environmental conditions, social work has a unique contribution to make toward the advancement of evidence-based practices. Given the transition from institutional to community services in many fields of practice, social workers can once again embrace their role as knowledge synthesizers and multiprofessional team leaders across all practice environments: mental health, substance abuse, child welfare, gerontology, forensic services, and others.

Because there is no universally accepted taxonomy of psychosocial problems, social work client groups tend to be represented in various texts by a hodgepodge of overlapping categories including psychiatric diagnoses, fields of practice, personal characteristics, referral source, and treatment environments. Although the helping professions must rely on psychiatric labeling for reimbursement, these categories are inadequate for defining complex problems that are largely psychosocial in origin (e.g., couple and family problems, childhood and adolescent behavior problems, adjustments to growing old, loneliness and homelessness, substance abuse, domestic violence). To accommodate this grab bag of client-defining characteristics, this book uses an amalgam of broad diagnostic and psychosocial problem categories that realistically reflect the way social work services are organized in the major fields of practice.

The purpose for writing this text was straightforward: *social workers need an organized evidence-based framework to help them conduct assessment, intervention, and evaluation with clients who have difficult and complex psychosocial problems.* Evidence-based practice (as defined in this book) requires critical thinking and flexibility guided by best evidence. The multidimensional and functional approach to assessment is designed to integrate knowledge of human behavior with an understanding of each client's experiences. Effective interventions require competence in evidence-based approaches combined with the ability to adapt core effective skills to each client's circumstances. Evaluation methods in this book address the need to monitor and evaluate interventions for each client as well as client data at the program level.

In part 1, the basic building blocks of evidence-based practice are defined and explained. In parts 2 and 3, these concepts and methods are applied to a range of serious psychosocial disorders of adults, children, and their families. Key theories, qualitative and quantitative assessment methods, intervention research, and descriptions of effective interventions are examined critically. Each chapter includes at least one case study to illustrate these principles and methods. These case studies are fictional, but inspired by real cases. They provide an opportunity for the student-practitioner to apply these concepts and methods as an intellectual exercise. The student should feel free to critique my analyses and intervention plans, and perhaps argue for alternative evidence-based strategies. Students are also encouraged to consider "what if" scenarios by making modifications to the client's psychosocial history or the presenting problem, or by including emergent crises that (as so often happens in real practice) occur in the middle of an otherwise well-planned intervention. To further their skills in assessment, intervention, and evaluation methods, however, student-practitioners must go beyond this text, and examine in greater detail many of the key references. As new evidence emerges, student-practitioners should also amend these findings and build upon these evidence-based models.

Parts 2 and 3 of this text include assessment instruments carefully chosen for their optimal balance of psychometric integrity and usefulness in practice. Although an array of other fine scales are available in the literature, most of those selected for this text are readily available in the public domain or from the cited authors for little or no fee. Additional instruments are in appendixes A–G. Appendix H contains details about where to obtain copies, scoring sheets, and other supporting materials as needed.

I do not claim to have the definitive view of evidence-based practice. Evidence-based practices and processes are emerging, and students, scholars, and practicing professionals should critique and debate the conceptualization of evidence-based practice put forth in this text. A basic assumption in this book is that open, honest, scholarly debate supported by testable and verifiable assertions is essential if evidence-based practice is to flourish. I feel privileged to have had the time to review, organize, and describe the contributions of many leading practitioner-researchers in social work and the allied helping professions. I consider all those contributors who respect the processes of practice scholarship to be colleagues. It was my purpose in writing this text to collate the best of the best, so that social work practitioners and others could apply these methods for the benefit of our clients in need. Lastly, since this text is the work of a single author, any inadvertent misrepresentations, omissions, or other errors are my sole responsibility.

Thomas O'Hare

PART ONE

DEFINING EVIDENCE-BASED PRACTICE
IN SOCIAL WORK

CHAPTER 1

DEFINITION, PROCESSES, AND PRINCIPLES

This first chapter provides an overview of some of the core concepts, processes, and principles that characterize evidence-based practice in social work (EBPSW). The key components of EBPSW at the clinical practice level are the main focus of this text and will be more thoroughly described in chapters 2–4, culminating in an outline of the critical EBPSW service plan.

THE TRADITIONAL PRACTICE-THEORY APPROACH TO SOCIAL WORK

Proponents of social work practice theories have struggled to one degree or another with three main questions. What is the nature of human problems and adaptation in the social environment? What interventions are most likely to ameliorate our clients' psychosocial problems and enhance their ability to cope? How can we tell if our efforts have been successful? Variants of practice theories (known as schools of thought, orientation) range from the conceptually specific to the general and abstract. They include psychodynamic and other personality theories, social cognitive theory and cognitive-behavioral interventions, various family systems theories and practices, general systems and ecosystems models, and, more recently, empowerment, solution-focused, and constructivist approaches. Students and practitioners typically use one or two preferred practice theories to guide assessment and intervention with their clients.

Practice theories vary considerably in the extent to which they address salient questions regarding human behavior theory, provide adequate detail to guide assessment and intervention methods, and use research and evaluation methods to support their theories and practices. For example, humanist, constructivist, empowerment, solution-focused, and strength-based models generally eschew human behavior research altogether, offer some practical techniques for enhancing client coping abilities, and have provided little evidence to support the effectiveness of their intervention methods. Psychodynamic theories of psychopathology have long lacked empirical support, and there is little evidence to support unique or specific aspects of psychodynamic techniques. Yet the emphasis on a strong therapeutic relationship in practice has been demonstrated through intervention-process research to be an essential ingredient for effective practice. Although family systems theories have highlighted the importance of understanding interactions among family members, evidence for the effectiveness of some popular family treatment models remains thin, with the exception of structural and behaviorally oriented family therapies. Lastly, social cognitive theory has produced a vast body of knowledge regarding psychosocial disorders, and cognitive-behavioral interventions for many disorders are now supported by an impressive body of outcome research. Some would argue, however, that a disproportionate emphasis has been placed on the role of cognition at the expense of other social-environmental determinants. *In brief, no single practice theory provides a sufficiently comprehensive and valid foundation for understanding and treating the full range of serious human problems confronted by social workers.*

EFFICACIOUS OR EFFECTIVE PRACTICE? THE PRESSURES FOR ACCOUNTABILITY

Although many social workers and practitioner-researchers in the allied professions have long endorsed the development and use of effective practices, there is a growing mandate from funding bodies, regulatory agencies, and other professional bodies to ensure accountability in service delivery. As a result of these influences, psychosocial interventions and programming are now increasingly guided by outcome research and program evaluation instead of theoretical, pragmatic, or ideological preferences (e.g., Howard, McMillen, & Pollio, 2003; Gambrill, 2004; Thyer, 2004). However, there are a number of interpretations among practitioners, policymakers, administrators, and academics as to what becoming more accountable means.

There have been two prevailing strategies in social work. The first emphasizes *efficacy,* that is, selecting and implementing interventions that have been shown to be efficacious in controlled practice research. In this approach, practitioners use the existing outcome research to help guide their selection of an intervention once they have conducted a thorough assessment. This approach might be called the outcome research or efficacy research approach to evidence-based practice. The effectiveness approach emphasizes the routine use of practice evaluation methods as part of practice to demonstrate practice effectiveness. In this approach, practitioners incorporate evaluation methods into practice and, based on feedback from the client, make incremental changes to the intervention in the hopes of achieving optimal client outcomes.

For the efficacy model, the body of research used to guide treatment selection is typically based on a series of randomized controlled trials conducted under relatively ideal circumstances. Practitioners are usually trained specifically in the interventions that are being tested, clients are often sampled by strict selection criteria, and multiple standardized measures are employed at assessment, at planned intervals during intervention, and at some follow-up period to measure client change. Controlled trials may be the best tool that researchers have to test whether an intervention model is more efficacious than no intervention or some alternative intervention (often some approach that has been employed as "treatment as usual" in the field). After several controlled trials have shown the intervention to be efficacious across different samples, the approach may be deemed a "promising" or "established" treatment by a committee of experts qualified to critically review outcome research. Practitioners can then learn these new approaches and implement them in their own practice. Many social work practitioners, researchers, and educators have endorsed the use of outcome research to guide the selection of social work interventions (J. Fischer, 1973; K. Wood, 1978; Reid, 1997a, 1997b; Gambrill, 2001; O'Hare, Tran, & Collins, 2002; Thyer, 2004).

By contrast, the effectiveness approach to evidence-based practice emphasizes the process of evaluating social work interventions in everyday practice. There are two variations of this process-oriented approach. First, earlier proponents of "empirical practice" social work focused almost exclusively on "evaluating one's own practice" (K. Corcoran & Gingerich, 1994; Bloom, Fischer, & Orme, 1999), where practitioners employ qualitative case analysis or single-subject designs (or both) to monitor and evaluate the intervention. However, early proponents of practice monitoring and evaluation paid little attention to a key question: what knowledge base and decision-making criteria guided the initial choice of intervention? More recently, a second process-oriented strategy has been promulgated in the social work literature. Although access to and use of existing outcome research is acknowledged as an important first step, it is also stressed that applying the findings of outcome research to unique cases requires a considerable degree of flexibility and "practice wisdom" in that practitioners need to adjust the intervention, based on recursive evaluation (Klein & Bloom, 1995; A. Rosen, 2003). In other words, iterative and reciprocal feedback between client and practitioner is needed to demonstrate whether treatment is going well, and this new information can be used to make adjustments that will lead to an optimal outcome for the client. Although few might argue with this model in principle, the iterative client-practitioner process is complex and not yet well understood. In addition, no empirically validated process models have been developed or evaluated to date for an array of serious psychosocial disorders. At this point, practitioners should be prepared to be flexible and rely on informed judgment, critical thinking, and the monitoring and evaluation of cases to guide the progress of their interventions.

In reality, the distinction between efficacy and effectiveness is far from absolute, and both concepts are essential to implementing EBPSW (O'Hare, 1991, 2002; A. Reid, 1997a, 1997b; Gambrill, 2001, 2004; Proctor, 2003; A. Rosen, 2003). In this text, the implementation of EBPSW emphasizes outcome research to help guide the initial choice of intervention, and monitoring and evaluation methods to facilitate optimal implementation. The use of knowledge gleaned from reviews of the research literature (based on controlled trials) is essential and increasingly required for providing clinical services. Because of considerable variability in client characteristics, client needs, and problem circumstances, however, flexibility and adjustments to the initial intervention plan are usually necessary to maximize optimal intervention.

Although current guidelines for decision making during the implementation process are far from clear, practitioners should consider themselves to be on very firm empirical grounds when they employ the core ingredients of effective helping: good listening skills, empathic attunement, positive regard, and motivational enhancement skills. In addition, the use of client self-monitoring techniques is often an effective way to engage many clients as collaborators and evaluators of their own intervention. Having clients test out the results of the intervention in their everyday environment is not only a powerful form of idiographic evaluation, but an empowering therapeutic tool that can enhance self-efficacy by putting the client in the driver's seat. Client engagement and self-monitoring skills are well-supported in the practice literature and will be examined in more detail in chapter 3. With a sound practitioner-client working relationship in place, both qualitative and quantitative evaluation methods can be seamlessly integrated into routine practice to help practitioners and clients collaborate on the optimal implementation of evidence-based practices.

DEFINING EBPSW: A COMPREHENSIVE STRATEGY FOR CONDUCTING ASSESSMENT, INTERVENTION, AND EVALUATION

Rather than continuing the search for one-size-fits-all practice theory, patching together eclectic models on an impromptu basis, or searching for the holy grail of evaluation methods, social workers need an operable framework for guiding assessment, intervention, and evaluation to accommodate a wide range of practice situations. In this text, EBPSW is defined as *the planned use of empirically supported assessment and intervention methods combined with the judicious use of monitoring and evaluation strategies for the purpose of improving the psychosocial well being of clients*. Here are the primary characteristics of EBPSW.

Conducting qualitative assessment informed by current human behavior research and accompanied by the use of reliable and valid quantitative assessment instruments (i.e., scales, indexes). These instruments also provide a baseline for further monitoring and evaluation.

Selecting and implementing interventions that have been shown to be efficacious in controlled outcome research. Reasonable flexibility in implementing evidence-based practices is usually necessary to accommodate client needs and situational factors.

Implementing evaluation methods as part of practice at the individual and program level.

Evidence-based practice is not a new practice theory. It is a procedural framework that emphasizes the use of current scientific knowledge to support assessment and intervention, and employs qualitative and quantitative evaluation methods that address the evaluative question at hand. When conducting *evidence-based assessment,* the practitioner

> goes beyond general theoretical perspectives to *use problem-specific knowledge,* such as research findings on schizophrenia or child abuse, to identify important biopsychosocial risk and protective factors that cause and maintain the client's problems;

> assesses clients' well-being on multidimensional levels (e.g., psychological, social);

> employs functional analysis to describe how more proximate cognitive, behavioral, physiological, interpersonal, and social factors interact over time and across situations;

> incorporates the client's unique understanding of the problem into the assessment;

> uses multiple methods of data collection from multiple sources;

> pragmatically emphasizes problems that are amenable to change; and

> employs scales and indexes to enhance the reliability and validity of the assessment and to provide a baseline for monitoring and evaluation.

In *intervention* the practitioner

uses representative research based on practice outcome;

accommodates clients' unique construction of the problem, individual differences, circumstances, preferences, and the unpredictability of day-to-day events and responses to the intervention;

gives priority to interventions shown to be effective in controlled trials; and

incorporates other methods as needed, preferably those supported by current outcome research.

Monitoring and evaluation methodologies are used to

incrementally adjust the interventions to optimally meet client needs;

measure client outcomes on an individual level; and

aggregate data for the purposes of quality assurance and program evaluation.

Although qualitative case analysis is important, quantitative data should also be part of individual and program evaluation. Routine aggregation of data is increasingly required by funding bodies as a condition of contracting for services in both the public and private sector.

A micromodel of EBPSW (fig 1.1) illustrates the relationships among assessment, intervention, and evaluation.

FIGURE 1.1   Micromodel of evidence-based practice

ASSESSMENT: informed by current human behavior research; emphasizes multidimensional and functional analysis; enhanced by qualitative and quantitative tools

EVALUATION: qualitative and quantitative methods used to update the assessment, adjust the intervention and measure client progress

INTERVENTION: methods guided by outcome research; eclectic combinations of supported methods

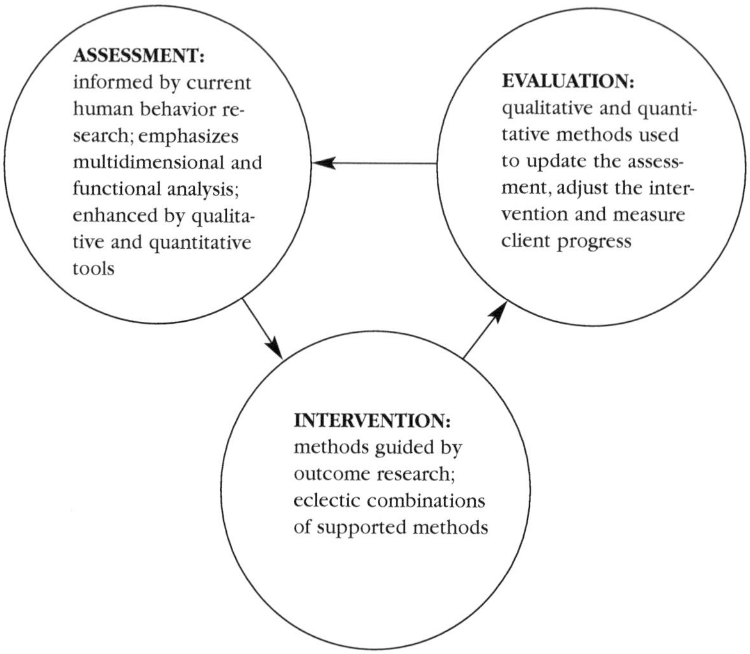

ASSUMPTIONS ABOUT VERIFIABLE KNOWLEDGE

EBPSW assumes that human experience and problem solving can be better understood through research (both qualitative and quantitative) to explain problems and evaluate ways of ameliorating them. People's problems are seen as complex (multidimensional, interactional, context-dependent), and, although the uniqueness of each person is understood, evidence-based practitioners believe that generalizations based on data derived from research with large groups of individuals can provide useful knowledge for assessment and intervention. Replication and generalization of important findings are seen as key to building a professional knowledge base, and employing such evidence is understood to be necessary for the conduct of ethical professional practice. Social scientists reject the notion that knowledge is merely the residue of the sociopolitical scene and believe that, with the use of adequate methods over time, useful knowledge can emerge to help practitioners better understand human problems and more effectively help individuals cope with them. Scientifically oriented practitioners tend to see claims of "intuition, deep and rich insights" as arbitrary (if not self-indulgent) and in need of some agreed-upon definitions and external empirical testing (Dawes, 1989).

EBPSW is clearly commensurate with the scientist-practitioner tradition. However, the implementation of evidence-based practices also requires empathic engagement with clients, keen judgment, good critical thinking, qualitative and quantitative data collection, and flexible response to pragmatic considerations through critical feedback loops with the client within the context of daily practice (Gambrill, 1990; Reid, 1997b; Klein & Bloom, 1995; Beutler, Clarkin, & Bongar, 2000; O'Hare, Tran, & Collins, 2002; A. Rosen, 2003; Thyer, 2004). Initiating and implementing assessment and intervention procedures that are not supported by research is no longer considered acceptable. Ultimately, professional decision making uses the best available evidence to guide the application of assessment, intervention, and evaluation methods.

THE ROLE OF CRITICAL THINKING

Practitioners must rely on good critical thinking skills to effectively apply the existing practice knowledge base for at least two reasons: First, scientific evidence does not speak for itself. Some inference and interpretation is involved in understanding and applying a professional knowledge base. Second, applying knowledge gleaned from research to individual cases and unique circumstances is not easy. Although generalizable findings from research are helpful (e.g., youthful conduct disorder is associated with future substance-abuse problems, cognitive-behavioral therapy works well with anxiety disorders), they provide probability estimates, not predictive guarantees.

All practitioners suffer from inherent limitations in clinical judgment to one degree or another. Social workers are human and therefore subject to the influence of personal life experiences, cultural background, preferred ideologies, political opinions, inadequate professional training, psychological and emotional problems, the seduction of practice fads, collegial peer pressure, money, ambition, and professional status-seeking. Some succumb to self-serving influences, (such as client exploitation for personal gratification or financial gain). But even assuming the best of intentions, practitioners should study carefully the systematic thinking errors that they should avoid (Tversky & Kahneman, 1974; Nurius & Gibson, 1990; Gambrill, 1990, 2004). These include

   confusing description with inference by substituting handy labels (e.g., she's a "borderline," he's an "Axis II") for a thoughtful analysis of the person and situation (e.g., client has suffered from many chronic and stressful experiences, and has not learned effective ways to cope with these troubling feelings);

   focusing on dramatic stereotypes (e.g., "she's just a lying drug abuser") rather than seeing client behavior in context (e.g., mom is trying to retain custody of children and avoid imprisonment);

   overreliance on easily accessible information (e.g., an emotionally compelling case study) to make practice judgments rather than acquiring a more representative view of the problem by using relevant research;

ascribing too much or too little importance to some data when formulating an assessment (e.g., an adverse childhood event) at the expense of other important influences (e.g., multiple chronic environmental stressors such as poverty or long-term psychological abuse);

failing to employ accurate base rates of a problem by becoming infatuated with rare phenomena (e.g., "multiple personality disorder") rather than first considering more common explanations (e.g., feigning mental illness, drug abuse, medical disorder);

engaging in dichotomous thinking (e.g., treatment success or failure) rather than measuring behavior on a continuum (e.g., client is now less anxious, demonstrates better communication skills, has lowered alcohol or drug consumption);

overgeneralizing ("all traumatized women develop post-traumatic stress disorder") rather than considering individual variability and accurate base rates;

engaging in hindsight bias to create the illusion of predictive expertise (e.g., "You should have known that client would attempt suicide!") when, in fact, predicting relatively rare events on a case-by-case basis has proven to be very difficult under the best of circumstances;

confusing correlation (e.g., co-occurring heavy drinking and depression) with causation, rather than considering a range of causal relationships that may involve multiple factors (e.g., client drinks heavily because he is depressed, or client is depressed because he drinks heavily, or client is depressed for reasons other than drinking);

engaging in circular reasoning (e.g., client can't remember incidents of child abuse because memories are repressed; repressed memories are an indication of childhood trauma, therefore, the client must have been sexually abused because she cannot recall the incident) versus examining multiple factors (including the possibility of trauma) and multiple sources of evidence as part of a thorough objective assessment;

selectively attending to evidence that confirms one's theoretical or practice opinions rather than considering alternative explanations (e.g., citing only studies that appear to support one's point of view rather than conducting a representative review of the existing research);

engaging in non sequiturs (e.g., some traditional mental health services have failed our clients; therefore, unconventional or alternative therapies will be more effective).

The implementation of evidence-based methods requires careful reasoning. Although all practitioners are susceptible to personal biases and logical failings, employing sound assessments based on well-founded human behavior theory, implementing evidence-based practices, and carefully monitoring and evaluating each case can go a long way to avoiding some of these pitfalls.

THE ETHICAL ARGUMENT FOR EBPSW

All social work practitioners, researchers, academics, and administrators should be familiar with and adhere to the NASW Code of Ethics. The code outlines the ethical duty of social workers to use and promote scientifically sound theories and practices, and engage in ethical research and evaluation activities. EBPSW not only conforms to the code, but enhances and facilitates its implementation by providing a rational framework for integrating and implementing it. The core ethical considerations for conducting both social work practice and research are quite similar (Reamer, 1995, 2000; Houston-Vega, Nuehring, & Daguio, 1997).

Three basic guidelines must be adhered to: client confidentiality, informed consent, and a mandate to do no harm as a result of intervention and evaluation activities. Confidentiality has always been one of the foremost ethical principles for social workers, and has been robustly supported in court decisions (see *Jaffee v. Redmond* in Appelbaum 1996) and in federal legislation, specifically the Health Insurance Portability Accountability Act of 1996. Practitioners and researchers also share the responsibility to get adequately informed consent from clients, by explaining the nature of the intervention or evaluation research project, and by indicating whether there is any potential for causing psychological distress. Practitioners and researchers are also required to be responsive should clients become distressed in the course of an intervention or research/evaluation procedure. With increasing frequency, practice and evaluation activities occur simultaneously (e.g., using clinical scales as part of assessment and clinical review procedures), often rendering the intervention *vs.* evaluation distinction moot for practical and ethical purposes. A sensible policy would be for social workers to concentrate on applying good ethical principles whether the professional activity is defined as practice, evaluation, research, or a combination of these.

Because few social workers engage in controlled experimental research projects with innovative or potentially controversial experimental treatments, such as drug trials or other medical research, most of the concerns about breaches of ethics, practically speaking, are relevant to social work practice activities, not to the conduct of social work survey or evaluation research. Generally, there has been an increase in malpractice claims in the past decade or so related to incorrect treatment, sexual impropriety, breaches of confidentiality, failure to diagnose correctly, client abandonment (i.e., terminating prematurely), and suicide attempts (Houston-Vega et al., 1997; Reamer, 1995). Although anyone can inadvertently breach ethical principles or be sued for malpractice, evidence-based practice can help mitigate these threats by providing a rational basis for assessment (including identifying high-risk behaviors), guiding choice of interventions that are supported by research, and providing a sound basis for evaluating cases at both the individual and aggregate levels.

PRINCIPLES OF EBPSW

The working principles of EBPSW are listed below. They will be examined further in subsequent chapters.

1.   Social work is a profession based on values, ethics, knowledge, and skills. Value-based professional decision making requires evidence-based knowledge and skills applied to assessment, intervention guided by critical thinking, and good judgment honed by practice experience.

2.   The knowledge base of social work is rooted in the social science disciplines. The causes of people's problems are understood to be complex and involve interacting biopsychosocial risks and resiliencies. These influences vary across time and situation, and have both remote and proximate effects on the cause and maintenance of a client's problems. Cross-sectional, longitudinal, and experimental research on human behavior and the social environment provide some understanding of the risks and resiliencies associated with client problems, and provide a foundation for valid assessment.

3.   Although clients' views of the problem, their coping capacities, and their suggestions for potential solutions should be given the utmost consideration in professional assessment and treatment planning, practitioners are primarily responsible for formulating assessment, intervention, and evaluation plans. Funding sources, regulatory agencies, and the courts recognize licensed social workers, not their clients, as the experts and hold the social workers accountable for these activities.

4.   Person factors such as age, gender, sexual orientation, race, ethnicity, and cultural identity interact in a complex and, sometimes, indeterminate manner. These factors are essential for developing and understanding valid human behavior theory, assessment, and practice principles.

5.   Outcome research provides substantial guidance for practitioners when developing effective intervention strategies. Nevertheless, interventions shown to be effective in controlled studies often require flexible, eclectic adaptation for the individual client, given their preferences, circumstances, and the unpredictable events that occur during intervention.

6.   Evidence-based practitioners have a number of evaluation research methods at their disposal. All have strengths and weaknesses based on their design. The evidence-based practitioner uses the design that best answers the evaluative question at hand.

7.   Above all, the development, teaching, and dissemination of evidence-based practice is guided by the time-honored tradition of rational, scholarly discourse. Critical thinking and peer-reviewed methodologically sound research are the currency of ethical, professional knowledge building and debate.

8.   The implementation of EBPSW in community service settings requires adherence to evidence-based protocol leavened with flexibility to adapt these practices to complex cases in fluid service environments.

9.   Assessment, intervention, and evaluation processes are integrated in EBPSW for the purpose of providing compassionate and effective care. Qualitative and quantitative evaluation methodologies are combined to demonstrate and improve quality of service.

10.   For social work to remain a vital profession well into the future, social workers must play an active role in the development, implementation, and evaluation of EBPSW.

CHAPTER 2

QUALITATIVE AND
QUANTITATIVE ASSESSMENT

Assessment in psychosocial practice is a form of problem analysis. It is an attempt on the part of the practitioner, client, and other collaborators to identify what biopsychosocial factors seem to have caused and currently maintain the client's problems, to assess client capacities for adaptation and change, and to specify those aspects of the client's problems that are amenable to change. Setting goals and objectives, selecting effective intervention methods, and designing the evaluation are inextricably linked to assessment as part of the intervention planning process.

This chapter examines the research that supports evidence-based assessment. It then examines the major components for applying this knowledge: the multidimensional functional (MDF) assessment, and the adjunctive use of measurement tools. The purpose of this chapter is to provide practitioners with an integrated assessment model that uses both qualitative and quantitative methods in a coherent and practical manner to guide intervention planning and evaluation, the subjects of chapters 3 and 4.

THE CONTEMPORARY KNOWLEDGE BASE OF
MULTIDIMENSIONAL/FUNCTIONAL ASSESSMENT

A valid assessment must consider a person's unique experience and the problem specific knowledge based on research. A body of contemporary research relevant to a specific problem is most likely to be a combination of cross-sectional and longitudinal surveys, experimental research, and case-study research. The use of relevant and methodologically sound research findings supports assessment by providing base-rate estimates (incidence and prevalence) of specific problems in the community, estimating the rates of co-occurring problems, identifying key risk and resiliency factors (both developmental and current) that are likely to contribute to the client's problems or predict recovery, providing estimates for the relative strength of risk and resiliency factors, explaining the multidimensional nature of client problems, providing support for some theories and invalidating others, and providing an empirical and theoretical foundation for instrument development.

To conduct an informed qualitative assessment, practitioners must choose a human behavior model that is relevant to the client's presenting problems and based on research specific to the relevant problem area (Wakefield, 1996). Currently, a wealth of problem-specific research is available to social workers to inform their practice. Highlights of research that supports the assessment of each problem area are summarized in the first parts of chapters 5–16.

Contemporary human behavior models that inform clinical assessment are multifactorial (often multitheoretical) and involve a range of developmental biopsychosocial processes mediated by a variety of individual person factors such as age, gender, race, ethnicity, and cultural background (Basic Behavioral Science Task Force, 1996). Person factors are not simply demographic categories, but represent essential characteristics that are inextricably related to biological, psychological, social-environmental, historical, cultural, and economic determinants of human experience and behavior. These factors often play an important role in the causes of human problems, in the epidemiology (prevalence and incidence) of psychosocial disorders, and in how problems are defined by the client, practitioner, or others, expressed by individuals, and treated by practitioners (Pinderhughes, 1989; Sue, Zane, & Young, 1994).

Although findings from research on white males have historically been overextended to assessment and intervention guidelines for women and people of color (Schliebner, 1994; Beckman, 1994; R. T. Carter, 1995), a rapidly expanding literature emphasizes differences associated with gender, race, and other person factors (Basic Behavioral Science Task Force, 1996). One example is the research on the impact of poverty and violence on racial minorities and their families (J. H. Williams, Stiffman, & O'Neal, 1998; Gorman-Smith & Tolan, 1998).

Although it is critical that person factors be taken into account in an assessment, overgeneralizations about women, broad ethnic-cultural groups, sexual orientation, or other differences should also be avoided (Gopaul-McNichol & Brice-Baker, 1998; Uba, 1994; Manoleas, 1996; Vasquez, 1994). For example, women of color may share a common bond in oppression, but they also manifest considerable differences between and within racial groups. Indeed, some theoreticians have suggested a more fine-grained assessment of group differences. Rather than emphasizing broad ethnic and racial glosses to describe culturally disparate peoples, for example, more fine-grained approaches may provide greater sensitivity (O'Hare & Tran, 1998; D. B. Heath, 1991; Trimble, 1990). Those assessments include identifying one's birthplace and that of other family members over two or three generations; analyzing ethnic-specific behavior patterns such as language use, ethnic identity of friends and acquaintances, use of various media, participation in ethnic-specific activities such as cultural and religious events, and music and food preferences; and exploring subjective assessments of ethnic identity, acculturation and assimilation status, value preferences, role models and preferred reference groups, and attitudes toward "out" groups.

These differences must also be seen in a temporal or developmental context. Rather than seeing acculturation as a linear transition from immigrant culture to the host culture, it may be better measured on a bidirectional continuum. Accordingly, multiple psychological and behavioral aspects of acculturation vary between both the immigrant and host culture. Various aspects of cultural identification may be acquired, retained, or discarded to one extent or another (J. Anderson et al., 1993; Marino, Stuart, & Minas, 2000). Berry (1986) conceptualizes four possible outcomes of the acculturation process: assimilation toward the dominant culture, integration of both cultures, reaffirmation of the traditional culture, and marginalization from both cultures. Characterizing large groups of people by gender, race, sexual orientation, and the like as though they share a common characteristic is fraught with peril, and only serves to blind practitioners to the uniqueness of clients' experiences, and how their experiences shape their view of themselves and others in their own reference groups over time.

Assessment instruments designed to be sensitive to person factors have been developed and tested with the following problems: race-related stress (Utsey & Ponterotto, 1996), language proficiency among recent immigrants (J. Anderson et al. 1993), mental health (Mollica, Wyshak, de Marneffe, Khuon, & Lavelle, 1987), and substance abuse (Saunders, Aasland, Amundsen, & Grant, 1993). Some attention has also been given to refining methodological processes for valid scale construction with people from different cultural groups (Tran, 1997).

Person factors are not confined to those that identify a client's gender, cultural background, or financial status. Other individual qualities relevant to assessment include the circumstances that brought the client to social work service (e.g., court-ordered or voluntary), and their motivation or readiness to change. These dimensions of assessment overlap with the subject of treatment engagement, and they are dealt with in chapter 3.

THE MULTIDIMENSIONAL/FUNCTIONAL APPROACH TO ASSESSMENT

Given the assumption that valid assessment must consider both generalizable knowledge and individual experience, a comprehensive assessment must incorporate two core organizing concepts: multidimensionality and functionality (table 2.1). Both concepts are at the heart of what is defined within this text as evidence-based assessment.

Multidimensionality requires judgments about the nature and severity of the client's difficulties, judgments supported by the best available scientific knowledge specific to the client's problems. Factors, both past and present, that contribute to clients' problems are understood to interact systemically over time and across situations. Multidimensionality also implies measurement of the

TABLE 2.1 Conceptual domains of evidence-based assessment

Multidimensionality	*Functionality*
Assess developmental and current causes of client difficulties and the trajectory of problems over time. Analysis is informed by valid human behavior theories;	Examine temporal sequencing and patterning of problem behaviors over time and across situations; focus on current functioning and key problems;
Analyze interactional/systemic influences and behaviors over time in family and social situations;	Measure important problems on a continuum (e.g., frequency, severity or duration) with either self-anchored indexes or dimensional scales;
Conduct a thorough examination of current biopsychosocial difficulties across multiple domains (e.g., mental status, relationships, work, health, etc. . .)	Identify important contingencies, that is, rewards and punishments that appear to maintain current conditions;
Carefully consider the role of person factors (e.g., gender, race, ethnicity, sexual orientation, spirituality, etc. . .) on the problems and potential solutions.	Set problem priorities and develop hierarchies for achieving objectives toward resolving those problems;
	Explore client's unique problem constructions and expectations toward resolving problems;
	Emphasize problems that are *amenable to change*, changes that can be measured incrementally over time for monitoring and evaluation purposes.

client's difficulties across multiple psychosocial domains in living. *Functionality* is assessed primarily through understanding the client's unique experiences based on reports from multiple sources including the client, family, collaborating professionals, and other collateral sources. These concepts are collectively reflected in the work of many practice scholars who have written lucidly about assessment (see, e.g., C. Franklin & Jordan, 2003; Karls & Wandrei, 1994; Hartmann, Roper, & Bradford, 1979; Haynes, 1998; O'Hare et al., 2003; Antony & Swinson, 2000; Persons & Fresco, 1998).

Assessment is multidimensional to the extent that it has the following characteristics: (1) The practitioner's understanding of the client's general psychosocial history and specific problem history is informed by contemporary human behavior research. Human development, problems, and adaptive capacities are understood to be caused by *reciprocally and systemically interacting biopsychosocial processes*. (2) It considers interacting influences over time. (3) It measures current client distress across multiple domains of psychosocial functioning or well-being. These domains minimally include mental status (psychiatric symptoms), substance abuse, social functioning in immediate social relationships with partners and family and extended (community) relationships, access and use of environmental resources such as housing, gainful vocational activity, general health status, leisure activities, criminal involvement, and sense of spiritual well-being. (4) The expression of a client's problems and life circumstances are recognized as mediated by gender, age, cultural identity, and other defining characteristics referred to above as "person factors."

Although human behavior research informs assessment, it must be coupled with a unique functional analysis of the individual's day-to-day experiences. Knowledge of schizophrenia, for example, is helpful for understanding the condition of clients who share this affliction. However, all people with schizophrenia are unique in many other ways. An MDF assessment reflects functionality to the extent that it provides an in-depth analysis of the unique patterning and sequencing of clients' experiences that interact with day-to-day events in their social environment. A functional assessment is by its nature idiographic; that is, it is unique to the individual. To the extent that a functional analysis considers the client's unique cognitive experiences, it is also commensurate with a constructivist view. Thus, the practitioner and client must work collaboratively to describe, explain, understand, and, build a detailed yet hypothetical working model of the client's problems.

The functional assessment emphasizes the importance of (1) *temporal sequencing and patterning* of thoughts, feelings, behaviors, and social-environmental events related to the problem; (2) measuring the *frequency, intensity, or duration* of specific problems in order to measure changes over time; (3) identifying salient *contingencies* (rewards and punishments) in the environment that appear to influence the client's behavior and overall well-being; (4) *setting of priorities* among different problems, and establishing progressive hierarchies to gradually address individual intervention objectives; (5) paying close attention to clients' unique *construction of the problem* and their *expectations* for change; (6) giving priority to problems that are *amenable to change*, and defining and measuring problems in a way that is sensitive to incremental change over time in order for practitioners to conduct meaningful monitoring and evaluation of each case.

Although most assessment models emphasize work with individuals, social workers are often required to assess couples, families, and other small groups. Conducting an assessment with clients in their immediate and extended social context often has distinct advantages over relying on self-report alone. Family systems assessment, for example, encompasses both multidimensional and functional aspects. The practitioner must provide an assessment for individual members while examining the interactional and temporal patterns among family members in order to understand *how the system functions.*

THE ROLE OF MEASUREMENT IN MULTIDIMENSIONAL/ FUNCTIONAL ASSESSMENT

Few practitioners would doubt that the severity of problems can vary between two different clients and within the same client over time as they become worse or improve. Practitioners are called upon to make frequent judgments regarding the severity of problems for purposes of treatment planning, referral, and evaluation. How reliable and accurate are those judgments?

Although much of the judgment that goes into a skilled assessment is qualitative, judgment can be improved when practitioners also incorporate reliable, valid, and practical standardized instruments into assessment, monitoring of client progress, and evaluation. These instruments can engender increased reliability and validity for the individual practitioner's assessment; accurately identify risks and ensure that all staff cover the bases on high-risk clinical concerns; help clients identify specific complaints, clarify their definition of their problems, and educate themselves about the problem; prompt more in-depth discussion about the problem with the practitioner and thus provide an opportunity for more targeted assessment; and provide a baseline for evaluating intervention effectiveness by measuring change across one or more domains of client well-being. Used consistently and skillfully, assessment tools can provide an important foundation for monitoring and evaluation.

Client problems are measured in a number of ways: by *classification* (e.g., diagnosis), *frequency* with which the problem occurs, *intensity*, or *duration*. Types of instruments also vary by degree of complexity from simple classification and single-item indexes, to unidimensional and multidimensional scales.

Continuous measures are useful for baselining and monitoring client change over time. They can be unidimensional *single-item indexes*, *unidimensional scales* that measure one problem using multiple indicators, or *multidimensional scales* that measure more than one aspect of a problem. Each approach has its advantages, and often these measurement tools are used in combination. For example, a practitioner working with a middle-aged woman who has been abused in her marital relationship may incorporate the following into the MDF assessment: simple index to measure the weekly frequency of suicidal thoughts, a unidimensional scale to measure depression or self-esteem, and a multidimensional scale to gauge her overall psychosocial well-being.

Diagnostic Classification

For many social workers, an assessment, by necessity, uses the *Diagnostic and Statistical Manual of Mental Disorders* (American Psychiatric Association, 2000). The *DSM* has contributed greatly to the recognition of serious mental disorders, provides a common nomenclature for practitioners, and has stimulated and guided much clinical research. Social work practitioners should be familiar with it, and know how to use it competently.

The *DSM* is limited as a tool for assessment, however. First, *DSM* diagnosis is premised on the notion that the locus of dysfunction is within the individual. "Whatever its original cause (the disorder) must currently be considered a manifestation of a behavioral, psychological, or biological dysfunction in the individual" (*DSM-IV-TR*, p. xxxi), an assumption that is increasingly at odds with knowledge regarding the influences of psychosocial stressors and other social-environmental factors. Second, *DSM* categories lack differentiation. As the authors of the current version of the *DSM* opine, classification systems work best when the categories are relatively homogeneous, there are clear boundaries between them, and they are mutually exclusive. Generally, homogeneity is more the exception than the rule in *DSM* diagnoses, because many symptoms and behaviors are common to more than one disorder. Practitioners often compensate for this limitation by applying multiple diagnoses to the same client.

Third, aside from determining the presence of serious mental illness presumably caused, in part, by some physiological dysfunction, the *DSM* is misapplied, in the view of many, to conditions in which psychosocial factors play a prominent if not dominant role. Many *DSM* categories also appear to be merely descriptions of behaviors that are sometimes troubling to the client or, especially, others (Kutchins & Kirk, 1997; Peele, 1989; Sroufe, 1997; Wakefield, 1997). The lack of empirical evidence for biological etiology of many disorders includes diagnoses applied to children with psychosocial or behavioral difficulties (e.g., oppositional-defiant disorder; Achenbach, 1995). However, even with disorders such as severe mental illness in which biological factors have been shown to play a dominant etiological role, social and environmental factors weigh heavily in the exacerbation of symptoms, access to treatment, and long-term outcomes.

Fourth, reviews of the field trials and data related to the development of the *DSM* have consistently concluded that the methods employed in reliability and validity testing are seriously flawed (Kutchins & Kirk, 1988, 1997). Although a few of the major diagnostic categories have been shown to be used reliably in normal interviewing situations, the reliability of childhood and personality disorders, among others, has been shown to be quite poor.

Lastly, aside from setting rather gross treatment expectations for practitioners, diagnosis provides relatively little guidance for treatment planning and evaluation, given that clients' problems are typically multidimensional and idiographic in nature, and diagnoses lack sensitivity to change.

Screening Devices

Screening devices in social work practice play an important role as prelude to more thorough assessment. Screening tools are scales that use a cut-off score to detect the likelihood that a client may have a particular problem. Instruments such as the Michigan Alcoholism Screening Test (Seltzer, 1971) or the Drug Abuse Screening Test (Skinner, 1982) use cut-off scores to identify people who may be at risk for a serious substance-abuse problem. Although some screening devices cannot be used as outcome measures because (due to the wording of items or scoring method) they cannot show change over short periods (e.g., three months), others are more sensitive to change and can be employed for both screening and evaluation. For example, the Geriatric Depression Scale (Yesavage et al., 1983) can serve as a screening device with elderly clients (see chapter 9). Because it is sensitive to change, it can also be used as an assessment/evaluation tool.

Before using screening devices, practitioners should be sure that the recommended cut-off score is based on research subjects similar to the client's reference group. As with all instruments, screening devices should be validated with samples that reflect the population for whom they are intended. In addition, the results of a screening instrument should not be considered a confirmation of the problem, but simply a warning light to induce a more detailed assessment.

Single-Item Indexes

Sometimes clients' most pressing concerns can be summed up in a simple index: number of drinks, frequency of panic attacks, severity of arguments, level of postoperative pain, degree of intimacy, number of suicidal thoughts, level of depression, days without a meal, level of hope for recovery, and so on. Single item indexes were originally associated with early behavioral interventions where "target" problems were the focus of treatment (Hersen, 1985; Bloom et al., 1999). For a child with severe autism, reducing repeated head banging or hair pulling may be used to judge the success of behavior modification. The intensity of flashbacks related to post-traumatic stress as measured by a client on a scale from 0 to 100 may be used to assess progress in response to stress management and guided imagery. Number of successfully completed homework assignments for a child struggling with ADHD can be logged on a brightly colored chart. When applied to more complex problems, the adjunctive use of unidimensional indicators as part of a comprehensive assessment and evaluation can help focus the intervention on key problems and provide a straightforward and substantive measure for idiographic evaluation.

Figure 2.1 provides a template for considering how to define target problems (thoughts, feelings, and behaviors) and how to measure them (frequency, intensity, and duration). For treatment planning, these indexes can also represent specific treatment objectives. How the problem or objective is defined and measured should be the result of client-practitioner discussion to maximize the salience for clients, encourage their willingness to participate, and reflect whatever seems most congruent with their situation. For example, for serious suicidal thoughts (cognition), frequency may be the main concern for one client, severity or intensity of the thoughts for another. For an assaultive adolescent, intensity of anger may be the main focus of change, rather than frequency. For the person with agoraphobia, the frequency of panic attacks may be most critical as well as the amount of time they can remain in the supermarket without "freaking out" and running outside. For a couple struggling to improve communications and intimacy, reducing the frequency of interruptions during conversations (behavior) may be their initial objective, and later, increasing the amount of recreational or romantic time spent together may become the new objective. As treatment objectives are accomplished, they can be modified to reflect improvement to focus on a different problem. When defining these indexes, careful attention should be given to the context within which the target symptom or problem occurs.

FIGURE 2.1   Template for defining and measuring target problems

	Frequency	*Intensity*	*Duration*
Cognitive (thoughts)			
Emotional (feelings)			
Physiological (symptoms)			
Behavioral (actions)			

Other single item indexes measure more general levels of client functioning rather than one discrete problem. Perhaps the most commonly used is the Global Assessment of Functioning (GAF), published in the *DSM-IV-TR* and derived from the original Global Assessment Scale (Endicott, Spitzer, Fleiss, & Cohen, 1976). This index is often required as part of routine diagnosis. The GAF is scored from 1 to 100, corresponding to global descriptions of clients' functioning ranging from "persistent danger of severely hurting self or others" (1–10), to "serious symptoms [and] impairment in social, occupational, or school functioning" (41–50), to "superior functioning in a wide range of activities" (91–100). Data suggest, however, that the GAF may correlate primarily with mental status symptoms, and not be a particularly valid estimate of broader social functioning (Roy-Byrne, Dafadakis, Unutzer, & Ries, 1996; Dickerson, 1997). As an evaluation tool, the GAF may be a useful adjunct, but should be augmented with measures of social functioning.

Unidimensional Scales

Although unidimensional (or narrowband) scales are typically constructed with at least five items, and may range up to thirty or more, they measure only one dimension of client well-being, such as depression, anxiety, self-esteem and so forth, but do so with multiple items. Although less flexible in use than simple single-item indexes, unidimensional scales have usually been tested for reliability and validity. Notable examples include the Beck Depression Inventory (Beck et al., 1961), the Hamilton Depression Rating Scale (Hamilton, 1960), the Obsessive-Compulsive Inventory (Foa, Kozak, Salkovskis, Coles, & Amir, 1998), and the Index of Marital Relations (Hudson, 1982a). although unidimensional scales can be a valuable adjunct to a comprehensive assessment, they are limited in focus. They can be used in specialized intervention settings (e.g., depression or anxiety clinic) or as a supplement to multidimensional (or broadband) instruments.

Multidimensional Scales

One remedy for dealing with a "jumbled array" (Hudson & McMurty, 1997) of single-measure scales is to employ multidimensional instruments that measure a number of important areas of psychosocial well-being. Multidimensional measures provide a quantitative counterpart to the multidimensional qualitative assessment. Such an assessment package can focus on the individual while providing a foundation for aggregating data for program evaluation. Reliable and valid instruments have been developed to measure clients' functioning across an array of psychiatric, psychosocial, and health-related domains (Dickerson, 1997; Srebnik et al., 1997). Many scales designed to balance reliability, validity, and utility will be highlighted throughout this text.

Although some practitioners might question the reason for measuring problems other than those "target problems" for which the client requested treatment, most intervention models in mental health, substance abuse, child welfare, and elderly services now require the measurement of multidimensional outcomes. For this purpose, there are a number of broadband scales developed for assessment and evaluation. Practitioners must choose those that best fit their assessment and evaluation needs.

The Psychosocial Well-Being Scale (PSWS; O'Hare, Sherrer et al., 2002; O'Hare et al., 2003) is an example of a broad-spectrum instrument. It was developed as a comprehensive yet easy-to-use debriefing tool or final "score card" to quantitatively summarize clinical judgments regarding problem severity on a range of important psychosocial domains. Clinicians are encouraged to use a broad array of sources (e.g., client self-report, clinical records, input from significant others and collaborating professionals) before making a final judgment about problem severity. Because the PSWS was developed for adults in a comprehensive community mental health center, it may have wide applicability.

The twelve items that make up the PSWS are rated by the practitioner on a five-point scale (see appendix A). They cover the following problem domains: Two four-item subscales include psychological well-being (cognitive mental status, emotional mental status, impulse control, and coping skills), and social well-being (immediate social network, extended social network, recreational activities, and living environment). The four items in each subscale can be totaled and divided by four to obtain a relative measure of severity. In addition, there are four single-item indexes, global measures of substance abuse, health, activities of daily living and work satisfaction. These four items can be used as stand alone indexes. The PSWS has been shown to have good reliability and validity in that its sub-scales have correlated well with other valid scales (O'Hare, Sherrer et al., 2002; O'Hare et al., 2003). No population norms are set for the PSWS, and the items are intended to be self-anchored. Thus, the PSWS is best used as part of a compre-hensive strategy of assessment, monitoring, and evaluation that incorporates the observations and judgments of client, practitioner, and other corroborating sources. After scoring each item on the scale, practitioners should briefly de-scribe the client's specific problem in the lines provided. In this way, the PSWS serves as both a quantitative and qualitative assessment/outcome instrument. The PSWS is available in appendix A and can be used without obtaining special permission from the author.

Broad-based scales for assessing children's disorders are also available. The Child Behavior Check List (CBCL; Achenbach, 1995; Lowe, 1998), a widely used and well-regarded multidimensional functioning scale, measures both social competence and behavior problems in children. Different versions have been developed for use by parents, teachers, and children themselves, and it has been validated by gender and race. The CBCL is proprietary, and requires special per-mission from its author (Thomas Achenbach) to use it.

The Shortform Assessment for Children (SAC; Glisson, Hemmelgarn, & Post, 2002; Hemmelgarn, Glisson, & Sharp, 2003) is a viable alternative to the CBCL. The SAC is a brief and reliable broadband scale that measures both internalizing (depression, anxiety) and externalizing (behavioral problems) in children. The SAC is a recent addition to a series of scales developed with the support of the National Institute of Mental Health (NIMH) from behavioral items created in the 1940s and 1950s (E. H. Tyson & Glisson, 2005). With a sample of 3,790 children (ages 5–18) served by the child welfare and juvenile justice systems, the SAC pro-duced stable factor structures across age, gender, and respondent groups (i.e., parents and teachers; Glisson et al.). Internal consistency reliability coefficients ranged between .86 and .96 for all groups using either parents or teachers as re-spondents, and subscales showed significant correlations with child placement decisions and other validity criteria. NIMH funded a subsequent study with a new sample to determine if the same short list of behavioral items included in the SAC could be used with equal validity by parents and teachers (Hemmelgarn et al.). Validity coefficients were equivalent for parents and teachers, and exter-nalizing scores showed good criterion validity for fighting, placement ejections, and time in custody. Furthermore, an additional independent sample of 1,252 children produced factor structures and validities that indicated the SAC to be equally valid with African-American and Caucasian-American children (E. H. Tyson & Glisson). The SAC can be completed by parents, teachers, or preferably both. The one-page scale has forty-eight items (twenty-four internalizing, twenty-four externalizing), and takes only a few minutes to complete. Each item is rated on a three-point scale (never, sometimes, often). Scores for both internalizing and externalizing dimensions are obtained by summing the twenty-four respective items, and a global score combines both subscales scores. The SAC is accompanied by software-based scoring guidelines normal for the child's age, gender, and respondent. A copy of the SAC appears in appendix B.

Other broadband scales are available to accommodate a range of assessment needs. The Family Adaptability and Cohesion Evaluation Scales (FACES), currently in its fourth revision, measures levels of cohesiveness and flexibility in family functioning (Olsen, Russell, & Sprenkle 1989; C. Franklin, Streeter, & Springer, 2001). It was developed from a systems perspective, and the scale is intended to be self-administered. The instrument may be obtained from David Olsen at the University of Minnesota, Department of Family Social Sciences. The Addiction Severity Index (McLellan, Luborsky, Woody, & O'Brien, 1980) measures degree of distress from alcohol and drug use across a number of problem domains, including legal, medical, family, social, and occupational functioning (see chapter 6). The Social Functioning Scale was developed to measure both general health and social functioning and is available from John Ware (New England Medical Center, Boston) without cost in a twelve-item version (Ware, Kosinski, & Keller, 1996). A. F. Lehman's Quality of Life Scale (1988) measures seven areas, including living situation, family and social relations, leisure, work and religious activity, finances, safety, and health. It is available from Anthony Lehman (University of Maryland) for a nominal cost. All of these instruments have been shown to be reliable and valid to one degree or another with specific populations, provide continuous measures to gauge treatment progress, and can usually be completed within an hour.

Basic Guidelines for Instrument Selection

A number of basic criteria should be considered before selecting and using a scale (O'Hare, Sherrer et al., 2002).

- It measures multiple dimensions of client well-being on continuous scales.
- It is part of the typical qualitative psychosocial and psychiatric assessment required in community programs.
- It is relevant to the treatment agenda of all members of an interdisciplinary team.
- It facilitates treatment planning by providing a template for measuring treatment goals and outcomes.
- It works as a summary assessment/evaluation instrument to synthesize data accumulated from numerous, interdisciplinary sources.
- It is reliable, valid, and relatively easy to use after some training.
- Its scoring methods have immediate face validity for practitioners (i.e., no complicated or cumbersome scoring guidelines).
- It produces scores (both individual items and aggregate scores) that have straightforward resonance with clients, practitioners, administrators, and policymakers.

Reliability and validity constitute the core psychometric criteria that must be considered when developing or choosing any quantitative evaluation instrument (Kazdin, 1994a; DeVellis, 2000). It should have *face validity* and be considered by both practitioners and clients to be relevant to the clients' overall problems. It should have a track record of research supporting its *internal consistency reliability* (items of the scale show good interitem correlation), *test-retest reliability* (scale is consistent when filled out at two different intervals), and *interrater reliability* (two observers who use the same scale with the same client show a high degree of agreement). Instruments should ideally meet criteria for three forms of validity: *construct validity* (the scale measures what it purports to measure), *criterion validity* (it correlates with similar measures concurrently and predicts relevant outcomes), and *content validity* (it includes a reasonably representative array of relevant items). Although ideally a scale should meet all of these standards, most published scales are considered acceptable if they meet at least one or two forms of reliability and show both construct validity and some form of criterion validity with relevant target populations.

A variety of statistical methods are used to demonstrate the degree of reliability and validity. For reliability measures, scores above .70 indicate adequate reliability, above .80 good, and above .90 excellent. Validity of scales is indicated by moderate to high correlations (>.50) between the scale score and another valid benchmark, or a lower correlation (<.50) to indicate discriminant validity. The construct validity of scales involves a more detailed analysis of the underlying factor structure, and requires advanced statistical techniques, known as exploratory and confirmatory factor analysis, to demonstrate that the scale items individually and collectively actually measure the theoretical construct of interest (such as anxiety, psychopathy, or alcoholism). In addition, these psychometrics should be demonstrated in the research literature with community and clinical samples reasonably similar to the clients with whom the practitioner intends to use the scale. Lastly, instruments intended to be used for monitoring and evaluation purposes should be sensitive to change in the client's target symptoms or overall well-being. Some scales may be useful as screening devices, but may not be suitable for use as evaluation tools because they are not sensitive to changes in problem severity. Although practitioners should be familiar with the basic concepts of reliability and validity, experts in instrument development and selection can provide helpful consultation.

Methods for Gathering Assessment Information

Qualitative and quantitative assessment information can be obtained in several ways, and, to some degree, the methods employed depend upon the situation. For the most part, social workers depend upon client self-report in *face-to-face interviews,* which may range from relatively unstructured to standardized formats. To obtain a more complete picture of the client's situation as well as ensuring accurate self-report practitioners may also need to obtain *collateral or corroborating information,* such as police records, physician exams, hospital records, and employer's report of job performance. Other methods include *observing clients in their natural environment* asking clients to *role-play a problem situation,* and requesting clients to *self-monitor* their thoughts, feelings, and behaviors in different circumstances for a week or two in order to develop a better working model of the problem. All of these assessment activities may include the collection of qualitative data, quantitative data, or preferably both.

Practitioner judgment is required to decide how to obtain the most accurate and representative information in order to conduct the optimal MDF assessment. In some instances, client self-report may be sufficiently valid if there appear to be no memory problems or compelling motive for misrepresenting the truth. When clients have cognitive impairments, or are likely to minimize a problem or lie, practitioners should obtain corroborating information. Given that effective intervention is in part contingent upon an accurate assessment, practitioners should be assertive about obtaining an accurate, through, and balanced view of the client's problems.

In the final analysis, assessment is both art and science, inductive and deductive, idiographic and nomothetic. Assessment is the thoughtful application of generalizable knowledge in the service of understanding a client's unique experience.

SUMMARY

MDF assessment in evidence-based practice is defined by the following characteristics: It is informed by current biopsychosocial research regarding risks and resiliencies related to clients' dysfunctions and strengths across multiple domains of well-being. It requires a systemic and functional analysis of client's problems within interactional social contexts, measuring the severity of problems across multiple psychosocial domains. The client's difficulties are also viewed in the context of person factors. MDF assessment incorporates clients' personal account of their difficulties as well as detailed idiographic functional analysis of their experiences to help understand the sequencing and patterning of factors related to the clients' present efforts to cope in their environment. It emphasizes the use of both idiographic and standardized dimensional scales to define specific problems in a way that is amenable to measuring change. Whenever possible data are collected with multiple qualitative and quantitative methods employed with multiple sources.

MDF assessment lends itself to intervention planning because problems are defined dimensionally on a continuum to reflect changes in client well-being across multiple problem domains. It also is well-suited to practice evaluation, because it can be accommodated to evaluate interventions for one client, groups of clients, or entire programs.

CHAPTER 3

SELECTING AND
IMPLEMENTING INTERVENTIONS

This chapter addresses the selection and implementation of evidence-based practices. It defines the intervention in EBPSW and identifies essential practice components. It addresses the debate over flexibility and manualization. A brief overview presents current finding in controlled outcome research. The chapter also summarizes basic guidelines for critically reviewing outcome studies, a key step in selecting evidence-based practices.

DEFINING INTERVENTIONS IN EBPSW

Interventions in evidence-based practice are activities engaged in by the practitioner, the client, and perhaps other collaborators for the purpose of solving specific problems, enhancing clients' psychological and behavioral coping abilities and modifying social-environmental contingencies to improve a client's psychosocial well-being. If *intervention* is the overarching term, skills are the most elemental component, and strategies or techniques are combinations of skills that constitute the intervention. It has long been understood that social work interventions often comprise various combinations of both basic and advanced skills, techniques, and strategies (Shulman, 1992; Hepworth, Rooney, & Larsen, 1997; B. R. Compton & Galaway, 1999). Novice social workers may initially focus on learning a few discrete basic skills, specific behavioral techniques, or case management methods.

Advanced evidence-based interventions, however, are combinations of skills and techniques that have been shown to be efficacious in controlled outcome studies with more serious and complex psychosocial problems. These interventions may include psychoeducation and behavioral family therapy for the mentally ill, community reinforcement and contingency management for paroled inmates chronically addicted to street drugs, interpersonal psychotherapy for depressed clients, exposure with response prevention for people with obsessive-compulsive disorder, cognitive-behavioral intervention for bulimia nervosa, dialectical behavior therapy for borderline personality disorder, and behavioral family therapy for conduct-disordered and delinquent adolescents. In addition, more difficult and complex problems often require the collaboration of multiple adjunctive practitioners (e.g., psychiatrist, school social worker, teacher, and coaches for work with a child with severe ADHD) as a part of broad-based approaches. Thus, many advanced interventions must be skillfully applied within a broader case management framework. Interventions that are sufficient to resolve mild to moderate psychosocial problems are considered basic whereas those required to ameliorate moderate-to-severe and more complex problems are considered advanced.

THE ESSENTIAL SKILLS OF EBPSW

It is difficult to define the actual skills and interventions employed by the practitioner without implying some intended response or change process in the client. *Skills, techniques* and *strategies* (collectively, the intervention) are terms that emphasize what the practitioners do. Change processes, however, are primarily psychological and emotional changes in the client that facilitate attainment of therapeutic goals. For example, a practitioner employs good listening and empathy skills with a mentally ill client, and as a result, the client responds with feelings of trust toward the practitioner and a degree of optimism that the practitioner will be helpful. The practitioner then uses cognitive techniques to help the client identify a consistent pattern of "expecting the worst" in social encounters, and with further discussion, the client reacts by remembering that, sometimes, social encounters in the past have gone well. The practitioner then role-plays with the client to practice asking someone out on a date. The client gains confidence that they just might be able to attempt it. These examples highlight the use of basic relationship-building skills, challenging dysfunctional beliefs, and rehearsing a change in behavior. Research on practice processes has demonstrated that many different practice methods, despite theoretical differences, share these and other "common processes" (Goldfried, 1980, 1995; Grencavage & Norcross, 1990; Orlinsky & Howard, 1986; Walborn, 1996; O'Hare, Collins, & Walsh, 1998; O'Hare, Tran, & Collins, 2002). These findings provide the basis for theoretical integration and practice eclecticism, two somewhat overlapping concepts relevant to EBPSW that will be addressed later in this chapter.

Although the common-processes approach implies that client change processes and intervention skills are overlapping constructs, *the emphasis in EBPSW is clearly on the eclectic application of intervention skills, techniques, and interventions.* Observable activities by the practitioner and client that collectively make up the intervention can be more readily defined than can underlying theoretical change processes. The pragmatic reason for emphasizing observable skills and interventions is so that practice methods can be more readily researched, taught, and evaluated. Based on reviews of both process and outcome research, practice skills can be subsumed under three major categories: *supportive and facilitative skills; therapeutic coping skills,* which include cognitive change techniques and behavior change techniques; and *case management skills,* which are essential for helping clients cope with social-environmental risks and barriers as well as for coordinating complex intervention plans (Lambert & Bergin, 1994; Orlinsky & Howard, 1986; Orlinsky, Grawe, & Parks, 1994; O'Hare et al., 1998; O'Hare Sherrer et al., 2002).

It is evident from both the process and outcome research literature that effective practices usually comprise some combination of intervention skills. The case for an eclectic, empirically based social work model that incorporates the use of the full range of psychotherapeutic and case management skills drawn from multidisciplinary sources is now stronger than ever. *Controlled practice research has produced an eclectic, multidisciplinary amalgam of supportive/facilitative, therapeutic coping skills and case management strategies that collectively have come to represent EBPSW* (J. Fischer, 1973, 1981, 1993; K. Wood, 1978; O'Hare, 1991; G. MacDonald, Sheldon, & Gillespie, 1992; Reid, 1997a, 1997b; O'Hare, Tran, & Collins, 2002).

Although not specifically considered part of the actual intervention, structural elements of treatment should be noted here because they define important parameters that affect service delivery. Structural elements include the programmatic context of care (e.g., inpatient, community agency, private practice); associated policies; bureaucratic, fiscal, and contractual conditions; the working contract with the client; and treatment planning and evaluation methods that may be incorporated into care (Orlinsky & Howard, 1986; K. Wood, 1978; B. R. Compton & Galaway, 1999; O'Hare, 1991; K. B. Wells, Astrachan, Tischler, & Unutzer, 1995).

Interacting structural and practice dimensions of effective care have been highlighted through research on brief treatments (Budman & Gurman, 1988; Eckert, 1993; Koss & Butcher, 1986; Koss & Shiang, 1994) and through exhaustive reviews of the clinical process and outcome research (Orlinsky et al., 1994; Lambert & Bergin, 1994). For example, despite the uncritical endorsement, by some, for employing long-term psychotherapy for moderate psychosocial conditions, mental health outpatient interventions with mild to moderate disorders have historically been relatively brief (average six to eight visits) in both public and private intervention settings (Koss & Shiang, 1994). Cost-effectiveness research suggests that programmers move beyond the simplistic short- versus long-term dichotomy, however, and emphasize developing optimal formats for type, frequency, and duration of the intervention based on clients' changing needs. Flexibility may prove to be a sensible approach leading to more ethical cost-effective care (K. B. Wells et al., 1995). Effective brief interventions are characterized by using evidence-based interventions, a sound collaborative working relationship, promptness in offering service, goal-oriented treatment planning, flexibility in scheduling visits, and using evaluation tools to monitor progress.

Cost-effectiveness research has already had profound effects on service policy. Although practitioners tend to assume that cost-effectiveness research uniformly endorses cuts in the amount of treatment, the evidence often supports more long-term care, varying the frequency and intensity in delivery of services.

Cost-effectiveness research is likely to continue to focus on identifying optimal service-delivery methods that are both effective and sensitive to cost. For example, although programs for assertive community treatment (PACT) have been shown to help reduce hospitalization among the mentally ill, the amount of service from which each client may benefit varies considerably. Rather than a use-it-or-lose-it approach to mental health program financing, evidence-based approaches should base the amount of care on need and the extent to which the client is likely to benefit (Essock, Frisman, & Kontos, 1998). Whether major service providers and managed-care organizations can move toward employing the best evidence in a cost-effective manner when defining "best practices" remains to be seen.

Supportive and Facilitative Skills

Supportive and facilitative skills include putting the client at ease; employing basic listening and communication skills; engendering trust; communicating empathy, genuineness, and positive regard; enhancing clients' confidence and morale and stimulating clients' motivation to engage in the intervention. Dimensions of the therapeutic relationship have been researched extensively in the counseling, psychotherapy, and social work literature for many years (e.g., C. Rogers, 1951; Barrett-Leonard, 1962; Truax & Carkhuff, 1967; Horvath & Greenberg, 1989; Duan & Hill, 1996; O'Hare, Tran, & Collins, 2002). Practitioners from different schools of thought may disagree about the nature of the relationship, the theoretical differences regarding the inferred change processes, and the associated therapeutic techniques employed. For example, theoretical explanations regarding how the working relationship affects change include the inherent curative effects of the human encounter, the collaborative problem-solving aspects of the relationship, and the creation of a psychological environment that facilitates the reexperiencing of childhood unconscious conflict. Although theoretical opinions vary regarding *how* the relationship helps, process and outcome research strongly supports the quality of supportive and facilitative skills as an essential dimension of effective psychosocial practice.

The therapeutic relationship provides other opportunities for change as well. Although social work practitioners have long been exhorted to "begin where the client is," only recently have practice researchers focused on the influence of clients' motivation and readiness to change. To underscore their importance, supportive and facilitative skills have taken on increased relevance as part of the growing interest in strategies that focus on motivating and engaging clients in the change process (W. R. Miller & Rollnick, 1991; Prochaska, DiClemente, & Norcross, 1992; O'Hare, 1996a). An empirical stage model of change has been developed by Prochaska and colleagues (Prochaska & DiClemente, 1984; Prochaska et al., 1992; McConnaughy, DiClemente, Prochaska, & Velicer, 1989) and stipulates five stages of change: *precontemplation,* when clients do not agree that they have a problem, may see others as the cause of their difficulties, or may feel coerced into treatment by the courts or significant others; *contemplation*, when a client is aware of a problem and may want to find out whether therapy can help; *preparation*, when the client is taking initial steps toward change; *action*, when a client may take more significant steps toward working on the problem and seek help in the change process; and *maintenance*, when clients have already made changes with regard to a problem and have sought treatment to consolidate previous improvements. Clients may cycle through these stages of change. A person with an addiction, for example, may consider change many times before taking action, and may relapse numerous times before stabilizing (DiClemente & Hughes, 1990). The stages-of-change model has been employed with a range of problems, including smoking cessation, substance abuse, and other mental health and health-related problems.

If stages of change suggest *when* clients are ready, motivational enhancement methods suggest *how* to help clients engage in the change process. Readiness to change is particularly relevant for working with clients who are more or less coerced into receiving social work services, and are often labeled by practitioners as resistant, hard to reach, hostile, and unmotivated (H. Goldstein, 1986; Rooney, 1992; W. R. Miller & Rollnick, 1991). The dichotomy of voluntary and involuntary is far from absolute, however. The findings of one investigation clearly demonstrated a tendency for voluntary clients to express much more engagement in the change process, but did not support the common generalization that all court-ordered clients are incapable or unwilling to change (O'Hare 1996b). Many involuntary clients can be engaged successfully through the skillful use of a number of strategies, such as accepting their initial reluctance, avoiding premature confrontation, clarifying one's dual role within the social service and criminal justice systems, providing some sense of control and choice in selecting treatment objectives and methods, avoiding overemphasis on irrelevant self-disclosure, anticipating obstacles to treatment compliance, employing behavioral contracting, involving significant others when at all possible, and actively enhancing motivation (Behroozi, 1992; Rooney, 1992; Meichenbaum & Turk 1987; W. R. Miller & Rollnick, 1991).

Although the supportive and facilitative skills are an essential dimension of effective intervention, they are also considered insufficient for establishing lasting change with more challenging psychosocial conditions (Lambert & Bergin, 1994). For more robust interventions, expert therapeutic cognitive and behavior coping skills are necessary.

Therapeutic Coping Skills

Empirically supported interventions that emphasize coping skills are used in every kind of contemporary cognitive-behavioral practice. Therapeutic coping skills are practitioner activities that help the client, the couple, or the family develop more effective ways of coping with psychosocial and environmental challenges. These skills may be initially promoted and taught by the practitioner, but it is an explicit goal of the intervention that clients will practice and incorporate them into their daily coping repertoire. Growth in understanding the interaction of cognitive, physiological, behavioral, and environmental elements of human experience has been largely driven by social-cognitive theory (Bandura, 1986), the foundation for cognitive-behavioral interventions (L. W. Craighead, Craighead, Kazdin, & Mahoney, 1994; Dobson & Craig, 1996). These skills and interventions are usually combined into an overall strategy, and implementation is guided by outcome research and tailored to clients' needs and treatment expectations. These skills include self-monitoring, psychoeducation, changing dysfunctional thinking, interpretation, behavioral coping, problem solving, contingency management, and stress management.

Self-monitoring techniques are self-assessment skills that clients use to learn about their problems and track progress in coping with them. This skill is highly flexible, can use qualitative (e.g., diaries) and quantitative (e.g., weekly charts) data collection, and should be crafted to precisely reflect the client's unique needs. Self-monitoring can be used to identify occurrences of psychological, physical, behavioral, interpersonal, or situational events that seem relevant to the cause or maintenance of the client's problem. Emphasis is placed on honing the client's skills in self-assessment by tracking the frequency, intensity, or duration of the problem, and by conducting a functional assessment that notes patterns, sequences, and psychosocial cues associated with the reoccurrence of the problem. These skills may include identifying triggers for substance-abuse relapse, anticipating events that provoke trauma-related flashbacks, learning to detect and recognize anger as a prelude to practicing constructive social responses, and identifying cues that trigger a child's obsessive-compulsive behaviors. Self-monitoring skills are key to connecting functional assessment with practice monitoring and evaluation. It thus combines assessment, intervention, and evaluation.

Psychoeducation can provide factual information to help inform clients about the nature of their problem and ways to cope. Often a preliminary and important component of intervention, psychoeducation can take many beneficial forms: to reduce self-blame in the families of people with severe mental illness; as a brief intervention for problem drinkers where feedback on medical and behavioral consequences is emphasized; as a basis for educating and reassuring anxiety-disordered clients that they are not "going to die" or "go crazy" as a result of their disorder; or to teach basic parenting skills to an overwhelmed, young, single mother. Psychoeducation, as with many of these skills, can be either a part of a multifaceted intervention or a stand-alone intervention.

Challenging and *changing dysfunctional thinking* has also become a prominent strategy for helping clients improve coping skills. Effective practice often operates on the assumption that client's difficulties are sometimes grounded in erroneous, distorted, or dysfunctional beliefs and thought processes regarding themselves, others, the world, and the future. Negative schemata can promote negative automatic thoughts and, subsequently lead to systematic thinking errors and poor coping abilities. It is essential to try to understand clients' unique view of themselves, others, and their world, challenge those views, and encourage creativity and resourcefulness in finding solutions. These techniques are also referred to in the practice literature as *cognitive restructuring*.

Helping clients learn from past experiences through *interpretation*, traditionally an approach associated with psychodynamic therapy, has come to be seen as a relatively generic aspect of other effective therapies as well (Lambert & Bergin, 1994; E. E. Jones & Pulos, 1993; Safran, 1998). Cognitive change is often focused on client's interpersonal relationships. In addition to providing support and facilitating change, the therapeutic alliance can serve as a proxy relationship for clarifying cognitive distortions regarding interpersonal conflict (past or present).

Practitioners can help clients clarify and disconfirm these interpersonal misattributions by examining the meaning of the interpersonal distortion or conflict, and then experientially testing the client's inferences. For example, if a young woman has been emotionally abused by important people in her life and continues to find herself in emotionally abusive relationships as an adult, it would be very helpful for her to identify what characteristics she looks for in an intimate relationship and reexamine those criteria. If these interpersonal distortions lead to repeated conflict though her misinterpretation of others' behaviors, testing her expectations may lead to "behavioral disconfirmation" of some of her more negative and distorted beliefs ("he is controlling and abusive because he really loves me," or "if I respond to his abuse with love, I know I can really change him!"). Behaviorally disconfirming these beliefs may lead to lasting change.

However, insight means more than understanding how past relationships affect current problems. Insight happens when clients make better cause-effect connections among their thoughts, feelings, behaviors, and interpersonal relations (past and present), and relate how these factors cause and maintain the problem (Cautela, 1993). An infinite array of "aha!" connections can constitute insight: when a client realizes that her excessive social drinking is exacerbating her depression and marital conflict; when an ambitious and overly competitive man realizes that his personal career is causing marital strain and alienation from his children; when a young mentally ill woman realizes that working part-time has given her a sense of accomplishment, and being around others has made her less afraid and mistrustful; when a young adolescent realizes that her mother's controlling behavior has more to do with her own anxieties than with her daughter's trustworthiness or lack of maturity; when a young couple realizes that their mistrust is based on prior failed relationships, and that frequent, open and honest communication diminishes mistrust. Although theories about how insight occurs may differ, most practitioners challenge clients to change the way they think about their own and others' behaviors, and help their clients understand the nature of their persistent difficulties in living. Obviously, insight can come in many forms, and coming to some understanding of the problem is *sometimes* a prelude to behavior change. In fact, insight may not occur primarily through verbal discussion of cognitive distortions and processes, but through behavior change that disconfirms distorted expectations (G. T. Wilson, 1995).

Once a good therapeutic alliance is established and the client has questioned some of her basic assumptions and beliefs about her problems, *behavioral coping skills* can help the client test those dysfunctional beliefs and establish more effective coping skills that may lead to lasting change (Thorpe & Olson, 1997; L. W. Craighead et al., 1994; Dobson & Craig, 1996). For many conditions, such as mental illness, addictions, marital and family problems, child abuse and neglect, and health-related disorders, behavioral coping skills and strategies have come to be seen as essential for competent social work practice, and are no longer dismissed as adjunctive means for enhancing "deep" therapy. These skills and techniques include *modeling, communication and problem solving, role-playing and rehearsal, graduated exposure* (i.e., graduated practice) of new behaviors in the "real world," and ongoing *practice*. Graduated exposure and ongoing practice in the client's own environment is the key to enacting intervention success, because without it there is little chance of generalizing the client's new skills across situations or maintaining therapeutic gains over time.

Problem-solving skills are often embedded in evidence-based intervention packages for both adults and children. Although there are slight variations on these models (e.g., D'Zurrilla & Goldfried, 1971; Meichenbaum, 1974), problem solving generally includes recognizing, exploring, and defining the problem; generating alternative solutions and developing a plan; anticipating consequences and obstacles to problem resolution; and performing, monitoring, and evaluating the problem-solving plan.

Contingency management techniques are also an essential component of many effective interventions. Implementing reinforcement procedures to reduce problem behaviors and increase adaptive and prosocial behaviors are an essential skill for many serious conditions, including self-regulation of health-risk behaviors, parenting skills to help children with internalizing and externalizing disorders, couples counseling, behavioral family interventions with adolescents, and social-skills training with the mentally ill and people with serious developmental disabilities. In addition, contingency management techniques have come to be seen as an essential component of interventions for court ordered and other involuntary clients. Outcome research should be referenced to help decide how and in what combination behavioral skills can be optimally used before applying them in practice. As will be seen in subsequent chapters, the empirical literature abounds in behavioral-skills methods (now most often packaged as cognitive-behavioral interventions). These are recognized as essential components of effective interventions for adults, children, and their families, spanning a wide spectrum of serious psychosocial disorders.

Therapeutic coping skills also include techniques for regulating physiological and emotional distress. These include various types of *stress-management* tools, including progressive muscle relaxation (Jacobsen, 1938), breathing and meditation techniques (Benson, 1975), and systematic desensitization (Wolpe, 1958, 1973) often accompanied by creative use of imagery to help clients confront their fears. Anxiety has long been a key concept in psychosocial theories, and the goal of regulating anxiety is common to most psychosocial change methods. Anxiety-reduction skills are also employed as part of successful interventions for the treatment of high blood pressure and pain control (Blanchard, 1994; Blechman & Brownell, 1998). Stress-management skills can be used alone for some clients, but are often part of an overall intervention package for more serious and complex disorders. They can be applied with unlimited creativity to accommodate client needs, preferences, and capabilities.

Although therapeutic coping skills can be used individually, they are typically used in combination as part of an overall cognitive-behavioral intervention designed to deal with more challenging psychosocial problems. For example, a young man with schizophrenia may learn to self-monitor delusional symptoms, engage in behaviors to disconfirm these frightening thoughts, participate in behavioral family therapy, and practice social skills in the community. A person suffering from agoraphobia will first establish control over anxiety symptoms through relaxation methods and imaginal exposure (i.e., gradually approaching the feared situation in her mind's eye), and then gradually spend increasing amounts of time outdoors or in a specific situation until the anxiety dissipates and her range of activities increases. Couples who argue destructively may work on basic communication skills, and then focus on clarifying interpersonal distortions that may have generalized from previous relationships. A single mom with a rebellious teenage son might benefit from learning better communication and negotiating skills, and setting better limits through the use of contingency management (i.e., rewards and sanctions). People with chronic addictions may learn to self-monitor triggers, use imagery to focus on negative consequences of use, and learn alternatives for dealing with negative or painful feelings that could precipitate relapse. How these therapeutic coping skills are combined as effective intervention methods will become increasingly evident in subsequent chapters.

Case Management Skills

Although many psychosocial difficulties can be effectively addressed through supportive, cognitive, and behavioral coping skills, these methods are often not robust enough to overcome the environmental pressures and barriers that weigh down many of our clients (O'Hare, 1996b; Bouton, 2000; Hopps, Pinder-hughes, & Shankar, 1995). Practitioners are remiss when they place disproportionate emphasis on psychological causes of clients' problems or focus solely on clients need to change. Evidence for the impact of social-environmental pressures such as homelessness, poverty, and discrimination on the psychological well-being of individuals is compelling (Dohrenwend, 1998; Avison & Gotlib, 1994; Moos & Moos, 1992). Although large-scale political and socioeconomic change may not be the primary target of the clinical or direct-practice social worker, evidence-based interventions demand a thorough assessment of social-environmental factors that affect the client directly. Some of these barriers and problems may be amenable to direct influence, or the client may be able to cope with them more effectively. If nothing else, an accurate and thorough assessment of social-environmental factors, even those beyond the client's direct influence, can provide an opportunity for psychoeducation, a reduction in self-blame, and a more realistic intervention plan that emphasizes the problems that are amenable to change.

Case management skills include an array of social work strategies that enhance client functioning through the coordination of complex interventions and improvement of access to other social, material, and environmental resources (Hopp et al., 1995; Woods & Hollis, 1990; Shulman, 1992; Rothman, 1991; Veeder, 2002). This role often requires a broad scope of knowledge concerning comprehensive assessment and treatment needs as well as a good degree of professional initiative, leadership, and communication skills to make interdisciplinary services and bureaucratic systems work in concert for clients. Beyond mere brokering of services, case management skills have come to be seen as essential for coordinating multiple services and enhancing instrumental and social supports with a range of problems, including mental illness (Mueser, Bond, Drake, & Resnick, 1998), child abuse and neglect (R. E. Lewis, Walton, & Fraser, 1995), conduct-disordered adolescents (Henggeler, Schoenwald, Borduin, Rowland, & Cunningham, 1998), and criminally involved people who abuse alcohol and other drugs (S. T. Higgins et al., 1993).

Enhancing social supports is one critical goal of case management. The quality of social supports is associated with a number of factors, including a sense of self-efficacy and personal empowerment (Gutierrez, 1990; Sarason, Pierce, & Sarason, 1994). Social supports can be either naturally occurring or orchestrated as part of formal social work interventions (Streeter & Franklin, 1992). They may include contact and emotional support from others and instrumental support, in the shape of concrete and tangible goods and services (Richey, 1994; Sarason et al., 1994). Social supports should also be understood both structurally (connections, networks, relations with different groups such as family, co-workers, and other social organizations) and functionally (availability, accessibility, and satisfaction with support received). Enhancing social supports may take many forms, such as encouraging clients to try out mutual-help groups like Alcoholics Anonymous (Humphreys, 1999), facilitating the development of a consumer group for people with mental illness (Heinssen, Levendusky, & Hunter, 1995), and providing social supports to buffer the stressful effects of grief on the elderly (Fitzpatrick, 1998). Practitioners may have to help clients optimize the potential benefits from social supports by helping them improve their social skills (Richey, 1994).

Case management methods have often been treated as a poor relative to psychotherapeutic skills, perhaps because using these skills is often associated with less attractive clients or less prestigious practice settings. For evidence-based

practitioners, it is understood that failing to provide effective coordination of services or ignoring social and environmental needs may preclude solid long-term
outcomes with even the most skillfully delivered intervention. Case management
skills, when used judiciously and assertively, can often be the most powerful
agent of stable change.

GUIDELINES WITH FLEXIBILITY

How the core skills and techniques of evidence-based practices are combined,
configured, and implemented in routine service is currently the focus of considerable debate. The major helping professions have only begun to struggle
with transferring psychosocial interventions shown to be efficacious in controlled trials into everyday practice. Two debates regarding implementation of
evidence-based practices are considered here: manualization versus flexibility,
and theoretical integration versus practice eclecticism.

Manualization versus Flexibility

The "manualization" of treatments derives largely from controlled practice research. Opinions vary regarding the use of treatment manuals to guide interventions (Mitchell, 2001; Kirk, 1999).

Some practitioners resist any perceived mandate to use interventions that
are not congruent with their own preferred approaches, feel that this movement
is a challenge to their professional autonomy, and consider manualization to be
little more than a cost-control strategy of managed-care organizations. Some
practitioners see that interventions for some mild conditions are often responsive to different approaches, and conclude that choice of intervention really
does not matter. Because *DSM* classifications drive outcome research, manualized interventions are designed for rather narrow clinical disorders. Social workers often address more complex psychosocial disorders, and clients' problems,
therapists' styles, and situational factors often preclude strict adherence to manualized approaches (Garfield, 1996).

Proponents of manualization respond to these criticisms by pointing out
that clinician preferences should not drive treatment selection, as there is no evidence that experience or "practice wisdom" alone is a sound basis for professional decision-making. Far from being cost-control measures, many manualized
guidelines are at odds with managed-care recommendations and call for two to
four times the number of sessions typically authorized by managed-care utilization review boards (J. R. Weisz & Hawley, 1998). Another point is that, although
basic counseling skills may be sufficient for many mild transitory problems-in-living, research demonstrates differential outcomes among intervention methods
with more serious psychosocial disorders.

Although diagnosis-driven practice guidelines are artificially narrow, there is
now a growing recognition that considerable flexibility is needed to apply in-

terventions optimally in everyday practice. This flexibility may be accommodated through advances in practice integration (i.e., reconciling underlying common change-processes, as noted above) and practice eclecticism (Garfield, 1996; Beutler, 1999; Scaturo, 2001; Reid, 1997b; O'Hare et al., 1998). The evidence-based practitioner should first learn effective interventions by the book and then adapt them to complex psychosocial problems with judgment, flexibility, and keen attention to the client's unique treatment expectations, goals, and circumstances. Although evidence for guiding flexibility in practice is currently sparse, practitioners should employ monitoring and evaluation methods to make incremental adjustments during the course of the intervention.

Initial investigations suggest that manualized care has been well-received by clients (Mitchell, 2001). Evidence also suggests that interventions conducted within the context of controlled investigations may often be quite comparable to "real" treatment conditions (M. E. Franklin, Abramowitz, Kozak, Levitt, & Foa, 2000). Manuals that guide research on and teaching of clinical practice can go a long way toward providing social work practitioners with the necessary expertise for intervening with serious psychosocial problems, and can reduce excessive variation in applying effective practices (G. T. Wilson, 1996).

Theoretical Integration versus Practice Eclecticism

Given that a variety of manualized intervention methods share a range of common skills and techniques, practitioners, in addition to specializing in one or two key manualized methods, should focus on learning core clinical skills that can be adapted to a range of client problems. The developments in theoretical integrations and practice eclecticism have illuminated many of these common processes and skills, and provide some guidance for improving the practical utility and transferability of manualized interventions.

Although *integration* and *eclecticism* are sometimes used interchangeably, they emphasize different aspects of theory and practice. Integrationists (e.g., Goldfried, 1980, 1995; Wachtel, 1977, 1987) are primarily concerned with reconciling theoretical explanations about how psychosocial interventions engender and facilitate change processes within the client or between the client and others (change-process theory). Thus, change processes are not the intervention skill itself, but are inferred cause-effect psychosocial processes that occur within the context of an intervention. (Human change processes can be studied outside the context of psychosocial interventions as well.) Change-process theory addresses questions at the very heart of practice theory and research. Research has identified a number of change processes common to different treatment approaches, such as the healing qualities of the interpersonal relationship (C. Rogers, 1951; Raskin & Rogers, 1995); insight and corrective reexperiencing to counter psychological harm associated with prior relationships (Brandel & Perlman, 1997; Ackerman, 1966; Scharff, 1995; J. Weiss, 1995; Henry, Strupp, Schacht, & Gaston, 1994; Henry, 1996); disconfirming dysfunctional thinking and increasing self-efficacy through behavior change (Bandura, 1986; G. T. Wilson, 1995); facilitating change in family structural and systemic processes (Nichols & Schwartz, 1995); and facilitating creative and spontaneous problem-solving activities through narrative, constructivist, solution-oriented, paradoxical, and strength-based approaches (Haley, 1976; Madanes, 1981; Saleeby, 1996; DeShazer, 1985; Granvold, 1996). Practice integrationists see theoretical common ground among the different practice models, and attempt to devise intervention strategies that optimally capitalize on them. Even where research has clearly demonstrated the efficacy of an intervention for certain psychosocial problems, however, little definitive evidence supports specific or unique underlying change processes as being the catalyst of change. This indeterminacy in the findings of change-process research extends to the treatment of depression (Oei & Shuttlewood, 1996), post-traumatic stress disorder (Tarrier, Sommerfield, Pilgrim, & Faragher, 2000), eating disorders (G. T. Wilson & Fairburn, 1993), and substance abuse (Mattson, 1994), among other problems.

While integrationists argue for common theoretical change processes, proponents of evidence-based eclecticism emphasize the optimal configurations of skills, techniques, and intervention strategies that are most likely to help clients solve problems, improve coping skills, and enhance psychosocial well-being. To clarify the difference between change processes and interventions, consider the following examples: if insight is the change process, interpretation would be the intervention; if altering dysfunctional thinking is change process, then Socratic questioning and behavioral disconfirmation (i.e., testing one's beliefs) are the interventions; if shifting power dynamics in a family is the change process, directed role-playing and practicing better communication skills among family members may help to achieve it; if feeling validated is an important change process, then empathic listening and communicating unconditional positive regard is the intervention; if a corrective emotional experience is the change process, then providing a good working alliance through empathic listening and a collaborative attitude is the intervention.

Change processes and practitioner skills are closely rated, but specific change processes and interventions are not necessarily linked in any unique combination. Different intervention strategies may activate the same change process, or an intervention may activate different change processes in different clients, or activate different change processes within the same client at different times over the course of the intervention. Obtaining insight, for example, may occur as a result of either verbal interpretation, behavioral practice, environmental changes, some combination of these, or some unknown serendipitous event. Perhaps the most obvious way of distinguishing change processes from psychosocial interventions is to point out that psychosocial changes occur in people all the time in the natural environment. The question for practitioners is whether they can effectively activate these change processes for the good of the client on a consistent basis through the use of formal psychosocial interventions. Thus, it is the actual intervention, not the inferred change process, that is the main focus of outcome research and practice evaluations in EBPSW.

Evidence-based practitioners give the highest priority to the use of existing outcome research to *guide* the choice and implementation of intervention, but employ flexibility to provide the optimal configuration of skills and interventions to accommodate the client's unique needs, expectations, and circumstances. Two of the better-known examples of formal eclectic models in psychotherapy practice include Arnold Lazarus's multimodal approach (1981, 1997) in which he uses a multidimensional assessment model (BASIC ID behavior, affect, sensation, imagery, cognition, interpersonal, drugs); and Beutler and Clarkin's systematic eclectic psychotherapy (1990), which attempts to tailor the intervention by using empirically guided considerations of patient's predisposing factors, relationship factors, treatment factors, and context. Both approaches rely first on empirical literature to guide treatment planning, but endorse considerable flexibility and judgment in dealing with specific cases. EBPSW incorporates the findings and strategies of eclectic psychotherapy, but adds case management skills to the mix to address more severe and complex psychosocial disorders than those typically addressed in psychotherapy practices.

A BRIEF OVERVIEW OF THE CURRENT FINDINGS OF OUTCOME RESEARCH

Up to this point, the discussion of EBPSW has focused mostly on specific skills, the essential components of effective interventions, and a rationale for flexibly combining them. Although articulating these skills is necessary in order to provide the practitioner with building blocks, or the ingredients to be eclectic, evidence-based practices are primarily delineated through studies demonstrating how combinations of these skills are efficaciously applied to serious psychosocial disorders. By necessity, these developments are the result of contributions from multiple disciplines, including social work, and are applied with clients in fields of practice where social workers have made substantial contributions: mental health, substance abuse, child abuse and neglect, and forensic services, among others.

Outcome research relevant to social work (i.e., psychotherapy, casework, psychosocial rehabilitation, and case management research) did not begin in earnest until after Eysenck (1952) in psychology and J. Fischer (1973) in social work posed the challenge to the helping professions to demonstrate the effectiveness of psychosocial interventions. By the early 1980s, a substantial body of clinical outcome research had emerged (Lambert, Shapiro, & Bergin, 1986). Traditional scholarly reviews (e.g., Luborsky, Singer, & Luborsky, 1975) and later meta-analytic reviews (e.g., M. L. Smith, Glass, & Miller, 1980) of the clinical research demonstrated the overall effectiveness of psychotherapy interventions. Reviews of the literature in social work, reported mixed results. (J. Fischer, 1973, 1981; K. Wood, 1978; Reid & Hanrahan, 1982; Rubin, 1985). Studies of outpatient treatment problems revealed comparable results for insight and behavior therapies (Sloan, Staples, Cristol, Yorkston, & Whipple, 1975; Lambert et al., 1986), but behavior therapies demonstrated superior outcomes with more serious disorders in both adults (Kazdin & Wilson, 1980) and children (J. R. Weisz, Weiss, Alicke, & Klotz, 1987). Positive findings for cognitive-behavior approaches continued to grow through the 1990s (Lambert & Bergin, 1994; Reid, 1997; Nathan & Gorman, 1998; J. R. Weisz, Donenberg, Han, & Weiss, 1995, B. Weiss, Catron, Harris, & Phung, 1999), and are often combined with case management skills for treating the most challenging client groups.

The most efficacious practices, in general, are more likely to be delivered effectively within the context of a competent and compassionate therapeutic alliance. In addition, psychosocial interventions for complex problems are more likely to be successful if delivered within a broader case management or multisystemic framework in collaboration with other professionals, in order to maintain psychosocial improvements over time and generalize results across different situations. Evidence supporting evidence-based practices for these problems (and more) will be examined in greater detailed in parts 2 and 3. What follows is a brief list of the outcome research that supports interventions for common and serious psychosocial interventions. The sources by no means list all the published research.

Cognitive-behavior approaches have been effectively implemented within a case management framework for helping people with severe and persistent mental illness (A. F. Lehman, Steinwachs, & Co-investigators of the PORT Project, 1998; Huxley, Rendall, & Sederer, 2000).

Interpersonal psychotherapy and cognitive-behavioral interventions have been shown to be comparably effective with depression (Weissman, Markowitz, & Klerman, 2000) and binge-eating disorder (G. T. Wilson & Fairburn, 1993; Shekter-Wolfson, Woodside, & Lackstrom, 1997; McIntosh, Bulik, McKenzie, Luty, & Jordan, 2000).

Cognitive-behavioral interventions have demonstrated clear superiority for serious anxiety disorders, including obsessive-compulsive disorders (Steketee, 1993; Abramowitz, Brigidi, & Roche, 2001), agoraphobia and panic attacks (Anthony & Swinson, 2999), and post-traumatic stress disorder (Rothbaum, Meadows, Resick, & Foy, 2000).

Cognitive-behavioral interventions have been shown to be effective with substance abuse and dependence (W. R. Miller, Meyers, & Hiller-Sturmhofel, 1999) and a positive addition to twelve step approaches (Humphreys, 1999; US-DHHS, 2000).

Cognitive-behavioral methods are very promising when incorporated into brief early intervention strategies with youthful substance abusers (Borsari & Carey, 2000).

Cognitive-behavioral interventions have been successfully applied to chronic adult behavioral disorders, including borderline personality disorder (Linehan, 1993a, 1993b; E. B. Simpson et al., 1998) and court-ordered offenders (McGuire & Hatcher, 2001), including those with chronic and severe drug addiction (S. T. Higgins et al., 1993; Abbott, Weller, Delaney, & Moore, 1998).

Emotion-focused therapy (Johnson & Greenberg, 1995), behavioral couples therapy (C. Thomas & Corcoran, 2001) and to a lesser extent insight-oriented couples therapy (Snyder, Wills, & Grady-Fletcher, 1991) have been shown to be effective for couples.

A large and growing body of research supports a range of cognitive-behavioral therapies for both internalizing and externalizing childhood and adolescent disorders (Kazdin & Weisz, 1998; Silverman & Berman; 2001; Farmer, Compton, Burns, & Robertson, 2002).

Cognitive-behavioral approaches for children's disorders are now increasingly implemented within the context of behaviorally oriented family therapies (S. N. Compton, Burns, Egger, & Robertson, 2002; Northey, Wells, Silverman, & Bailey, 2003). They are often incorporated into ecological and multisystemic frameworks to deal with complex and serious behavior problems such as youthful delinquency (Henggeler, Schoenwald, Borduin, Rowland, & Cunningham, 1998).

Although there have been serious methodological problems with much of the research on child-abuse and neglect interventions, some interventions have been shown to be more effective than others, particularly those that incorporate parenting skills and behavioral family therapies to prevent and reduce child abuse and neglect (Smokowski & Wodarski, 1996; Kazdin & Weisz, 1998; Lutzker, Bieglow, Doctor, Gershater, & Greene; 1998).

REVIEWING OUTCOME RESEARCH

Although reviews of the outcome research in journal articles and a growing array of texts on evidence-based practices are available to students and practitioners, social workers should be prepared to critically review outcome research themselves in order to stay abreast of state-of-the-art practices. This skill uses basic research methodology to access data bases through digital library resources and ability to distinguish true outcome research from marketing ploys. Although authors differ somewhat on the level of methodological rigor that should be employed in determining efficacy and effectiveness (see, e.g., Kazdin & Kendall, 1998; Chambless & Hollon, 1998; Thyer, 2001), the guidelines below should be considered minimal considerations when judging the quality of outcome studies. Their order reflects the organization of a journal research article. Some of the design terminology referred to below will be examined in chapter 4.

For an original research article, the literature review should be representative of the current available research and cover a range of refereed journals from social work, clinical psychology, psychiatry, marriage and family publications, as well as other relevant specialty journals. Review articles, which critically review and summarize previously published research, should cover all the available evidence.

The purpose of the study should be made clear. Is it an examination of the predictive validity of client, clinician, or practice processes, or does it primarily test the effectiveness of a specific treatment approach?

The author should clearly define client descriptors (e.g., age, sex, ethnicity), sources of referral, and diagnostic and other formal selection criteria. Client problems should be clearly defined, with valid baseline measures taken prior to the intervention.

If the article is a controlled outcome study, clients should be randomly assigned to treatment conditions or specifically matched to different interventions on a number of variables, such as age, gender, or problem severity. The intervention should be compared with some alternative treatment (or no treatment). Replication of controlled studies by independent research groups substantially strengthens an argument for efficacy. If the evaluation study has no control or comparison group, statistical controls can be used to help identify client and treatment factors that predict outcomes. Although these designs are not as strong, such studies are valuable because they sometimes reflect everyday practice conditions (effectiveness) more realistically than do some controlled investigations.

Single-subject designs, particularly ABAB and multiple baselines designs (described in chapter 4), may provide strong support for treatment efficacy if they are replicated on at least three study participants. Again, replication by other researchers strengthens the argument for efficacy.

If the study is testing the linkage between specific intervention components and client outcomes, clear linkage must be established between the intervention component and changes in client functioning in one or more areas. If the study is an investigation of theoretical change processes that are hypothesized to be activated by a specific intervention, a clear theoretical rational must be defined before casual inferences can be made regarding the effect of a specific intervention component on client outcomes. Demonstrating *how* the treatment works is much more difficult than demonstrating that the intervention *does* work.

The investigators should employ at least one standardized scale (preferably more) with a history of adequate validity and reliability for the subject population. Simple indexes with clear face validity (e.g., number of panic attacks or days in the hospital) are also useful. Measures should ideally focus on target problems and on broader measures of psychosocial well-being.

What practitioners and clients actually do should be clearly described. Vague references made to perspectives, orientations, or practice theories are not good enough. Treatment manuals, evidence of close supervision, adequacy of therapists' training in the specific interventions employed, and use of fidelity measures (scales that demonstrate the faithful implementation of the model; see chapter 4) are a plus.

Outcome data should include baseline measures, and additional measures taken at regular intervals that make sense given the duration of the program, at termination, and at follow-up at a reasonable time after service ends.

Discussion should examine methodological flaws as well as alternative explanations for outcomes. To argue that results can be generalized beyond the study participants, evidence that the intervention methods can be transferred and implemented in typical community service settings after some training of staff is essential.

SUMMARY

Effective social work interventions are likely to be defined by some optimal amalgam of supportive and facilitative skills, therapeutic coping skills, and case management strategies. Practitioners should initially consult the published outcome research and available clinical manuals and texts describing a method, obtain adequate training and supervision in the use of the method, and be prepared to apply the interventions with cautious flexibility within an eclectic practice framework.

CHAPTER 4

EVALUATING INTERVENTIONS
AND PROGRAMS

Interventions shown to be efficacious in controlled trials may not be implemented effectively due to a number of factors, including lack of training in specific practices, poor transfer of training, lack of funds for professional staff development, organizational structures and processes that militate against the implementation of evidence-based practices, and inadequate supervision. Evaluation is thus a key part of EBPSW. This chapter examines a number of evaluation designs to determine their relative strengths, weaknesses, and suitability for ensuring the effective implementation of evidence-based practices. The emphasis is on the use of naturalistic monitoring and evaluation methods that are integrated at both the individual practice and program levels. The chapter ends with a description of the complete service plan, from assessment to evaluation.

DESIGNS USED IN EVIDENCE-BASED PRACTICE RESEARCH AND EVALUATION

Social workers and allied professionals have been trying to bridge the gap between practice and research for some time. Many practice scholars have engaged in spirited debate regarding what the "best" evaluation design is, and whether qualitative or quantitative methods are superior. Before proceeding with an examination of the roles of different research and evaluation designs relevant to social work practice, some basic clarification is required.

As noted in chapter 1, practice research and practice evaluation have two somewhat overlapping purposes. Practice research tests whether interventions work under controlled conditions (to demonstrate efficacy), and practice evaluation is used to test whether interventions work under everyday practice conditions (to demonstrate effectiveness; Hargreaves, Shumway, Hu, & Cuffel, 1998; O'Hare, 2002). Now, this distinction is not always very neat. Some well-designed outcome studies can closely replicate "real-world" treatment conditions, and evaluation designs can range from *naturalistic evaluation*, where few efforts are made to control or manipulate treatment conditions, to controlled *evaluation research*. Thus, the differences between controlled outcome research and naturalistic evaluation may best be understood on a continuum from a high level of control of client and intervention variables to no controls. Controlled evaluation research is somewhere in the middle of the continuum. This gradation of control applies to both single-subject and group designs, and both qualitative and quantitative data can be used to measure outcomes in any design (although qualitative data becomes somewhat unwieldy with larger groups of clients). This continuum of control roughly corresponds to the classic distinctions among "preexperimental," "quasiexperimental," and "experimental" designs (see table 4.1).

Distinguishing controlled outcome research, evaluative research, and naturalistic monitoring and evaluation is a matter of degree, and it is a distinction that should become increasingly blurred as agency-based evaluation improves in methodological quality. However, in addition to pragmatic considerations (cost, feasibility of the design, purpose of the research or evaluation project), the differences among the different research and evaluation designs can be explained as differences in balancing internal and external threats to validity.

The many potential sources of error should prevent practitioners and evaluators from being supremely confident in assuming that their positive treatment outcomes are the direct result of the intervention. These threats to drawing valid conclusions are problems of *internal validity*. One has to consider whether the

TABLE 4.1   Evaluation and outcome research designs

High control	Moderate control	Low control
Efficacy		Effectiveness
Experimental design	*Quasi-experimental design*	*Preexperimental design*
Controlled outcome studies (either groups of clients or single-subject).	Evaluation research	Naturalistic program evaluation.
Clients are carefully selected.	Clients may be selected or matched across two different approaches, or two programs are compared and statistical controls are used to determine treatment effectiveness.	Monitoring a single case, using qualitative or quantitative methods to measure outcomes.
Practitioners are trained to the treatment manual.		
Clients are matched or randomly assigned to the experimental and comparison (control) groups.	Outcome measures are used.	No design or statistical controls used.
In single-subject studies, clients serve as their own control.		
Multiple outcome measures are used.		

intervention was implemented faithfully (treatment fidelity), whether the client would have improved with no treatment or some alternative intervention, whether other factors such as the client's history, maturational, or other external factors played a role, whether "good" clients are being self-selected by the practitioner-evaluator, whether there were problems in using the instruments to collect data, and whether statistical analysis (when data are aggregated) was done correctly.

Practitioners should also be concerned with how well the intervention will replicate in similar practice environments with other client groups. These ambiguities are caused by threats to *external validity*. For many reasons, one cannot assume that a successful intervention with one person or even a whole program can be successfully exported to other situations. As noted earlier, practitioners often feel that interventions shown to be effective in well-controlled outcome studies don't seem to fit their own practice situation. This transition from efficacy studies to effectiveness gets to the heart of generalization, that is, external validity. What is certain is that all approaches to evaluation research have their share of strengths and weaknesses, as well as their place in the seamless continuum of reasoned inquiry into matters of practice efficacy and effectiveness.

The commonalties and shared purposes of clinical social work practice and evaluation methods have long been recognized (Siegel, 1984; O'Hare, 1991; K. Corcoran & Gingerich, 1994; K. Cocoran, Gingerich, & Briggs, 2001). Both activities require that clients and practitioners make judgments about the nature of the client's problem, determine what kind of intervention should be used, measure whether the client's problems are improving, and whether the intervention had anything to do with the outcome. Although it may seem to some practitioners that drawing conclusions about the effectiveness of their practice with a specific case should be relatively straightforward, such conclusions can often be misleading. In addition, when one has to answer the same question regarding 10, 100, or 1000 clients in a program, evaluation becomes even more challenging. Nevertheless, practitioners and evaluators must begin in the same place: define the problem, define the intervention, and establish some criteria and a method for judging success. What follows is a review of the more common designs used in evaluation and outcome research, and their relative strengths and weaknesses in providing sound answers to matters of efficacy and effectiveness.

QUALITATIVE APPROACHES

Qualitative evaluation employs an array of observational data-collection techniques and methods of analysis to obtain detailed, highly textured descriptions of human behavior, including making cause-effect inferences about the efficacy of social work practice interventions. Qualitative methods have long been commensurate with traditional methods of social science. They similarly require review of the existing literature and sampling strategies, and often include quantitative data collection. Qualitative researchers investigating social work practice may employ focus groups, in-depth interviews, case studies, and structured or semistructured questionnaires. Qualitative methods provide nuance, detail, and exploratory flexibility not usually obtainable with experimental or most large-sample survey methods. Although there is often a heavier emphasis on thick description in qualitative case studies, this approach also requires making cause-effect linkages between interventions and outcomes, based on one's observations. Case studies are a unique complement to experimental research, often spawning innovative assessment or intervention hypotheses. Qualitative methods are good for studying rare phenomena, can provide some degree of disconfirmation of a prevailing theory or claims of practice effectiveness (through counterinstance), and have persuasive and motivational value (Kazdin, 1998; C. Marshall & Rossman, 1995).

In response to the romanticizing of qualitative methods in social work literature (Heineman-Pieper, 1985; K. B. Tyson, 1992), some authors have highlighted considerable liabilities in the use of qualitative methods (Gambrill, 1995; Mullen, 1995; Stake, 1995). Qualitative inquiry is highly susceptible to personal bias. The tendency to force-fit observations to one's preferred theories provides a weak basis for drawing conclusions, often raises more questions than it answers, is extremely labor intensive, and yields few generalizable results, resulting in relatively little overall contribution to the social science knowledge base. Drawing cause-effect conclusions from qualitative research or evaluation requires extreme caution, and often begs alternative explanations. Nevertheless, qualitative evaluation can provide excellent detailed idiographic (naturalistic) analysis of unique cases, and is an essential beginning point for developing a more systematic evaluation protocol.

Although qualitative *research* can be highly controlled, qualitative *evaluation* is typically used in uncontrolled designs to assist practitioners in evaluating their own practice (i.e., the standard case study). However, conclusions about treatment effectiveness from single-case analyses should be taken with a grain of salt. Observing that the client has improved, stayed about the same, or deteriorated since the initial assessment is the main function of monitoring and simply tells us how the client is doing. Given the limitations of qualitative evaluation with single cases, drawing the conclusion that the intervention was the primary cause of client change should be done cautiously.

SINGLE-SYSTEM DESIGNS

Single-system design (also called single-subject, $n = 1$) in social work practice generally refers to evaluation of an intervention with a client or a family. In single-system design, the baseline measure is typically represented as A (which provides a measure of current performance and a criterion against which one predicts change in the client's problem), and the intervention is represented as B (C, and D, etc., for multiple interventions). Although single-system designs are typically used for uncontrolled (naturalist) monitoring of cases, some are referred to as "experimental" because the underlying logic of control is similar to that of classic group experimental designs: the design compares intervention effects under different treatment conditions, and the client serves as his own control. Variations on experimental single-system designs include withdrawal and reintroduction of the intervention (ABAB design, called the reversal design), introduction of an alternative intervention (ABAC), and combinations of interventions (ABCA). Obviously, many other design variations are possible (Kazdin, 1978, 1992; Hersen, 1985; Bloom et al., 1999).

Given that the baseline constitutes the criteria against which the success of treatment is judged, a stable baseline (with several observations) is preferred, because an improving baseline makes it more difficult to argue that a successful outcome was the result of the intervention and not just the result of spontaneous improvement or other nontreatment factors. The new level of performance provides a new baseline for future changes in the treatment condition. Treatment can be withdrawn to see if performance deviates from the predicted level under treatment, or to see if the original baseline would have continued. Baselining is often done retrospectively when collecting baseline data and withholding the intervention is either impractical or unethical. In actual practice, intervention withdrawal can happen spontaneously, as clients sometimes unexpectedly drop out of treatment and return at a later date.

There are a number of benefits to employing $n = 1$ methodology. First, simple designs are relatively easy to implement as a monitoring and evaluation tool. Second, single-system designs are quite flexible and can be designed to fit unique practice situations. Third, they provide some degree of structure for treatment planning by necessitating clear definitions of problems, interventions, and goals. Fourth, clients often see the utility of evaluation and are willing to use self-monitoring devices to baseline their problems and track their own progress. Defining a particular problem becomes a self-monitoring tool in addition to providing baseline data for tracking progress and outcomes. Although (as with qualitative evaluation) conclusions about the effectiveness of the intervention with a single case should be made cautiously, replication with similar cases using controlled experimental single-system designs can provide some basis for generalization regarding the efficacy of an innovative intervention method.

Methodological problems with single-system designs can be formidable, however (Kazdin, 1978; Bloom et al., 1999). These include several threats to internal validity. Obtaining stable baselines is often impractical. Altering phases or conditions during intervention can cause ambiguity in the interpretation of outcomes. Clients often do not improve in linear, incremental fashion, but take two steps forward, one step back. It is difficult to attribute changes in the client to specific interventions when multiple interventions are employed (ABCA). And cause-effect reasoning can be confounded by "history" or "carry-over effects" because clients' recollections of previous events affect their future behavior (Wakefield & Kirk, 1995).

Originally employed to evaluate behavior-modification methods with the most severely disordered populations, single-system design is less useful with more-complex cognitively based or eclectic interventions because it is more difficult to link client improvements to specific treatment methods or different phases of treatment. In addition, aside from naturalistic monitoring and evaluation in which no treatment conditions are altered, it is unrealistic to expect busy practitioners to employ well-planned single-system designs in everyday practice, and it is unethical to manipulate treatment conditions without clients' informed consent. Every case subjected to a new design would have to be approved by an institutional review board . . . a prospect that is not likely to be welcomed by busy administrators. Unless the administrative permissions were expedited, clients would have to wait, perhaps unnecessarily, for the intervention to commence. Perhaps the most serious problem with single-system designs is that they can be applied to only a handful of cases at one time, and generalizing results to other clients or treatment situations is impractical. The question is, beyond simple monitoring and evaluation, what can be inferred about the effectiveness of the intervention? Some social work commentators have suggested that social work go beyond the limitations of idiographic evaluation and emphasize program evaluation instead (Benbenishty, 1996).

Others have argued that $n = 1$ evaluation has advantages over group designs because, first, problems and interventions can be more specifically defined for the individual client, and second, making causal linkages between interventions and outcomes appears to be more straightforward (Bloom et al., 1999; Ivanoff, Blythe, & Briar, 1987; Mattaini, 1996). Ambiguity in defining the intervention is not an inherent weakness of group designs, however, and making causal connections between treatment and outcomes is certainly no easier in single-system design than in group designs. The use of treatment manuals and intervention process measures can capture many of the salient dimensions of the intervention in group designs, and group designs can provide a stronger basis for inferring causality between intervention and outcome along with a stronger case for generalization. In addition, the use of single-system designs without reference to treatment selection presents a more fundamental dilemma for social work practitioners: what criteria do we use to guide our choice of intervention in the first place? In summary, single-system designs provide a sound basis for routine monitoring and evaluation and, when used as a controlled experimental design with several cases, serve as a valuable tool for investigating the efficacy of innovative treatments, an important first step on the path to controlled outcome research.

GROUP DESIGNS

Controlled group designs are not typically employed in the routine evaluation of social work interventions, but constitute a methodological gold standard for conducting efficacy studies. More advanced group designs (randomized experimental designs) do a good job of controlling for internal threats to validity, although generalizing to everyday practice environments must be done with caution. In group designs, relationships among intervention and outcome variables are examined in a number of configurations (Kazdin, 1994a, 1998; Campbell & Stanley, 1963; Royse, Thyer, Padgett, & Logan, 2001). These strategies include larger numbers of clients (at least ten under each condition, although more is preferable) and may compare the experimental treatment to intervention (control group) or an alternative intervention (comparison group, often treatment as usual in the community). The basic models of group designs are considered here.

The elements of experimental design include the initial observation (O1) of the client's difficulties, the intervention (X), and a subsequent measure of the client's problem (O2) to determine some degree of change. If only these basic elements are employed with no comparison or control group, this design is a preexperimental or prepost design. As noted in table 4.1, this design reflects a low level of control. The model conceptually can be portrayed as

$$O1 \qquad X \qquad O2$$

This design illustrates the basic components of controlled research but is itself a weak argument for drawing conclusions regarding the efficacy of the intervention, because there is no basis for comparison (clients could improve for reasons other than the intervention).

A typical quasi-experimental design compares the original intervention to some alternative treatment.

$$O1 \qquad X1 \qquad O2$$
$$O3 \qquad X2 \qquad O4$$

This design provides a stronger basis for inferring treatment efficacy or effectiveness than the first design, because of the presence of a comparison group. But it is still difficult to draw firm conclusions. How clients are assigned to the different groups also matters considerably. If clients chose their own treatment condition (perhaps by seeking help in two different mental health agencies, X1 and X2), then the design would be considered quasi-experimental. The weakness in this design, of course, is that little consideration is given to the impact of differences in the agencies themselves of the effect of clients' treatment expectations or other factors (such as socioeconomic status or location) that may have influenced their decision to select one agency over another. This model reflects a moderate degree of control, although alterations in the design could strengthen the level of control (e.g., matching clients in both groups on selected demographic variables through client selection or through statistical controls).

If clients are randomly assigned to these different treatment conditions, however, the design becomes experimental, and can be depicted as

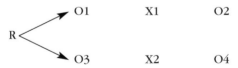

The R represents random assignment to these two groups. Purists might contend that the above design is still quasi-experimental. The classic experimental design

compares the effects of one intervention with a "placebo" or no intervention at all (usually a waiting-list control group), and would be illustrated as

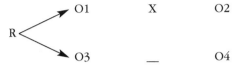

The __ represents the control group.

One way to strengthen this design would be to collect follow-up data to see how stable the changes are over three to six months or more. With that addition, the previous model would like

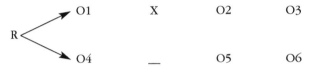

Although not foolproof, random assignment tends to reduce the likelihood that outcomes would be affected by client differences such as client-selection factors or treatment expectations rather than the effects of the intervention.

Experimental designs can become increasingly complex. For example, researchers may decide to measure two variations of an experimental treatment with a comparison or control group. To maintain the experimental quality, cases would have to be randomly assigned to three treatment groups. If researchers wanted to compare the effects of treatment on equal numbers of men and women across all three groups, the participants would also have to be randomly assigned to both treatment groups and the "treatment as usual" comparison or control group. When specific client or practitioner factors are controlled for, these are referred to as factorial designs.

Controlled comparisons have the potential to provide robust evidence to support whether an intervention is efficacious. Depending on design complexity, they can also account for the role of client and practitioner factors, the effects of individual treatment components, and interactions among these factors. They have other advantages as well: pretesting allows for better client matching and accounts for different pretest performance levels among clients; data allow for measures of change both within and between the treatment groups; and controlled studies can control for the effects of attrition. Controlled experimental designs can make a strong case for treatment efficacy when clients are well-chosen, practitioners are well-trained, and the instruments employed are reliable and valid. Results can also be sufficiently robust to justify the claim of superiority of one treatment over the alternative treatment or control group, particularly if several similar studies replicate these findings.

These approaches are not without limitations, however. Drawing conclusions about the relationship between the interventions and changes in clients' problems can still be difficult due to a number of threats to validity (Kazdin, 1994a).There may be variations and inconsistencies in the way the interventions were provided; disproportionate or excessive attrition; aspects of the intervention that are unaccounted for in the design; unintentional cues that the participants in the experimental group were getting the "better" intervention; low statistical power; and use of instruments that have poor reliability, validity, or sensitivity to change. Perhaps one of the most difficult problems is in generalizing the results of controlled trails to real practice situations. Despite the limitations, however, replicated controlled trails provide the strongest basis for establishing intervention efficacy, and provide the foundation for intervention planning in EBPSW.

NATURALISTIC PROGRAM EVALUATION

Although controlled designs provide valuable guidelines for choice of intervention, they are rarely used as a method of routine evaluation in human service agencies, due to their exacting requirements. One strategy for evaluating whether evidence-based practices are implemented effectively accommodates the demands of day-to-day agency practice.This approach is naturalistic evaluation (also known as passive-observational designs; Kazdin, 1998; Hargreaves et al., 1998; Rossi & Freeman, 1993).

Naturalistic evaluation strategies can accommodate the classic organizational model that integrates agency structure, service processes, and client outcomes (Donabedian, 1980; Salzer, Nixon, Schut, Karver, & Bickman, 1997). Structurally, programs should be well-designed, with a clear organizational mission and goals that support the administration, training, implementation, supervision, and evaluation of evidence-based interventions. Naturalistic designs employ assessment and evaluation methods that can be readily integrated into normal clinical and administrative functions of human service agencies. As the term *naturalistic* implies, no extraordinary means (such as random assignment, or control groups) are used to manipulate the treatment conditions. Agencies function as usual in terms of general service delivery, but great emphasis is placed upon developing quality programming based on careful reviews of the relevant practice outcome literature; training staff in best practices; and integrating the use of brief, reliable, and valid measures into assessment and evaluation procedures to capture pretest, posttest, and (in sampled cases) follow-up data over time.These data collectively link client characteristics, elements of the intervention, outcomes, and (with increasing emphasis) service costs in one coherent model (Salzer et al., 1997; Newman, Howard,Windle, & Hohmann, 1994; O'Hare et al., 1998; Lyons,J. S. Howard, O'Mahoney, & Lish, 1997; G. R. Smith, Fischer, Nordquist, Mosley, & Ledbetter, 1997). Meaningful and useful reports can then be designed to enhance administrative decision making and respond to accountability expectations of insurers, funding agencies, and quality-assurance organizations.

Although the ideal scenario for developing such systems would be to start from scratch, evidence-based practices and evaluation procedures can be implemented at any time, often in fluid and contentious service environments. Achieving a reasonable measure of both practicality and scientific validity is a constant balancing act when conducting program evaluation. The intervals for data collection during the intervention and at some follow-up period will vary based on the treatment environment. For outpatient mental health programs that provide brief interventions of generally less than eight visits, data may be collected at baseline, termination, and (with sampled clients) at three-month follow-up as indicated in the paradigm O1 X O2 ... O3). For a program that serves people with severe mental illness, the design would likely require repeated measures over longer periods during which different components of intervention are offered: O1 X1 X2 O2 O3 X3 O4 and so on. In addition to basic univariate data reports (i.e., baseline and outcome data periodically reported for groups of clients), more sophisticated statistical techniques should be provided by expert consultants to examine the relationships among several types of variables, including client characteristics, intervention type, frequency of visits, service cost, and client outcomes.

Because naturalistic evaluation is based on the preexperimental paradigm, there are inherent threats to validity. Nevertheless, selection and development of key measures can strengthen the design. A data-collection package should minimally include key client characteristics; brief, reliable, and valid assessment and outcome measurers that are sensitive to detecting changes in client functioning and well-being over the course of the intervention; consumer satisfaction measurers; fidelity measures (discussed below) that can capture key aspects of the interventions employed; and a range of other indexes that may be useful for other external reporting requirements. At the individual case level, the combination of qualitative and quantitative data provides the basis for monitoring and evaluating intervention. Quantitative data aggregated from scales and indexes provide the basis for program evaluation. The combination of client, intervention-process, and assessment and outcome measures provides a comprehensive system for naturalistic program evaluation that can be seamlessly integrated into the delivery of evidence-based practices (J. S. Lyons et al., 1997; Salzer et al., 1997; Newman et al., 1994; Royse & Thyer, 1996; [Joint Commission on the Accreditation of Healthcare Organizations], 2004; Yates, 1996).

Although naturalistic designs reflect considerable external validity in their real-world application, this approach incurs some degree of threats to internal validity even when they are well-designed and carefully implemented. Potential problems include the inability to consider other explanations for client improvement (e.g., alternative programming), substandard implementation of the intervention methods, poor data-collection procedures, moderating effects of repeated data collecting, history and maturational affects of the clients, and client-selection factors (Rossi & Freeman, 1993; Hargreaves et al., 1998; J. S. Lyons et al., 1997; K. Corcoran & Vandiver, 1996). The strength of the naturalistic evaluation is its external validity. The quality of practice and service delivery is being judged within the context of the typically messy, complex, and unpredictable environment of the human service agency.

FIDELITY ASSESSMENT

Simply because an agency or an individual practitioner claims to use evidence-based practices does not mean that they are implemented with a high degree of skill. Although evaluation usually brings to mind client outcomes, measuring various aspects of the intervention is becoming increasingly important and, in some instances, is mandated by funding sources. The main purpose for measuring the intervention process itself is to ensure that evidence-based interventions are being implemented with fidelity, that is, actual service delivery is faithful to the intervention as described in "the manual." In an agency setting, three methods are available to achieve this end: qualitative case analysis in supervision or supervised focus groups; direct observation (e.g., the one-way window); and fidelity and other process measures completed by staff and/or clients as part of routine clinical documentation. These data can be entered into a data base, aggregated, and linked to client characteristics and client outcomes to enhance the program evaluation.

Qualitative process evaluation (case-study analysis) is an invaluable tool for examining implementation up close and personal. Through supervision or focus groups, practitioners can examine the intervention process through case discussions and scenario building as a brainstorming method to discuss how to deal with more challenging and less predictable cases. This constructive sharing of practice experience can help staff learn to anticipate problems that may arise and address them in a way that maintains the essential integrity of an evidence-based approach. Under selected circumstances, practitioners can be observed in vivo with clients (with clients consent) in order to compare the practitioner's intervention approach with the model, and to help the practitioner deal with unanticipated occurrences. As with program monitoring and evaluation in general, these activities should be undertaken in a context of mutual support to help refine methods and learn to adapt evidence-based practices creatively to complex client problems. However, case studies must be balanced against larger data bases compiled from fidelity scales and other intervention-process indicators such as type, frequency, and duration of service. One way to ensure reasonable congruency between the model and actual implementation is to allow for some degree of flexibility in the application of evidence-based approaches, so practitioners can adjust manualized approaches to the needs of more complex cases. The thoughtfully planned application of both qualitative and quantitative methods for measuring intervention fidelity can help ensure high-quality services.

A number of process instruments measure different dimensions of psychosocial interventions (Hill, Nutt, & Jackson, 1994; O'Hare & Collins, 1997). Most of these focus on the interpersonal aspects of psychotherapy, an important but incomplete view of psychosocial interventions. Recently, a number of promising initiatives have demonstrated that the implementation of practice skills for social work practice can be measured reliably. These scales include the Inpatient Measure of Adolescent and Child Services and Treatment (Pottick, Hansell, & Barber, 1998), the Hospital Social Work Self-Efficacy Scale (Holden, Cuzzi, Rutter, Rosenberg, & Chernack, 1996), the Dual Disorder Treatment Fidelity Scale (Mueser et al., 2003), the Practice Skills Inventory (O'Hare & Collins, 1997; O'Hare et al., 1998; O'Hare, Tran, & Collins, 2002), the Substance Abuse Treatment Self-Efficacy Scale (Kranz, 2003; Kranz & O'Hare, in press), and a fidelity measure of service delivery with people who have severe mental illness and substance-abuse problems (Teague, Bond, & Drake, 1998).

Fidelity instruments vary in the level of service delivery being measured. Variations include measurement of service-program processes (such as indicators that assessments were conducted, and clients referred for treatment), the use of certain "packaged" intervention models (such as motivational interviewing, and behavioral family therapy), the use of practice skills, and basic administrative aspects of service delivery.

The Practice Skills Inventory (PSI) is one process measure that could be adapted for use as a fidelity scale. Theoretically based on broad reviews of the practice literature, the PSI measures three major categories of intervention skills: supportive skills that focus on facilitating a sound working relationship, coping-skills interventions that include a range of problem-solving and cognitive-behavioral methods shown to be essential for moderate to severe psychosocial disorders, and case management skills, which are essential for coordinating complex cases. One study with experienced practitioners also supported the use of an "insight facilitation" skill (O'Hare et al., 1998), a subscale that represents more interpersonal approaches to psychosocial treatment. The PSI has been shown to have good-to-excellent internal consistency reliability for all its subscales, and has demonstrated a good factor structure with both student and experienced social work practitioners (O'Hare & Collins, 1997; O'Hare, Tran, & Collins, 2002).

The PSI has a number of potential uses that social work students, practitioners, researchers, and evaluators can explore. These include examining patterns of skill application in practice; measuring the implementation of evidence-based guidelines; examining whether skill application varies with different types of problems or severity of problems presented by clients; examining variations in skill application over time within the same case; and linking processes with outcomes. A slightly modified version of the PSI is included in appendix C to be used as an exploratory device by students and practitioners with individual cases. (It may be reproduced without permission.) The instructions direct the practitioner to indicate the number of client contacts on which completion of the scale is based. The number of contacts could range from one to several, depending on service-delivery patterns. Respondents then report the frequency with which they used certain skills with a particular client during that period of time. Respondents can describe in more detail the particular skill used. Students and practitioners could use the scale for self-review or in supervision to compare the configuration of practice skills they relied upon with those recommended in the literature. At the program level, evaluators could aggregate data with the PSI to determine whether the proper category of skills generally conform to best practices, and use the results of such a report as a basis for providing feedback to staff. These data could prompt further supervision, consultation, or staff development.

The individual items of the PSI were designed to be somewhat general so the scale could have broad application to social work service settings. Practitioners estimate the frequency with which they used these general skills, and describe more specifically what skill they actually used with their client. In this way, the PSI can serve as a tool for both qualitative and quantitative analyses. For an item on the coping-skills subscale, for example, the practitioner could specifically define the intervention skill used with that client (in parentheses under the specific item). For a conduct-disordered adolescent, it might read "taught and role-played anger management skills." Although more validity work is required for the PSI, students and practitioners are encouraged to use the scale in an exploratory way to examine practice patterns relative to guidelines provided in evidence-based practice texts and treatment manuals.

The Substance Abuse Treatment Self-Efficacy Scale was designed to measure practitioners' confidence in carrying out substance-abuse intervention skills. This scale appears in appendix D and may be used without permission. The scale has thirty-two items and measures five domains of substance-abuse skills employed by social workers: assessment/treatment planning, individual counseling, group counseling, case management, and ethics. The instructions direct practitioners to rate their level of confidence in using specific skills for working with substance-abusing clients. The scale can be used to evaluate practitioners' training needs or, with minor modification, as a fidelity tool in environments where it is important to measure how consistently practitioners are using core substance-abuse intervention processes and skills. To be used as a fidelity scale, the instructions could be modified to have respondents measure "how confidently they applied each skill with a particular client." The instrument was validated through exploratory and confirmatory factor analysis, and showed excellent internal consistency reliabilities for all subscales (.89–.96). Further field testing across an array of service environments is needed to strengthen its external validity.

THE EBPSW SERVICE PLAN

The key link between individual service delivery and program evaluation is the qualitative/quantitative service delivery plan. Most practitioners and agencies are required to document their services to clients. This documentation takes many forms and is far from standardized. The format varies by funding source, accreditation organizations, and state and federal regulatory agencies. Although documentation varies considerably, some basic assumptions are suggested here. First, documentation is required, necessary, and important for a variety of contractual, legal, risk management, and ethical reasons. Second, although service documentation is often (and sometimes justifiably) seen as a time-consuming and expensive nuisance, documentation can be an essential part of delivering and evaluating evidence-based practices for a number of important reasons: when conceptually well-designed, service plan documentation can improve the validity and reliability of assessment; clarify the goals, objectives, and methods used in the intervention; and detail the methods used for monitoring and evaluation. Third, a well-conducted assessment, intervention, and evaluation plan is essential for guiding individual service for clients, and when data from individual service plans are aggregated, they can provide a sound basis for program-level evaluation.

The Assessment

As outlined in chapter 2, the assessment should include a number of basic considerations: a thorough psychosocial history and problem formulation that is informed by contemporary human behavior theory, assessment of the severity of client problems across multiple problem domains, and a detailed functional assessment of psychosocial factors that affect the client's main difficulties. This detailed MDF assessment should be supported by thoughtfully chosen instruments that can also serve as outcome measures. These instruments are likely to be a combination of individual indexes specific to client problems and standardized instruments that provide a foundation for naturalistic evaluation.

The Intervention Plan

Once the assessment data have been collected, practitioners and clients need to collaboratively define problems and goals. This process includes, first, developing a *definition of the client's problem(s)* based on the MDF assessment. Although the assessment may provide a somewhat complex understanding of the factors involved in the client's problems, the final problem definition should be relatively straight-forward.

Second, practitioner and client should *decide on reasonable intervention goals,* that is, achievable resolution of problems or acquisition of certain coping abilities. Goals can be stated somewhat generally, although they should represent a reasonable and clinically significant improvement in the client's condition and ability to cope.

Third, practitioners should *reference evidence-based practices,* discuss them with the client, and discuss how they can collaboratively and flexibly implement the intervention to accommodate the client's needs and circumstances. Interventions should be defined by the formal title of the approach, the details of actual implementation should be spelled out.

Fourth, practitioner and client must *define intervention objectives,* that is, short-term and hierarchically ranked stepping stones that lead toward the ultimate treatment goal. Objectives are a critical linchpin between the practitioner's intervention skills and the client's efforts at problem-solving and strengthening coping skills. Objectives are likely to unfold and change as the client improves, as new problems arise, or if a new approach is taken. Treatment plans should be updated as objectives are achieved.

Objectives may be defined as "incremental steps toward a treatment goal," but they may also overlap with the interventions for one simple reason: an intervention is not something that is *done to the client.* The objectives are often the main vehicle by which the client implements the intervention. So, for example, the practitioner might provide psychoeducation and a brief intervention to encourage a client to try out an Alcoholics Anonymous meeting (the objective) in the coming week. A traumatized young woman who has become agoraphobic may benefit from an intervention that includes support, psychoeducation, anxiety-management skills, and practice to gradually confront the anxiety. The objective may be for her to walk down the street a quarter mile to mail a letter or pick up a few groceries every day for the next two weeks. For a child struggling with shyness and depression, the intervention may emphasize couples therapy to reduce marital conflicts that affect the child's emotional well-being. The objective may be for the couple to encourage the child to attend a birthday party unaccompanied by the parents.

The interventions are the skills and techniques the practitioner brings to the table. The objectives are intermediate goals for the client to achieve, and they should be thoughtfully chosen in collaboration with clients in a way that helps them progress toward their treatment goals. Intermittent and meaningful successes increase clients' self-efficacy and their chances of coping successfully with their difficulties. Achieving meaningful objectives is empowering for clients and helps them enhance their adaptive strengths.

The Evaluation Plan

The evaluation plan should be briefly described in the service plan. It includes the standardized measures and idiographic indexes that were used in the assessment. It should also include a brief description of data collection (who will collect the data, at what intervals, under what circumstances). The evaluation plan serves two purposes: it is a foundation for individual qualitative and quantitative evaluation, and if broad spectrum measures are also used, the data are aggregated as part of program evaluation.

Linking well-chosen, clear problem definitions with intervention goals, choosing the intervention, constructing key objectives, and implementing clinically useful evaluation tools require considerable skill. When done well, the service plan can reduce complex information regarding the client's problems and recommended interventions to a relatively simple plan focused on problem-solving and improving a client's ability to cope. The client service plan serves many useful purposes: it is a necessary bureaucratic tool used for meeting contractual and regulatory obligations, it is a blueprint for clinical intervention that should reflect expertise in clinical assessment and intervention (often in collaboration with both the client and other helping professionals), and it stipulates the assessment and evaluation tools to be employed. The complete service plan should thoughtfully reflect all three components of EBPSW: assessment, intervention, and evaluation.

PART TWO

PSYCHOSOCIAL PROBLEMS
OF ADULTS

CHAPTER 5

SCHIZOPHRENIA

People with schizophrenia struggle with one of the most challenging of psychosocial disorders. Much of what is discussed in this chapter regarding assessment and intervention with this disorder is also relevant to other serious mental illnesses such as bipolar disorder, schizoaffective disorders, severe chronic depression, and, to some extent, co-occurring personality disorders. In addition to biological causes, many psychosocial risks, resiliencies, and person factors such as gender, race, and socioeconomic conditions affect the course of schizophrenia and its response to treatment. This chapter also highlights a key co-occurring problem that may affect up to half of clients with major mental illnesses: the abuse of alcohol and other drugs. A number of assessment instruments are available to reliably measure key psychosocial symptoms of schizophrenia. This chapter highlights the Brief Psychiatric Rating Scale, a well-established and widely used measure of serious psychiatric symptoms.

In addition to a range of medications that have been shown to be effective for reducing the severity of major symptoms, research on effective psychosocial interventions has grown considerably and offers much hope for improved functioning and quality of life for these clients. These interventions include cognitive-behavioral coping skills, social skills training, psychoeducation and behavior therapy with the families of mentally ill people, and assertive case management.

ASSESSMENT

Background Data

Schizophrenia covers a spectrum of related diseases marked by thought disorders (hallucinations, delusions), disorganized speech and behavior, flattening of emotional response, and deterioration in social functioning. The disorder occurs in about 1% of the general population, and is more or less evenly divided between genders. Clients with schizophrenia often have little awareness of being ill and needing treatment. The course of schizophrenia is quite variable and defies easy summation. Although many clients face considerable psychosocial deterioration over many years, some may experience early remission, manage the disorder quite well, and see their symptoms level off rather than face inexorable deterioration and decline (*DSM-IV-TR*; H. I. Kaplan & Saddock, 1998; D. L. Johnson, 1997). Women with later and acute onset, good predisease functioning, and good social supports appear to have a better chance of recovery. When young people who experience their first psychotic episode are treated in a timely manner with both medication and psychosocial interventions, the prognosis for recovery improves (Falloon, Roncone, Malm, & Coverdale, 1998). In addition, larger social networks and more social supports have been shown to be associated with less inpatient treatment and better outcomes (Albert, Becker, McCrone & Thornicroft, 1998). Nevertheless, as many as 10–15% of people with schizophrenia will commit suicide during the course of their lives.

People with schizophrenia are far from all alike. In addition to individual differences, person factors such as gender and race are related to variation in the onset, course, and outcomes for schizophrenia. Women generally have later onset than men (late twenties to early thirties versus late teens to early twenties, respectively), better premorbid history, fewer negative symptoms, and better outcomes, social adjustment, and response to medication overall. It has been suggested that differential response to family interventions between men and women may be due to different gender-role expectations (men are expected to demonstrate more "independent" behavior) (J. M. Goldstein & Tsuang, 1990; Angermeyer, Kuhn, & Goldstein, 1990). Men also tend to show more recidivism than women (Test, Burke, & Wallach, 1990). Although there are few differences overall between men and women in hospitalization, treatment utilization, and aftercare (Klinkenberg & Calsyn, 1998), women who are seriously mentally ill incur additional risks, including a greater chance of contracting HIV as a result of having been sexually victimized, a risk compounded by associated substance abuse and poverty (Cournos & McKinnon, 1997; Carey, Carey, & Kalichman, 1997; Otto-Salaj, Heckman, Stevenson, & Kelly, 1998). Many women with mental illness also struggle to retain custody of their children, a monumental challenge given the adversities they face (Mowbray, Oyserman, Bybee, McFarlane, & Rueda-Riedle, 2001). Although there is relatively little research on gender differences of mentally ill people who abuse substances, research has revealed similar rates of abuse between men and women, but differences in associated risk factors such as better social supports among women, more criminal involvement for men, and more victimization of women (M. F. Burnette & Drake, 1997; L. A. Goodman et al., 2001). Women with bipolar disorder, however, may be disproportionately at greater risk for alcohol dependence than men (Frye et al., 2003). With regard to treatment, preliminary evidence suggests that women may do at least as well as men in programs that address both substance abuse and mental illness (Jerrell & Ridgely, 1995).

Although schizophrenia has been shown to occur at similar rates across different ethnic and racial groups, cultural biases and racism have been noted as mediating factors in the application of certain diagnostic labels (*DSM-IV-TR*) and in service-delivery patterns. For example, Whaley (1998) notes a tendency of practitioners to see the guarded behavior of their African-American clients as "paranoid." Other evidence suggests more difficulty in procuring aftercare housing for mentally ill black men (E. S. Uehara, 1994). There is also higher risk for contracting HIV among African-American mentally ill males (Cournos & McKinnon, 1997; Carey et al., 1997). Clearly, risk factors associated with racism, poverty, and mental illness may reciprocally interact. On the other hand, some research reports comparable service utilization patterns and outcomes for mentally ill black and white men in a Veterans Administration residential program (Leda & Rosenheck, 1995), perhaps underscoring the positive association between outcomes and comparable health benefits. People with schizophrenia also experience a disproportionate degree of psychosocial stressors that increase the risk for the development of post-traumatic stress disorder (Harris, 1996; Drake, Green, Mueser, & Goldman, 2003; Osborn, 2001). For the mentally ill in general, there is also negative stigma, particularly in regard to the exaggerated perception of a propensity toward violent behavior (T. Ryan, 1998; Monahan, 1996).

Schizophrenia and Substance-Abuse Problems

Considerable evidence from both epidemiological studies and surveys of clinical populations show roughly half of all clients with serious mental illness (including schizophrenia, bipolar disease, and major depression) are likely to have been identified at some time in their lives as abusers of psychoactive chemicals (Helzer & Pryzbeck, 1988; V. B. Brown, Ridgely, Pepper, Levine, & Ryglewicz, 1989; Drake & Wallach, 2000; Hilarski & Wodarski, 2001). Overall estimates in the research range from 20% to 85% (Hilarski & Wodarski, 2001; Mueser, Noordsy, Drake, & Fox, 2003). Six-month incidence rates are somewhat lower and range from 25% to 35% (Graham et al., 2001; S. D. Rosenberg et al., 1998). Numerous studies support the view that when mentally ill people abuse alcohol and other drugs, they increase their risks for exacerbated psychiatric symptoms, hospitalization, poorer treatment compliance and outcomes, polysubstance use, risky sex and increased likelihood for HIV infection, and other health difficulties. Additional risks include homelessness, financial problems, and involvement with the criminal justice system (Drake et al., 1998; Drake, Mueser, Clark, & Wallach, 1996; Drake, Alterman, & Rosenberg, 1993; R. E. Clark, Ricketts, & McHugo, 1999; Drake & Wallach, 2000). The findings on long-term outcomes for substance-abusing mentally ill people are ambiguous, but evidence suggests that they are at considerable risk of remission and recidivism (Turner & Tsuang, 1990; Drake & Meuser, 1996; Drake, Osher, & Wallach, 1989).

It is understood that the relationship between substance abuse, mental illness, and a host of other psychosocial factors is complex, and simple cause-effect explanations (e.g., self-medication) for their relationship lack explanatory power (Turner & Tsuang, 1990). At the pharmacological level, the interaction among alcohol and other drugs, schizophrenic disease processes, and medications is not well understood. Current theories of co-occurring substance-use disorders and serious mental illness posit a range of explanations that include the existence of common biopsychosocial factors or the potential of one condition to increase risk for the other. At the practice level, the use of alcohol or other drugs may precipitate or exacerbate symptoms and behavior problems as well as interfere with assessment and the effects of psychotropic medication.

Theories

Before conducting a formal assessment with a person who suffers from schizophrenia, it is critical to have a basic understanding of both the biological nature of the disease and the relevance of environmental stressors in the exacerbation of symptoms and behavior problems. Decades of research have produced an abundance of evidence establishing biological explanations as the primary cause of schizophrenia (H. I. Kaplan & Saddock, 1998; Bogerts, 1993; E. H. Taylor, 1987; D. L. Johnson, 1997), although the exact nature of these processes is still not known. Much of the research has focused on the limbic system of the brain as the primary site of dysfunction. A review of over fifty brain-imaging and post-mortem brain studies (Bogerts, 1993) strongly suggests abnormal brain development, physiological dysfunction, and neuroanatomical anomalies that cannot be accounted for by psychosocial influences. These physiological changes occur at the higher integrative and associative (cortical) brain functions as well as in basic drives and emotions (Bogerts, 1993). Because the exact organic etiology is not known, schizophrenia is considered a functional psychosis. Research suggesting that schizophrenia is related to temporal-lobe dysfunction extends back over a century. Technological advances in the form of computer tomography research in the 1970s and, currently, magnetic resonance imaging (MRI) provide more clearly delineated structural differences in the brains of people with schizophrenia. These problems are primarily located in the temporal lobe, which is closely related to other brain functions. Psychotic symptoms caused by temporal-lobe abnormalities are presumably the result of genetic mechanisms or physical trauma (Shenton, 1996).

Other theories, most notably the dopamine hypothesis, have focused on dysfunction in neurotransmitter production and/or reuptake of dopamine and serotonin as the cause of schizophrenic symptoms. It appears more likely that multiple interacting neurotransmitter systems are implicated (H. I. Kaplan & Saddock, 1998). There is also growing evidence to support the hypothesis that schizophrenia "may be the consequence of anomalous synaptic reorganization" caused by brain abnormalities (again, primarily in the limbic system) stimulated by hormone surges during late adolescence (Stevens, 1992). Hemsley (1996) suggested that because perception depends on the interaction between context-related stimuli and stored memories, behavioral abnormalities in schizophrenia are the result of a breakdown in the normal relationship between memory and sensory input. Brain-imaging research, particularly more recent developments with MRI, have revealed abnormalities in the size of cerebral ventricles in many schizophrenic patients. The higher concordance rates between identical twins raised apart and the higher rate of schizophrenia (by a factor of ten) in first-degree relatives with the disease has, perhaps, provided the strongest evidence to date for biogenetic influences as the primary cause of the disease (*DSM-IV-TR*; H. I. Kaplan & Saddock, 1998; Kety, 1996). Although environmental stress is seriously considered to be a precipitating factor in the etiology of schizophrenia, no specific environmental factor (including the postulated "schizophrenogenic mother") has ever been shown to play a significant role (Erlenmeyer-Kimling, 1996). Some environmental stressors may, however, increase risk for organic causes such as viruses, prenatal trauma, and autoimmune disorders.

Although schizophrenia is now presumed to have a strong biological basis, an array of psychosocial factors exacerbate the condition, and, reciprocally, psychosocial consequences result from symptoms and behaviors associated with this disease. Stress-environment models have also provided important insights into the course and outcomes of schizophrenia, although the interactions of biological processes and environmental stressors are not yet thoroughly understood. Once the disease process begins, however, understanding and mitigating the impact of environmental stressors becomes critical to the psychosocial assessment and intervention with people who suffer from schizophrenia. It has been long recognized that people in the lowest socioeconomic stratum are much more likely to suffer from serious psychopathology, schizophrenia included (Dohrenwend & Dohrenwend, 1974; Kohn, Dohrenwend, & Mirotznik, 1998). Two prevailing theories attempt to account for this situation: The social causation hypothesis suggests that "rates of psychiatric disorders are higher in the lower socioeconomic strata because of greater environmental adversity. The selection theory argues that rates are higher in the lower strata because pre-disposed individuals drift down to or fail to rise out of the lower social strata" (Kohn et al., p. 275). In the case of schizophrenia (more so than other disorders, such as depression, where the cause of the disorder appears to be more reactive to social stressors), the selection theory ("downward drift") seems to account for the reasons that people with schizophrenia are incapacitated in ways that prevent them from advancing socioeconomically (Dohrenwend et al., 1998). Although one cannot argue that schizophrenia is caused primarily by social factors, the social work practitioner must be acutely aware of how living in poverty and high-crime areas, living in substandard housing, experiencing stigma, and an inconsistent work history can adversely affect the client. Schizophrenia therefore, for all practical purposes, becomes not only a mental disease, but also complex disorder-in-living on every level.

Key Elements of Multidimensional/ Functional Assessment

The diagnostic criteria for schizophrenia (*DSM-IV-TR*) are widely considered to be both reliable and valid. The main criteria are two or more symptoms (for at least one month's duration) including delusions, hallucinations, disorganized speech, grossly disorganized or catatonic behavior, or negative symptoms (e.g., flat affect). If delusions or hallucinations are severe, then one symptom may suffice. In addition to active symptoms, there must be some evidence of serious social or occupational dysfunction, and continuous signs of the disorder for at least six months (including one month of active symptoms). Other causes such as other mood disorders, substance abuse, or medical conditions must be ruled out as the primary cause of the client's symptoms.

Providing a diagnosis for schizophrenia is an important part of an overall assessment. However, given that the primary impact of medication is on "positive symptoms" (i.e., hallucinations, delusions) of schizophrenia, but only limited benefits accrue for "negative symptoms" (i.e., emotional withdrawal, interpersonal functioning), an MDF assessment is essential (Bedell, Hunter, & Corrigan, 1997; O'Hare et al., 2003). It should cover the following domains:

psychiatric symptoms, including hallucinations, delusions, disorganized thinking, depression, anxiety, social withdrawal, motor retardation, and blunted affect;

highly stressful or traumatic events;

use of medications and other substances;

social functioning in proximate relationships and extended relationships;

ability to negotiate daily living activities;

access and use of environmental resources;

money management and gainful vocational activity;

general health status;

leisure activities; and

civic responsibilities.

In conducting the MDF assessment, it is important to collate data from multiple sources, including other mental health professionals, primary physicians, case managers, counselors, community members, law enforcement, and family members.

In addition to assessing the client's well-being over multiple domains, it is essential to conduct a careful functional assessment. Examining the day-to-day experiences of the client during a "typical" week is likely to reveal circumstances under which the client is likely to do particularly well or to experience stressors that may be associated with crises or deterioration in well-being. Antecedents to potential problems may include conflict with family members, acquaintances, work mates, or others in the community; depression or anxiety associated with trauma-related symptoms; abuse of alcohol or other drugs; or exacerbation of symptoms due to noncompliance with medication regimen. These difficulties can easily escalate into serious crises that require emergency intervention, police involvement, or hospitalization. By learning self-monitoring skills as part of the ongoing assessment, clients can begin to link these experiences with the potential for decompensation, and perhaps identify emotional upset, discouragement, suicidal thoughts, anger, conflict, or other troubling experiences as a "warning signal" to seek social supports or to contact someone on their mental health team to reduce the likelihood of further problems. The functional analysis can also identify areas of opportunity where clients can practice their social skills and stress management to reduce the likelihood of crises and enhance their sense of self-efficacy, confidence, and overall well-being.

Instruments

The MDF assessment should use instruments to enhance the qualitative assessment and provide a baseline for evaluation. A number of brief scales measure psychiatric symptoms and social functioning in people with serious mental illnesses. Some focus on one specific domain, such as mental status or social functioning, while others cover a variety of domains, including mental status, social well-being, community functioning, health, and other important areas. Some of these instruments can be used repeatedly to track changes and monitor progress over time, say every six months.

Suitable instruments include the Brief Psychiatric Rating Scale (BPRS; Lachar et al., 2001) and the Brief Symptom Inventory (BSI; Derogatis & Melisaratos, 1983), both of which focus primarily on psychiatric and psychological symptoms. The Behavior and Symptom Identification Scale (BASIS-32; S. V. Eisen, Dill, & Grob, 1994) gauges a client's well-being across psychological and social domains, including interpersonal relations, daily living and role functioning, depression and anxiety, impulsive and addictive behaviors, and psychosis. All three scales have been extensively tested for reliability and validity. The Role Functioning Scale (RFS; S. H. Goodman, Sewell, Cooley, & Leavitt, 1993) measures client well-being in four distinct areas: work productivity, independent living and self-care, immediate social-network relationships, and extended social-network relationships. Results of preliminary psychometric testing with seventy-nine low-income African-American women revealed excellent internal consistency, and adequate test-retest reliability for this brief four-item scale. The RFS also predicted the diagnostic status of the client, and correlated in the expected direction with other psychiatric and role-functioning scales.

Other important measures include quality-of-life questionnaires (see Nieuwenhuizen, Schene, Boevink, & Wolf, 1997, for a review). Quality of life is understood to be a multidimensional concept that includes access to resources, fulfillment, and satisfaction in various social roles. One well-regarded example is A. F. Lehman's Quality of Life Interview (QLI; 1988). It has 143 items covering the following domains: living situation, family and social relations, leisure, work, religious activity, finances, safety, and health. The QLI takes about forty-five minutes to complete, and it can be used with relatively little training. Subsequent confirmatory factor analysis strongly supports both the reliability and validity of the scale (A. F. Lehman, McNary, & O'Grady, 1997).

Perhaps the benchmark instrument for psychiatric assessment is the BPRS (Overall & Gorham, 1962; Woerner, Mannuzza, & Kane, 1988; Roy-Byrne et al., 1995; Lachar et al., 2001). The BPRS-A (anchored version; instrument 5.1) has acquired a solid record of reliability, validity, and utility in assessing clients for psychiatric symptom severity. A recent study with 3,000 hospitalized psychiatric clients (Lachar et al.) demonstrated that the BPRS has good factorial validity, internal consistency, and interrater reliabilities for each of the subscales. Subscales of the BPRS also add significantly to predictions of hospital length to stay (Hopko, Lachar, Bailley, & Varner, 2001), and scores are sensitive to clinical change (Bailley et al., 2004).

INSTRUMENT 5.1   Brief Psychiatric Rating Scale–Anchored (BPRS-A)

Date of 24-48 Hours Rating: _____

The BPRS-A will be completed within 48 hours of admission (rate from initial interviews). Place one check mark to indicate the most descriptive BPRS-A level (1 through 7) for each dimension.

1. Somatic Concern: Degree of concern over present bodily health. Rate the degree to which physical health is perceived as a problem by the patient, whether the complaints have a realistic basis or not. Do not rate mere reporting of somatic symptoms. Rate only concern for (or worrying about) physical problems (real or imagined). [Rating based primarily on verbal report.]

1____**Not reported**.
2____**Very mild**: Occasionally is somewhat concerned about body, symptoms, or physical illness.
3____**Mild**: Occasionally is moderately concerned about body, or often is somewhat concerned.
4____**Moderate**: Occasionally is very concerned, or often is moderately concerned.
5____**Moderately severe**: Often is very concerned.
6____**Severe**: Is very concerned most of the time.
7____**Very severe**: Is very concerned nearly all of the time.

2. Anxiety: Worry, fear, or over-concern for present or future. Rate solely on the basis of verbal report of patient's own subjective experiences. Do not infer anxiety from physical signs or from neurotic defense mechanisms. Do not rate if restricted to somatic concern.

1____**Not reported**.
2____**Very mild**: Occasionally feels somewhat anxious.
3____**Mild**: Occasionally feels moderately anxious, or often feels somewhat anxious.
4____**Moderate**: Occasionally feels very anxious, or often feels moderately anxious.
5____**Moderately severe**: Often feels very anxious.
6____**Severe**: Feels very anxious most of the time.
7____**Very severe**: Feels very anxious nearly all of the time.

3. Emotional Withdrawal: Deficiency in relating to the interviewer and to the interview situation. Overt manifestations of this deficiency include poor/absence of eye contact, failure to orient oneself physically toward the interviewer, and a general lack of involvement or engagement in the interview. Distinguish from BLUNTED AFFECT, in which deficits in facial expression, body gesture, and voice pattern are scored. [Rating based primarily on observation.]

1____**Not observed**.
2____**Very mild**: E.g., occasionally exhibits poor eye contact.
3____**Mild**: E.g., as above, but more frequent.
4____**Moderate**: E.g., exhibits little eye contact, but still seems engaged in the interview and is appropriately responsive to all questions.
5____**Moderately severe**: E.g., stares at floor or orients self away from interviewer, but still seems moderately engaged.
6____**Severe**: E.g., as above, but more persistent or pervasive.
7____**Very severe**: E.g., appears "spacey" or "out of it" (total absence of emotional relatedness), and is disproportionately uninvolved or unengaged in the interview. (Do not score if explained by disorientation.)

4. Conceptual Disorganization: Degree of speech incomprehensibility. Include any type of formal thought disorder (e.g., loose associations, incoherence, flight of ideas, neologisms). DO NOT include mere circumstantiality or pressured speech, even if marked. DO NOT rate on the patient's subjective impressions (e.g., "My thoughts are racing. I can't hold a thought." "My thinking gets all mixed up."). Rate ONLY on the basis of observations made during the interview.

1____**Not observed**.
2____**Very mild**: E.g., somewhat vague, but of doubtful clinical significance.
3____**Mild**: Frequently vague, but the interview is able to progress smoothly; occasional loosening of associations.
4____**Moderate**: E.g., occasional irrelevant statements, infrequent use of neologisms, or moderate loosening of associations.
5____**Moderately severe**: As above, but more frequent.
6____**Severe**: Formal thought disorder is present for most of the interview, and the interview is severely strained.
7____**Very severe**: Very little coherent information can be obtained.

5. Guilt Feelings: Over-concern or remorse for past behavior. Rate on the basis of the patient's subjective experiences of guilt as evidenced by verbal report. Do not infer guilt feelings from depression, anxiety, or neurotic defenses. [Rating based primarily on verbal report.]

1____**Not reported**.
2____**Very mild**: Occasionally feels somewhat guilty.
3____**Mild**: Occasionally feels moderately guilty, or often feels somewhat guilty.
4____**Moderate**: Occasionally feels very guilty, or often feels moderately guilty.
5____**Moderately severe**: Often feels very guilty.
6____**Severe**: Feels very guilty most of the time, or encapsulated delusion of guilt.
7____**Very severe**: Agonizing constant feelings of guilt, or pervasive delusions(s) of guilt.

6. Tension: Rate motor restlessness (agitation) *observed* during the interview. DO NOT rate on the basis of subjective experiences reported by the patient. Disregard suspected pathogenesis (e.g., tardive dyskinesia).

1____**Not observed**.
2____**Very mild**: Occasionally fidgets.
3____**Mild**: E.g., frequently fidgets.
4____**Moderate**: E.g., frequently fidgets. Wrings hands and pulls clothing.
5____**Moderately severe**: E.g., constantly fidgets. Wrings hands and pulls clothing.
6____**Severe**: E.g., cannot remain seated (i.e., must pace).
7____**Very severe**: E.g., paces in a frantic manner.

7. Mannerisms and Posturing: Unusual and unnatural motor behavior. Rate only abnormality of movements. Do not rate simple heightened motor activity here. Consider frequency, duration, and degree of bizarreness. Disregard suspected pathogenesis. [Rating based on observation.]

1____**Not observed**.
2____**Very mild**: Odd behavior but of doubtful clinical significance, e.g., occasional unprompted smiling, infrequent lip movements.
3____**Mild**: Strange behavior but not obviously bizarre, e.g., infrequent head-tilting (from side to side) in a rhythmic fashion, intermittent abnormal finger movements.
4____**Moderate**: E.g., assumes unnatural position for a brief period of time, infrequent tongue protrusions, rocking, facial grimacing.
5____**Moderately severe**: E.g., assumes and maintains unnatural position throughout interview, unusual movements in several body areas.
6____**Severe**: As above, but more frequent, intense, or pervasive.
7____**Very severe**: E.g., bizarre posturing throughout most of the interview, continuous abnormal movements in several body areas.

8. Grandiosity: Inflated self-esteem (self-confidence), or inflated appraisal of one's talents, powers, abilities, accomplishments, knowledge, importance, or identity. Do not score mere grandiose quality of claims (e.g., "I'm the worst sinner in the world." "The entire country is trying to kill me.") unless the guilt/persecution is related to some special exaggerated attributes of the individual. Also, *the patient* must claim exaggerated attributes: e.g., if patient denies talents, powers, etc., even if he/she states that others indicate that he/she has these attributes, this should not be reported. [Rating based primarily on verbal report.]

1____**Not reported**.
2____**Very mild**: E.g., is more confident than most people, but of only possible clinical significance.
3____**Mild**: E.g., definitely inflated self-esteem or exaggerates talents somewhat out of proportion to the circumstances.
4____**Moderate**: E.g., inflated self-esteem clearly out of proportion to the circumstances, or suspected grandiose delusion(s).
5____**Moderately severe**: E.g., a single (definite) encapsulated grandiose delusion, or multiple (definite) fragmentary grandiose delusions.

6_____**Severe**: E.g., a single (definite) grandiose delusion/delusional system, or multiple (definite) grandiose delusions that the patient seems preoccupied with.

7_____**Very severe**: As above, but nearly all conversation directed towards the patient's grandiose delusion(s).

9. Depressive Mood: Subjective report of feeling depressed, blue, "down in the dumps," etc. Rate only degree of reported depression. Do not rate on the basis of inferences concerning depression based upon general retardation and somatic complaints. [Rating based primarily on verbal report.]

1_____**Not reported**.

2_____**Very mild**: Occasionally feels somewhat depressed.

3_____**Mild**: Occasionally feels moderately depressed, or often feels somewhat depressed.

4_____**Moderate**: Occasionally feels very depressed, or often feels moderately depressed.

5_____**Moderately severe**: Often feels very depressed.

6_____**Severe**: Feels very depressed most of the time.

7_____**Very severe**: Feels very depressed nearly all of the time.

10. Hostility: Animosity, contempt, belligerence, disdain for other people outside the interview situation. Rate solely on the basis of the verbal report of feelings and actions of the patient toward others. Do not infer hostility from neurotic defenses, anxiety, or somatic complaints.

1_____**Not reported**.

2_____**Very mild**: Occasionally feels somewhat angry.

3_____**Mild**: Often feels somewhat angry, or occasionally feels moderately angry.

4_____**Moderate**: Occasionally feels very angry, or often feels moderately angry.

5_____**Moderately severe**: Often feels very angry.

6_____**Severe**: Has acted on his/her anger by becoming verbally or physically abusive on one or two occasions.

7_____**Very severe**: Has acted on his/her anger on several occasions.

11. Suspiciousness: Belief (delusional or otherwise) that others have now, or have had in the past, malicious or discriminatory intent toward the patient. On the basis of verbal report, rate only those suspicions which are currently held whether they concern past or present circumstance.

1_____**Not reported**.

2_____**Very mild**: Rare instance of distrustfulness which may or may not be warranted by the situation.

3_____**Mild**: Occasional instances of suspiciousness that are definitely not warranted by the situation.

4_____**Moderate**: More frequent suspiciousness, or transient ideas of reference.

5_____**Moderately severe**: Pervasive suspiciousness, frequent ideas of reference, or an encapsulated delusion.

6_____**Severe**: Definite delusion(s) of reference or persecution that is (are) not wholly pervasive (e.g., an encapsulated delusion).

7_____**Very severe**: As above, but more widespread, frequent, or intense.

12. Hallucinatory Behavior: Perceptions (in any sense modality) in the absence of an identifiable external stimulus. Rate only those experiences that have occurred during this rating period. DO NOT rate "voices in my head" or "visions in my mind" unless the patient can differentiate between these experiences and his or her thoughts. [Rating based primarily on verbal report.]

1_____**Not reported**.
2_____**Very mild**: Suspected hallucinations only.
3_____**Mild**: Definite hallucinations, but insignificant, infrequent, or transient (e.g., occasional formless visual hallucinations, a voice calling the patient's name).
4_____**Moderate**: As above, but more frequent or extensive (e.g., frequently sees the devil's face, two voices carry on lengthy conversations).
5_____**Moderately severe**: Hallucinations are experienced nearly every day, or are a source of extreme distress.
6_____**Severe**: As above, and has had a moderate impact on the patient's behavior (e.g., concentration difficulties leading to impaired work functioning).
7_____**Very severe**: As above, and has had a severe impact (e.g., attempts suicide in response to command hallucinations).

13. Motor Retardation: Reduction in energy level evidenced in slowed movements. Rate on the basis of observed behavior of the patient only. Do not rate on the basis of the patient's subjective impression of his or her own energy level.

1_____**Not observed**.
2_____**Very mild** and of doubtful clinical significance.
3_____**Mild**: E.g., conversation is somewhat retarded, movements somewhat slowed.
4_____**Moderate**: E.g., conversation is notably retarded but not strained.
5_____**Moderately severe**: E.g., conversation is strained, moves very slowly.
6_____**Severe**: E.g., conversation is difficult to maintain, hardly moves at all.
7_____**Very severe**: E.g., conversation is almost impossible, does not move at all throughout the interview.

14. Uncooperativeness: Evidence of resistance, unfriendliness, resentment, and lack of readiness to cooperate with the interviewer. Rate only on the basis of the patient's attitude and responses to the interviewer and the interview situation. Do not rate on the basis of reported resentment or uncooperativeness outside the interview situation.

1_____**Not observed**.
2_____**Very mild**: E.g., does not seem motivated.
3_____**Mild**: E.g., seems evasive in certain areas.
4_____**Moderate**: E.g., monosyllabic, fails to elaborate spontaneously, somewhat unfriendly.
5_____**Moderately severe**: E.g., expresses resentment and is unfriendly through-out the interview.
6_____**Severe**: E.g., refuses to answer a number of questions.
7_____**Very severe**: E.g., refuses to answer most questions.

15. Unusual thought content: Severity of delusions of any type—consider conviction, and effect on actions. Assume full conviction if patient has acted on his or her beliefs. [Rating based primarily on verbal report.]

1____**Not reported**.
2____**Very mild**: Delusion(s) suspected or likely.
3____**Mild**: At times, patient questions his or her belief(s) (partial delusion).
4____**Moderate**: Full delusional conviction, but delusion(s) has little or no influence on behavior.
5____**Moderately severe**: Full delusional conviction, but delusion(s) has only occasional impact on behavior.
6____**Severe**: Delusion(s) has significant effect, e.g., neglects responsibilities because of preoccupation with belief that he/she is God.
7____**Very severe**: Delusion(s) has major impact, e.g. stops eating because believes food is poisoned.

16. Blunted affect: Diminished affective responsivity, as characterized by deficits in facial expression, body gesture, and voice pattern. Distinguish from EMOTIONAL WITHDRAWAL, in which the focus is on interpersonal impairment rather than affect. Consider degree and consistency of impairment. [Rating based on observations made during interview.]

1____**Not observed**.
2____**Very mild**: E.g., occasionally seems indifferent to material that is usually accompanied by some show of emotion.
3____**Mild**: E.g., somewhat diminished facial expression, or somewhat monotonous voice or somewhat restricted gestures.
4____**Moderate**: As above, but more intense, prolonged, or frequent.
5____**Moderately severe**: E.g., flattening of affect, including at least two of the three features: severe lack of facial expression, monotonous voice, or restricted body gestures.
6____**Severe**: E.g., profound flattening of affect.
7____**Very severe**: E.g., totally monotonous voice, and total lack of expressive gestures throughout the evaluation.

17. Excitement: Heightened emotional tone, including irritability and expansiveness (hypomanic affect). Do not infer affect from statements of grandiose delusions. [Rating based on observations made during interview.]

1____**Not observed**.
2____**Very mild** and of doubtful clinical significance.
3____**Mild**: E.g., irritable or expansive at times.
4____**Moderate**: E.g., frequently irritable or expansive.
5____**Moderately severe**: E.g., constantly irritable or expansive, or at times enraged or euphoric.
6____**Severe**: E.g., enraged or euphoric throughout most of the interview.
7____**Very severe**: As above, but to such a degree that the interview must be terminated prematurely.

18. Disorientation: Confusion or lack of proper association for person, place or time. [Rate based on observations made during interview.]

1_____**Not observed**.
2_____**Very mild**: E.g., seems somewhat confused.
3_____**Mild**: E.g., indicates 1996 when in fact it is 1997.
4_____**Moderate**: E.g., indicates 1991.
5_____**Moderately severe**: E.g., is unsure where he/she is.
6_____**Severe**: E.g., has no idea where he/she is.
7_____**Very severe**: E.g., does not know who he/she is.

Individual subscale scores (rather than a global score) should be used for assessment and evaluation purposes. Based on an examination of factor structure (Lachar et al., 2001), these four subscales included resistance (grandiosity, hostility, uncooperativeness, excitement), positive symptoms (conceptual disorganization, suspiciousness, hallucinatory behavior, unusual thought content, disorientation), negative symptoms (emotional withdrawal, motor retardation, blunted affect), and psychological discomfort (somatic concern, anxiety, guilt feelings, tension, depressive mood). "Mannerisms and posturing" is not currently factored into any subscale. (Each item of the scale is scored 1–7 not reported/ not observed to very severe.)

Assessment with Mentally Ill Clients Who Abuse Alcohol and Other Drugs

Reviews of the assessment literature for people who experience both mental illness and substance abuse reveal a pattern of underdetection in daily practice (Drake et al., 1993; Drake & Meuser, 1996; Drake & Wallach, 2000). Since most assessment strategies and techniques have both strengths and limitations, a multidimensional approach including qualitative interviewing and quantitative instruments is recommended. The following areas should be investigated thoroughly during the clinical interview: determine the type, quantity and frequency of specific substances used; examine the temporal history related to the course of both substance use and the onset of schizophrenia; take a detailed family history of mental health problems and substance abuse, and tentatively sort out any cause-effect relationships between substance-abuse and mental health problems up to the present. Although this can be a time-consuming and difficult task, one can look for psychosocial and physiological correlates of substance use and important psychosocial problems or crises. Other important factors associated with abuse may include demographics, alcohol expectancies (i.e., strong beliefs that alcohol or drugs are helpful for alleviating tension or other problems), physiological and health indicators, social and environmental difficulties, abuse of prescription medication, trouble with the law, and other impulse-related problems. In general, accurate retrospective information can be difficult to come by, and a period of abstinence may be illuminating when sorting out the complex interplay between drugs and other psychiatric symptoms (Brems & Johnson, 1997; Buckstein, & Brent, & Kaminer, 1989).

Given the critical importance of assessing and monitoring substance abuse, it is important for practitioners to incorporate brief measures to gauge the client's involvement with alcohol and other drugs. Although lab tests, self-report, observing physical signs and symptoms, and collateral information are also valuable sources of assessment data, practitioners should not overlook one of the most effective methods of detecting substance-abuse problems in people with mental illness: the use of simple paper-and-pencil screening tools (Wolford et al. 1999). The Alcohol Use Scale (AUS) and the Drug Use Scale (DUS) are single-item clinician-rated indexes of alcohol and drug abuse that mirror *DSM* diagnostic criteria (Carey, Cocco, & Simons, 1996; Drake, McHugo, et al., 1998; Mueser et al., 2003). Responses to the one-item AUS and DUS (done separately for alcohol and drugs) are: abstinent, use without impairment, abuse, dependence, and dependence with institutionalization. Recent evidence suggests that the use of simple substance-abuse indexes by case managers correlates well with more extensive batteries (Carey et al.; Drake, McHugo et al.), and should be included as part of a brief, multidimensional assessment.

Recently, there has been a growing interest in assessing "readiness to change" in clients who abuse alcohol or other drugs (O'Hare, 2002). This assessment model has been accompanied by gradual and flexible approaches to setting treatment goals through motivational interviewing and harm-reduction approaches (Drake, Rosenberg, & Mueser, 1996; Osher & Kofoed, 1989). This staged assessment approach to intervention is reflected in the Substance Abuse Treatment Scale (SATS; see McHugo, Drake, Burton, & Ackerson, 1995), which can also be used to monitor the client's treatment progress. These stages include pre-engagement, engagement, early persuasion, late persuasion, early active treatment, late active treatment, relapse prevention, and remission or recovery. Psychometric evaluation of the SATS reveals good to excellent test-retest and interrater reliabilities, concurrent validity for the SATS between researchers and case managers, and concurrent validity between case-manager ratings of substance abuse and the SATS. Revised versions of the AUS, DUS and the SATS are available to clinicians in Mueser et al. (2003).

In addition to these brief indexes, other "mainstream" substance-abuse instruments have been shown to be reliable when used with mentally ill people. The Alcohol Use Disorders Identification Test (AUDIT [Saunders, Aasland, Babor, de la Fuente, & Grant, 1993] which will be discussed in chapter 6) has been shown to be valid when used with people who have serious mental illnesses, although cutoff points lower than the standard score of eight have been suggested for this population (e.g., O'Hare, Sherrer, LaButti, & Emrick, 2004).

In summary, conducting a through and valid assessment with people who suffer from severe mental illness presents a considerable challenge to the clinical social worker, given the multiplicity of interacting factors to be considered.

Many types and sources of data are required in both qualitative and quantitative methods. A thoughtful summarizing of the information also requires considered judgment regarding which problems are to be addressed first and which intervention methods are to be employed.

SELECTING EFFECTIVE INTERVENTIONS

Despite advances in medications for the mentally ill, pharmacotherapy alone is often not sufficient to increase a client's overall psychosocial well-being or improve overall adjustment in the community (H. I. Kaplan & Saddock, 1998; D. L. Johnson, 1997; Mueser, Drake, & Bond, 1997). The preponderance of outcome research on psychosocial interventions with people suffering from schizophrenia can be roughly classified into three categories that reviewers have collectively deemed efficacious practices (A. F. Lehman, Steinwachs, et al., 1998; Huxley et al., 2000; Falloon et al., 1998): coping skills and problem-solving approaches, psychoeducation and behavior therapy with families, and variations on assertive case management. Because there is a robust body of research in these areas, summaries of findings from controlled investigations are presented here along with exemplar studies to illustrate representative research strategies. A number of comprehensive critical reviews of the literature have been used as sources for this summary, with the emphasis on controlled studies, although findings are supplemented with uncontrolled studies when randomized designs are sparse.

Coping-Skills Approaches

Generally, coping-skills methods for people with severe mental illness cover a variety of cognitive-behavioral and problem-solving interventions that focus on psychosocial adjustment problems. These approaches include social-skills training, cognitive-behavioral interventions, and eclectic combinations of coping-skills approaches such as personal therapy. Embedded within general coping-skills strategies are traditional behavioral techniques such as communication and problem-solving training, and stress-management techniques. More recently, cognitive-behavioral therapies represent a new approach within the coping-skills repertoire.

Cognitive-Behavioral Therapy.   There has been growing interest in the use of cognitive-behavior therapy (CBT) with people who have schizophrenia (Alford & Correia, 1994; Kingdon & Turkington, 1991). These approaches help the client directly analyze the dysfunctional cognitions (e.g., delusions, other anxieties), and test the validity of these dysfunctional beliefs within the context of a supportive and collaborative relationship with the practitioner. Preliminary results are promising, and these approaches may be an effective part of an overall coping-skills strategy. Alford and Correia (1994) summarize the basic steps:

1. Identify the problematic belief.

2. Encourage the client to keep a log and further examine the belief, and rate the level of conviction for this belief.

3. Examine beliefs for content, and discuss the reasons and plausibility of the beliefs.

4. Encourage "distancing" to help the client see the disturbing thought more objectively.

5. Encourage the client to consider another perspective or alternative reaction to the specific belief.

6. Explore alternative explanations for the belief.

7. Perhaps encourage the client to test out these beliefs, and examine evidence that confirms or disconfirms the belief.

8. Monitor and evaluate the client's progress.

Kingdon and Turkington (1991) conducted an exploratory (qualitative) investigation of the effectiveness of cognitive therapy with sixty-four patients with schizophrenia. The intervention focused on psychoeducation to help clients rationally examine some of their psychosocial experiences; normalize some of these perceptions, thoughts, and experiences; correct faulty cognitions (e.g., I am being controlled by alien beings); and use homework assignments to test out the validity of some of these troubling beliefs. Stress-management techniques were taught to deal with anxiety and to help decatastrophize specific fears. Clients were helped to cope with family emotional responses, use support groups, and accept medication. Although not a controlled comparison, results were quite promising. Clients achieved good results, and showed genuine acceptance of the treatment. The intervention was used safely with relatively low doses of medication. Hospitalization was used less often, and clients reported acceptable levels of psychological symptoms and social well-being.

Recently, some randomized trials were conducted with CBT. A controlled trial of 144 people with schizophrenia (or related disorder) was carried out for a twelve-month period (Gumley et al., 2003). During that time, a five-session engagement phase was introduced, followed by two or three sessions per week when the client showed evidence of possible relapse. The CBT intervention (combined with treatment as usual and compared to a separate treatment-as-usual control condition) focused on an examination of cognitive and emotional "triggers" associated with possible relapse. It helped the client increase self-efficacy through enhancement of coping skills to maintain medication compliance and avoid relapse. After twelve months, it was evident that those in the CBT condition were about half as likely to relapse or be hospitalized, and general psychosocial well-being improved significantly. Rector, Seeman, and Segal (2003) carried out a randomized control trial with a smaller sample ($n = 42$) by similarly adding CBT to treatment as usual, yet failed to demonstrate significant effects posttreatment for CBT. Lastly, meta-analysis underscores the early stage of research with cognitive therapies for seriously mentally ill people yet suggests, that results to date should be considered promising (Pilling, Bebbington, Kuipers, Garety, Geddes, Orbach, et al., 2002).

Social-Skills Training.   A considerable amount of research has been conducted on social-skills training, a behavioral intervention that focuses on clients' ability to appraise and respond to social situations in a way that enhances their relationship to others and their adaptation to the community. The need for improved social skills is based on the premise that one of the more debilitating problems for the mentally ill person is the inability to relate to others effectively. Reviews of the literature (Liberman, Kopelowicz, & Young, 1994; T. E. Smith, Bellack, & Liberman, 1996; Penn & Mueser, 1996; Mueser, Drake, & Bond, 1997; Pilling. Bebbington, Kuipers, Garety, Geddes, Martindale, et al., 2002) reveal that social-skills training yields significant improvements in assertiveness, anxiety, and other problems. These interventions produce better social functioning with increased benefits over time. Positive results were found for both improved social adjustment and decreased symptom severity, but mixed results were revealed for reducing rehospitalization rates. People with schizophrenia can successfully learn a wide range of social skills, from simple changes such as maintaining eye contact during conversations to more complex skills such as assertiveness and communication skills. More research is needed on integrating social-skills approaches into community-based programs. Although behavioral changes in social skills can be readily demonstrated in controlled trials, generalization of these improvements to day-to-day use in the community has been more challenging. More research is needed to show how changes can extend to community living and be maintained over time.

Exemplar Study: A Controlled Trial of Coping-Skills Training. Hayes, Halford, and Varghese (1995) compared social-skills training for sixty-three people with schizophrenia to a supportive discussion (control) group. Patients were assessed for level of social skill and anxiety in standardized role-playing in different interpersonal situations, and community functioning was assessed through the coding of client diary entries. Assessment also included the BPRS, the Global Assessment of Functioning and a quality-of-life scale. Both treatments were conducted for thirty-six sessions of seventy-five minutes each over the course of eighteen weeks. The skills group focused on standard behavioral approaches, including instructions in social skills, modeling, rehearsal, feedback, and structured homework tasks to generalize the results outside of the sessions. Therapists received ten hours of specific instruction on the intervention methods. Thirty-seven clients completed the intervention, and thirty-four were assessed at follow-up. Although both groups showed improvements in psychiatric symptoms and quality of life, the social-skills group showed greater improvements on some social-skills measures. However, generalizations of gains were somewhat limited.

It is important to note the lack of research and evaluation on social-skills training with clients from other cultures. The assumption that treatment goals are intended to result in independent living may be presumptuous in a culture where better integration with the family, extended family, and immediate community may be considered preferable. Behaviorally oriented social-skills interventions can be modified for use with Hispanic families, for example, by incorporating culturally congruent staff and other indigenous helpers to facilitate better family and social adjustment (Kopelowicz, 1997). The goals may emphasize interdependence among family and other social supports rather than the independent functioning of more highly valued in "Anglo" families.

Assuming the practitioner has conducted a thorough multidimensional assessment, a more focused functional assessment is in order, to specifically ascertain clients' strengths and deficits in interacting comfortably and competently with others in their social sphere. Bellack, Mueser, Gingerich, and Agresta (1997) posit four questions to guide this functional assessment. (1) Does the client manifest some dysfunctional interpersonal behavior? This can be determined through observation of the client in various social circumstances, and can be guided by common sense regarding normal social behavior and discourse. (2) What are the specific circumstances in which the dysfunction occurs? Ideally, assessment should cover a range of circumstances, for example, with familiar acquaintances in a social club to more stressful circumstances such as waiting on a long line in the supermarket. (3) What is the probable source of the dysfunction? These could include severe shyness, depression, a lack of effective conversational skills, or distraction from obsessional thoughts or hallucinations. (4) What specific skill deficits does the client have? Is there difficulty in listening attentively or responding in a congruent way to "keep the conversation going"? Assessment interviewing techniques should include a good detailed history, observation of role-playing situations, and observation of the client in vivo, if possible.

Mueser et al. (1997) enumerated core intervention steps typically applied in social skills training. The practitioner should provide a clear rationale for learning the skill; demonstrate the skill in role-playing with the client; collaborate with the client in role-playing the skill; provide positive and corrective feedback about how well the client performed the skill; engage the client in more role-playing, followed by positive and corrective feedback; and assign homework for the client to practice the skill in real-life situations. These processes should be repeated and advanced gradually as the client gains confidence and demonstrates mastery of the technique.

There are a range of variations on effective social-skills training. Some social-skills interventions may also include live modeling of the skill, videotape modeling, assertiveness training, communication and problem-solving skills, and increased social supports (Bedell et al., 1997; Liberman et al., 1994). Providing homework assignments is essential, so that clients can practice on their own. But evidence has not been strong for generalization of gains from social-skills training, perhaps due to a lack of direct guidance and reinforcement by case managers in community settings. Certainly, enhancing social skills in people with schizophrenia is challenging, and results will depend on the client's level of social deficit as well as the seriousness of co-occurring problems such as substance abuse. Rather than broad-based efforts, practitioners might focus on one or two specific circumstances where the client would likely benefit most from improvement (e.g., engaging in light conversation on the job or reducing argumentative interactions with acquaintances in a social club). Details for starting and maintaining social-skills groups and trouble-shooting specific problems can be examined in more detail in evidence-based practice guides (e.g., Bellack et al., 1997; Mueser et al., 2003).

Personal Therapy.   Personal therapy (Hogarty et al., 1995; Hogarty, 2002) is a multifaceted coping-skills approach that addresses mentally ill clients' problems in thinking, expressing emotions, and behavioral deficits. Commensurate with the long-term goals of psychiatric rehabilitation, personal therapy is a long-term commitment to a client, and works best when implemented in stages. Personal therapy incorporates a range of coping skills, including psychoeducation, self-monitoring, problem solving, communication skills, rehearsal, feedback, and homework (in vivo practice). One of the more important dimensions of personal therapy (not always made explicit in the literature on other coping-skills interventions) is the gradual cultivation of a strong therapeutic relationship as a foundation for teaching a variety of coping skills. The practitioner also encourages medication compliance when indicated. Intervention is based on the premise that the mentally ill person must deal directly with cognitive dysfunctions and with the regulation of emotional reactions in a social context. Behavioral progress should gradually move forward as the client masters each of the following phases: Phase 1 includes relationship building and psychoeducation about the disorder and the intervention. Phase 2 develops self-awareness of cognitive, affective, and behavioral skills, and uses self-monitoring to learn self-regulation of cues and symptoms. Phase 3 applies coping skills in the social environment. These approaches include a range of standard CBT skills: self-monitoring, modeling, rehearsal, feedback, and in vivo practice. Skills are tailored to the client's unique treatment needs. Although few controlled studies have been done on what is specifically referred to as "personal therapy," qualitative evaluation seems to indicate that the interventions are well accepted by clients with severe mental illness, and similar skills have been supported in controlled studies with similar approaches.

By now it should be clear that there is no uniform coping-skills approach, but rather a collection of intervention skills and strategies built upon a sound therapeutic alliance and applied in a number of different configurations. The ideal combination of skills may vary from program to program, from client to client, and even from time to time for the same client.

Exemplar Study: Evaluation of an Eclectic Coping-Skills Program. A controlled study of a structured group intervention with people with schizophrenia provides a good example of one coping-skills approach (Bradshaw, 1996). This eclectic intervention consists of four modules: physiological arousal management, time management, cognitive restructuring, and social-skills training. The rationale of the intervention was to improve overall psychosocial functioning and prevent relapse (including rehospitalization). Sixteen clients (two later dropped out) were randomly assigned to two interventions: the experimental (coping-skills) group and a comparison or control (problem-solving) group.

The experimental intervention included the development of treatment goals specific to each client; physically oriented relaxation methods to reduce anxiety; time management (self-monitoring to identify stressful situations and pleasurable activities); planned activities intended to be constructive and enjoyable, and geared toward increasing social supports that would mitigate stress; cognitive restructuring such as thought stopping, and developing constructive self-statements in response to troubling thoughts; learning additional coping skills to deal with anticipated stressful situations through modeling, role-playing, practice, and self-reinforcement techniques; and learning social skills. The intervention was conducted within the context of a structured group approach, in part, to take advantage of socialization aspects of group interaction. The problem-solving control group, in contrast, required more initiative from clients to develop problem-solving methods, and group process methods were not emphasized. Both groups met for ninety-minute sessions for twenty-four weeks. Global attainment scaling, Global Assessment of Functioning, rehospitalization, and time in the hospital were used as outcome measures.

The coping-skills group showed better goal attainment and fewer hospitalizations than the problem-solving group. Results, however, were only suggestive. The small sample size and an inability to infer which specific skills in the overall treatment package had the most impact preclude firm conclusions about the effectiveness of the treatment. Nevertheless, the study illustrates a thoughtful and innovative multimodal approach to a coping-skills intervention for people who have schizophrenia.

Applying Coping-Skills Approaches to Mentally Ill Clients Who Have a Co-occurring Substance-Abuse Problem

Given that a large proportion of clients in treatment are likely to have a co-occurring substance-abuse problem, it is essential to give it priority in the treatment plan. Fortunately, many of the intervention strategies and skills outlined above can be readily adapted to the client who also abuses alcohol and other drugs, with the understanding that a thorough assessment of substance abuse has been conducted. In addition, interventions with mentally ill people who have substance-abuse problems are better implemented if both conditions are addressed simultaneously in well-integrated treated programs rather than treated sequentially or in parallel programs (Mueser et al., 2003; Minkoff, 2000).

Helping the client reduce their abuse or dependence on substances is a goal that can be directly and effectively addressed by interventions that use coping skills, family psychoeducation, and case management. The results of studies that have focused on the integration of these effective methods into an assertive case-management framework appear promising. The few controlled investigations provide initial support for behaviorally oriented, long-term, integrated programs for reducing substance abuse and recidivism among the mentally ill (Jerrell & Ridgely, 1995; Blankertz & Cnaan, 1994; RachBeisel, Scott, & Dixon, 1999; S. E. Herman et al., 2000). Integrated substance-abuse programs have resulted in better treatment engagement, housing, and overall adjustment when compared with standard case management approaches (Drake, Yovetich, Bebout, Harris, & McHugo, 1997; Drake, McHugo, et al., 1998; Drake, Mercer-McFadden, Mueser, Hugo, & Bond, 1998; Mueser et al., 1997). A recent meta-analysis of fifteen controlled studies of interventions for people with co-occurring disorders (Dumaine, 2003) provided good support for combined intensive case management and psychopharmacology.

Based on the accumulated findings to date, the essential program elements in an integrated co-occurring mental illness/substance-abuse program should include integration and coordination of mental health and substance-abuse treatments within an assertive community treatment model, routine assessment of substance-abuse problems, flexibility in treatment, helping to match and involve clients in choice of treatment goals, use of persuasion-engagement, motivational interviewing and "staged" approaches (Osher & Kofoed, 1989; Bellack & DiClemente, 1999; Mueser et al., 2003), use of specialized substance-abuse interventions based on social-skills training, family psychoeducation and behavioral family therapy, supported employment, increased social supports, and residential stability (Mercer, Mueser, & Drake, 1998; Carey, 1996a, 1996b; Smyth, 1996; Drake & Mueser, 2000; Mueser et al., 2003).

The following skills should minimally be included in an integrated program to address co-occurring substance abuse and serious mental disorders:

Develop a good working alliance that is marked by a nonjudgmental attitude about the use of substances.

Identify and monitor problematic thoughts, feelings, and situations that are associated with increased risk for drug use.

Help the client *make consistent connections between their psychosocial complaints and their substance use.*

Gauge the client's level of engagement and self-confidence (self-efficacy) in dealing with risky situations.

Use motivational interviewing to engage the client in constructive change.

Apply interventions in a staged format (see the SATS noted above).

Provide psychoeducation to teach the client about the negative consequences of use and to challenge beliefs and expectancies regarding substance use.

Role-play new skills with the client and have them practice in vivo.

Provide constructive feedback.

Enhance available social supports.

Generalize improved skills in the community to reduce and prevent
relapse.

Teach the client to monitor and evaluate their own progress by keeping a
chart, log, or diary and by reviewing actual problem situations, their
responses to them, and the outcomes of their efforts.

It is understood that there may be a considerable amount of two steps forward,
one step back on the road to stable moderation or abstinence. As opposed to
dichotomous goal setting (i.e., abstinence versus failure), partial successes are
encouraged and rewarded (Drake, Rosenberg, & Mueser, 1996; Osher & Kofoed,
1989). Clinical guidelines are now readily available to help guide practitioners in
implementing evidence-based strategies for their mentally ill clients who abuse
substances (Bellack et al., 1997; L. J. Roberts, Shaner, & Eckman, 1999; Mueser et
al., 2003).

An Integrated Overview of Coping-Skills Interventions

Coping-skills approaches have evolved from a number of therapeutic traditions:
basic counseling, educational methods, cognitive and behavioral therapies, and
psychosocial rehabilitation models. Coping-skills approaches can be used eclec-
tically as long as core ingredients, identified in the summaries above, are used
in the approach. Why do they work when they are applied effectively? Underlying theoretical processes may suggest any number of factors: a corrective
emotional experience via the therapeutic alliance; changing one's beliefs and
expectations about other people's reactions or behaviors in social circumstances; reducing client anxiety in social situations; increasing the client's sense
of mastery, self-efficacy, and self-esteem as a result of accomplishing something
rewarding; or perhaps as a result of some combination of change processes. Although it is difficult to know how and why clients change, it is known that combinations of these intervention skills are more likely than other approaches to
be effective.

These skills can be creatively and pragmatically combined as needed by the
evidence-based practitioner. A number of intervention ingredients appear to be
essential: nurturing a sound therapeutic relationship over time; problem identification and self-monitoring skills; appraisal of cognitive dysfunction; role-playing, rehearsal, and corrective feedback; graduated exposure and practice to disconfirm irrational or unfounded beliefs and expectancies; stress management;

skill development in dealing with interpersonal and community relationships; and community-based support, reinforcement, guidance, and consistent follow-up coordinated by skillful case management. It should also be noted that, while interventions with mentally ill clients who abuse alcohol and other drugs have been discussed within the context of a coping-skills approach, elements of these methods should also be combined with other effective interventions, including family approaches and case management.

Family Interventions

Over the past decades, many families of mentally ill people have been subjected to ineffective interventions based on invalid theories regarding the causes of schizophrenia (such as inadequate mothering, or confusing family communications; Rubin, Cardenas, Warren, Pike, & Wambach, 1998; A. F. Lehman, Steinwachs, et al., 1998). Noting the extensive research on expressed emotion in families of schizophrenic people and its role in prediction of relapse, Lefley (1992) points to a substantial body of research supporting the view that high levels of "expressed emotion" (i.e., criticism, hostility, or emotional overinvolvement) may be a predictor of relapse in mentally ill persons. However, she cautions practitioners to avoid blaming family members for "causing" the patient's relapse. The fact that the exacerbation of a client's symptoms may *correlate* with dysfunctional family behaviors does not mean that a dysfunctional family *causes* schizophrenia, or that the family conflict is necessarily the primary cause of the client's relapse.

Family psychoeducation and behavioral family therapy (somewhat overlapping categories) share several assumptions: schizophrenia is regarded as an illness; family members' behaviors do not cause schizophrenia; families may be considered therapeutic agents; and interventions are not intended to stand alone, but are part of an overall approach to treatment that includes medication (Dixon & Lehman, 1995; Dixon et al., 2001). Basic family approaches include, in some configuration, psychoeducation about mental illness and its effects; family support; behavioral problem solving, and crisis interventions. These approaches may differ in modality (single family or family groups); whether the patient is included or not in each session; whether treatment is conducted in the home, professional setting, or elsewhere; and the phase of the illness during which the intervention is provided.

Narrative and meta-analytic reviews of mostly controlled studies of family interventions (Mueser et al., 1997; Bedell et al., 1997; Penn & Mueser, 1996; Lieberman et al., 1994; M. J. Goldstein & Miklowitz, 1995; Tarrier, & Barrowclough, 1995; Falloon & Coverdale, 1994; C. E. Simon, McNeil, Franklin, & Cooperman, 1991; W. R. McFarlane et al., 1995; Dixon & Lehman, 1995; Dixon, Adams, & Lucksted, 2000; Dixon et al., 2001; Pilling, Bebbington Kuipers, Garety, Geddes, Orbach, et al., 2002) have collectively shown robust outcomes in reducing family stress, reduction in caregiver burden, reducing symptoms, improving coping skills and social functioning, and reducing relapse and recidivism.

It appears that variations of family interventions and modalities are effective whether they be single- or multiple-family, supportive, or behaviorally oriented. Some have suggested that multiple-family therapy (MFT) may have advantages over single-family therapy (SFT; W. R. McFarlane et al., 1995). In one study, MFT was shown to be superior to SFT in a number of outcomes, including reduced relapse, reduced symptoms, improved medication compliance, reduction in the amount of medication required, and improved employment. In addition, several reviews support the conclusion that longer-term family interventions are more effective than individual treatments in delaying relapse and improving social functioning (Tarrier & Barrowclough, 1995; W. R. McFarlane et al.; Hogarty et al., 1995).

Based on these reviews, a number of common effective ingredients among family therapies for the mentally ill have been identified:

Employ both multidimensional and functional assessment to better tailor treatment to the family's needs and goals and foster the development of all family members.

Obtain detailed assessment information about each family member's thoughts, feelings, and behaviors in the situation.

Instill optimism, but anchor expectations realistically.

Offer emotional support, reframe the problem, and give advice when it seems needed.

Develop good working relationships with the families, respecting the families as experts for their experience and point of view.

Provide psychoeducation about the illness, including not blaming families for causing it or characterizing their attempts to cope as pathological.

Encourage medication compliance.

Identify interactional patterns among family members, and weigh the strengths and weaknesses of the family as a unit.

Monitor indicators of possible relapse.

Conduct treatment for long periods rather than attempting short-term therapy.

Work with multiple families when it is practical.

Improve communication and problem-solving skills in all family members.

Use homework to practice skills learned in sessions.

Use stress-management techniques.

Cope with special problems as they arise.

Focus on current problems of the patients and their families.

Employ crisis intervention when needed.

Family therapy should be implemented as part of a comprehensive approach that includes psychiatric consultation for medication, crisis management, and case management of other services such as facilitating employment, maintaining residential stability, and cultivating additional social supports.

Although there are variations in the way effective family interventions are conducted, a brief overview of behavioral family therapy (Mueser & Glynn, 1999) is presented here as an example of the most effective common ingredients found across several review of controlled studies. Ideally, adolescent and adult family members and the client should be included, although practitioners should be prepared, at times, to work with only the non–ill members. Initially, one should conduct weekly visits, gradually tapering off to monthly over the course of one to two years.

Several major components that are loosely sequenced include engagement, assessment, education, communications training, problem solving, and dealing with special problems. During engagement, practitioners should apply their general knowledge and skills in basic counseling and make an effort to engender hope and motivate clients. After a brief period of joining, practitioners should augment their multidimensional assessment and history taking by conducting functional analysis of their clients' specific complaints. This analysis looks at problem events and patterns of family members' reactions in sequence to determine factors that reinforce problem behaviors. Practitioners may also introduce and use standardized scales or client-specific indexes at this point to enhance the assessment and provide a baseline for evaluation. After the practitioner summarizes a case assessment and sets goals with the client and family, education about the nature of the disease is conducted to help families better understand positive and negative symptoms, and how all members can positively affect the family situation.

Communications training is then commenced, to reduce negative emotional states in the family, help them communicate more effectively with the mentally ill member (who may have serious problems processing information, especially under stress or when emotions are high), and improve interpersonal skills. Demonstrating basic listening skills and social skills can help family members relate more effectively and reduce negative emotional states. Standard problem-solving methods can be effective in helping families cope with a variety of specific problems as they arise. These well-known steps include (1) defining the problem, (2) brainstorming potential solutions, (3) evaluating alternative solutions, (4) choosing an agreed upon "best" solution, (5) planning an implementation, and (6) reviewing and revising, as needed, based on the family's evaluation of their "homework" efforts.

When working with families coping with a member who has a severe mental illness, practitioners should recognize that family support should take place in the context of the family's culture (Finley, 1998). Assessment should note kinship relationships, communication and problem-solving styles, various role expectations, attitudes about help seeking, attributions about illness and its meaning, the role of spirituality and indigenous healers in the community, and level of acculturation. Preliminary empirical evidence suggests that these differences may be more than theoretical. A recent exploratory survey (Guarnaccia & Parra, 1996) of ninety families of mentally ill people (45 Latino, 29 African-American, and 16 European-American) demonstrated differences by culture: Latinos and African Americans were much more likely to have the mentally ill family member living with them, and they were more involved in kinship networks. The European-American mentally ill family member was more likely to be in a residential treatment facility. Families expressed a variety of views regarding the causes of the problem, and African-American families expressed more distrust of mental health professionals. In one recent randomized controlled trial in six rural communities in China, where many people see the symptoms of mental illness as the work of witchcraft, family psychoeducation and medication were shown to be superior to medication alone in increasing knowledge about mental illness, and somewhat more effective in engendering in family members more understanding and caring, and less negligent attitudes toward the mentally ill member (Ran et al., 2003). More research is needed to delineate cultural differences in assessment and intervention with families who have a member with a serious mental illness.

Research on the needs of family caregivers of people with schizophrenia is also growing. Winefield and Harvey (1994) conducted a series of structured interviews to collect a combination of qualitative and quantitative data from 121 family caregivers of people with schizophrenia to describe the "nature and demands of the caring work." They also asked about professional sources of assistance, and obtained information about the caregivers' perceptions of their own needs. About three-quarters of caretakers were female. Caregivers reported a considerable level of burden particularly around holidays and significant impact on their social relationships, including family life. The burden was directly associated with more frequent contact with the mentally ill person. A large majority of caretakers said they would prefer that the clients live in a supervised arrangement other than their home or have their own residence. Caretakers saw little reciprocity in caring for the mentally ill relative. They felt that the client gave little emotional support in return. However, about two-thirds felt that the mental health system was available to them if they needed help in dealing with the client in crisis.

Psychoeducation and behavioral therapy with families with a mentally ill member are among the most effective strategies for helping the seriously mentally ill. For the mentally ill family member who also abuses substances, coping-skills approaches can be readily integrated into family approaches (R. E. Clark, 2001). Social workers who plan to work with the mentally ill need to learn these methods, and more research is needed to generalize these approaches to families from diverse cultural groups.

Case Management

The case management movement has developed in response to National Institute of Mental Health initiatives in the 1960s (Drake, 1998), and has evolved into a number of variations on the programs for assertive community treatment (PACTs) model (L. I. Stein & Test, 1980). These different versions include mobile treatment teams and intensive community treatment programs. These programs are typically marked by a coordination of comprehensive services provided by a multidisciplinary team, with twenty-four-hour coverage for open-ended treatment, and ideally a low (ten to one) client-to-staff ratio. PACTs were conceived as comprehensive community-based systems meant to prevent relapse and rehospitalization and to enhance psychosocial functioning in seriously mentally ill clients. Case management was seen as the coordinating element in the system, meant to orchestrate a seamless integration of mental health care for vulnerable clients. During the history of the case management movement, the system has been marked by various degrees of fragmentation (Drake, 1998; P. Solomon, 1992; Mueser et al., 1998; Mechanic, 1996).

Reviews of case management literature in the 1980s concluded that research efforts were in their infancy, and relevant data were characterized as "sparse and contradictory" (Anthony & Blanch, 1989). However, there is now a substantial body of controlled evaluation research on case management with the mentally ill. Although there are considerable methodological weaknesses, some relatively consistent findings are based on numerous reviews of controlled studies (Mueser et al., 1997; Mueser et al., 1998; Draine, 1997; Rubin, 1992; B. Burns & Santos, 1995; Scott & Dixon, 1995; P. Solomon, 1992). In general, case management programs (mostly based on the PACT model) have been shown to reduce hospitalization. There is some additional, but more modest, evidence that case management has resulted in increased employment, increased social contact, increased satisfaction with life, some reduction in symptoms (perhaps through medication compliance), increased family and patient satisfaction, improvements in social functioning, and improvements in residential stability and independent living. Some limited evidence suggests that time in jail may also be reduced.

Results of controlled studies of case management in general must be viewed with caution since methodological weaknesses abound (see McHugo et al., 1998). These problems include poor model conceptualization, inadequate sample size, lack of pretreatment data on clients, problems with random assignment of cases, high rates of attrition, poor sensitivity to measuring changes over time, poor utilization of existing standardized instruments, violations of statistical assumptions and a lack of multivariate analysis, vague definitions of the interventions resulting in a lack of distinction among treatment conditions, and lack of attention to faithfulness to the practice model.

Despite some evidence that intensive or assertive case management reduces hospitalization and, in some cases, improves levels of functioning, evidence suggests that cost-effectiveness advantages may be realized only if assertive case management is targeted at those clients *most at risk,* or those most likely to benefit from the service (Essock et al., 1998). In addition, despite some general positive effects of case management programs, it has been difficult to sort out the specific contributory effects of case management activities from overall treatment effects. Some correlational evidence strongly suggests that case managers themselves have a positive effect on client outcomes, suggesting that the worker's relationship with the client may make a discernable difference even when types of service and client characteristics are statistically controlled (C. S. Ryan, Sherman, & Judd, 1994).

Exemplar Study: An Experimental Comparison of PACT Versus Brokered Case Management.   In one experimental study (Morse et al., 1997), 135 of 165 originally selected clients were randomly assigned to three treatment groups. The treatments were two types of assertive case management and brokered case management. The experimental treatment was a form of assertive case management in which workers were responsible for treatment coordination with assertive follow-up, treatment was conducted in the community with a ten to one client-to-staff ratio, and no time limits were placed on services. Practitioners cultivated a positive working relationship with clients, emphasized practical problem solving, enhanced community living skills, provided supportive services, assisted with money management, and facilitated transportation. One type of assertive case management included the use of paraprofessional community workers who spent additional time with clients. In contrast, brokered case management (the comparison group) focused on developing treatment plans and purchasing services from various agencies. Client-to-staff ratio was eighty-five to one.

All subjects had serious mental illnesses and were eligible for social service benefits. Treatment process measures accounted for service activities in housing, employment, job training, financial assistance, and legal, mental health, substance-abuse, health, and supportive services. Outcome measures included client satisfaction, income, stability of housing, psychiatric symptoms, and substance abuse. A three-by-three factorial design was employed; that is treatment conditions with outcome measures taken over three time periods (six, twelve, and eighteen months). Overall, assertive case management groups provided considerably more assistance (housing, finances, health, and support), and both assertive community treatment conditions resulted in greater satisfaction and better psychiatric ratings. There were no differences among the groups in substance-abuse outcomes. It is worth noting that 33% of clients in the brokered group received no services at all, the addition of paraprofessionals in one assertive case management group made little difference overall, and cost differentials among groups were not calculated. The authors pointed out that this study was one of only a few that showed improvement in psychiatric symptoms in the experimental group.

Increasing Environmental Supports for Seriously Ill Clients

The most skillfully applied psychosocial interventions, however, will be of limited use if a client's living conditions and financial supports are not adequate or stable. Researchers have long understood that people with schizophrenia experience difficulties maintaining steady residences and employment (Anthony & Blanch, 1989; D. B. Herman, Susser, & Struening, 1998). A recent review of the literature estimates that lifetime prevalence of serious mental illness and substance abuse is more than twice as high for the homeless as for the general population (D. B. Herman et al.). In addition, when homelessness is associated with the loss of familial and social support, there appears to be greater risk of depression. Therefore, homelessness must be understood as a pronounced stressor associated with the loss of critical social and emotional supports (D. B. Herman et al.). In response to deinstitutionalization and subsequent homelessness, residential programs grew rapidly in the 1980s. By the end of that decade, the majority of state-affiliated community residential programs across the nation included group homes (23%), supervised apartments (21%), board and care homes (10%), and supportive housing (9%) (Randolf, Ridgway, & Carling, 1991). One recent survey of 158 mostly African-American adults in the Washington, DC, area provided suggestive evidence that housing stability was associated with reduced substance abuse (Bebout, Drake, Haiyi, McHugo, & Harris, 1997). Other data have shown that among the mentally ill, blacks, the poor, and those with substance-abuse problems are most at risk to be homeless (Kuno, Rothbard, Averyt, & Culhane, 2000). Given that homelessness remains a significant national problem, schizophrenia must continue to be assessed and treated within the context of substantial social, environmental, and economic risk factors.

Recent reviews of controlled and uncontrolled studies of supported employment provide substantive evidence that direct placement into real paying jobs (without pretraining), ongoing support, attention to client preferences, and integrating vocational services into the service model appear to result in superior rates of job placement, time worked, and wages earned in contrast to the use of traditional train-and-place approaches or sheltered workshops (Bond, Drake, Mueser, & Becker, 1997; A. F. Lehman, 1995; Bond et al., 2001). Bond et al. (1997) found that, across six experimental studies, almost three times as many clients who received supportive employment services achieved competitive employment as opposed to those who received traditional vocational services. Mueser et al. (1997) concluded from a review of seven controlled studies that supportive approaches are more effective when clients are *given direct assistance in finding and maintaining employment* (as opposed to general job counseling). However, more research is needed to determine whether benefits of employment generalize to other areas of psychosocial functioning.

There has also been an increase in awareness of the rates of mental illness and substance-abuse problems among those in prison and otherwise involved in the criminal justice system. Because mentally ill people are arrested more often than others, are often held without formal charges being filed, and are not adequately treated for their mental illnesses during incarceration, there have been increasing calls to integrate services across mental health, substance-abuse, and criminal justice systems (Rock, 2001; H. R. Lamb & Weinberger, 1998; Godley et al., 2000; Fisher, Packer, Grisso, McDermeit, & Brown, 2000). Some have argued convincingly for more research and consistent implementation of civil commitment procedures to help clients comply with treatment on an outpatient basis (as opposed to forced incarceration in mental hospitals or prison; Geller, 1995; Swartz et al., 1995). Considerable debate is likely to accompany these developments with respect to balancing the civil rights of clients who refuse treatment and the implementation of more humane alternatives to mental health care for those who commit crimes.

Although media depictions of mentally ill people as violence-prone have unfairly stigmatized this group, a number of factors independently and additively increase the relatively low risk that a mentally ill person will commit a serious violent act. These include a history of conduct disorder (as a child), antisocial personality disorder (as an adult), and a co-occurring substance-abuse disorder (Fulwiler & Ruthazer, 1999; Eronen, Angermeyer, & Schulze, 1998; Tehrani, Brennan, Hodgins, & Mednick, 1998). Being a victim of family and community violence in childhood and adulthood also appears to predict future violent behavior among mentally ill people, although this factor is not as strong a predictor as having a co-occurring substance-abuse problem (Hiday, Swanson, Swartz, Borum, & Wagner, 2001). In addition, a combination of substance abuse and noncompliance with medication has been shown to be associated with serious violent actions in the community (Swartz et al., 1998). However, most violence by mentally ill people is not directed at the general public. The victims are likely to be the person's family members (Eronen et al.) The use of contingency management strategies for mentally ill people who commit crimes has been suggested as a form of "therapeutic jurisprudence," that is, the application of legal contingencies to enhance the client's psychosocial well-being and to protect the community (Elbogen & Tomkins, 2000; D. B. Wexler, 1991). Although there have been few controlled trials, the results are promising for mandatory outpatient treatment (Gerbasi, Bonnie, & Binder, 2000; Appelbaum, 2001) and will, hopefully, lead to more humane alternatives to treating people with major mental illness who commit crimes.

Antipsychotic Medications

Social workers who treat people with serious mental illnesses need to be familiar with antipsychotic medications and their therapeutic effects and side effects, so they can conduct accurate assessments and collaborate knowledgably with psychiatric physicians and nurses. Reviews of the research on these drugs have summarized the most salient data regarding the effective use of antipsychotic medication (Dixon, Lehman, & Levine, 1995; Bentley, 1998). For three decades, the standard antipsychotic medications (e.g., chlorpromazine, haloperidol) have been the dopamine antagonists. These drugs are useful in reducing positive symptoms such as thought disorders, but less effective with negative symptoms (such as social withdrawal, and flattened affect). They often result in long-term negative extrapyramidal (nervous system) side effects (e.g., muscle rigidity, psychomotor retardation, restlessness, tremors, shuffling gait). Tardive dyskinesia can result from long-term use of these drugs, and may produce involuntary muscle movements, particularly in the face. These medications can also cause uncomfortable anticholinergic effects such as blurred vision, dry mouth, constipation, and urinary retention.

Newer serotonin-dopamine antagonists have proven to be as effective as standard neuroleptics but with fewer extrapyramidal symptoms overall. For patients who have not responded well to conventional antipsychotic medications, clozapine has been shown to be helpful in 30–60% of cases for reducing positive symptoms, and has garnered some evidence for improving social functioning, quality of life, negative symptoms, and risk of tardive dyskinesia. However, there is an increased risk of agranulocytosis and seizures (dangerous lowering of white blood cell count with potentially fatal results; Buchanan, 1995). Another relatively recent arrival, risperidone, has also been shown to be at least equally effective in reducing positive symptoms as other conventional antipsychotics, but it appears to have fewer extrapyramidal symptoms at lower doses (Umbricht & Kane, 1995).

On the whole, medications have been shown to be effective with most patients when they adhere to the treatment regimen, although noncompliance remains a persistent problem. Over 70% of clients show improvements in positive symptoms, and these drugs also substantially reduce risk of relapse for at least the first twelve months after the initial psychotic episode. Results, however, are not as good for negative symptoms or other social adjustment outcomes. Depot medication reduces risk of relapse better than oral medication, but many other factors that influence effectiveness in clinical application include accurate dosing, medication compliance, long-term outcomes, and the interrelationship between pharmacotherapy and other psychosocial interventions. Most of the therapeutic gains are realized within the first few weeks and months after initially prescribing medication. Regarding various prescribing practices, "rapid neuroleptization" (aggressive use of large doses) has not been shown to yield superior results, and the use of clinical judgment in dosing is apparently no more effective than standard dosing. After clients' symptoms stabilize, many can be maintained on lower standard doses (not intermittently targeted doses) without increased risk of relapse (Dixon et al., 1995). In addition to medication prescribed primarily for antipsychotic symptoms, other adjunct medication may be prescribed to offset side effects, enhance the effects of the primary medication, or deal with other related psychiatric symptoms such as depression, and anxiety (Bently, 1998)

IMPLEMENTING AND EVALUATING THE EVIDENCE-BASED INTERVENTION PLAN

CASE STUDY: MARTIN

Martin, a twenty-six year old African-American man, was referred to a social worker because he had not shown up at his maintenance job at a fast-food restaurant for four days, and had not returned home during that time. This was the third time that his supervisor had referred Martin for help. The assessment revealed that Martin had been diagnosed with schizophrenia in his late teens, had been hospitalized several times since then, but had not become consistently engaged in a community support program. It also became clear that Martin did not take his medication regularly, and periodically abused street drugs, most recently crack and amphetamines during his hiatus from work. He often did this when he became paranoid and experienced command hallucinations to hurt people around him, particularly when he was at work. These voices frightened him, and he felt that drugs temporarily quieted down the voices and took his mind off them. His live-in girlfriend, Maria, worried about him, and came with him to the consultation with the social worker. After Martin's parents divorced when he was in his teens, he ran away from home. He did not finish high school and had been living on his own much of the time for the past ten years. He presented as friendly and cooperative, but appeared suspicious, depressed, and remorseful about his recent absences from work. He was appreciative of his girlfriend's and his employer's continuing faith in him. Martin was willing to take his medication and go back to work, but was afraid that he would slip again and that people would lose patience with him.

Multidimensional/Functional Assessment: Defining Problems and Goals

Martin presented as soft-spoken and willing to engage with the social worker, Jim, although he seemed at times suspicious and a little guarded. Nevertheless, he was reasonably forthcoming and occasionally remorseful about running away from his girlfriend and abandoning his boss again. Face-to-face interviewing provided a good deal of information, but it seemed likely that his girlfriend and his boss would also be good sources of corroborating data. They would provide further insight into his behavior at home and at work.

Historically, Martin's family life was relatively uneventful. Neither parent had a major mental illness, although his father had a drinking problem. His paternal uncle and grandfather had psychiatric hospitalizations, but it was not clear what the specific diagnoses were. His parent divorced when he was about sixteen years old. He has a brother and a sister with whom he has had little contact. He did not report having been abused, although he remembered having been afraid of his father when his father was drinking heavily. His father disappeared for days at a time when he went on a drinking binge.

Martin often went for relatively long periods without displaying overtly psychotic symptoms. Although he was usually "standoffish," acted suspicious, and muttered to himself at work, his auditory hallucinations were generally tolerable as long as he stayed on his antipsychotic medication. He often seemed depressed, edgy, and anxious, and spent most of his time alone. He took his coffee breaks and lunches alone, and went outside to smoke behind the restaurant when he had a chance. When he stopped taking his medication (sometimes because he felt he was being poisoned by the government as "part of a conspiracy to make black Americans insane"), he became hostile, lashed out at his coworkers verbally, responded loudly to command hallucinations to "kill the white devils," and generally was uncooperative at work. Once he yelled at and pushed a young white man (an "enemy agent") who, Martin claimed, put "poison" in his lunch. He told his African-American boss about the incident. His boss often mediated arguments among his young staff, and was aware of racial tensions among them and occasions when racial epithets had been exchanged. His boss was having difficulty sorting out how much of the racial content was real and how much was in Martin's imagination.

After consulting with Maria, his Latina girlfriend, it seemed to Jim that Martin was usually able to trust her. She described Martin as being "sweet to me . . . he does stuff for me," but added that he sometimes went for days without speaking to her, and was preoccupied with watching the news. He seemed very interested in computer technology, talked about Internet security features a lot, and worried about whether the government was monitoring his Internet browsing. She said that she was afraid for him when he disappeared for days, did not know where he went, was afraid that he might get infected with AIDS if he was having sex in crack houses, and was afraid that he might infect her. She said she loved him, and felt that she could help him. She worried about him a lot and felt that she needed help to deal with his problems.

To date, Martin seemed to have avoided any serious encounters with the police, although they were aware of him because he appeared from time to time in the local hospital emergency room. He had never been caught in possession of drugs, and usually didn't carry any with him or use them except for the occasional binges when he would disappear for three or four days. His health was reported as good, he worked for three or four months at a time with good attendance and performance at work, and generally took care of his hygiene and appearance, although his hygiene deteriorated when he was going through his more paranoid phases. He stopped showering during those times, and his coworkers and customers would complain. His boss seemed to be the only person from whom he would take constructive criticism of his appearance and hygiene when these matters were brought to Martin's attention.

Although Martin was (based on previous diagnoses) apparently suffering from schizophrenia, he had been doing reasonably well over the past few years.

Aside from periodic hospitalizations when his symptoms become acute, he had been able to maintain a job and a relationship for more than two years. As he became more suspicious and hostile to those around him, however, they responded more negatively to him, thus increasing his feelings that others didn't like him or were out to harm him. The flashpoint in this sequence of events could have been a relatively innocuous event: a nasty look, an innocent laugh of a colleague, a news report on the television in the back room regarding war, a terrorist attack, or the arrest of a black media personality.

Jim worked with Martin to keep the problems well-defined, the goals reasonable, and the treatment plan manageable. He also arranged for psychiatric consultation to manage Martin's medication. Working together, Jim and Martin agreed that some folks at work probably were racist, but that Martin's reactions may have worsened his paranoid delusions. He spent a lot of time withdrawing from those around him, and the estrangement from his coworkers left room for his imagination and delusions to "fill in the gaps." It appeared that, as he became more wary of others, including his white therapist and white female psychiatrist, he sometimes stopped taking his medication because he felt that they are tying to "control my mind." As his delusions increased in intensity, and his command hallucinations grow louder, he became increasingly frightened and belligerent, which led eventually to a crisis at home or at work, and the possibility of a crack binge.

In brief, Martin appeared to suffer from paranoid delusions and occasional hallucinations that had a persecutory quality, but seemed to worsen within a context where racial tensions add to their plausibility. At some point, he would stop taking his medication regularly, and his paranoid delusions and hallucinations would subsequently increase. His behavior would become more belligerent, and those around him would respond and reinforce this behavior accordingly. Things would escalate into a crisis. This sequential pattern played out several times within the previous year, and provided a good, workable functional assessment to guide part of the intervention plan.

Martin had other difficulties as well. He was chronically depressed and anxious, did not sleep well, and felt that the medications he took occasionally interfered with his lovemaking when he and his girlfriend felt intimate. He also had real strengths in that he was diligent in his work, related well to Maria from time to time, and received considerable social support from both her and his boss. Preliminary intervention goals included improved medication compliance to reduce symptoms, improved social supports and coping skills at work, and abstaining from alcohol and other drugs.

Selecting and Designing the Intervention: Defining Strategies and Objectives

Jim and Martin worked out an intervention plan (table 5.1) that initially included the following approaches: CBT was initiated to test out and gain some control over the paranoid delusions, particularly at work. Social-skills training

TABLE 5.1   The client service plan for Martin

Problems	Goals	Sample Objectives	Interventions	Assessment, Tools
Frightening paranoid delusions; feels the government and coworkers are out to harm him	Reduce the frequency and intensity of fearful delusions; gain better cognitive understanding of link between symptoms and exaggerated fears	Monitor, identify, and record daily level of intensity of delusions; think about alternative interpretations and record them	Cognitive therapy to examine and challenge delusional thinking; testing alternative interpretations Social-skills training; role-playing and in vivo practice of basic communication skills; focus on clarifying meaning of others' communications and responding in a friendly manner Psychoeducation for client and girlfriend to help her cope Assertive case management; consultation with MD to ensure medicine compliance; coaching client's boss to monitor and assist client; support for girlfriend and her "cotherapist" role Self-monitoring and related coping skills: identifying triggers associated with thinking about drug use; written crisis plan that he can put into effect; paycheck deposited directly to joint account; "persuasion" group for co-occurring mental illness/substance-abuse clients	BPRS to monitor changes in mental status BASIS-32 to measure psychological and social functioning RFS to measure social and occupational functioning AUS and DUS to monitor involvement with drugs SATS as a gauge of level of involvement in dealing with episodic but risky drug problem Credibility index (5-point, low to high) for paranoid delusions Weekly count of frequency of positive interactions at work (have boss keep a log); qualitatively review their meaning and salience Weekly count of conversations he initiates at home (have girlfriend keep score); record successful medication administrations
Withdrawal from others; failure to communicate his fears; lashing out angrily when he feels threatened	Improve his ability to reach out to social supports when he feels the need	Initiate at least one conversation daily at home and work; when confused by someone's comment, ask other person to clarify meaning		
Inconsistent medication use	Improve medication compliance close to 100%	Take meds daily in front of girlfriend (after she is given instructions by nurse, case manager)		
Occasional drug binges, which lead to risky sexual behaviors	Eliminate binges; develop an alternative to running away when he is in a crisis; join "persuasion" group at mental health center	Identify thoughts of bingeing and other related thoughts daily; note feelings or situations that provoke bingeing for discussion with social worker		

was employed to help Martin cope better with interpersonal exchanges at work (e.g., communicate better with his boss when he was feeling angry or frightened, engage in friendly conversation with some of his coworkers). Psychoeducation and behavioral couples therapy was implemented with Martin and his girlfriend together. This approach was intended to engage Maria as a therapeutic ally, help her better understand Martin's condition, teach her to deal with him more effectively, and provide support for her as well. Martin focused on self-monitoring and coping skills to identify triggers and seek help before taking off on a binge. Lastly, assertive case management was initiated to coordinate psychiatric care and enhance social supports in the community.

A number of specific objectives were designed to help engage Martin in treatment and move him toward his goals in a step-by-step approach. Jim helped Martin examine some of his delusions carefully and distinguish those aspects that might have had some validity (blacks and whites are often hostile to one another in our society, the government does monitor Internet communications) from overgeneralizing (not *every* white person is out to hurt him because he is black, the government is not necessarily out to get *him*, in particular). Jim then tried to help Martin see that, when he kept to himself and acted unfriendly or was angry toward others at work, his coworkers might have thought he did not like them, or they might have felt threatened by him. Considering these alternative explanations seemed to be helpful in encouraging Martin to test his more troubling beliefs. Martin and Jim role-played a typical situation at work. Martin was gradually able to consider that perhaps some of his suspicious were blown out of proportion. With some practice, Martin was later able to better identify his reactions to some of these relatively minor incidents at work and, by talking with his coworkers and his boss, was able to clarify some matters before he responded angrily or in a threatening manner. His communication skills seemed to improve a bit on the job, at least enough to forestall further serious conflict.

A similar application of self-monitoring and coping skills was used to identify precipitating factors for drug use. These triggers were often associated with anxiety or emotional distress at work. A crisis plan was developed and written down with important phone numbers (to be kept in his wallet), so that Martin would pause and consider more constructive alternatives before taking off from work impulsively. Jim taught Martin how to stop and review a list of potentially negative consequences he might bring upon himself and others if he gave into the impulse to run away and use drugs, such as becoming a victim of violence, contracting HIV, losing his girlfriend, losing his job, getting arrested, and going to prison. Through couples therapy, Martin agreed to have his paycheck deposited directly to his account to reduce the chances that he would impulsively go off on a binge. He knew from experience that he needed cash to buy drugs. Martin also agreed to attend a treatment group for co-occurring disorders.

Couples psychoeducation helped Maria to better understand Martin's problems, to recognize when he was becoming "symptomatic," and to intervene before his condition deteriorated. Maria also monitored his medication regimen more carefully. She practiced role-playing and communication skills that Martin had learned with Jim. Those skills were reinforced during couples visits. Maria also appeared to benefit from the support provided during couples sessions. In addition, both agreed to undergo physical exams to test for sexually transmitted diseases.

Selecting Scales and Creating Indexes to Monitor and Evaluate Client Progress

Several scales are suitable for assessment and evaluation in this case (table 5.1). The BPRS subscales for positive and negative symptoms, resistance, and psychological distress were used to target Martin's mental-status symptoms; the AUS, DUS, and SATS, for tracking his substance use and engagement in treatment; and the RFS, for monitoring his social and work functioning. These measures could have been supplemented with specific indexes to measure and track individual problems unique to Martin's immediate concerns. For example, employing a five-point severity scale to have him judge the intensity of his suspiciousness that others were out to harm him specifically; how strongly he felt about taking his medication according to prescription; how strong his urges were to run away and go on a crack binge; and how frequently he constructively used social supports.

SUMMARY

Given the multidimensional nature of problems experienced by people with serious mental illnesses such as schizophrenia, an eclectic evidence-based strategy can help clients improve their cognitive, emotional, behavioral, and interpersonal skills; make better adjustment to family life; and function more effectively in the community. Comprehensive reviews of the research have concluded that psychosocial interventions should emphasize the use of cognitive-behavioral coping skills, family psychoeducation and behavioral family therapy, and supported employment, all delivered in the context of integrated assertive case management. The skills for working with mentally ill people who also abuse alcohol and other drugs can be readily integrated into the psychosocial interventions reviewed above. Together these evidence-based strategies can empower the person with mental illness to make a more satisfactory adjustment to life in the community.

CHAPTER 6

SUBSTANCE ABUSE AND DEPENDENCE

Millions of Americans abuse alcohol and other drugs. Other drugs include "recreational" or "street drugs" and prescription medications. These problems cost many billions of dollars and inflict enormous human costs on the health and psychosocial well-being of the nation (U.S. Department of Health and Human Services [USDHHS], 2000). No single theory dominates the current scientific understanding of the causes, course, or consequences of substance abuse. Research has demonstrated a range of moderately effective interventions, including brief psychoeducation, motivational enhancement therapy, behavioral coping skills, behavioral couples and family interventions, traditional recovery programs, and community reinforcement strategies. Often these methods are used in eclectic combinations. Practitioners have become more flexible with regard to treatment goals which range from harm reduction and moderation to abstinence and long-term recovery. Efforts to predict choice of treatment based on client characteristics have not produced substantive results, but research in this area continues.

This chapter provides an evidence-based overview of assessment and interventions that social workers can either provide as primary treatments or integrate into practices where substance abuse co-occurs with other problems. Adults are the main focus of this chapter. Adolescents who abuse substances often have other behavioral difficulties as well, and thus will be addressed in chapter 13. Older adolescents and young adults (roughly ages eighteen to twenty-five) who abuse substances will be addressed in chapter 16.

ASSESSMENT

Background Data

Definitions of substance abuse and dependence cover a continuum from experiencing moderate distress in daily life (e.g., work, mood, relationships) to developing some degree of physiological dependence on one or more substances. Although current diagnostic nomenclature will be examined in more detail below, the dividing line between abuse and dependence remains unclear. MDF assessment of substance abuse and dependence is critical, given that the problem manifests itself quite differently depending on person factors and individual

cognitive, physiological, behavioral, and situational differences. This approach requires an examination of the quantity and frequency of substances used and
measurement of psychosocial, physiological, and clinical health consequences
on a continuum of severity.

Most Americans drink alcoholic beverages with few associated problems for
the most part. Another large proportion also use illegal drugs, and many others
abuse prescription medication. Although epidemiological data for alcohol and
other drugs vary from year to year, overall Americans use more substances than
in the past, and the traditional gap between men (who generally use more substances) and women has been closing. Although whites traditionally consumed
more alcohol per capita than Hispanic Americans and African Americans, risks
for these minorities have shown increases in recent years. Data from the National Longitudinal Alcohol Epidemiologic Survey (NLAES; Grant & Dawson,
1999; Grant et al., 1994) indicated that 66% of adults (eighteen or older) were
lifetime drinkers who had consumed at least twelve drinks of an alcoholic beverage during any twelve-month period of their life. In addition, almost half
(44.4%) had consumed twelve or more drinks in the preceding year. Almost one-
quarter were classified as lifetime heavy drinkers, and about 9% were classified
as heavy drinkers within the past year. Using *DSM* diagnostic criteria, the NLAES
survey showed that 4.9% of the total U.S. population meet lifetime criteria for alcohol abuse and 13.3% for alcohol dependence. Three percent met the criteria
for alcohol abuse over the previous year, and 4.4% met criteria for alcohol dependence over the previous year. The highest rates of abuse and dependence
over both lifetime and previous year were in the 18–24 age group, with rates declining with age. Men showed over double the rates compared with women for
abuse and dependence over both lifetime and in the previous year. Men were almost three times as likely to drink heavily during their lifetime and within the
previous year as women, a profile similar by gender among youthful drinkers
(18–29). For both men and women, rates of heavy drinking in the previous year
declined after age 30. College students and their noncollege cohorts continue to
drink prodigious amounts of alcohol on average, and a sizeable proportion also
use illegal drugs during their young adult years. Over twenty years of college-
drinking research shows that more than two-thirds of college students drink alcohol, 40% are considered binge drinkers (consumed five or more drinks at one
sitting within the past two weeks), and rates of alcohol use have not changed
substantially since the 1950s (O'Malley & Johnston, 2002).

There are variations in alcohol consumption patterns among racial groups
in the United States. Between 1984 and 1995, rates of abstinence from alcohol
increased somewhat among both men and women within white, black, and Hispanic groups. However, frequent heavy drinking declined among white men and
women, stayed about the same in black men and women, and increased among
Hispanic men and women. Current rates of frequent heavy drinking among
these three racial groups (by men and by women, respectively) are whites (12%,
2%), blacks (15%, 5%), and Hispanics (18%, 3%). Problems related to alcohol

either declined or stayed about the same for whites and blacks, but problems showed a notable increase for Hispanic males and females (Caetano & Clark, 1998; Galvan & Caetano, 2003).

Perhaps most of the research regarding the negative consequences of substance abuse and addiction is based on alcohol use. The consequences to health and psychosocial well-being are considerable. It is now well recognized that, although light to moderate drinking among otherwise healthy adults has significant cardiovascular health benefits, excessive bingeing and chronic abuse significantly increases the likelihood of serious illnesses such as heart disease and various cancers (Rehm, Gmel, Sempos, & Trevisan, 2003). The more prominent consequences include 20,000 alcohol-related deaths due to traffic accidents, 25,000 deaths due to cirrhosis, and increased risk of death by other traumatic events, including fires, falls, drowning, and interpersonal and domestic violence (USDHHS, 1997, 2000; Rehm et al., 2003). Males between the ages of twenty-two and forty-five are at greatest risk of driving under the influence and being involved in fatal alcohol-related accidents. The risk of an alcohol-related fatal crash is dose dependent (i.e., the higher the blood alcohol level, the greater the risk of an accident). Although drinking-related fatalities leveled off in the mid-1990s, they have increased in recent years (Hingson & Winter, 2003).

The NLAES data also revealed that 15.6% of the U.S. adult population reported having used illicit drugs at least twelve times in their lifetime, mostly marijuana (13.9%), amphetamines (4.1%), cocaine (3.7%), and about 2% each for tranquilizers, hallucinogens, opioids, and sedatives. Those in the 18–29 age range used almost twice as much as those over 30, men used more than women by a margin of 19.5% to 12.0%, and men used more drugs than women in all drug categories. The percentage of past-year use was 4.9% for any drug, with marijuana topping the list at 3.9% and all other drugs rated below 1%. Past-year drug use for men was almost twice that for women, and those 18–29 were more than three times as likely to use as those over 30.

The National Household Survey on Drug Abuse (USDHHS, 1998) estimated the proportions of people who have *ever used* an illicit drug in the following age groups: ages 12-17, 23.7%; 18-25, 45.4%; 26-34, 50.8%; and over 35, 31.5%. Rates of drug use among males tend to be higher than for females in a range of approximately 1% to 10%, with differences increasing with age. The following proportions are for people who have used an illicit drug in the past year: ages 12-17, 18.8%; 18-25, 25.3%; 26-34, 14.3%; and over 35, 6.1%, again with comparable differences between males and females.

In 1998, cocaine (including crack) was the drug most frequently reported in emergency-room visits, according to the Drug Abuse Warning Network, and injection-related AIDS cases accounted for 32% of total adolescent and adult cases (USDHHS, 1999a). Overall, the use of illicit drugs has remained relatively stable over the past several years (USDHHS, 1999b).

Racial differences from the National Household Survey on Drug Abuse revealed that whites have a higher lifetime rate of marijuana use (35.6%) than

Hispanics (22.3%) or African Americans (28.5), and both whites and African Americans showed comparable rates of marijuana use in the previous year (9.1% versus 9.9%), which exceeded that of Hispanics (7.5%). Whites also had higher rates of lifetime cocaine use (11.8%) than Hispanics (7.3%) and African Americans (6.5%), but were slightly less likely to have used in the past year (1.9%) when compared with Hispanics (2.0%) or African Americans (2.4%). Whites' rates of drug use in both lifetime and past-year categories for inhalants, hallucinogens, stimulants, tranquilizers, and analgesics also exceeded the rates for both Hispanics and African Americans. Other researchers have compared data on whites, African Americans, Hispanics, Asian Americans, and Native Americans, and have drawn similar conclusions (Kitano, 1989; Caetano, Clark, & Tam, 1998).

In the NLAES study (Grant & Dawson, 1999; Grant et al., 1994), high rates of co-occurring abuse of alcohol and other drugs were also demonstrated. Sixty-nine percent of those with any drug-use disorder also were classified with an alcohol-use disorder. Those classified with an alcohol-use disorder were about ten times as likely to have a drug-use disorder as those with no alcohol-use disorder. Results were fairly consistent over the different major classes of licit and illicit drugs (Grant & Pickering, 1996).

The abuse of illicit drugs, particularly marijuana, cocaine, and amphetamine "designer" drugs, is relatively common among adolescents and young adults. According to the Monitoring the Future survey (USDHHS, 1999c), although there were some variations in types of drugs used and in their rates of use, drug-abuse rates continue to be relatively stable among 19–28–year-olds. Recently there has been an increasing trend among college students in the use of marijuana, MDA/MDMA (ecstasy), and cocaine. Between 1991 and 1998, the rates of marijuana use among eighth graders nearly tripled from 6% to 17%, among tenth graders nearly doubled (15% to 31%), and among twelfth graders grew by 80% (22% to 38%). Among high school seniors, the use of any illicit drug rose from 15% to 21% since 1992. Although brief trends have emerged in the data, no steady downward trends have been recorded in drug use overall in recent decades. Among young people (USDHHS, 1999c), African-American students use drugs at significantly lower rates than whites and, binge-drink less (12%) than Hispanic students (28%) or whites (36%). Whites use other drugs at higher rates, including marijuana, inhalants, LSD, heroin, barbiturates, amphetamines, and tranquilizers. However, Hispanics in their senior year showed the highest rates of use for some of the most dangerous drugs, including cocaine and crack.

Problems That Co-occur with Substance Abuse and Addiction

Substance abuse co-occurs with the full range of psychosocial and health problems encountered by social workers in their daily practice. These problems include mental health disorders (Kessler et al. 1996; Petrakis, Gonzalez, Rosenheck, & Krystal, 2002; Drake & Mueser, 2002), health problems (USDHHS, 2000), child and family disruptions (Orford, 1990; Azzi-Lessing & Olsen, 1996), domestic violence (Gmel & Rehm, 2003), and the full range of other psychosocial disorders commonly seen in social service environments (Weisner & Schmidt, 1993; O'Hare, 1993; USDHHS, 2000). National epidemiological surveys of co-occurring mental health and substance-abuse problems have revealed generally consistent findings. The Epidemiological Catchment Area survey (Helzer & Pryzbeck, 1988), the National Comorbidity Survey (Kessler et al., 1994), and the (Grant & Harford, 1995) have shown significant correlations among anxiety, depression, and antisocial behavior with substance abuse and addiction. Women have consistently shown a disproportionate degree of co-occurrence between substance abuse and emotional distress such as anxiety, and depression, whereas substance-abusing men are more likely to engage in antisocial behaviors. People with serious mental illnesses also show a disproportionate degree of substance abuse (as reviewed in chapter 5). The Methods for the Epidemiology of Child and Adolescent Mental Disorders study (Kandel et al., 1997) also demonstrated that the use of alcohol, cigarettes, and other illicit substances, even at relatively low doses, were significantly associated with anxiety, mood, and disruptive behavior disorders in young people, with gender differences essentially mirroring adult data.

Prominent Risk Factors Associated with Substance Abuse and Addiction

Although substance abuse has been correlated to or predicted by many risk factors, only some of the more prominent empirically validated risk factors are noted here. In addition to the forms of psychopathology noted above, these include age, gender, alcohol expectancies, family history, and culture. It should be understood that these risk factors may be associated with interacting biological, psychosocial, and cultural processes.

As noted above, young adults are among the highest consumers of alcohol and drugs in the nation and consequently run relatively high risks of psychosocial problems such as depression, anxiety, suicide, contracting HIV, accidental injury, and death often associated with drinking and driving (USDHHS, 2000; L. D. Johnson, O'Malley, & Bachman, 1996; Quigley & Marlatt, 1996; O'Hare, 1997b). Although most youthful substance abuse is transitory, the earlier young people begin to abuse drugs, the more likely they are to have long-term problems (K. Chen & Kandel, 1995). By comparison with their younger counterparts, the elderly drink considerably less (Liberto, Oslin, & Ruskin, 1992) but suffer greater risks of cognitive and health-related problems, in part because of inherent vulnerabilities of aging as well as interactions with medications. An elderly person may have been struggling since early adulthood (early onset) or may have begun to abuse alcohol more recently (e.g., after retirement or after loss of a spouse). Late-onset drinkers, however, are more likely to respond positively to an intervention (Brennan & Moos, 1996; Liberto et al., 1992).

Although substance-abuse research has been traditionally male-focused (Wilk, 1994; A. S. Floyd, Monahan, Finney, & Morley, 1996), research on women has steadily increased. Despite using lower amounts of alcohol and street drugs than men, women suffer higher risks due to associations between alcohol and health risks, depression, anxiety, polydrug use (including prescription medications), the consequences of sexual abuse, role disruption, and domestic violence (Corrigan, 1985; Klee, Schmidt, & Ames, 1991; Wilsnack, Wilsnack, & Hiller-Sturmhofel, 1994; Gomberg, 1994, 1999; O'Hare, 1995b; Hurley, 1991; Norris, 1994; Lex, 1994; L. W. Bennett, 1995; Project Worth, 1997; USDHHS, 2000).

Research related to the social-cognitive context of drinking (Abrams & Niaura, 1987; Critchlow, 1986) has emphasized the importance of alcohol expectancies, that is, beliefs in relatively specific types of reinforcement from drinking (S. Brown, Goldman, Inn, & Anderson, 1980; O'Hare, 1998a). Expectancy constructs as measured by the Alcohol Expectancy Questionnaire have been shown to predict drinking patterns and associated problems (S. A. Brown, Christiansen, & Goldman, 1987), and appear to add to the predictive value of general attitudes toward drinking (Wall, Hinson, & McKee, 1998). They include beliefs that drinking will enhance sexual relations, add warmth and pleasure to celebratory occasions, increase social assertiveness, increase aggression, and reduce physical tension. Alcohol expectancies correlate with problem drinking (S. Brown et al., 1980) and may vary by race and ethnicity (O'Hare, 1995a). Higher alcohol expectancies also appear to be related to coping with negative emotions (Evans & Dunn, 1995; O'Hare, 2001a).

In addition to genetic influences from biological parents, children (and those children as adults) who grew up with substance-abusing parents incur some degree of increased risk for emotional, behavioral, and social problems. The level of risk, however, is likely to be predicted by a range of interacting factors including genetic influences on both substance abuse and psychopathology, quality of parenting, level of marital conflict, degree of job-related problems, and role modeling with respect to drinking practices (J. L. Johnson, Sher, & Rolf, 1991; Zucker & Fitzgerald, 1991; Sher, 1997; Pandina & Johnson, 1990; Windle, 1996). Not all adult children of alcoholics share the same experience or list of pathologies (caricatured in popular self-help books) as a result of their experiences with problem-drinking parents.

Differences in substance-use patterns do exist among Americans from different cultural and ethnic backgrounds. However, generalizations about the drinking patterns of broad racial groups should be made cautiously, given the high degree of heterogeneity of interethnic subgroups (D. B. Heath, 1991; Caetano et al., 1998). Asian Americans, for example, generally consume the least alcohol overall, but, as with other cultural groups, acculturation pressures have resulted in higher alcohol consumption (Kitano, 1989). Native Americans' use of alcohol varies widely from tribe to tribe, some being relatively abstemious, and others showing profound alcohol problems that account for death rates in excess of five times the national norm (Beauvais, 1998). Culture is a risk factor, but a complex one in which ethnic identity and degree of assimilation and acculturation to American drinking norms need to be considered.

Theories

Assessment models of substance abuse necessarily reflect theoretical assumptions. Although a number of competing theories purport to account for the causes of alcohol abuse and dependence, the major dialectic in substance-abuse research has been between predominantly disease-oriented explanations (biological causes) and learning-based theories (beliefs, behavior, and sociocultural factors). Modern biological explanations for the causes of alcoholism have focused on studies of heredity and associated vulnerabilities to alcohol abuse, including central nervous system (CNS) response to alcohol ingestion, temperament, and related forms of psychopathology (A. C. Heath, 1995; Pickins & Svikis, 1991; Hesselbrock, Hesselbrock, & Epstein, 1999). Genetic researchers have most prominently employed studies of children of alcoholic parents who were adopted and raised by presumably nonalcoholic parents (to control for environmental factors), and studies of identical and fraternal twins (identical twins should have higher rates of alcoholism). Both avenues of research have supported the theory of heritability, and results for both men and women appear to be comparable (A. C. Heath, 1995). Disease proponents acknowledge no clearly identified etiology, but maintain that

> At the heart of the disease model is the fundamental tenet that alcohol and drug dependence is a physical illness. The disease is neither the end result nor the symptom of another disorder, but a primary, progressive, chronic illness. Rather than a singular personality disorder or maladaptive learned behavior, alcohol and drug dependence involves the biological fabric of the individual and eventually impacts every phase of the afflicted person's life. (Sheehan & Owen, 1999, p. 269)

Biological models incorporate learning processes as well, but subordinate them to neurological functioning. Drug addiction is understood to be primarily a response of the brain to the reinforcing qualities of drugs, a key to the process of addiction (Gold, 1994).

Social-cognitive theorists, by contrast, assert that biological vulnerabilities or processes provide only partial explanations for addiction, and learning plays a more prominent role in abuse, addiction, and coping or recovery. Contemporary social-cognitive analysis (Bandura, 1986, 1999; Abrams & Niaura, 1987; Maisto, Carey, & Bradizza, 1999) emphasizes interacting physiological and psychosocial influences on the initiation and course of abuse and addiction, and personal agency (volition, choice, self-efficacy, decision making) and self-regulatory strategies (coping skills) as mechanisms of change. Although early stimulus-response theories continue to resonate through modern addictions theory and treatment models, research has shifted to cognitive mediating factors such as alcohol expectancies and self-efficacy. A contemporary social-cognitive view, however, incorporates behavior and physiological factors as they interact with cognitive expectancies. Social and environmental influences including family, peers, culture, and the environmental context of use also play a significant role. Cultural factors have long been recognized as powerful predictors of problematic use (Vaillant, 1983; Amodeo & Jones 1997), although definitions of problem use vary widely by culture (L. A. Bennett, Janca, Grant, & Sartorius, 1993).

In a similar vein, other researchers have conceptualized the development of substance abuse and addiction in a contemporary transactional model in which biological temperament associated with early behavioral problems is hypothesized to interact with a host of social and environmental risk and resiliency factors (such as stressful events, family relations, and academic and peer experiences) to predict future substance abuse (Wills, Sandy, & Yaeger, 2000; Tarter et al., 1999). Given the growth in biopsychosocial evidence concerning the causes, course, and consequences of addiction in recent years, a contemporary addiction model has become increasingly heterogeneous (Zucker & Gomberg, 1986; Abrams & Niaura, 1987; Schuckit, 1998; Pattison, Sobell, & Sobell, 1977; Finney & Moos, 1991; Wills et al.; Tarter et al.). It is also more commensurate with social work's person-in-environment paradigm (Freeman, 1991) than is the traditional disease model.

In summary, a contemporary evidence-based model reflects the following findings: Rather than being a dichotomous phenomenon, substance abuse spans a continuum from mild to severe. The causes, course, and consequences of substance use and abuse vary widely, according to a host of interacting physiological, psychological, interpersonal, and environmental risks and resiliencies. Substance abuse usually follows a variable course over time and does not necessarily follow a predictable trajectory of a progressive, irreversible disease. Substance abuse and addiction may improve or worsen with or without formal treatment through self-directed moderation, elective abstinence, or self-regulated recovery, perhaps as a response to the assistance of normal social supports or to negative social consequences. The type, severity, and interpretation of substance-abuse problems vary by situational factors as well as by age, gender, race, and culture. Substance abuse and dependence are typically intertwined with co-occurring health, mental health, and other psychosocial problems, and severity is only partly related to consumption level and symptoms of physiological dependence such as craving or loss of control. The consequences of illicit drugs are often determined by the illegal context of use, rather than to the expected pharmacological characteristics of the drugs themselves.

Prelude to Assessment: A Basic Knowledge about Drugs and Their Effects

Because social workers treat many people with primary or co-occurring substance-abuse problems, a basic knowledge of the pharmacology of alcohol and other drugs, prescribed or otherwise, is essential for conducting a competent assessment. Such basic information includes the main chemical actions of drugs; the various routes of transmission and use patterns; their acute and long-term cognitive, physiological, and behavioral effects; risks for overdose and withdrawal; and the potential for physical addiction and psychological dependence. Knowledge of the actions and effects of these drugs not only identify risks of overdose and withdrawal, but also help differentially assess mental health and assorted behavioral problems from drug-related symptoms. The information for major drug groups including sedatives (alcohol, benzodiazepines, barbiturates), stimulants (cocaine, amphetamines, related "designer" drugs such as MDMA, caffeine), narcotics (heroin, methadone, codeine, oxycodone), and others (hallucinogens, marijuana, PCP, inhalants, over-the-counter drugs) can be found in an array of sources (e.g., Ray & Ksir, 1999; Frances & Miller, 1998; McCrady & Epstein, 1999).

Important pharmacological concepts include knowing the effective dose; being aware of dangerous drug interactions (such as when CNS depressants are mixed); recognizing behavioral tolerance, demonstrated when a substance user can control behavioral manifestations of being intoxicated; and physiological tolerance. Practitioners should also be aware of the various routes of transmission: drugs may be taken orally, insufflated (sniffed), injected, or smoked.

Tolerance and withdrawal are important considerations when determining whether a person is drug dependent, and whether a person needs medical assistance to stop using the drug and avoid potentially dangerous effects of withdrawal. Interventions for serious withdrawal symptoms include initial medical detoxification either on an inpatient basis (for those with potentially dangerous withdrawal symptoms or other compromising health conditions) or outpatient basis (for those with mild to moderate withdrawal symptoms). Detoxification may be followed up with aversive medications (e.g., disulfiram) or anticraving medications (e.g., naltrexone; Hayashida, 1998; Litten & Allen, 1999; Myric & Anton, 1998). In addition to social and psychological supports, clients may also need medication (e.g., antianxiety drugs) to help reduce withdrawal symptoms, and may be given intravenous fluids and vitamin supplements. Although drugs may be helpful for blocking cravings or as treatment for secondary psychiatric symptoms such as depression, and anxiety, medication is not yet considered a primary form of treatment for addictions. However, research efforts are currently being directed toward this goal. Beyond detoxification, substance-abuse intervention remains a primarily psychosocial endeavor.

The risks of overdose and withdrawal are a critical concern for the practitioner because both conditions can be fatal. Advising clients to decrease or abstain from use without medical supervision carries risks. Clients may suffer convulsions when detoxifying from alcohol, benzodiazepines, barbiturates, and other CNS depressants. Although the elimination of some drugs (e.g., marijuana, cocaine) poses little risk of serious physiological withdrawal, psychological consequences such as depression may require acute mental health intervention. For clients who are willing to discuss openly their history of alcohol and drug use, questions about prior treatment and incidents of overdose or withdrawal may be very telling in this regard. For those clients in the light-to-moderate abuse range, specific questions about "how much" and "how often" are also critical. As noted above, many clients may be vulnerable to acute negative effects of substances even at low to moderate doses, particularly if multiple substances are involved.

Although all drugs are different in dosing, effects, interaction effects with other drugs, side effects, time needed to metabolize (half-life), and withdrawal symptoms, four classifications will be employed here for heuristic purposes: CNS depressants (alcohol, sedatives, hypnotics), stimulants (amphetamines, cocaine), opioids (heroin, narcotics), and other commonly abused illicit drugs (marijuana, hallucinogens, PCP, inhalants, etc.). Again, it is emphasized here that social workers should make liberal use of medical consultation in regard to detoxification, an often necessary step before psychosocial interventions can be employed.

CNS Depressants.   Alcohol is the most widely used psychoactive drug, and causes the greatest amount of psychological, social, and long-term health problems in the United States. Although use patterns and responses to alcohol vary based on gender, age, weight, cultural expectancies, drinking experience (e.g., behavioral and physical tolerance), and drinking context, generally low-to-moderate doses (a couple of drinks) are considered pleasantly relaxing and are associated with sociability in most societies. After three to six drinks, the drinker is likely to experience impaired motor functioning, and gradually worsening cognitive functioning. After seven to fifteen drinks (depending on level of tolerance), the drinker is probably quite drunk, or unconscious. These large amounts of alcohol can be lethal. Signs of alcohol intoxication include slurred speech, loss of coordination, unsteadiness on one's feet, difficulty focusing, impaired attention or memory, stupor, and coma. Persons sometimes die from rapid ingestion of high doses of alcohol, and withdrawal after long-term heavy drinking can be dangerous or even fatal.

In the alcohol-dependent person, withdrawal symptoms may begin a few hours after the last drink and last up to five days, usually peaking somewhere between twenty-four to forty-eight hours. Nervous-system hyperactivity resulting from a rebound effect of alcohol's depressant effects can be marked by moderate-to-severe anxiety, increased heart rate, hand tremor, blood pressure, nausea, and insomnia, and may result in an alcohol-withdrawal seizure. At the severe end of the spectrum, delirium tremens (the d.t.'s) may occur within two to three days, and the person has a 10–15% chance of dying if withdrawal symptoms are left untreated. Long-term effects of heavy alcohol abuse include damage to virtually all major organ systems, most prominently liver damage resulting in cirrhosis, heart damage and other circulatory problems, severe cognitive impairments including organic brain disorders (e.g., Bernice and Korsakoff syndromes), and gastrointestinal disorders.

Sedatives and hypnotics are also CNS depressants. At lower doses they are meant to have a calming effect; at higher doses, they are used to induce sleep. Barbiturates also can induce general anesthesia, although benzodiazepines do not. These drugs are also used as anticonvulsive medications. Sedatives and hypnotics vary in both half-life and their specific therapeutic effect. Benzodiazepines, alleged by some to be widely overprescribed, have a more specific antianxiety effect, whereas barbiturates have a more general sedating effect on the nervous system. Signs of intoxication are very similar to those related to alcohol. Dangers of lethal overdose are more prominent with barbiturates than with benzodiazepines. Sedative effects of both types of drugs are magnified when mixed with alcohol, and a mix of alcohol and barbiturates may be fatal. Withdrawal symptoms will vary depending on the specific drug, but care should be taken to refer clients who have a history of sedative-hypnotic use to a physician if they are considering discontinuing use. Withdrawal symptoms can begin anywhere from one to three days (for shorter half-life drugs) to four to seven days or longer. Most people who withdraw from sedative-hypnotic drugs under medical supervision experience mild to moderate anxiety. For more severely dependent people, however, withdrawal can be very similar to withdrawal from alcohol and may include increased pulse rate, insomnia, hand tremors, nausea and vomiting, transient hallucinations, anxiety, and grand mal seizures. For some clients, distinguishing between withdrawal symptoms and the reemergence of anxiety symptoms can be difficult.

Most people who take these drugs under prescription do not abuse them; however, those who do tend to abuse other drugs as well, and often use them to regulate the withdrawal symptoms associated with other drugs. Long-term abuse can be associated with common mental health symptoms including depression and anxiety. Newer classes of benzodiazepines (e.g., buspirone hydrochloride) appear to have lower risks for abuse.

Stimulants.   Stimulants generally refer to cocaine and amphetamine-related products. Cocaine has a shorter half-life than most amphetamines. Stimulant use can be a problem even if the client does not use these drugs daily. Abusers often go on binges or "runs" for days at a time, marked by a cycle of craving, bingeing, withdrawal and depression, more craving, and resumption of use. General effects of these drugs include CNS arousal, increased libido, feeling energetic, decreased appetite, hyperalertness, increased self-confidence, talkativeness, and repetitive behavior. Intoxication results in increased heart rate, dilation of pupils, elevated blood pressure, chills, nausea, vomiting, psychomotor agitation or retardation, cardiac arrhythmia, muscular weakness, confusion, and seizures, among other signs and symptoms. Chronic abuse can result in depression, fatigue, and poor concentration.

Despite the reinforcing qualities of amphetamines and cocaine, relatively few of the many people who try these drugs develop a serious problem or an addiction to them (less than 15%). Methamphetamines and related designer drugs such as ecstasy (MDA, or methylenedioxyphenylisopropylamine) combine the effects of amphetamines and hallucinogens: general arousal, and feelings of well-being and intimacy with others. Although in higher doses these drugs share some of the potentially toxic effects of other amphetamines, users also run the risk of dehydration and hyperthermia from prolonged frenetic activity. Although injection produces the quickest high, smoking results in full absorption as well. Snorting is the least-efficient method to absorb these drugs.

An overdose on stimulants can result in a cardiac emergency, stroke, convulsions, and toxic "psychosis," which can last for hours with longer-acting amphetamines. Withdrawal symptoms commence soon after stimulant abuse ends. The user experiences the rapid reduction in mood and energy, and chronic abusers may experience anxiety, depression, and paranoia. Symptoms may last for a few days. Depression, boredom, memory problems, and malaise (perhaps accompanied by suicidal ideation) may continue for a few days or weeks. If abusers do not relapse during this period, they may experience cravings for months or years after they have stopped using stimulants. Other specific long-term effects of abuse include damage to the heart (e.g., cardiomyopathy), "crack lung" (a chronic cough producing black sputum), or damage to nasal membranes from snorting powdered cocaine.

Opioids.   Opium-based drugs such as morphine and its derivative heroin, originally designed for pain relief, can result in a dependence syndrome when abused. Intoxication from abuse can produce euphoria, and relief from anxiety, followed by apathy, depression, psychomotor agitation or retardation, "nodding" or dreamy twilight state, constriction of pupils, lowered respiration, slurred speech, and impaired judgment. Although many occasional users of opioids do not develop dependence, tolerance can develop with repeated use and the concomitant withdrawal syndrome. Severe intoxication or overdose may present a medical emergency, indicated by pinpoint pupils, depressed respiration, and coma. Withdrawal from opioids is considered generally safe, assuming that the user is not cross-addicted to CNS depressants. Withdrawal symptoms may begin within a few hours of the last dose, and last up to a few days. Symptoms are similar to those of a twenty-four-hour bout with influenza: depressed mood, nausea and vomiting, muscle aches, runny nose, watery eyes, gooseflesh, dilation of pupils, diarrhea, yawning, fever, and insomnia. Withdrawal is also likely to be accompanied by craving for the drug which often leads to relapse and drug seeking. Treatment of withdrawal often includes use of opioid agonists (e.g., methadone), antagonists (e.g., naltrexone), or some combination of drugs.

Other Commonly Abused Drugs.   The active ingredient of marijuana (*Cannabis sativa*) is delta-9-tetrahydrocannabinol (THC). The percentage of this active ingredient ranges from 5% to 15%. Hashish is more potent, and the THC content in hashish oil may be as high as 60%. Most cannabis users report the subjective experience of being high as mild euphoria and relaxation, but effects vary considerably depending on the user's mood, state of mind, and social context, among other factors. Abuse of cannabis can result in panic reactions among inexperienced or anxious users, a problem addressed effectively with calming reassurance and the passage of time. In other respects, immediate overdose risks from marijuana abuse are minimal. Negative effects can include short-term memory loss and attention lapses, and disjointed thought patterns, symptoms that may be problematic depending on the context of use (e.g., driving a bus versus listening to music at home). A subgroup of heavy regular users of marijuana can develop some degree of tolerance, but withdrawal symptoms are generally mild and may include some sleep disturbance, nervousness, moodiness, and appetite changes. Chronic heavy use poses a serious risk to the health of the lungs. Amotivational syndrome is not unique to the abuse of marijuana, and marijuana has not been empirically demonstrated to be a gateway drug for any pharmacological reasons. Because of its current status as an illegal substance, however, it may increase the likelihood of other drug use by exposing users to a wide array of products available on the illicit drug market.

Hallucinogens come in more than one hundred types with varying molecular structures. The better-known are LSD (lysergic acid), mescaline, and psilocybin (magic mushrooms, peyote). These substances produce physiological effects such as elevated blood pressure and temperature soon after ingestion, and hallucinogenic effects within a couple of hours. Visual hallucinations are the most commonly cited effects, although all senses may be affected. These effects may last for several hours after ingestion. Users report alterations in aesthetic experience, slowing of time, synesthesia (mixing of senses such as "hearing colors" or "seeing musical tones," etc.), fluctuation of emotional states, increased vividness of memories, and a perception of deep insight regarding philosophical or spiritual matters. There are no risks of serious overdose from LSD, although a lethal dose of mescaline is estimated to be about ten to thirty times higher than the effective dose. Some users have reported ingesting and surviving prodigious amounts of hallucinogens, while others have reported "bad trips" or panicky feelings that can make the experience seem endless. Tolerance to these drugs develops rapidly and dissipates as rapidly. There is little danger of physiological withdrawals from hallucinogens and little risk of physiological dependence. For some, hallucinogen abuse has resulted in long-term psychological problems.

PCP, often misrepresented as THC or LSD on the street, is not a true hallucinogen but at lower doses can produce feelings of relaxation or numbness, confusion, disorientation, and distortions of body image. Higher doses can result in depression, anxiety, confusion, and paniclike states. PCP use is often associated with people who become belligerent or out of control. It is often sprinkled into a marijuana joint or a standard cigarette. PCP effects begin within about five minutes, plateau within thirty minutes, and may last for several hours, with effects lingering for up to two days. An overdose can result in coma.

Inhalant abuse is associated with hundreds of chemicals often easily available in the home or workplace. These products include gasoline, cleaning solvents, glues, and aerosol products (e.g., toluene in spray paint). They are sniffed through a rag soaked in the chemical or from some kind of container. Those who use inhalants (any use should be considered abuse) anticipate the "rush," that is, feelings of euphoria, floating, hallucinations, and other perceptual distortions. Repeated use often leaves the user with a characteristic smell and a rash around the mouth. CNS damage and occasionally seizures can result. Long-term use of some of these chemicals can lead to damage to organ systems and increased risk for serious diseases. Death can result from sniffing certain products, and some children have died when the products were inadvertently ignited (they tend to be highly inflammable). Tolerance can develop, and withdrawal may include cramps, nausea, vomiting, diarrhea, tremors, and irritability.

Having a familiarity with the basic effects, patterns of use, routes of transmission, and risks of tolerance and withdrawal of these substances is key to conducting evidence-based assessment for the abuse of alcohol and other drugs. Although most social workers are not employed in primary addictions facilities, conducting routine screening and assessment for substance abuse and addiction is essential for all clients, given high rates of co-occurrence with other psychosocial disorders and problems in living.

Key Elements of Multidimensional/ Functional Assessment

Substance abuse is diagnosed when maladaptive use has occurred over the previous twelve months in at least one of the following areas: failure to fulfill major role obligations at work, school, or home; recurrent use in hazardous situations; recurrent legal problems; and continued use despite persistent or recurrent social or interpersonal problems (*DSM-IV-TR*). Dependence is diagnosed when three or more of the following conditions have been met: tolerance; withdrawal symptoms; use of more of the substance than intended; difficulty cutting down; frequent drug-seeking behavior; impairment of social, occupational or recreational activities; and continued use despite persistent or recurrent psychological or physical problems. *Physiological dependence is not required to make a diagnosis of substance dependence.* Lengthy diagnostic instruments have been developed to confirm a substance-dependence diagnosis. These include the Structured Clinical Interview for the DSM (SCID; Hasin, 1991) and the Alcohol Use Disorders and Associated Disabilities Schedule (Grant et al., 1994). Although essential to research, routine use of these extensive instruments in treatment is not considered practical.

The call for practitioners to conduct routine assessment of substance abuse has been well articulated (Griffin, 1991; Carey & Teitelbaum, 1996; Sobell, Toneatto, & Sobell, 1994; Donovan, 1999). Although a brief screening tool may be helpful initially, a more thorough MDF assessment is required if there are positive indications that the client is experiencing significant problems with alcohol or other drugs. Although the diagnostic criteria for substance abuse and dependence touch on the major points of a multidimensional assessment, the practitioner should examine each of these domains of living (e.g., psychological, family, interpersonal, work, health) in more detail, and employ multiple sources of data as needed.

Assessment should be seen as an ongoing process that serves multiple purposes. Given the demonstrated effectiveness of self-monitoring in substance-abuse assessment and treatment (Annis & Davis, 1991; Carey & Teitelbaum, 1996), the client's collaboration with data collection also becomes an effective therapeutic tool in the following ways: it helps clients to specify what substances they use, how much, and how often; it assists them in making connections between substance abuse and variations in other health or psychosocial complaints; it provides therapeutic structure and clarity concerning treatment goals and objectives; it confirms their motivation; it signals inconsistencies in self-report; and it provides clear evidence of improvement or the need to reassess and alter the treatment plan.

Five major questions frame the substance-focused assessment: (1) What substances (legal and illicit, prescribed or nonprescribed) are used? (2) How much of the substances (estimated ounces, grams, milligrams, joints, hits, lines, etc.) are used? (3) how often are they used? (4) What precipitating factors (negative mood, cravings, situational factors, etc.) appear to be associated with problem use? (5) What are the consequences (acute and chronic) of substance use across physiological, psychosocial, and health domains?

Although some have overgeneralized the impression that "you can't trust alcohol and drug abusers," the overwhelming body of evidence on self-report of alcohol and drug use refutes this contention (Hesselbrock, Babor, Hesselbrock, Meyer, & Workman, 1983; Babor, Stephens, & Marlatt, 1987; Sobell et al., 1994). Under some circumstances, clients may be inclined to lie, deny, or minimize their use and related consequences, but clinical research has consistently demonstrated that the self-report of substance use and abuse is relatively valid and reliable in the hands of a skilled interviewer. Clients are often relatively forthcoming when confidentiality is assured and they are not threatened with negative consequences. An evaluation of the client's relative veracity should also take into consideration the client's referral source and level of motivation for seeing the practitioner. The techniques listed here can improve the accuracy of self-report.

> Desensitize clients to a discussion of the use of psychoactive chemicals rather than approaching it in an accusatory, judgmental manner (don't ask, "Are you a drinker? A drug abuser?").
>
> Clients who are guarded may be more responsive when questions are approached in the context of health concerns: ("Do you smoke? . . . use alcoholic beverages? . . . take medication? . . . non-prescription, recreational or street drugs?").
>
> The practitioner can express concern about being able to help the client if she or he is not honest about drug use and abuse.

Assure confidentiality to the extent that one can.

Reduce or eliminate negative program contingencies for honest reporting at assessment, ongoing evaluation, and follow-up.

Anchor the client's recent and long-term memory with important life events.

Use clear and specific terminology regarding what constitutes a drink, and the types of drugs, routes of transmission, dosage, and so on.

If necessary, inform the client that collateral sources of information can be obtained from significant others or other agencies.

Discuss preliminary causal associations between drug use and presenting complaints.

Tactfully confront contradictory information.

Estimate acute physiological risks associated with potential overdose or withdrawal, and arrange for medical consultation if any risks seem apparent. Share these concerns with the client.

Once preliminary drug-use data have been collected, practitioners can conduct a more detailed functional assessment by helping the client make connections between drug use and other problematic psychological, social, and health-related experiences that have occurred over time. *This cause-effect sequencing of antecedent events, drug use, and consequences is at the heart of a good functional analysis.* Research findings have suggested that people concerned with their substance use and abuse tend to make changes by weighing the pros and cons of using, and many decide to reduce or eliminate use on their own because (in their estimation) the cost of using has become too high (J. A. Cunningham, Sobell, Sobell, & Kapur, 1995). Focusing on a nonconfrontational approach that appeals to clients' self-interest and to their sense of autonomy is commensurate with what is now referred to as motivational interviewing (W. R. Miller & Rollnick, 1991; DiClemente, Bellino, & Neavins, 1999). Emphasizing clients' self-interest rather than "extracting a confession" through aggressive confrontation seems to be a more constructive way to engage them in the initial stage of intervention.

Setting Intervention Goals

The assessment is not complete until tentative treatment goals have been negotiated. Given the heterogeneity and range of seriousness of substance abuse, abstinence is no longer considered the only treatment goal (H. Rosenberg & Davis, 1994). The range of possibilities now includes harm reduction, moderation, and abstinence. A review of the empirical literature for alcohol treatment goals (Ambrogne, 2002) summarizes the findings of more than two decades of research: reduced-risk drinking as an intervention goal is a viable option for some problem drinkers and some dependent drinkers; abstinence and non–abstinence-based interventions are comparably effective; those with moderate to severe dependence should be advised to achieve abstinence; providing clients with some choice in treatment goals promotes treatment effectiveness. Given that clinician-recommended treatment goals are generally not good predictors of outcome (Finney & Moos, 1991; Nordstrom & Burglund, 1987), a collaborative approach to goal setting may enhance the client's engagement and commitment to treatment from the start.

A few basics should be considered before goals are established. Clients enter treatment at different stages of readiness to change, and a clinician's ability to meet clients where they are can get treatment off on the right foot. Practitioners should be familiar with the stages of change defined in chapter 3: precontemplation, contemplation, preparation, action, and maintenance. For many substance abusers, the insistence on abstinence may set up a series of failure contingencies referred to as the abstinence violation effect (Marlatt & George, 1984; Marlatt & Gordon, 1985; Larimer, Palmer, & Marlatt, 1999), in which a "slip" is equated with failure. Depending on the client's readiness to make some changes, social workers should help abusers experiment first with cutting down or trying periodic abstinence, make tentative changes in the context of use to minimize serious consequences (e.g., drinking on the job or while driving), or eliminate one or two substances if the client is using multiple drugs (with consideration given to risks during withdrawal). Inclusion of the client in formulating the treatment plan and selecting treatment goals has been shown to contribute to treatment retention and positive outcomes (W. R. Miller, 1992; Sanchez-Craig & Annis, 1982; Sanchez-Craig & Lei, 1986; Sanchez-Craig, 1980).

Although practitioners do not want to unwittingly engage in enabling clients, caution must be used when imposing treatment goals that reduce the likelihood of even partial improvement. While a client's response to the initial assessment may be negative, resistance can be approached constructively by accepting initial reluctance, avoiding unnecessary confrontation, and working collaboratively with the client by providing choice in treatment methods and goals (W. R. Miller & Rollnick, 1991). However, equivocal outcomes of controlled drinking studies suggest a conservative approach to setting treatment goals (Nathan & McCrady, 1987; Ambrogne, 2002). Clients who appear to have trouble with loss of control or abstaining from use, have serious psychiatric disorders, few social supports, a history of treatment failure, or health problems resulting from substance abuse, should be strongly encouraged to make abstinence their goal. Nevertheless, any cutting down or reduction of harm on the way toward elective abstinence should be considered progress.

A graduated self-testing approach in the initial stages of treatment may help the client decide on optimal treatment goals. Although complete problem-free abstinence will always be an ideal goal for many clients, maximizing harm reduction for all clients may represent a more flexible and realistic clinical strategy (Marlatt, 1996). Once treatment goals have been negotiated, the clinician needs to consistently associate reduction of alcohol or other drug use with progress in the client's major complaints. Since substance abuse and other psychosocial difficulties exacerbate one another, progress in one area is often associated with progress in the other (Brownell, Marlatt, Lichtenstein, & Wilson, 1986; Rounsaville, Dolinsky, Babor, & Meyer, 1987).

Instruments

Many tools that assess substance use are available to clinicians (Hasin, 1991; Allen & Mattson, 1993; Carey & Teitelbaum, 1996; Donovan, 1999). These include brief screening devices, simple indexes for tracking changes and treatment progress, and multidimensional scales that measure problems, consequences, or other psychological aspects of substance abuse and dependence. Assessment tools are best used when they are incorporated into the comprehensive psychosocial assessment. Paper-and-pencil brief screening devices have been shown to be reasonably sensitive to the detection of substance abuse (Babor, Kranzler, & Lauerman, 1989), and have good clinical utility in that they signal the need for early intervention.

The Alcohol Use Disorders Identification Test (AUDIT; Babor & Grant, 1989; Saunders, Aasland, Amundsen et al., 1993; USDHHS, 2003), developed in ten countries under the auspices of the World Health Organization, was designed to detect harmful or hazardous drinking in addition to alcohol dependence (instrument 6.1). The ten-question AUDIT includes questions on alcohol consumption, along with four questions on dependence, and three on consequences. The AUDIT is scored on a frequency continuum (rather than dichotomously), requests measures over the last year (rather than lifetime), and appears to have broader applicability by discriminating hazardous and harmful drinkers rather than just those who are alcohol dependent (Bohn, Babor, & Kranzler, 1995). The AUDIT appears to have good potential as a brief screen in mental health and other social service environments where problem drinking frequently co-occurs with other complaints.

The Drug Abuse Screening Test (DAST; Skinner, 1982) is a twenty-eight-item self-report screening instrument intended to measure the extent of involvement with drugs other than alcohol. It uses a cutoff score of six or more to indicate a level of clinical concern. It provides a global measure of drug abuse, distinguishes drug abusers from those with mixed alcohol and other drug problems, and correlates well with a diagnosis of substance abuse. The DAST discriminated drug-abusing psychiatric patients with a primary *DSM-III* diagnosis of substance abuse, and showed excellent internal consistency (.94; Staley & El-Guebaly, 1990). Although it constitutes a valid screening tool for detecting drug abuse and dependence, the DAST is designed to diagnose lifetime dependence rather than actual consumption, and thus is not useful as an outcome measure. A ten-item version of the DAST (DAST-10) has been developed and correlated very highly with the full DAST in a population of mentally ill people with co-occurring substance-abuse disorders (Cocco & Carey, 1998; Maisto, Carey, Carey, Gordon, & Gleason, 2000). In the same study, the DAST-10 showed good interrater reliabil-

INSTRUMENT 6.1   Alcohol Use Disorders Identification Test (AUDIT)

Please circle the answer that is correct for you.

1. How often do you have a drink containing alcohol?

| Never | Monthly or less | Two to four times per month | Two to three times per week | Four or more times per week |

2. How many drinks containing alcohol do you have on a typical day when you are drinking?

| 1 or 2   3 or 4 | 5 or 6 | 7 to 9 | 10 or more |

3. How often do you have six or more drinks on one occasion?

| Never | Less than monthly | Monthly | Two to three times per week | Four or more times per week |

4. How often during the last year have you found that you were not able to stop drinking once you had started?

| Never | Less than monthly | Monthly | Two to three times per week | Four or more times per week |

5. How often during the last year have you failed to do what was normally expected from you because of drinking?

| Never | Less than monthly | Monthly | Two to three times per week | Four or more times per week |

6. How often during the last year have you needed a first drink in the morning to get yourself going after a heavy drinking session?

| Never | Less than monthly | Monthly | Two to three times per week | Four or more times per week |

7. How often during the last year have you had a feeling of guilt or remorse after drinking?

| Never | Less than monthly | Monthly | Two to three times per week | Four or more times per week |

8. How often during the last year have you been unable to remember what happened the night before because you had been drinking?

| Never | Less than monthly | Monthly | Two to three times per week | Four or more times per week |

9. Have you or someone else been injured as the result of your drinking?

| No | Yes, but not in the last year | Yes, during the last year |

10. Has a relative, friend, or doctor or other health worker been concerned about your drinking or suggested you cut down?

| No | Yes, but not in the last year | Yes, during the last year |

Procedures for scoring the AUDIT: Questions 1–8 are scored 0, 1, 2, 3, or 4. Questions 9 and 10 are scored 0, 2, or 4 only. The minimum score (for nondrinkers) is 0, and the maximum possible score is 40. A score of 8 or more indicates a strong likelihood of hazardous or harmful alcohol consumption.

ity, very good internal consistency, and good concurrent validity with other substance-abuse measures. With yes = 1 and no = 0, the recommended cutoff for detecting a probable drug problem is ≥3. The DAST-10 is reprinted here (instrument 6.2).

Multidimensional measures are recommended so practitioners can evaluate assessment and treatment outcomes in a number of problem domains. One example is the Addiction Severity Index (ASI; McLellan et al., 1980; Stoffelmayer, Mavis, & Kasim, 1994), a well-regarded multidimensional assessment instrument that is sensitive to change and can therefore be used to measure treatment outcomes. Because the ASI takes about an hour to complete, it should be used after the client has met initial screening criteria for substance abuse. It provides sub-

---

INSTRUMENT 6.2   Drug Abuse Screening Test-10 (DAST-10)

The following questions concern information about your possible involvement with drugs *not including alcoholic beverages* during the past 12 months. Carefully read each statement and decide if your answer is "yes" or "no." Then, circle the appropriate response beside the question.

In the statements "drug abuse" refers to (1) the use of prescribed or over-the-counter drugs in excess of the directions and (2) any non-medical use of drugs. The various classes of drugs may include cannabis (e.g., marijuana, hash), solvents, tranquilizers (e.g., Valium), barbiturates, cocaine, stimulants (e.g., speed), hallucinogens (e.g., LSD), or narcotics (e.g., heroin). Remember that the questions *do not* include alcoholic beverages.

Please answer every question. If you have difficulty with a statement, then choose the response that is mostly right.

These questions refer to the past 12 months	Circle your response	
1. Have you used drugs other than those required for medical reasons?	Yes	No
2. Do you abuse more than one drug at a time?	Yes	No
3. Are you always able to stop using drugs when you want to?	Yes	No
4. Have you had "blackouts" or "flashbacks" as a result of drug use?	Yes	No
5. Do you ever feel bad or guilty about your drug use?	Yes	No
6. Does your spouse (or parents) ever complain about your involvement with drugs?	Yes	No
7. Have you neglected your family because of your use of drugs?	Yes	No
8. Have you engaged in illegal activities in order to obtain drugs?	Yes	No
9. Have you ever experienced withdrawal symptoms (felt sick) when you stopped taking drugs?	Yes	No
10. Have you had medical problems as a result of your drug use (e.g., memory loss, hepatitis, convulsions, bleeding, etc.)?	Yes	No

jective (severity) ratings to determine need for treatment as well as composite scores for seven areas of functioning: psychiatric status, physical health, employment, legal status, alcohol and drug use, and family and social functioning. Evidence obtained with substance-abusing men and women supports interrater and test-retest reliability, good concurrent and discriminant validity, and good stability when used in longitudinal evaluations (McLellan et al.; Stoffelmayer et al.). A copy of the ASI appears in appendix E.

An indirect approach to measuring problem drinking emphasizes the respondent's ability to resist drinking under "at risk" circumstances. One such effort is the Inventory of Drinking Situations (Annis, 1982), which was designed to estimate the likelihood of relapse for people struggling with alcoholism. The eight dimensions include unpleasant emotions, physical discomfort, pleasant emotions, testing personal control, urges and temptations to drink, conflicts with others, social pressure, and pleasant times with others. In a treatment population (Isenhart, 1993), high scores on some of these subscales (unpleasant emotions, social pressure, testing control, pleasant emotions, and physical discomfort) were associated with heavy drinking. Similar instruments include the Situational Confidence Questionnaire (Kirisci, Moss, & Tarter, 1996) and the Alcohol Abstinence Self-Efficacy Scale (DiClemente, Carbonari, Montgomery, & Hughes, 1994).

Node-link mapping is a promising qualitative technique for helping clients create visual maps or schematics of the thoughts, feelings, and situations that can lead to substance abuse. For many clients, particularly those with modest verbal skills, this may be a more nonthreatening way of describing and explaining the processes that often lead to relapse. Some evidence has associated the use of this technique with better communication between practitioner and client (Dees, Dansereau, & Simpson, 1994).

SELECTING EFFECTIVE INTERVENTIONS

Treating substance abuse in the United States costs billions of dollars per year in a combination of private and public treatment facilities, and billions more in treating related illnesses (USDHHS, 2000). On any given day, more than 700,000 people are receiving alcoholism treatment (about one-forth women, almost two-thirds white, 86% on an outpatient basis; USDHHS, 1997, 2000). A considerable amount has been learned about the effectiveness of substance-abuse treatment from uncontrolled naturalistic evaluation data and matched treatment and community samples. Early detection of substance abuse and access to a range of intervention options and treatment goals appears to be the best course for making a positive impact on a substance user's long-term well-being (Finney & Moos, 1991; Finney, Moos, & Timko, 1999). Although treatment may shorten the trajectory of substance-abuse and addiction, psychosocial pressures and health consequences also play a powerful role in modifying substance-abuse behavior for the better. Treatment and policy initiatives should capitalize on these naturally occurring social factors (Finney et al.).

A few large uncontrolled evaluation studies of drug-treatment facilities in the United States have been conducted over the past thirty years: Drug Abuse Reporting Program Treatment Outcome Prospective Study, and Drug Abuse Treatment Outcome Study. Results suggest that treatment is modestly successful in helping clients overcome their addictions *when they remain in treatment for three months or longer.* These positive outcomes included reduced heroin and cocaine abuse and decreased criminal activity. Nevertheless, effective treatment components are often poorly defined, so it is difficult to say exactly what was helpful or effective. In addition, high treatment dropout rates make it difficult to determine whether the positive outcomes were due to effective treatment or to more highly motivated clients remaining in treatment (Hubbard, Craddock, Flynn, Anderson, & Etheridge, 1997; Fletcher, Tims, & Brown, 1997). Nevertheless, when representative samples of addicted people in the community are matched with those in treatment, evidence suggests that treatment shows positive results at twelve-month follow-up for both abstinence and nonproblematic use. Poorer outcomes are associated with co-occurring psychiatric disorders, drug abuse, and more negative social consequences (Weisner, Matzger, & Kaskutas, 2003).

Traditional psychotherapy has not been shown to be particularly effective in helping clients who have problems with substance abuse (Emrick, 1974, 1982; W. R. Miller, 1992). An array of effective interventions are now available, however, and social workers who do not work in facilities that primarily treat substance abuse can integrate these methods into their practice repertoire. These interventions help clients reduce or eliminate consumption, reduce harm, recover, and prevent relapse. Based on an extensive analysis of controlled studies for alcoholism treatments, it is clear that expensive inpatient services are no longer assumed to be the gold standard of treatment and do not generally result in superior outcomes (W. R. Miller & Hester, 1986; Holder, Longabaugh, Miller, & Rubonis, 1991). Critical reviews of controlled outcome studies demonstrate that there are a range of effective interventions available for people who abuse alcohol and other drugs. Briefly, these include

> brief interventions where practitioners provide a few psychoeducational and motivational enhancement sessions focusing on negative health-related consequences of drinking (Heather, 1995; DiClemente et al., 1999; USDHHS, 1997, 2000);

> cognitive-behavioral coping-skills strategies that emphasize learning to self-monitor, detect, and avoid urges and situations that increase risk of drinking or drug use, and replace substance abuse with more adaptive coping skills and healthier lifestyles (Kadden, 1994; W. R. Miller, 1992; Longabaugh & Morgenstern, 1999);

> behavioral couples and family therapies that include communications, problem-solving, contingency management, and coping skills (E. J. Thomas & Santa, 1982; O'Farrell & Fals-Stewart, 1999, 2003; Stanton & Shadish, 1997);

community reinforcement and contingency management strategies that combine coping-skills interventions with positive payoffs for abstinence and negative sanctions for relapse (Azrin, Sisson, Meyers, & Godley, 1982; S. T. Higgins et al., 1993; Acierno, Donohoe, & Kogan, 1994; S. T. Higgins, Wong, Badger, Ogden, & Dantona, 2000);

twelve-step facilitation by substance-abuse professionals to encourage and guide the addicted person through the first few steps of twelve-step programs (Humphreys, 1999; Nowinski, 1999).

Brief Interventions

Brief interventions are a collection of strategies used to ameliorate problem drinking and perhaps interrupt the trajectory of a more serious problem with alcohol dependence (Heather, 1995; DiClemente et al., 1999; USDHHS, 1997, 2000). The crux of the brief intervention is a thorough assessment accompanied by informed, structured feedback about the consequences of the client's drinking, including data from medical tests, advice on methods for avoiding drinking situations, and psychoeducation about the effects of alcohol. This approach can be provided over a few visits, and may include two or three sessions of assessment, psychoeducation, and advice, often accompanied by reading materials. Given the wide range of problems treated by social workers, they are in an ideal circumstance to screen, diagnose, assess, and provide early intervention or referral. Goal setting is oriented toward moderation or initial moderation with the intent of pursuing more extensive intervention for long-term abstinence, if needed. For problem users, brief interventions may be sufficient to help them modify their use and forestall more serious problems.

Motivational enhancement therapy (MET) is an elaboration on earlier work in motivational interviewing (W. R. Miller & Rollnick, 1991; DiClemente et al., 1999; USDHHS, 2000). Clients typically come to intervention at different levels (stages) of readiness to change (DiClemente & Hughes, 1990; Prochaska, DiClemente, & Norcross, 1992; O'Hare, 1996a). Many minimize or outright deny the existence of a substance-abuse problem, have little intention of changing, and may see others as being the source of the problem. Given the number of dropouts from treatment, initial efforts to meet clients where they are have focused on initially motivating clients in a nonconfrontational manner. This approach can be part of a brief intervention (as described above) or a prelude to a more lengthy engagement process (DiClemente et al.). In some respects, motivational interviewing reflects the basics of good client-centered counseling techniques, and reemphasizes the importance of employing a nonjudgmental approach, good listening skills, engaging clients in a process of gradually weighing the benefits and costs of their substance use, and ultimately relying on clients' ability to make decisions in their own best interest. In addition to providing psychoeducation, the practitioner helps the client compare personal goals with the actual situation, especially the problems incurred due to abuse of alcohol and other drugs. MET combines motivational interviewing with brief structured intervention and, after extensive assessment, gives the client feedback that may include the results of other tests, including health measures (in collaboration with a physician), and data comparing the client's substance use and consequences with population norms. Practitioners then focus on engaging and motivating the client, developing a specific plan of change, and examining ambivalent feelings and other potential roadblocks to change (DiClemente et al.).

Coping-Skills Approaches

Coping skills encompass an array of cognitive-behavioral methods that can be employed with those experiencing substance abuse or dependence. A range of goals are considered, including harm reduction, moderation, abstinence, and relapse prevention, as well as improvements in related psychosocial problems (W. R. Miller, 1992; Acierno et al., 1994; Nunes-Dinis & Barth, 1993; Kadden, 1994; Monti & Rohsenow, 1999). These skills have been incorporated into efforts to assist substance abusers who also are at risk for other serious problems such as HIV transmission (Schilling, El-Bassel, Hadden, & Gilbert, 1995; El-Bassel et al., 1995; Pomeroy, Kiam, & Abel, 1999). An impressive body of outcome research has accumulated in support of these strategies and skills. The best data appear to support the use of cognitive-behavioral coping skills when they are used as part of a comprehensive treatment strategy that includes motivational interviewing and twelve-step approaches (Longabaugh & Morgenstern, 1999). Coping-skills interventions were derived from a number of related approaches, including cognitive therapy (Beck, Rush, Shaw, & Emery, 1979; Moorey, 1989), self-monitoring and cue exposure (Monti & Rohsenow, 1999), social-skills training and stress management (Kadden 1994), and relapse prevention (Marlatt & Gordon, 1985; Larimer et al., 1999). CBT methods have also been incorporated into behavioral couples and family therapy and community reinforcement approaches, both of which are discussed below.

Core coping-skills strategies include:

developing rapport, assessing, and engaging motivation;

reviewing dysfunctional thinking regarding denial, rationalization, or hopelessness about the client's situation;

assessing high-risk situations, where clients are most likely to use drugs;

teaching self-monitoring of positive or negative thoughts, feelings, behaviors, and situations that could enhance or hinder moderation or sobriety;

identifying and learning to cope with cravings;

coping with intense or troubling thoughts and feelings;

practicing assertiveness and social skills when confronted with at-risk circumstances;

practicing stress-management skills to cope with daily stressors (use of imagery, self-desensitization skills, physical exercise, non–drug-centered recreation);

learning and sharpening problem-solving skills such as brainstorming and, considering alternatives;

teaching and practicing drink-refusal skills through the use of modeling, role-playing, rehearsal, and in vivo practice;

teaching communications skills to help the client deal with a wider variety of social situations.

The last skills include learning to give and take positive or negative criticism, improving conversational skills, using conflict-resolution techniques, developing sober social supports, and enlisting the help of friends, family members, romantic partners, workmates, employers, and other social supports such as AA buddies or sponsors.

Coping-skills methods have been packaged for clients who have made considerable progress in treatment, but whose current goal is to prevent relapse (Marlatt & Gordon, 1985; Daley, 1987; Annis & Davis, 1991; Larimer et al., 1999). Relapse prevention increases the client's self-efficacy in the use of these specific skills, and reduces the chances of relapsing in at-risk situations. The overall strategy includes cognitive self-assessment (e.g., pausing to think, reviewing the negative consequences of using and the positive consequences of abstaining or moderating use, taking one's mind off the urge to use), behavior change (e.g., seeking alternative activities, avoiding or leaving high-risk situations, planning healthier stress-reducing activities), coping with distressing or negative emotions (e.g., letting go of things that can't be controlled or changed, emphasizing positive feelings), and environmental changes (e.g., spending more time with family and friends who are supportive of non–substance-related activities). Homework helps clients practice self-monitoring skills and increase their confidence ability to cope with at-risk situations. These homework assignments can include self-rewards for dealing effectively with risky situations, rehearsal and role-playing of coping skills with the clinician and significant others, and gaining practice experience in the community. The level of challenge should be gradually increased to promote self-efficacy in high-risk situations. If the person does relapse, coping skills can also help mitigate the abstinence violation effect by preparing the client to interrupt the slip as soon as possible with a minimum of negative consequences. Long-term gains are encouraged by developing a healthier and preventive lifestyle to maintain gains over the long run.

Behavioral Couples and Family Therapy

Family members often play an important role in the recovery of a person addicted to alcohol or other drugs. A number of different approaches to dealing with couples and families have been developed. The family disease model (based on the Minnesota model developed at Hazelden; (V. W. Johnson, 1973) considers alcoholism a "family disease." The family systems model (Steinglass, Bennett, Wolin, & Reiss, 1987) is built on the premise that substance abuse developed or was maintained as part of an interactional family process, and both the drinker's behavior and the compensatory behaviors of other family members helped to maintain a homeostatic equilibrium. In both the family disease and family systems approaches, the practitioner attempts to help the family members reduce their overinvolvement in the drinker's behavior, and take a more adaptive stance for their own sake and for the health of the drinker. Little research, however, has been conducted to establish the effectiveness of the family disease model or family systems model.

Behavioral couples and family therapy is grounded in the premise that substance abuse, dependence, and associated maladaptive behaviors are learned, and that other family members (including spouses, generally referred to as "concerned significant others" or CSOs) sometimes unwittingly get caught up in attempts to cope with, ameliorate, cover up, or compensate for the drug user's behavior (McCrady et al., 1986; Noel & McCrady, 1993; O'Farrell, Choquette, Cutter, Brown, & McCourt, 1993; O'Farrell & Fals-Stewart, 1999, 2003). Often CSOs will reinforce the abuser's drinking by shielding, caretaking, or punishing the abusing member (e.g., refraining from talking, intimacy, sex). In behavioral couples and family approaches, the practitioner works with the CSOs to lessen these behaviors and to help them capitalize on opportunities to engage the drinking client in productive problem solving and improved communication. For example, rather than arguing with a husband who comes home intoxicated, the wife is encouraged to refrain from addressing it at the time, and to deal with it the next day when the husband is sober and, perhaps, in a better state of mind to discuss his drinking. If someone calls to inquire why the husband did not come into work that day, the wife will refrain from covering for her husband. No doubt there are risks, including potential retribution from the husband, suspension from work, or loss of a job. These matters need to be discussed thoroughly with family members. Although behavioral therapists share the view that family members' behaviors interact reciprocally, they do not contend that the person abusing substances has a disease, nor do they hold to the belief that other family members caused the drinker's problems or are "codependent." In addition, because they assume that substance abuse and related behaviors are primarily learned (and thus can be changed), behaviorally oriented practitioners assert that non–substance-abusing family members can help themselves cope better and have a positive impact on the family member's drinking.

Behavioral couples therapy (BCT) is the most strongly supported approach for substance-abusing couples, and has been shown to be among the most successful methods for treating substance abuse in general (McCrady et al., 1986; O'Farrell & Fals-Stewart, 1999, 2000, 2003; Noel & McCrady, 1993; O'Farrell, Choquette, & Cutter, 1998). Research repeatedly shows more positive outcomes in reduced drinking days and reduced drug use, improved marital relationships, reduced domestic violence, and improved psychosocial functioning in children (O'Farrell & Fals-Stewart, 2003). These approaches have been shown to be cost-effective as well (Fals-Stewart, O'Farrell, & Birchler, 1997; O'Farrell & Fals-Stewart, 2003). Behavioral contracting, particularly with the use of disulfiram, has been shown to be an especially effective component of BCT. Key components of BCT include seeing the couple, family, or individuals alone or together as needed; conducting a thorough MDF assessment of marital and family problems; engaging in crisis intervention as needed; using an (optional) disulfiram contract, where the drinking spouse agrees to take daily disulfiram accompanied by the nonabusing spouse's observation and reinforcement; implementing homework assignments and behavioral rehearsal; learning to deal with urges to drink; identifying at-risk interventions; incorporating coping-skills methods discussed above; practicing daily caring behaviors between spouses, and planning rewarding activities together; practicing better communications and problem-solving skills for the actual substance abuse as well as related problems; and incorporating relapse-prevention strategies into behavioral marital and family methods.

Exemplar study: Behavioral Couples Therapy.   In a key study, O'Farrell et al. (1993) recruited fifty-nine couples with husbands who had recently become abstinent. They agreed to participate in behavioral marital therapy weekly for five months, and were then randomly assigned either to receive fifteen sessions of conjoint relapse-prevention (RP) treatment over the course of a year, or to a control group. In addition to baseline and outcomes measured before and after BCT, couples also reported results at three, six, and twelve-month followups. The intervention included several pregroup sessions that included a thorough assessment, crisis intervention, disulfiram contract, feedback about the assessment of alcohol and marital problems, and efforts to enhance motivation. The couples group sessions consisted of ten weekly meetings of four to five couples and emphasized homework assignments and behavioral rehearsal. The intervention plan was designed to maintain abstinence, decrease arguments, maintain the disulfiram contract, provide crisis intervention for drinking episodes, monitor and initiate interpersonal caring behaviors, plan and share recreational activities, work on communication skills, and practice problem solving.

After the couples groups were completed, the couples were randomly assigned to RP or non-RP treatment conditions. Couples with RP went to fifteen sessions with decreasing frequency over the following year, and RP skills focused on maintaining drinking gains, in part, by continuing the disulfiram contract for several months along with Alcoholics Anonymous (AA) or Al-Anon. They also practiced behavioral skills to reduce marital problems, improve their relationship, and increase problem-solving skills. The couples practiced and rehearsed the RP plan by identifying high-risk situations and deciding on how to respond to them successfully when they occurred. Those who received the additional RP sessions demonstrated more days abstinent, fewer days drinking, and better marital adjustment than those who received BCT alone, although drinking measures were comparable between groups at further follow-up. RP subjects were also more likely to use specific treatment-targeted behaviors (i.e., disulfiram contract, marital improvements) at follow-up.

A follow-up study (O'Farrell et al., 1998) reported the results of twelve additional months of RP with eighteen-month follow-up after termination of treatment. The RP sessions were conducted jointly and had three major goals: to maintain the behavioral gains targeted by BCT (reduction in drinking, improvement in marital relations), to deal with unresolved marital problems, and to rehearse standard RP methods. Well-established standardized questionnaires measured both drinking and relational outcomes. Results demonstrated that the combination of BCT and RP resulted in somewhat better marital adjustment overall for the full thirty-month period, and alcoholic men (in both treatment groups) remained significantly improved after that time.

When the Drinking Spouse Is Reluctant to Participate.   A number of interventions have been developed to help CSOs either to persuade the substance-abusing spouse to engage in treatment, or to cope better on their own because their partner refuses treatment. A number of somewhat similar approaches generally referred to as unilateral family interventions (E. J. Thomas & Santa, 1982; Sisson & Azrin, 1986; E. J. Thomas & Ager, 1993) have been designed and evaluated for this situation. Two unilateral approaches that have produced promising results in successfully engaging reluctant spouses and/or improving the coping abilities for the nonabusing spouse include the Pressures to Change model (Barber & Gilbertson, 1996, 1997) and the Community Reinforcement and Family Training approach (Sisson & Azrin, 1986; W. R. Miller, Meyers, & Tonigan, 1999). In these unilateral approaches, the practitioners generally work with the CSOs over several months, provide psychoeducation about the nature of addiction, and try to help CSOs understand the futility of some of their compensatory behaviors (enabling). They may also develop and rehearse a plan to move the abusing spouse toward treatment. Specific supporting skills are enhanced to help CSOs cope with their emotional distress in trying to tolerate or influence the substance-abusing spouse. The major intervention steps include variations on the following key elements: CSOs learn about the nature of the intervention, its methods, purposes, and goals. They participate in an extensive assessment of the drinker's behaviors and the partner's response to them. The therapist acts as a coach to help the CSO understand the nature of the substance-abusing partner's behaviors, learn ways of enhancing the relationship (when the spouse is sober), and reduce behaviors that may be inadvertently reinforcing, such as shielding or nagging. Specific contracts may be developed to reinforce sober behaviors versus drinking behaviors (i.e., contingency management skills). A plan may be developed and rehearsed to enlist others to participate in the persuasion activities or, to prepare family members to participate in a confrontation in which the CSO (and perhaps others) expresses concern for the drinker, but demands certain changes, such as specific drinking-reduction goals or abstinence and, participation in treatment. The practitioner also provides an intervention focused exclusively on supporting the CSO, and helping the CSO deal with the emotional distress of living with an addicted or substance-troubled person. Some psychoeducation may be included to help CSOs deal with dangerous or potentially abusive situations (toward themselves or their children). RP methods are applied if the drinking spouse makes improvements. If the drinker fails to change, the focus of intervention may become more exclusive to the CSO who needs further support in dealing with the current situation or who decides to leave the relationship. Although these approaches are quite similar in methods and purpose, practitioners should consult specific models and accompanying treatment manuals before implementing unilateral approaches, because they do vary in technique and specific treatment goals.

Behavioral family methods have been used successfully where a family member had a serious primary addiction with drugs other than alcohol. A meta-analysis of controlled trials covering 3,500 clients and significant others showed that marital and family interventions produced superior outcomes compared with individual, peer group, or family psychoeducation (Stanton & Shadish, 1997). Family interventions also appear to be a cost-effective adjunct to methadone maintenance. These strategies appear to work equally well for both adolescent and adult abusers, and demonstrate relatively higher levels of client retention. Given the relatively small number of studies, however, no definitive conclusions can be drawn regarding the relative efficacy of different family approaches.

Community Reinforcement and Contingency Management Approaches

Although community reinforcement approaches (CRA) were originally developed and tested successfully with some of the most debilitated alcohol-dependent people (Azrin, 1976; Azrin et al., 1982), they have been largely overlooked until recently. CRA were originally designed to help the severely alcoholic person maintain sobriety through the use of community-based rewards (e.g., social connections, family relations, jobs, supported housing), and were later adapted to include the use of disulfiram and coping skills. CRA have come to be seen as one of the most effective substance-abuse interventions (W. R. Miller, Meyers, & Hiller-Sturmhofel, 1999).

Assessment in CRA emphasizes functional analysis of the client's drinking problem, that is, the identification of behaviors and situation-specific reinforcers and consequences that appear to maintain substance abuse. Clients are taught to engage in sobriety sampling (experimental periods of abstinence or reduced use) in order to better understand the relationship between substance use and its consequences, and they are urged to gradually extend the duration of sobriety with each effort. The goals of CRA are to reduce or eliminate substance use and improve overall lifestyle and social supports. Practitioners who use CRA may incorporate some of the coping-skills methods discussed earlier, but must link the client's performance directly to concrete rewards (R. J. Meyers & Smith, 1995; S. T. Higgins & Petry, 1999).

As with many effective treatments, CRA may begin with frequent visits and gradually increase the time between sessions as the client gains confidence in self-management methods. Outcomes for CRA have been very positive. Overall, results have shown that clients reduce their substance use substantially more than do counseling controls, need fewer days of institutionalization, work more days, and demonstrate greater social stability. CRA provide a flexible framework, can be used on an outpatient basis, can be integrated into a family treatment model and twelve-step approaches, and can incorporate disulfiram or similar medications. Although flexible in format, the core components are essential: a thorough MDF assessment and specific and valued concrete and social rewards for sobriety.

Contingency management (CM) approaches are similar to CRA, but are often used in the context of interventions for court-ordered drug offenders. CM is structured around two basic principles: withholding of incentives or punishment if drug use is detected, and positive reinforcers for sobriety and related positive treatment activities, such as taking medication, attending treatment sessions and, twelve-step participation. Although CM may incorporate the positive reward aspects of CRA, the threat of punishment (e.g., return to prison) due to failed drug tests is often an inherent element of the conditions for receiving the intervention (S. T. Higgins & Petry, 1999; S. Higgins et al., 2000). It has also been demonstrated that rewards alone are not as effective overall in reducing substance use or maintaining paid employment as when rewards are contingent on clean urinalysis (S. Higgins et al., 2003). CRA and CM approaches are commensurate with social work approaches, given that many of our clients are court-ordered (Rooney, 1992) and because case management is a critical element in co-ordinating and optimizing complex and interdisciplinary efforts to treat substance abuse (W. P. Sullivan, Hartmann, Dillon, & Wolk, 1994).

Exemplar Study: Combining Community Reinforcement Approach with Contingency Management.   One randomized controlled study of co-caine-addicted people recruited through newspaper advertisements compared a combined CRA and CM approach to a twelve-step counseling model based on the disease model (S. T. Higgins et al., 1993). CRA+CM comprised stimulus avoidance and community reinforcement for clean drug screens (i.e., vouchers for up to $1,000.00 of approved purchases); self-monitoring of cognitive, emotional, and situational antecedents; relationship counseling; skills training for drug refusal; problem solving; recreational counseling; AIDS-prevention counseling; and job training for drug abstinence. Fifty-eight percent of clients in the CRA+CM group remained in treatment compared with 11% of the comparison group. Forty-two percent of the CRA+CM group also received disulfiram, an important component in this approach. Sixty-eight percent maintained eight weeks of cocaine abstinence compared with 11% of the controls. Forty-two percent of the CRA+CM group achieved sixteen weeks of cocaine abstinence versus 5% for the comparison group. In a subsequent controlled study (Higgins et al., 1994), cocaine-dependent individuals were randomly assigned to CRA+CM using vouchers or CRA alone. Clients in the CRA+CM treatment showed a higher retention rate by completing the twenty-four-week treatment (75% versus 40%) and achieved a greater proportion of sobriety at five weeks (70% versus 50%), ten weeks (55% versus 15%), and twenty weeks (30% versus 5%). The CRA+CM group also demonstrated almost twice the duration (11.7 versus 6.0 weeks) of continuous cocaine abstinence as the CRA group.

CM has also been shown to have comparable success with alcohol abuse when it is added to standard treatment that includes RP and twelve-step groups. Treatment completion at eight weeks was almost four times greater for the CM group, and abstinence rates were significantly improved as well in a group of alcohol-dependent veterans (Petry, Martin, Cooney, & Kranzler, 2000). Similar CRA programs have been shown to have robust effects for opiate-addicted people (Abbott et al., 1998).

Twelve-Step Facilitation

The twelve-step model is essentially a spiritual model of recovery and mutual help. Although no scientific theory is explicitly endorsed, the twelve-step model has traditionally been associated with the disease model of alcoholism and recovery (W. R. Miller & Kurtz, 1994). The Minnesota model has become widely recognized as traditional alcoholism treatment in the United States. The traditional recovery model typically employs a multilevel approach, including initial detoxification, education about alcohol addiction and the associated psychosocial and medical consequences, the use of family and group therapy, nutrition and recreational counseling, and regular attendance at twelve-step meetings. Outpatient follow-up and continued involvement with AA (Al-Anon, Alateen for other family members) is typically emphasized (Nowinski, 1999). Similar programs have evolved, including Narcotics Anonymous, Cocaine Anonymous, Gamblers Anonymous, and the like. AA rightfully boasts tens of thousands of registered groups and two million or more members worldwide. Non–spiritually oriented recovery groups include Rational Recovery, SMART Recovery, and Moderation Management, which focuses on drinking reduction, not abstinence.

Pioneering efforts to assist alcohol-dependent people and their families were developed by the Johnson Institute (V. W. Johnson, 1973). The primary strategy, known as the intervention, involves development of a team of professionals and concerned others in the client's life, and a well-planned confrontation to persuade the alcohol-dependent person to enter treatment (Liepman, 1993). This approach is firmly embedded in the traditional disease/recovery model and incorporates concepts about resistance and denial, as well as some concepts commensurate with family systems theory, including the "codependence" of the other family members. Not only can the family wield considerable leverage to help the alcohol-dependent person come to a better understanding about their drinking and its consequences, but it can also be an important source of social support during recovery. In addition, family members often need assistance themselves in overcoming many of their "enabling" behaviors. Preparation for the intervention includes a thorough assessment of the problem, analysis of family structure and function, and selection of "team" members. Training for the actual confrontation includes psychoeducation about alcoholism and the family disease concept, an examination of members' feelings and experiences, negotiation of desired outcomes, an examination of members' willingness to follow through on their commitment to helping the drinker, and rehearsal of the confrontation. Assuming the confrontation is successful, assessment and evaluation of the situation continues, further adjustments to the family system are examined, and additional plans for recovery are pursued. The popularity of the Minnesota model is largely based on tradition and anecdotal reports, and there is limited evidence of effectiveness to be gleaned from controlled trials. Nevertheless, clinicians should be familiar with this popular model.

Some mostly uncontrolled research supports the efficacy of AA for many people (Emrick, 1993), but few studies have evaluated this approach adequately (Morgenstern, Labouvie, McCrady, Kahler, & Frey, 1997). Although most people who initiate contact with AA drop out within a few months, evidence suggests that those who progress through the steps are more likely to do well than those who drop out prematurely. Perhaps those who do well are those motivated to stick with it. In addition, clients who combine AA with another professional treatment program do better than those who do not attend AA (Emrick, 1993). AA is a free and worldwide fellowship available to any person who wishes to stop drinking and maintain sobriety. On any given day, millions of people worldwide are in attendance at an AA meeting (USDHHS, 2000). Since AA is a voluntary mutual-help group, it is not dealt with in this text as a formal intervention. It is not provided by licensed professionals and thus not subject to the same accountability standards. Nevertheless, helping clients to engage in twelve-step programs is often an essential component of effective practice, and clients should be introduced and educated about this valuable option.

Some clinician-researchers have noted the compatibility of coping skills and the self-help wisdom accrued in twelve-step programs. Morgenstern et al. (1997) demonstrated that one-hundred posttreatment AA participants showed increased self-efficacy, coping, and commitment to sobriety as a result of their affiliation in AA. These findings suggest the importance of encouraging clients to try mutual-help groups as well as the potential effectiveness of combining coping-skills interventions with mutual-help approaches. Coping-skills approaches and mutual help may have similar change processes. Clients in recovery often demonstrate self-monitoring skills when they talk about identifying "people, places, and things" and "stinkin' thinkin'," situations that increase risk for relapse.

Taking "one day at a time," putting "first things first," and complying with the exhortation of twelve-step colleagues to "take it easy" seem comparable to CBT practitioners' efforts to help the client reduce stress, set problem priorities, and strive for a healthier lifestyle. Other comparisons can be made, including the enhancement of communications and interpersonal skills that come with consistent attendance at twelve-step or similar mutual-help meetings. Going beyond rigid distinctions between "professional" and "practice wisdom" jargon can help practitioners integrate effective approaches with clients' understanding of the problems and their potential solutions.

Professionals can effectively promote the use of AA by encouraging and guiding their clients through the first few steps, but practitioners should be cautious not to confuse incongruent treatment goals (Humphreys, 1999). For example, CBT methods should be employed in conjunction with twelve-step approaches only when the common goal is abstinence, not moderation. At the very least, all practitioners should have a sound working knowledge of AA's twelve steps (1981):

1. We admitted we were powerless over alcohol—that our lives had become unmanageable.
2. Came to believe that a Power greater than ourselves could restore us to sanity.
3. Made a decision to turn our will and our lives over to the care of God as we understood Him.
4. Made a searching and fearless moral inventory of ourselves.
5. Admitted to God, to ourselves, and to another human being the exact nature of our wrongs.
6. Were entirely ready to have God remove all these defects of character.
7. Humbly asked Him to remove our shortcomings.
8. Made a list of all persons we had harmed, and became willing to make amends to them all.
9. Made direct amends to such people whenever possible, except when to do so would injure them or others.
10. Continued to take personal inventory and when we were wrong promptly admitted it.
11. Sought through prayer and meditation to improve our conscious contact with God as we understood Him, praying only for knowledge of His will for us and the power to carry that out.
12. Having had a spiritual awakening as the result of these steps, we tried to carry this message to alcoholics, and to practice these principles in all our affairs.

Person and Treatment Factors That Affect Treatment Outcomes

Because of the heterogeneity of treatment and variation in effectiveness, researchers have long wondered to what extent matching client factors with specific treatments would enhance outcomes. A major controlled comparison study

(Project Match) compared the relative effectiveness of twelve-step facilitation (TSF), motivational enhancement therapy (MET), and cognitive behavioral therapy (CBT), and identified client factors that predicted positive outcomes for one approach or another. A year after treatment, comparable results were found for the three treatment groups with slightly higher rates of abstinence reported for the TSF group. TSF showed some slight advantage for severely dependent individuals whose social networks supported drinking (Project Match Research Group, 1997; Fuller & Hiller-Sturmhofel, 1999). This link between level of client psychopathology and the need for more intensive treatments and social supports has been well-established for some time (e.g., McLellan, Luborsky, Woody, & O'Brien, 1983). On the whole, Project Match revealed relatively little new information to help guide treatment matching (USDHHS, 2000).

Other studies have shown positive correlations of client factors and treatment process with client outcomes. Some of these include client's insurance coverage or other funding constraints (Lordan, Kelley, Peters, & Siegfried, 1997), pretreatment motivation and the quality of the client-worker relationship (D. D. Simpson, Joe, Rowan-Szal, & Greener, 1997; Raytek, McCrady, Epstein, & Hirsch, 1999), the use of legal coercion and history of positive treatment experiences (Hser, Maglione, Polinsky, & Anglin, 1998), the use of CBT processes (Ogborne, Wild, Braun, & Newton-Taylor, 1998), and using a twelve-step treatment philosophy (Moos & Moos, 1998). Despite this smattering of findings, however, few definitive conclusions can be drawn regarding client and process factors and positive outcomes (Mattson et al., 1994; Saxon, Wells, Fleming, Jackson, & Calsyn, 1996).

One area of the research that has been generating positive results regarding client-treatment factors concerns the needs of women. It has long been recognized that substance-abuse treatment designed primarily for men fell short in addressing specific needs of women. Barriers to women's receiving adequate care include a lack of consideration for reproductive health, pregnancy, and child care; additional stigma for women who abuse substances; and lack of insurance coverage, (Haskett, Miller, Whitworth, & Huffman, 1992; Beckman, 1994; Schliebner, 1994; Nelson-Zlupko, Dore, Kauffman, & Kaltenbach, 1996; Carten, 1996). A recent review of the literature, which included seven randomized controlled trials, demonstrated that when specific components of women-oriented programs were included (e.g., prenatal services, child care, mental health and psychoeducational services geared to women), more women successfully completed treatment with lower rates of substance abuse and mental health problems, improved health and reduction in HIV risk (Ashley, Marsden, & Brady, 2003). Although some individual studies have shown no advantage for programs designed specifically for women (e.g., Bride, 2001), evidence in support of gender-specific interventions appears to be growing.

Although it has often been assumed that cultural congruity between treatment approaches and the clients' racial, ethnic, and cultural background would produce superior results, there is little hard evidence to date to support this view. Research suggests that practitioners need not reinvent the wheel when designing interventions for every individual ethnic group. Caetano (1993) points out, for example, that American cultural minorities have shown substantial acceptance of twelve-step programs. Another study demonstrated that, although Hispanic and non-Hispanic whites in alcohol treatment used somewhat different routes to recovery, outcomes were comparable and differences may have been largely due to income level, not cultural difference (Arroyo, Westerberg, & Tonigan, 1998). With some Hispanic families, however, one might find that family and kinship relationships are especially important, the family is reluctant to address problems in the family, family roles are culturally defined, and spirituality is important in the family (Gloria & Peregoy, 1996). Other uncontrolled evidence suggests that Asian Americans have found psychoeducational and coping-skills–oriented approaches to be acceptable, given their cultural expectations for professional advice and problem-oriented recommendations in treatment (O'Hare & Tran, 1998). Given the current state of the research, it may be reasonable for practitioners to assume that standard treatments will be acceptable to most clients, but should make efforts to adapt them to the client's or family's cultural expectations.

IMPLEMENTING AND EVALUATING THE EVIDENCE-BASED INTERVENTION PLAN

CASE STUDY: CARLA

Carla, a practicing nurse in her midthirties, had been using cocaine and drinking excessively for about six to nine months. She said she did so as a way of "dealing with my stressful job." After her divorce from a man who had a serious substance-abuse problem, she moved in with a new boyfriend, who also used drugs. One day Carla was accused of making a minor procedural error on her unit at the hospital. She became very upset and was referred by her supervisor to a social worker who did employee-assistance contract work for the hospital. The supervisor, a divorced mother of three, was sympathetic to Carla's situation, valued her work, and was willing to give her an opportunity to "to get herself together."

Carla told the social worker during the assessment that she "was depressed and having a relationship problem," and was now worried about losing her job. During a detailed evaluation over the next few weeks, Carla gradually revealed that she had been abusing alcohol and cocaine. She was snorting cocaine in the evening, having four to five "stiff" drinks per night to get to sleep, and using cocaine in the morning to energize herself for work. She was readily able to recognize and admit the "possible" role substance abuse played in her apparent depression, anxiety, problems in her relationship, and compromised attention at work. The therapist offered to continue to work with her and help her maintain her employment if Carla were willing to further explore the possible links between her substance abuse and other problems in her life.

Multidimensional/Functional Assessment: Defining Problems and Goals

Employing a multidimensional framework, the social worker, Anne, reviewed with Carla how things were going in the other areas of her life. Because Carla was primarily concerned about her job, she agreed that she had not been at "her best," but felt that much of her upset was due to her difficult relationship with her boyfriend. Upon further investigation, it became clear that her boyfriend, Terry, was involved with a group of people who were dealing cocaine. When she went home at night to her apartment, there was usually a group of "six or eight people sitting around doing lines of coke." Carla was simply expected to join in. On one recent occasion when she felt that she needed to slow down her "partying" because it was affecting her mood and job performance, she said she did not feel like using that night. Terry pulled her aside in the bedroom, pushed her down on the bed, and in a threatening tone, queried whether she wanted to be "part of things" any more. At that point, Carla felt that Terry could be potentially violent. She knew that he kept a gun in the apartment, and sometimes carried it with him when he went out on "business." She was experiencing that "here I go again" feeling with another abusive man in her life. She felt that joining in with routine cocaine use, for the time being, was the only way she could cope with the situation.

This was not the first time she had felt trapped and somewhat hopeless about her relationship. Upon further exploration, she reflected that she had always been attracted to men who were a "little dangerous," but this time it appeared that she had gotten herself in more deeply than she wanted, and was involved in illegal activities that could threaten her career. Her previous marriage was to a similar kind of guy, and although he was verbally abusive, he had never hit her, was not involved in illegal activities, and usually just got drunk and did not bother her. She thought about her parents, with whom she was not currently close, who seemed to be locked in an unhappy marriage. Her dad drank and hung out with his buddies at the local tavern. Her mom stayed home most of the time, and was usually in treatment for some kind of health-related problem that Carla felt was mostly related to anxiety. Her mom took prescribed tranquilizers, and had been getting them (without prescription) from friends as well. Although Carla said she missed her parents sometimes, she found it too depressing to go home and was afraid she would end up in a relationship like theirs. She said she wanted to have a family sometime, but did not want to be trapped in a relationship with a "loser."

Anne examined the depth of Carla's mood disturbance and found it difficult to sort out the factors related to her depression and anxiety. Since Carla had been abusing alcohol off and on for years since college, abusing cocaine (up to a gram per day) more recently, and had been unhappy in her relationships for some time, it was hard to pinpoint when the anxiety and depression began and whether it was the cause or result of the substance abuse. As a working hypothesis, the social worker suggested that the only way to find out would be to attempt some period of cutting down and, eventually, abstaining, at least for a while. Carla was concerned that she would not be able to do this.

Carla was particularly concerned about the status of her job. She was going to work on the 7:00 a.m. shift after snorting some cocaine in her car in the parking lot. She had become upset when she thought one of the doctors had seen her snorting some lines of coke off her pocket mirror. Generally, she felt pretty good for the first couple of hours on her floor, but by late morning would become exhausted and often went into the bathroom to snort some more cocaine. She had been feeling increasingly anxious about getting caught, and with this recent incident on her floor, she was becoming very anxious about losing her job.

Her health was good, and she did not have any pressing financial problems. Her boyfriend liked paying for things and "taking care of her," but she was beginning to feel that this arrangement was part of a deal, and not due to genuine caring for her.

After three or four visits, Carla begrudgingly began to agree that her drug abuse was in some way connected with her other concerns: anxiety and depression, job performance, and relationship problems. As she felt more comfortable and was more forthcoming with Anne about her problems, Carla began to see that dealing with her drug problem might help her get a handle on her life in many ways. The social worker assured Carla that she was willing to do her best to help her maintain her job (after a two-week "vacation"; that is, a leave of absence), but Carla would have to be completely forthright in her reporting of drug use and related problems.

To help Carla get a handle on the tentative links between her alcohol and cocaine use and her other symptoms, they developed a seven-day diary with which Carla would track the thoughts, feelings, and situations that stimulated her desire to use, the intensity of her desire to use, the type and quantity of substances used, and any consequences of use (fig. 6.1).

The social worker and Carla began to work immediately on developing alternative ways of coping in order to cut down and eventually eliminate her use of alcohol and other drugs. Given her history, it appeared that Carla was unlikely to experience dangerous withdrawal symptoms from her drinking. Five or six drinks (each drink probably larger than the "standard drink" of 1.5 ounces of 86-proof liquor) was a considerable amount of alcohol, but she had not been drinking that much for a long time, had never consumed more than that for any regular period of time, and never suffered from serious withdrawal symptoms. However, she would probably experience some anxiety and perhaps disrupted sleep for a while. The social worker suggested a medical consultation, but Carla knew that tranquilizers would probably be prescribed (she could get them for free if she wanted them), and (ironically, perhaps) did not want to use prescription medications since it conjured up images of becoming "like my mother": hopeless, helpless, and unable to extricate herself from a failed, unhappy relationship. Withdrawal from cocaine did not pose any physical threat either, but

FIGURE 6.1   Diary for substance use

	Monday	Tuesday	Wednesday	Thursday	Friday	Saturday	Sunday
Thoughts, feelings, situations							
Amount of coke used							
Number of drinks							
Consequences of use							

Anne noted that Carla would likely feel even more depressed for a time, and Anne let Carla know that she could call her once a day at an agreed-upon time if she needed to talk. A psychiatric consultation was arranged for possible prescription of antidepressants.

After using the diary for a couple of weeks while she began to cut down on her alcohol and drug use, Carla began to see for herself the day-to-day links among her depressed mood, negative outlook, edginess, poor quality of sleep, and drug abuse. Whereas she would normally fall asleep after two or three drinks, the cocaine would stimulate her and keep her awake in the evening and, thus drinking more than she normally would. To get up in the morning, she would use or want to use more cocaine. She felt depressed and anxious beginning her day like this, and since she had not been working for a couple of weeks, did not really know what to do with herself. She became more despondent thinking about feeling trapped in what was becoming apparent to her—a dead-end relationship with someone who really didn't care about her. She was feeling exploited. Her mood worsened during the day, but as she and her therapist agreed, she would leave the apartment for a while every day, and find constructive things to do: errands she had neglected such as taking care of her dry cleaning, getting her hair done, scheduling her car maintenance, or going to the dentist.

Her boyfriend became suspicious about her not working, and he began to query her about what she was telling her social worker. Since Terry was involved in dealing cocaine, he became angry when he realized Carla had been talking about him, felt betrayed that she did not want to live this lifestyle anymore, and became belligerent. He smacked her hard across the face, making her nose bleed profusely. She became angry and, after he went out, packed her belongings and left the apartment. She was somewhat afraid that he would come after her, but afterward mostly felt depressed about her circumstances and a little panicked. She decided to look up her old friend, Tara, whom she had been neglecting, and to stay with her for a few days to get reacquainted. Her friend agreed and told Carla that she had noticed changes in her over the past year or so, and had been worried about her. She invited Carla to stay with her a while, and meet some of her other women friends.

During this time, Carla (more or less) kept up with her diary and noticed that, despite her decrease in drinking (and lack of cocaine use in the past three days), she felt depressed and was crying a lot. Tara called the social worker, and told her that Carla had expressed some desire to "end it all," but that she did not feel there was any imminent danger. Tara accompanied Carla to her next session which included further assessment of her depression. Carla's drinking had been reduced to one or two per day ("to take the edge off at night"), but her cocaine use had been eliminated. Anne and Tara agreed, however, that if Carla moved back in with her boyfriend (who had located her by calling friends of Carla's at work), she would probably begin to use again. The substance abuse appeared to be somewhat contextually dependent, linked closely to her involvement with her drug-abusing boyfriend. Although Carla was depressed about her relationship (or unhappy about it ending, she wasn't sure which), the depression was exacerbated significantly by withdrawal from her daily gram of cocaine. She was sleeping more and feeling little energy during the day. Nevertheless, she forced herself to go out and do something, or at least help out around her friend's apartment. Carla was now convinced about the linkages among her drug use, negative mood, relationship problems, and dissatisfaction with her life. She and her social worker both agreed that, she needed first, to remain sober and drug-free, and then to make decisions about her relationship and how she would extricate herself from it. She also needed to meet with her supervisor and discuss her progress and a timetable for returning to work. Carla agreed that she should establish a goal of abstaining completely from illicit drug use, but was less sure about abstinence from alcohol at this point.

Selecting and Designing the Intervention: Defining Strategies and Objectives

As the assessment period blended into the beginning stages of intervention, it became apparent that a solid working alliance had been developed. Anne had employed good motivational enhancement methods to help Carla examine the role of drugs as a factor in her presenting problems and test out her own commitment to change. She had, in four weeks, moved from being rather ambivalent (the contemplation stage) about whether substance abuse played a role in her difficulties to feeling that she had proven the links between her problems and drugs to herself, and she was now prepared to take action. As she gradually began to sleep better and feel more optimistic about getting her job back on track, she moved into a more self-motivated, action-oriented stage of change.

Her social worker now began to introduce coping-skills methods in a more formal way (table 6.1). After her psychiatric consultation and decision to begin a trial of antidepressants, Carla's energy gradually began to improve, and she returned to work. She was still staying with Tara, felt she was becoming an imposition, but did not want to go back to her boyfriend's apartment. Since she had taken most of her things when she packed and left, she did not want to go back and recover the few things that she had left behind.

She and Anne focused on improving her day-to-day coping skills. First, her negative thinking about ever having a good relationship was addressed. A brief history-taking revealed that she previously did have a good relationship with a man, but she had decided to leave him for the person who became her husband. She recalled that she had wanted someone "stronger," but as this was examined further, it appeared that her boyfriend simply wanted to control the relationship. The more they examined her cognitive schema around "caring," the more it became apparent that Carla equated "caring" with "control." As a result, she engaged in relationships with men who were more likely to tell her what to do, and they become angry when she didn't comply. Anne noted that, early on, Carla also expected much direction from the social worker as well.

As a result of reviewing her diary for a few weeks, they both agreed that there were a number of specific high-risk thoughts, feelings, and situational triggers that Carla would have to watch out for if she was going to maintain long-term sobriety, maintain good job performance, and develop healthier relationships. These included some exaggerated negative expectations of relationships (I'll *never* find someone who will love me, I'll *never* have a family, I'll *never* feel good about myself), lack of confidence in herself on the job, and doubts about her ability to feel ok about living by herself for a while without jumping into a relationship with someone or making a sudden commitment to live with them. In response to these thoughts, Carla worked on labeling them as "old thinking" and countering them with more optimistic and realistic alternatives; for example, "I am attractive and I am a good person to be with, but I must use better judgment and get to know the person I want to be with. I will do well at work if I stay clean and sober, and if I take work one day at a time. When I am depressed about what is going on or scared of what lies ahead, these feelings will pass. In the meantime, I can talk to people, and find other ways to enjoy my life as I work on making things better. I know that all of this will not be easy, it will take hard work and patience, but I know that there are people who can help me."

Occasionally when Carla felt cravings to buy cocaine or have a drink, she distracted herself with television, read, called a friend, took a walk, or engaged in some other constructive activity. She drank some wine now and then, but had not consumed more than two drinks on any given occasion. She discussed this with her social worker and her psychiatrist, who both advised against it, at least for now. She felt that knowing she might be able to have a glass of wine or two in the future made her feel better by not having to commit herself, at this point, to lifetime abstinence. The social worker agreed that she was making great progress, but that she should be careful right now about tripping herself up. She agreed to put off social drinking for a while. In social situations, she also had the opportunity to successfully turn down offers of drinks, and she felt that she could manage this challenge for now. Sometimes she would dwell on regrets and guilt about lost opportunities or the time she had spent in bad relationships. Sometimes she felt that she would like to have been a better daughter and, perhaps, to have visited her parents more often. She discussed these feelings with her social worker, who pointed out that she seems to take on a disproportionate amount of the responsibility in relationships, and blames herself when things don't go well. Anne and Carla discussed various scenarios with her boyfriend and parents, and role-played alternative ways that Carla might deal with others when they are laying blame on her.

After a couple of months, it became apparent that Carla was doing much better at work, sleeping better, and coping adequately living alone, although this was distressing for her at times and she missed being in a romantic relationship. She was, however, coming home and feeling alone and stressed, and began to think about drinking excessively again, or even getting back together with her old boyfriend to patch things up. She was feeling vulnerable. She and Anne discussed this, and carefully reviewed what had led up to her crisis a couple of months ago, and where she was now. Carla decided to stay the course, but felt she needed to do more in her life right now to keep it from going "backwards." She joined an exercise group, and began to meet different people who had interests other than drinking and drug use. Carla did not have much experience with regular exercise such as biking, aerobics, or jogging. She fell in with a "beginner" group, and started meeting people that she felt pretty comfortable with. In collaboration with her social worker, she developed her own daily coping strategies by continuing to reflect upon her self-monitoring chart daily (it appealed to her familiarity with nursing protocol and her sense of "healing thyself"), used meditation to counter some of her fears and replace them with more constructive and goal-oriented thinking, and used relaxation (stretching) exercises that she learned in her workout group to relieve tension. Ann encouraged her to continue with her exercise and new social group because it could help her deal with the physiological stressors that she often interpreted as fear and depression, and helped her get involved with people who had more constructive and healthful lifestyles. She began to increase the amount of time between visits to the social worker. Together they developed a plan where Carla would develop goals in her personal and work life and report back periodically (every month, then three months) to see how she was doing.

The social worker regularly conferred with the nursing supervisor, and without going into too much detail (to respect the client's privacy, although all informed-consent procedures were in order), she informed her that Carla was making good progress. Given the possibility of relapse, they all agreed that the contingency management plan should remain in place. The terms were not written down, but were discussed with Carla: as long as her performance remained acceptable and there was no further evidence of drug relapse, her job was secure. Carla expressed relief in knowing that she was valued by her supervisor, and felt a sense of comfort knowing that she had a very compelling incentive to continue to take care of herself, and to watch out for situations where she might become vulnerable and slip.

Selecting Scales and Creating Indexes to Monitor and Evaluate Client Progress

The AUDIT and the DAST-10 both served as excellent screening tools during the preliminary assessment (table 6.1). In addition, the AUDIT provided a baseline assessment and was repeated periodically (every three months) to measure changes. The instructions were modified from "past year" to "the last 3 months." In addition, individual indexes were employed to help Carla measure the frequency or intensity of key triggers. These included level of depression, anxiety, or simply the urge to use. The ASI was used to provide baseline and outcome measures across multiple domains of well-being.

SUMMARY

Substance abuse and addiction present complex challenges across all social work fields of practice. These problems vary by types of substances used, range of co-occurring problems and consequences, and a host of person factors that affect the client's response to intervention. Effective substance-abuse interventions represent an array of supportive, coping-skills and case management interventions that can be employed as specific strategies, as complete "treatment packages," or in eclectic combinations. A sound working relationship is essential, as process research substantiates, and clients are more forthcoming and better engaged if practitioners emphasize motivational enhancement, accommodate the client's readiness to change, and exercise flexibility in methods and treatment goals. Even with court-ordered clients, some flexibility can be exercised within the context of mandated treatment. Coping-skills efforts have been demonstrated repeatedly to be effective for clients who want to reduce the harm of substance abuse through moderation or abstinence. Delivering effective behavioral couples and family work or providing services to court-ordered clients requires the skillful implementation of key effective elements including disulfiram and behavioral contracts, problem-solving and communication skills, and coping-skills and contingency management techniques to reduce substance use and improve interpersonal and social functioning at home and in the community. Coordination of multiple services through case management is often essential in substance-abuse treatment, and may include active facilitation of the client's involvement in mutual support groups such as Alcoholics Anonymous.

TABLE 6.1   The Client Service Plan for Carla

Problems	Goals	Sample Objectives	Interventions	Assessment Tools
Daily abuse of alcohol (8–10 oz. of liquor) and about 1 gram of cocaine of fairly high purity	Reduce her use and abuse of alcohol and other drugs; eliminate cocaine use permanently; abstain from alcohol for the time she is in treatment; revisit this goal on termination	Engage in daily self-monitoring: record thoughts, feelings, situations related to substance use, exact amounts of substances used, consequences of use	Motivational enhancement therapy to begin the engagement process and help client "own" her intervention goals and methods	AUDIT and DAST-10 as initial screens
				Daily self-monitoring chart to record triggers and level of substance use; rate intensity of triggers on self-anchored scale (1–10)
			Coping-skills interventions tailored to her specific needs: self-monitoring skills (daily charting); cognitive reappraisal of her dysfunctional thinking regarding her own worth and expectations in relationships, and her negative view of the future; daily alternative ways of coping with depression, anxiety, and urges to drink or use drugs; tension-reducing healthful exercises alone and with others	
Depression symptoms: negative view of self as hopeless in relationships and failing at work; guilt, remorse, lack of self-confidence; sleep disturbance	Alleviate depressive symptoms: improve self-image and negative view of herself in relationships; build self-confidence by accomplishing her treatment goals; improve sleep through improved health habits	Identify and provide counterargument to daily negative thoughts about herself, her value in a relationship or as an employee; challenge her negative outlook for the future		Recommended: weekly use of the Inventory of Drinking Situations (modify for both alcohol and drugs) or the Situational Confidence Questionnaire
				AUDIT to track alcohol use every 3 months
Anxiety symptoms: worried about losing job, concerned about getting caught with drugs; muscle tension, nervousness, sleeplessness	Similar to above: alleviate anxiety symptoms through abstinence and improved health habits	Engage in daily reflection on her chart combined with 10 minutes of meditation on positive planning and stretching/relaxation exercises to reduce tension		ASI as a multidimensional measure for assessment and evaluation
			Later, focus these self-monitoring and lifestyle changes on relapse prevention when she feels discouraged again	
Poor relationship with abusive boyfriend; relationship lacks intimacy, based on common interest in drug use	Improve her judgment in partner selection and social supports	Reach out to healthful social supports: friend and acquaintances in social support/health activities group; initiate a conversation with one of them daily	Contingency management: progress linked to job performance through liaison and consultation with her supervisor	
Work performance suffering: client "on probation" informally; will be closely evaluated on return	Achieve and maintain satisfactory work performance	Keep in touch with supervisor; after returning to work, meet with her weekly to review her performance on the job	Social supports enhanced through continued contact with health activities group	
			Medication consultation with psychiatrist to monitor use of antidepressant medication	

CHAPTER 7

PANIC DISORDER WITH AGORAPHOBIA AND OBSESSIVE-COMPULSIVE DISORDER

Anxiety disorders cover a wide array of disabling conditions that may be accompanied by dreadful and terrifying thoughts, uncontrollable physiological symptoms, and avoidance behavior. Although diagnoses depict anxiety disorders as discrete syndromes, different anxiety disorders share many symptoms. In addition, over time a client may experience signs and symptoms related to more than one anxiety disorder. So, for example, a person who experienced specific phobias as a child and suffered from long-standing generalized anxiety may, at other points in life, also experience problems with obsessional thinking or panic attacks with avoidance of important activities such as driving, flying, or going out in public. To fully appreciate the suffering of a person with a serious anxiety disorder, it is necessary to go beyond diagnosis, and understand how the anxiety-related thoughts, feelings, and behaviors vary over time and across situations, and how these debilitating conditions can affect other areas of people's lives.

Decades of extensive clinical research has confirmed that CBT has become a first-line treatment for anxiety disorders in general and for panic with agoraphobia and obsessive-compulsive disorder (OCD), specifically. These interventions include developing a sound working alliance with the client, challenging dysfunctional thinking regarding the perceived threat, teaching physiological coping mechanisms to mitigate anxiety and counter feelings of losing control, and engaging in graduated, frequent, and prolonged exposure to the feared thoughts or situations. Over time this process has a high likelihood of helping the client gain a sense of mastery over anxiety and improving general psychosocial well-being. Case management skills are also invaluable in coordination of care and engendering social supports to aid the client.

ASSESSMENT OF PANIC DISORDER WITH AGORAPHOBIA

Background Data

A considerable amount of research has provided understanding of debilitating anxiety (DSM-IV-TR; Antony & Swinson, 2000; Barlow, 1997; Craske, 1999). Panic

146

attacks are marked by feelings of overwhelming fear accompanied by very distressing physiological symptoms, including racing heartbeat, shortness of breath, dizziness, and nausea. Panic disorder often makes people avoid situations where they believe panic attacks are more likely to occur, such as supermarkets, driving, and other public places. The disorder may begin with a panic attack in a stressful or relatively arbitrary situation; people gradually avoid more and more situations where they feel vulnerable to another attack. In the extreme case, they may become virtually immobilized and homebound.

Experts have described three types of panic attacks: (1) unexpected, (2) responsive to specific situations, and (3) situationally predisposed. In the last type, a person may experience panic associated with the situation, but the connection is not predictable. Cues relevant to the attack can be internal (e.g., physical symptoms or frightening thoughts) or external (e.g., being on a bus, in an elevator, in a grocery store). The frequency and severity of panic attacks vary widely, but the associated fears can be quite persistent, despite much reassurance. Fears about the next attack often lead to avoidance behaviors, as in agoraphobia. People with panic disorder may be generally anxious about other matters, including health, work, finances, and life changes such as separations and sudden losses. Panic disorder may be associated with depression or substance abuse and may co-occur with other anxiety disorders.

Agoraphobia can exist without panic disorder, but they co-occur in about 95% of cases.

> The essential feature of agoraphobia is anxiety about being in places or situations from which escape might be difficult (or embarrassing), or in which help may not be available in the event of having a panic attack or panic-like symptoms. The anxiety typically leads to a pervasive avoidance of a variety of situations that may include being alone outside the home or being home alone, being in a crowd of people, traveling in an automobile, bus or airplane, or being on a bridge or in an elevator. (*DSM-IV-TR*, p. 432)

Lifetime prevalence of panic disorder is estimated to be between 1% and 2%, although some estimates have been higher (3.5%; see Kessler et al., 1994; Antony & Swinson, 2000; Craske, 1999), and prevalence of agoraphobia has been estimated at 6.7% (Magee, Eaton, Wittchen, McGonagle, & Kessler, 1996). Onset for panic disorder may be bimodally distributed, with peaks in the late teens and early thirties. Panic disorder seems to be somewhat chronic, with some waxing and waning (*DSM-IV-TR*). The relationship of agoraphobic symptoms to panic attacks is also variable, with some predictable development of symptoms following panic attacks, but in other cases, agoraphobia may persist despite a lessening of attacks (possibly due to clients' avoiding specific situations, however).

Onset of panic disorder may be associated with periods of stress. Stressful life events such as unemployment, divorce, deaths, and positive events such as weddings, births, and graduations may increase the likelihood of onset (Antony & Swinson, 2000; Barlow, 1988). Women appear more likely to be diagnosed with panic disorder and are more likely to develop agoraphobia and require companions to accompany them in public. When researchers examined the assumption that men are more likely to exercise greater bravado when approaching fear-inducing situations, one recent gender comparison found no differences in men and women in the amount of courage or coping self-efficacy displayed when dealing with phobic avoidance (N. B. Schmidt & Koselka, 2000). People with histories of childhood separation anxiety, first-degree relatives with anxiety disorders, and medical illness are more likely to have panic disorder.

Fokias and Tyler (1995) addressed an often overlooked factor that appears to play a compelling role in the development and maintenance of agoraphobia: the quality of social support as a buffer against environmental stressors. They argued that a conceptualization of social support should include the perception of support, a range of different types of support covering a range of situations and activities, degree of satisfaction with these supports, and the identification of a confidante within the social support network. They suggested that reviews of research showed consistent correlation between the absence of social support and level of psychological distress. The marital relationship may also constitute an important factor in the etiology, maintenance, or successful intervention with agoraphobia, although their review showed conflicting evidence in this regard. Situational stressors may not be the primary cause of debilitating anxiety but can exacerbate an existing anxiety disorder and can be mediated (for better or for worse) by the quality of available social supports.

Prevalence appears to be relatively similar across racial and ethnic groups (Antony & Swinson, 2000; E. Horvath & Weissman, 1997). However, there do appear to be some differences in the meaning of anxiety (Guarnaccia, 1997). For example, *ataques de nervios* in some Latino communities seem to include behaviors such as screaming uncontrollably or having attacks of crying. Although this concept in similar to panic attack as defined in the *DSM-IV*, it also appears to be associated with a specific upsetting event, and there may not be the signature dread of future panic attacks. *Ataques de nervios* may also be associated with affective disorders, anger, loss of impulse control, and possible dissociative features. Other symptoms may include verbal or physical aggression and suicidal gestures—a general feature of being out of control (*DSM-IV-TR*). Caution and a familiarity with cultural norms are important when interpreting or judging the clinical relevance of some culturally based ritualistic behaviors.

Hispanic Americans are less likely to access mental health services, because of cultural and language barriers (M. Friedman, 1997). Some feel great stigma associated with being perceived as "loco." Those with a higher level of acculturation are more likely to use mental health services. Some Hispanic Americans seek help though normal medical and social service channels; others may seek assistance through indigenous healers in their community (*curanderas*). Overall, Hispanic Americans tend to be less informed about American mainstream views of mental health problems and available services. Ultimately, however, outcomes for treatment of panic disorder with agoraphobia show little variation by gender or culture (Steketee & Shapiro, 1995).

People with anxiety disorders, including panic disorder and agoraphobia, appear to have higher than usual rates of alcohol abuse and dependence (Bibb & Chambless, 1986; Kessler et al., 1996), although no clear causal direction has been established. People with serious alcohol-abuse problems are likely to experience more anxiety-related symptoms from withdrawal as well as the psychosocial stressors caused by drinking (e.g., legal and occupational problems, marital difficulties, medical concerns), and conversely people with anxiety disorders may be more likely to use alcohol as a coping mechanism to dampen the effects of anxiety (Sher, 1987). The link between panic with agoraphobia and alcohol abuse suggests that improvement in one problem can improve treatment outcomes in the other (C. Lehmen, Brown, & Barlow, 1998). Panic attacks also co-occur with other disorders, including OCD and major depressive disorders (Steketee, Chambless, & Tran, 2001; M. Fava et al., 2000). Assessment of other problems is important because evidence suggests that co-occurring problems such as major depression can have a direct negative effect on outcomes with otherwise effective interventions (Steketee et al.).

Theories

A range of theories have been offered to explain the development of debilitating anxiety including panic disorder. Historically, the two most prominent theories evolved from early psychoanalytic explanations such as abandonment fears and early classical and operant conditioning theories such as generalization of a frightening experience. Contemporary scientific theories tend to look at a complex and reciprocal interplay of inherited temperament, developmental learning experiences (e.g., innate inhibitions having been reinforced or challenged), the persistence of anxiety-driven cognitive schemata, misinterpretation of physiological cues, and behavioral avoidance in part related to specific sociocontextual or other situational factors.

Biological inheritance appears to play a role in enduring traits such as hyperarousal, neuroticism, chronic worrying, and shyness, and may predispose some people to anxiety disorders including panic disorder (e.g., Kagan, 1997). Although the inborn propensity for nervousness may provide a foundation for many of the anxiety disorders, development of more specific anxiety disorders, such as social anxiety and OCD, is likely to be shaped by a host of other learning experiences that are responsive to interpersonal and other situational factors (Craske, 1999; see also Barlow, 1988; Zinbarg, Barlow, Brown, & Hertz, 1992). Barlow (1997), for example, conceptualizes this biobehavioral link as the genesis of panic disorder. Occurring within the context of life stressors, the initial panic attack acts as a possible "false alarm" because it happens at an inappropriate, coincidental, or unnecessary time rather than at a time of actual mortal danger.

This false alarm may become associated with internal bodily cues (e.g., rapid heart rate, dizziness), leading to additional learned panic responses. The possible reexperiencing of that initial panic may become a source of genuine dread. Some people begin to avoid situations that they feel with trigger another false alarm, and by reinforcing their anticipatory anxiety, they become increasingly agoraphobic.

There is little reason to believe, however, in a simple relationship between biological tendency and the development of an anxiety disorder (Barlow, 1988). Cognitive appraisal and interpretation (in other words, perceptions, attributions, and expectancies) give meaning to events and interact with anxious feelings. Cognitive theories emphasize the role of dysfunctional attributions or appraisals via automatic thoughts rooted in negative schemata and information-processing errors (Beck, 1976, 1996). Beck and associates see cognitive, emotional, behavioral, and physiological dimensions of behavior as interactive, and understand biological processes as essentially innate. Cognition is the primary activating agent, however, in that the appraisal of threat gives it meaning and subsequently determines, to some extent, the type and severity of physiological response. In the anxious person, the cognitive schema is defined by an overvigilant expectation of risk or danger, and these distortions extend through a person's view of herself, the world, and the future. Thus anxiety-tinged automatic thoughts will precipitate anxious responses through physiological arousal and avoidant behavior. Cognitive models (see Beck, 1976, 1996; Bandura, 1986) emphasize beliefs centered around danger (danger schemata), which

> serve as pre-dispositional cognitions, leading to processing of information about the world, self and future in a framework of automatic thoughts and images of danger. Danger-related schemata contrast with negative self-evaluation and schemata related to loss, a cognitive style typical of depressed mood. Schemata are posited to cause preferential encoding of threatening, or schema-congruent, information that produces cognitive biases, which in turn are responsible for initiating an anxious state. (Beck & Emery, 1985, p.64)

Other researchers stress the interaction of cognitive, physiological, behavioral, and situational factors. Craske (1999) points out that parental behavior can contribute to the development and shaping of specific anxiety problems by sending out excessive danger signals to a child, but it is not clear whether parents are primarily causing the anxiety or merely responding to an already anxious child. Genetic predisposition to anxiety is probably nonspecific, and is likely to be mediated by environmental experiences (Craske, 1999; Barlow, 1988), including appraisal of stressors as determined by cognitive schemata, and the ability of the person to cope with those stressors (R. S. Lazarus & Folkman, 1984; Holahan & Moos, 1994; Beck & Emery, 1985; Bandura, 1986). Stressful life events can shape the development of anxiety disorders as well as precipitate relapse. These effects may vary by the type, frequency, and severity of the event; other circumstantial and interpersonal factors; and degree of controllability, among other variables. Although what constitutes stress is certainly subject to one's unique appraisal, stressful conditions associated with lower socioeconomic status have been shown to predict higher rates of panic disorder (Kohn et al., 1998; Kessler et al., 1994). It should come as no surprise that poverty, homelessness, and exposure to violence, among other serious stressors, should provide fertile ground for being on alert and at risk for developing panic disorder.

Given the combined risk factors of temperament, stressful environmental factors, compromised coping skills, and limited social supports, acute stressors are likely to be appraised as uncontrollable and unpredictable, resulting in subsequent dread and avoidance of these seemingly related events. The focus of fear may narrow to a certain thought, feeling, or circumstance, and the resulting anxiety may increase in intensity and generalize to other areas of the person's life (Barlow, 1988, 1997; Craske, 1999). One can easily imagine how the confluence of these risk factors could increasingly immobilize an anxious person. For example, an innately "nervous" girl grows up in an uncertain, unsupportive, unpredictable environment, struggles with shyness and low self-confidence throughout adolescence, and is thrust suddenly into the challenges of adulthood as a single parent. She experiences an initial panic attack while waiting in line in a grocery store, trying to finish the shopping with not enough in her checkbook, knowing that she will be late for the third time this week to pick up her daughter from day care. She is afraid she will again be asked to remove her daughter after she has once again adjusted to a new set of friends and caretakers. With racing heartbeat, feeling as though she is about to faint, she rushes to the day-care center, almost has an accident along the way, and is told at the center that she can no longer bring her daughter. She seats her daughter in the car and has her first full-blown panic attack. This episode of feeling as though one has almost "lost one's mind" can launch a period of incapacitating dread as the client faces each new day uncertain when these feelings will return and whether she will be able to cope sufficiently to survive the day. It appears that the etiology and development of panic disorder is a complex interplay of biological predisposition, developmental learning experiences, life circumstances, and environmental stressors, with the development of panic disorder hinging on the psychological interpretation of these interacting internal and external stimuli.

Key Elements of Multidimensional/ Functional Assessment

DSM-IV-TR diagnosis of panic disorder and agoraphobia has been well researched, and is considered reasonably reliable and valid. To meet the diagnostic criteria, the client must experience recurrent unexpected panic attacks. Symptoms of panic attack may be one of more of the following: pounding heartbeat or accelerated heart rate, sweating, trembling or shaking, shortness of breath, feelings of smothering, a choking sensation, chest pain, nausea, feeling faint or experiencing feelings of unreality or depersonalization. The client may also experience an intense fear of losing control, "losing my mind," or "going crazy," a fear of dying, paresthesia (numbness or tingling sensations), and either chills or hot flushes. At least one of the attacks must have been followed by at least one month of one (or more) of the following: the client has persistent concerns about having another panic attack or the consequences of having another attack (i.e., anticipatory dread), or demonstrates a significant change in behavior related to the attacks. To meet the full diagnosis, the client must experience agoraphobia as indicated by anxiety about being in places or situations from which escape might be difficult (or embarrassing), or in which help may not be available in the event of having a panic attack. Clients avoid situations that may trigger an attack; if they do not limit their movements, they endure the experience with marked distress about having a panic attack, or require a companion. Agoraphobic fears are usually related to being alone in situations outside the home, such as being in a crowd, standing in a line, being stuck in traffic on a bridge, or traveling in a bus, train, airplane, or automobile.

As outlined above, *DSM-IV-TR* provides a well-researched list of symptoms associated with panic disorder with agoraphobia. The multidimensional assessment should include a careful review of these problems with analysis of the frequency, severity, and duration of the symptoms. However, these signs and symptoms need to be understood within the broader context of the client's psychosocial well-being. Many people struggle on their own with anxiety disorders, may not be aware of what is happening to them, and do not bring their concerns to the attention of professionals until a crisis such as a suicide attempt, "nervous breakdown," or false heart attack has occurred.

This assessment should include other aspects of the client's mental status and co-occurring problems, including depression and any suicidal thoughts, impulsive behaviors, and substance abuse. A routine health screening is also important, given the significant rates of co-occurrence between anxiety disorders and other health-related problems. Further health assessment should be conducted by a physician. A thoughtful examination of important relationships is crucial, because important people in the client's life may be exerting stress on the client and exacerbating the anxiety, or preventing the person from getting and benefiting from psychosocial interventions. For example, a young woman with a history of trouble with anxiety may be trapped in an abusive relationship, perhaps living day-to-day with the realistic fear of being physically assaulted. She may be exerting much of her energy just getting through the day and protecting her children, and may be too frightened to go for help. Substance abuse may be a readily available coping mechanism for dealing with her fears. The existence of other co-occurring problems such as depression, serious interpersonal conflicts, traumatic events, changes, losses, or other stressful changes (e.g., marriage, relocation) should be examined carefully as precipitants or as factors that exacerbate the existing condition. A thorough history can provide clues regarding when the problems with severe anxiety began, including panic attacks or agoraphobic behavior, and what circumstances may have precipitated the attack.

A careful analysis of clients' living circumstances, safety of their environment, working conditions, and financial well-being is essential. Any or all of these common life stressors—being evicted, losing one's job, a child's heath crisis, or violence and other crimes in the neighborhood—can increase the client's day-to-day anxiety. In brief, *no potential sources of acute or chronic stressors should be overlooked.* Although the causes of panic and agoraphobia are mixed and not always clearly linked to situational factors, daily stressors in clients' lives can make their struggle much more difficult and become a barrier to successful coping with panic and related avoidance behaviors. Practitioners should also carefully consider the cultural significance of the client's beliefs or fears.

An accurate functional assessment is essential to helping the client implement coping skills as part of the intervention. Practitioners should focus on the specifics of clients' thoughts, feelings, behaviors, and circumstances and work with them to describe a detailed patterning and sequencing of these various manifestations of anxiety and related problems. Practitioners should also examine the day-to-day impact of other related situational stressors such as marital and family problems, substance abuse, community stressors such as poverty, safety, and other social factors that may be exacerbating the problem. Panic attacks can be measured in a number of ways. Most clients are terrified of any attacks, but practitioners should teach clients to measure at least the frequency of occurrence, intensity on a self-anchored scale (0–10), and duration in minutes. It is also important for clients to note what the circumstances were at the time, what they were thinking and feeling, what they did in response, and other factors that may have made the situation more stressful (or less stressful, should they initiate their own coping responses). Asking clients to collect this data in a seven- or fourteen-day diary gets them quickly involved in their own treatment, and can provide some sense of clinical perspective and control over the problem. This functional analysis also provides rich clues and useful benchmarks to help develop the intervention plan. In addition to the face-to-face examination, practitioners could enhance the assessment by acquiring the observations and insights of significant others who may accompany the client, if possible. Antony and Swinson (2000) suggest capturing data on these key points:

development and course of the problem

impact on functioning

pattern of physical symptoms

cognitive factors such as general beliefs, expectancies, dysfunctional thinking, and cognitive biases

focus of apprehension (internal versus external)

patterns of overt avoidance as well as subtle avoidance strategies such as distraction, overprotective behaviors, or safety signals

variables affecting fear

family factors and social supports, such as family history of the problem, family accommodation, and potential for family and friends to help with treatment

treatment history

skills deficits in communication skills, driving, and so on

medical history and physical limitations

In addition to identifying the characteristics of panic symptoms and avoidance, the practitioner and the client should collaborate on development of a list of situations from least fear-inducing to most fear-inducing and a graduated hierarchy for gradually confronting each fear. For example, a client may be afraid of a number of situations (in ascending order) such as going outside the house, driving, being in a crowd, and standing in line in a grocery store. Although the first two problems may be more manageable and may be dealt with directly through graduated daily practice, a more challenging problem such as going into a grocery story and patiently standing on line may have to be broken into smaller steps as part of a thorough assessment (e.g., driving to the store; going inside; spending two, five, ten, then (eventually) twenty minutes shopping; standing on line; and checking out). Since it is unlikely that a seriously agoraphobic person who has not shopped in years is likely to accomplish this in one session, breaking the process into increasingly challenging smaller steps (i.e., an ascending hierarchy of objectives) provides a clear plan where the client can gain control gradually instead of feeling pressured to accomplish the final goal at once. The details of developing such a hierarchy are key to developing a good functional assessment, because during the discussion of each step, clients provide important clues about symptoms, specific frightening thoughts, and likely behavioral responses that can be discussed early on. This information can help the practitioner and client anticipate problems and tailor the intervention to obtain maximum effect. The Subjective Units of Distress Scale (SUDS), a self-anchored 0–10 anxiety scale developed as an assessment tool for systematic desensitization (Wolpe, 1973), can be used to help clients gauge their anxiety level during the development of the hierarchy. It also provides a baseline by which clients can judge their progress when they implement in vivo exposure. The SUDS is a useful tool that can be employed with other anxiety disorders, or any problem where overcoming anxiety is a key component to achieving therapeutic goals. The details of developing a graduated hierarchy will be examined more thoroughly following, when effective intervention for panic disorder with agoraphobia is described.

Instruments

Although a detailed functional assessment of the frequency, severity, and duration of panic symptoms and the circumstances of avoidance behavior provide important measurable benchmarks for assessment and evaluation, standardized scales are an important adjunct to the overall assessment process. A number of scales are available for measuring panic symptoms and agoraphobic avoidance. The Panic Attack Symptoms Questionnaire (PASQ) measures the duration of autonomic symptoms associated with panic. The Panic Attack Cognitions Questionnaire (PACQ), a companion scale, measures how thoroughly catastrophic cognitions dominate a client's thinking (Clum, Broyles, Borden, & Watkins, 1990).

Clum et al. (1990) examined ninety-three individuals (ages 18–57; thirty males) with various anxiety diagnoses. In addition to the PASQ and PACQ, clients completed well-established measures of general anxiety and depression. Items from the PACQ were generated from *DSM-III* criteria as well as items from client input and other scales. Each item is rated on a four-point scale (1 = not at all, 4 = totally dominated) indicating the degree of preoccupation with each cognition during a panic attack. The subject rates the severity of the thought before, during, and after an anxiety episode. Scores are summed across individual items. Those who experienced panic attacks scored higher on eight of twenty-five items on the scale. Internal consistency for the PACQ was .88. PASQ items were generated from *DSM-III* descriptors of panic symptoms, from interviews with clients, and from another standardized scale. Each item is rated on a six-point scale indicating duration of symptoms ranging from 1 (do not experience this) to 6 (protracted period from twenty-four hours to two days or more). Results of the analysis indicated that all eighteen items of the PASQ significantly differentiated people who had a diagnosis of panic disorder. Internal consistency for the PASQ was .88. The PASQ appears to be a more accurate measure of panic attacks than the PACQ.

Although the PASQ and the PACQ are both well-regarded scales, the Agoraphobia Scale (Ost, 1990) is recommended here for practical reasons. With only twenty items, it measures two primary symptoms of agoraphobia: fear and avoidance (instrument 7.1). The patient rates a variety of situations for anxiety and avoidance after reading brief descriptions of potential fear- and avoidance-inducing inducing situations, and rates each item from 0, no anxiety whatsoever, to 4, very much anxiety. The same situations are then rated for avoidance: 0 = do not avoid at all; 1 = avoid if possible; 2 = always avoid. Two samples of agoraphobic and community clients were obtained to validate the instrument along with *DSM* diagnosis, other validated agoraphobic questionnaires, results from behavioral tests (i.e., the percentage of hierarchically ordered anxiety-provoking tasks completed), and other standardized measures of anxiety and depression. Results of the analysis showed the Agoraphobia Scale to have high internal consistency (.87 for the anxiety subscale, .89 for the avoidance subscale). It significantly correlated with other agoraphobia scales, but discriminated from other general psychopathology scales, including the Beck Depression Inventory and the Hamilton Anxiety Scale. In addition, both the anxiety and avoidance subscales predicted the client's degree of avoidance based on the behavioral-avoidance test. Both subscales also showed good sensitivity to client change during treatment.

An evidence-based assessment of a client with panic disorder with agoraphobia combines the best of an MDF qualitative analysis with simple indexes and standardized scales. These complementary approaches will provide the

INSTRUMENT 7.1   Agoraphobia Scale

Anxiety level: 0 = no anxiety whatsoever, 1 = a little, 2 = moderate, 3 = much,
4 = very much anxiety
Avoidance: 0 = do not avoid at all, 1 = avoid if possible, 2 = always avoid

	Anxiety	Avoidance
1. Being alone in your home		
2. Shopping unaccompanied in small shops (e.g., grocery, tobacco shop or pharmacy)		
3. Crossing a street in the city alone		
4. Being in a crowd without the company of a friend		
5. Unaccompanied, riding the bus at rush hour		
6. Walking straight across large open spaces in the city (e.g., a square)		
7. Driving a car alone through a long tunnel		
8. Walking away from your home alone		
9. Going by train or subway unaccompanied, when it is crowded		
10. Standing in long lines in the post office, bank or department store, unaccompanied		
11. Sitting in a chair for a long time, in the company of other people		
12. Eating at a restaurant or lunch bar		
13. Going to a cinema or theater and sitting in the middle of a row		
14. Shopping unaccompanied in a department store full of people		
15. Crossing a bridge where there is a lot of traffic, unaccompanied		
16. Driving a car alone over a viaduct or bridge		
17. Having a haircut at the hairdresser, unaccompanied		
18. Shopping unaccompanied in a large supermarket, crowded with people		
19. Unaccompanied walking in crowded streets		
20. Riding in an elevator alone		

practitioner and client with a unique portrait of the client's strengths and vulnerabilities for dealing with a potentially incapacitating disorder.

SELECTING EFFECTIVE INTERVENTIONS

It has long been established that, for panic disorder with agoraphobia, prolonged exposure accompanied initially by a practitioner (or other trained assistant) is the most effective approach. Although earlier reviews of the literature (e.g., Marks, 1987; Jansson & Ost, 1982) almost exclusively emphasized the importance of in vivo exposure as the intervention of choice for panic disorder with agoraphobia, more recent evidence provides some tentative support for adding cognitive techniques to the overall intervention package (Craske, 1999). Cognitive therapy appears to enhance treatment for panic disorder by helping clients change their cognitions about bodily sensations that are misinterpreted as potentially catastrophic and that often provoke panic and subsequent avoidance. Treatments may include some combination of breathing retraining to reduce hyperventilation, cognitive restructuring to correct catastrophic misinterpretations of harmless bodily sensations, and exposure to somatic cues (Zinbarg et al., 1992; Emmelkamp, 1994; Chambless & Gillis, 1996; Craske, 1996a, 1996b). Effective interventions often require an eclectic blend of treatment ingredients tailored to clients' needs. Antony and Swinson (2000) categorize CBT methods for panic disorder with agoraphobia into four types of strategies. These are in vivo exposure to feared situations such as driving on busy highways; interoceptive exposure exercises such as repeatedly spinning in a chair to overcome a fear of becoming dizzy; cognitive strategies such as examining evidence that supports or contradicts anxious beliefs; and relaxation-based strategies such as learning to breathe more slowly and in a more relaxed way. They also suggest that adjunctive interventions such as using a cell phone to communicate during graduated exposure tasks and self-guided instructional manuals may be helpful.

Critical reviews of the outcome literature have established that cognitive-behavioral treatments are the most effective interventions for treating panic disorder and agoraphobia, and result in lasting positive outcomes for many sufferers, although some continue to struggle with relapses of panic (Emmelkamp, 1994; Hollon & Beck, 1994; Zinbarg et al., 1992; Barlow, 1988, 1997; Craske, 1999; Antony & Swinson, 2000). About three-quarters of participants can expect to be virtually free of panic at completion and at six-month follow-up (for up to two years and more). Long-term outcomes appear to include improvements in overall quality of life with relatively low attrition rates. More seriously debilitated clients may benefit from booster interventions to maintain gains over time. Nevertheless, about half of clients with more severe agoraphobia achieve substantial improvement. No other psychosocial interventions for panic with agoraphobia have been shown to be nearly as effective in the short- or long-term as cognitive-behavioral methods.

Medications Used with Panic Disorder

Four types of medications are potentially helpful in the treatment of panic disorder (H. I. Kaplan & Saddock, 1998; Sundel & Sundel, 1998): selective serotonin reuptake inhibitors (SSRIs), tricyclic antidepressants (TCAs), benzodiazepines (BZDs), and monoamine oxidase inhibitors (MAOIs). Among the available medications for panic disorder, SSRIs have emerged as the first-line medical intervention. However, more research on long-term outcomes is needed (Sundel & Sundel, 1998). SSRIs have the benefit of being effective for reducing depression (which often accompanies panic disorder) as well as the occurrence of panic attacks. They have also been shown to be effective with OCD and eating disorders. In addition, they are usually effective at lower starting doses, have low risk of causing dependence or withdrawal, and may cause fewer and less serious side effects than TCAs. They are not free of adverse side effects, however, including lowered sex drive and impaired sexual functioning, gastrointestinal irritation, insomnia, and irritability. SSRIs usually take two or more weeks for the therapeutic effects to take hold.

BZDs are also helpful in the treatment of panic disorder (Sundel & Sundel, 1998; H. I. Kaplan & Saddock, 1998), and come in both short-acting and longer-acting forms. They are marked by a rapid onset in dampening anxiety symptoms, but can cause drowsiness. Clients risk dependence and withdrawal symptoms upon discontinuation of use. Generally it is recommended that BZDs be prescribed for only a few to several weeks, but there is evidence that they can be taken relatively safely for more than a year. There is, however, considerable risk for a relapse of panic symptoms upon their discontinuation.

MAOIs, although no longer considered a first-line treatment, may also be helpful in a panic attack. They do not have the disadvantage of causing an initial spike in anxiety (as do the SSRIs and TCAs), but they must be taken within strict dietary guidelines. Reviews of the literature have shown few differences in overall effectiveness between antidepressants and anxiolytics (Antony & Swinson, 2000).

Cognitive-Behavioral Therapy versus Medication

CBT is likely to improve the performance of medications, but not vice versa (Craske, 1999). Although medication may be of assistance, CBT alone may be as effective as a combination of CBT and medication (Barlow, 1997). Others have suggested that medication may actually interfere with the long-term effectiveness of CBT because clients attribute their progress to the use of medication rather than efforts exerted toward psychosocial and behavior change (Antony & Swinson, 2000). In practice, pragmatism may dictate combining medication with cognitive-behavioral treatments because many managed-care organizations see medication as cost-effective (Mitchell, 1999).

Exemplar Study: Comparing Medication Alone to Medication plus CBT in a Managed-Care Setting.   Mitchell (1999) examined the following question: "Do cognitive-behavioral interventions for panic disorder have an effect that goes beyond the effect of medication alone?" To answer this question, a quasi-experimental design was employed. Fifty-six adults diagnosed with panic disorder were free to select either group CBT and medication or medication alone. Medication regimens followed standardized dosing protocol for either BZDs or SSRIs, and those who also received CBT participated in one of four separate therapy groups (all run by the same therapist who followed the same eight-week protocol of weekly 1.5-hour sessions). The intervention is summarized as follows: week 1, psychoeducation about panic disorder and breathing retraining; week 2, development of a personal anxiety-management program; week 3, progressive muscle relaxation and physical exercise; week 4, imaginal relaxation techniques; week 5, desensitizing to interoceptive cues (i.e., internal physiological symptoms); week 6, phobic desensitization (covert and in vivo); week 7, countering cognitive distortions related to anxiety; and week 8, examining core beliefs regarding anxiety, plus a final review and discussion of posttreatment follow-up.

A multidimensional scale that measured cognitive, behavioral, and physiological symptoms of anxiety was used at baseline and at posttreatment. Clients chose either medication alone or medication plus CBT. Findings significantly demonstrated that clients who received the medication plus CBT intervention fared better on all three outcome measures than those who received only medication. Although this particular investigation demonstrates the superior effectiveness of providing CBT with medication, the study has some limitations. The fact that clients chose their intervention protocol suggests that client treatment expectancies may have affected the outcome. In addition, the study does not provide evidence for maintenance of gains at follow-up.

Including Partners in Evidence-Based Interventions with Panic Disorder and Agoraphobia

Although there is little evidence for the effectiveness of family or couples therapy when panic disorder or agoraphobia is treated as a "symptom" of family dysfunction, there is a growing consensus in the evidence-based literature that partner participation in BCT can help effect positive outcomes. In their review of the literature on BCT and implications for treatment of agoraphobia, Daiuto, Baucom, Epstein, and Dutton (1998) suggested that partner-assisted exposure treatment may enhance maintenance of gains in relatively healthy couples who demonstrate adequate communication and problem-solving skills. However, partner-assisted exposure treatment may be countertherapeutic for more seriously troubled couples. In otherwise well-functioning couples, the assisting partner can help the identified client by providing support, acting as coach, and otherwise assisting the client in following through on homework exercises, actively discouraging avoidance behaviors, praising and supporting intervention efforts and client progress, countering the client's dysfunctional anxiety-producing cognitions, problem solving with the client, and facilitating better communications (Baucom, Mueser, Shoham, Daiuto, & Stickles, 1998; Antony & Swinson, 2000). By working with the couple, the practitioner can also identify otherwise unhelpful partner behaviors that interfere with therapeutic progress. Although some evidence supports couples work with agoraphobic clients (e.g., Jacobson, Holz-worth-Munroe, & Schmaling, 1989), others contend that the evidence is mixed (Fokias & Tyler, 1995).

Description of Effective Psychosocial Intervention for Panic Disorder with Agoraphobia

Cognitive-behavioral interventions for panic disorder accompanied by agora-phobia include several components (Barlow, 1997; Craske, 1999; Antony & Swin-son, 2000): psychoeducation regarding the nature of the disorder and the basic components of the intervention; cognitive reappraisal skills to challenge dys-functional thinking that reinforces panic and avoidance; development of self-monitoring skills to assess the patterning of anxiety and specific situational fac-tors related to implementing the new techniques; anxiety-reduction skills, including breathing retraining and perhaps imaginal exposure (desensitization) to frightening thoughts and images; in vivo graduated exposure to the feared sit-uation; life-style changes to help clients maintain their gains and prevent relapse. A more detailed breakdown is presented below. Although published protocols vary somewhat, core effective elements in the CBT literature are similar, and practitioners tailor a treatment plan to the client's needs, preferences, and cir-cumstances.

Psychoeducation. The practitioner provides didactic information regarding the nature of fear and anxiety (e.g., "fear of the fear" model, anticipa-tory dread) and false beliefs about the harmful nature of the physical symptoms themselves (assuming the client has received a clean bill of health in a medical exam). Psychoeducation also examines other erroneous cognitions and thinking errors that often accompany panic attacks, to help the client understand that these physical symptoms can be brought under control through the use of CBT methods and that these fears often lead to avoidance behaviors. The practitioner explains how the biopsychosocial aspects of the symptoms work. This education helps the client understand the sequencing and patterning of thoughts, feelings, behaviors, and situations and how these factors can be modified to reduce dis-tress associated with the disorder. The practitioner overviews the specific treat-ment strategies to be employed.

Cognitive Restructuring. Cognitive reappraisal helps clients identify and challenge core cognitions and common thinking errors associated with dys-functional misinterpretations of bodily sensations such as heart palpitations and frightening thoughts ("I'm going to faint in front of everyone"). Practitioners help clients identify and challenge their overestimations of danger, catastrophic thinking, overgeneralizing ("I'm afraid of *everything*"), and dichotomous think-ing ("I'm either going to die or get better"). In short, they help clients consider more realistic and plausible interpretations. Clients revise their overall appraisal of their symptoms as a danger to their health and future well-being.

Cognitive restructuring should focus on (1) teaching the client to identify the anxiety-producing belief; (2) generating alternative explanations; (3) examining the respective evidence for the original belief and the alternative belief; and (4) choosing a more realistic interpretation or prediction.

Self-Monitoring Skills.   Other cognitive tasks can facilitate the intervention: using self-monitoring strategies (practicing between visits), and developing exposure hierarchies (a scenario of approaching the feared situation broken into gradual steps). These skills will be used later for either in-session (imaginal) exposure or in vivo exposure.

Anxiety-Reduction Skills.   Managing physiological symptoms centers on breathing retraining. The practitioner teaches diaphragm breathing to reduce hyperventilation often associated with panic attacks, and demonstrates hyperventilation to help correct misconceptions about anxiety symptoms as being very dangerous. Clients learn about physiology of respiration and that over-breathing leads to feelings of dizziness and lightheadedness that often trigger panic but can be controlled through deep, slow breathing. Clients practice holding deep breaths and letting them out slowly.

Imaginal exposure methods help clients focus on interoceptive sensations that have become associated with panic attacks. Using the hierarchy developed earlier for a feared situation, clients gradually confront the feared thought and situation in their mind's eye (i.e., covertly), and learn to maintain exposure until the anxiety is reduced substantially. Have clients fill in the details and help them make the imaginal scenario as salient and as emotionally compelling for them as possible.

Perhaps the most common form of imaginal exposure is systematic desensitization. After the practitioner assists the client in developing a fear-inducing hierarchy from low anxiety to high anxiety, the client practices basic relaxation techniques, and learns how to use the SUDS, which the client scores verbally when prompted by the practitioner during the desensitization procedure. After the client is relaxed, the practitioner introduces images from the hierarchy that increase incrementally from low to higher anxiety. Periodically the practitioner asks how anxious the client is on a scale from 0 to 10. As the client begins to report some degree of discomfort, the client is asked to hold the image and use relaxation exercises at the same time. This may be repeated several times, until the client can move up the hierarchy. This approach gradually helps the client reach a point where they can imagine being in a high-anxiety situation, perhaps rated 8 on the SUDS, and maintain imaginal exposure until the score drops to a 4. Imaginal exposure is not typically used as the core intervention for agoraphobia, but may be helpful as a warm-up before beginning in vivo sessions.

In Vivo Exposure.   During in vivo graduated exposure, clients incrementally confront the frightening situation, and remain in that situation for a prolonged time while practicing their anxiety-reducing coping skills (e.g., breathing, self-soothing talk, reassuring images). In vivo sessions are carefully planned and structured down to details about what the client will do and how long it will take. The sessions are behavioral experiments designed to challenge clients' dysfunctional beliefs about their fears and the potential effects of anxiety. They create a cognitive "contest" whereby clients' catastrophic anxieties are pitted against the reality that, if they remain long enough in the situation, they will be able to maintain control and the anxiety will dissipate, thus "disproving" that their terrifying expectations are justified. With practice, the belief that they can cope with these situations increases and provides clients with a more assured sense of empowerment and self-control.

Graduated exposure is generally recommended over rapid exposure (flooding), but progress should be made expeditiously. The pace of exposure should be gradual, but the tasks should be at least moderately fear-inducing. The practitioner should challenge clients to do a little more than they think they can at each threshold. Exposure practices should be fairly frequent and spaced close together, and duration should be enough to achieve a significant decrease in anxiety. The client should expect to feel uncomfortable, and not to obtain quick and easy results.

The practitioner should encourage clients to *give in to the fear*, and not to fight it. They need reassurance that at worst they will feel uncomfortable, but their catastrophic fears will not be realized. Clients should be directed to use their cognitive coping strategies to challenge negative automatic thoughts during the exercise, but not to use subtle avoidance strategies such as drinking beforehand, arriving late, and leaving early.

Clients can engage in self-directed exposure, be accompanied by a practitioner, or have a trained significant other coach them. Agoraphobic self-help groups have become increasingly sophisticated in using behavioral techniques, and often provide "buddy systems" to help newer members overcome their fears. Use of technologies such as virtual reality may be helpful where in vivo practice is not practical. Cell phones may be useful to assist an agoraphobic person who is engaged in exposure therapy. Socially phobic clients may also benefit from social-skills training.

Lifestyle Changes.   Depending on the situation, clients should attempt to generalize the exposure to other relevant situations. Although therapist-directed exposure is important in the beginning, clients should be encouraged to practice on their own, and to continue practicing as treatment contacts are reduced or terminated.

Follow-up sessions are encouraged to help maintain gains. Clients should also leave treatment with a plan to maintain positive changes such as consistently exposing themselves to the anxiety-inducing situation if it is practical (so they don't backslide), and to maintain other positive habits such as anxiety-management techniques and abstinence or moderation in substance abuse, as is warranted.

IMPLEMENTING AND EVALUATING THE EVIDENCE-BASED INTERVENTION PLAN

CASE STUDY: MILAGRA

Milagra, a seventeen-year-old Latina woman, was brought to an outpatient mental health clinic by her mother and a local parish priest. Although she had experienced "nerves" in the past, she recently began experiencing panic attacks several times a week. As a result, she was terrified of driving, and did not even want to think about leaving her immediate neighborhood for any reason whatsoever. Since her mother (who had never learned to drive) had come to rely on her to run errands now that Milagra had her license, this turn of events was disruptive for the entire household. In addition, Milagra shared some of the parenting responsibilities for her two younger siblings, Raul, age ten, and Pablo, eight. The family immigrated from Mexico twelve years before, and moved into a community that strongly held to its heritage, language, and customs. Because of her early school experiences, Milagra gew up speaking excellent English, thus acquiring much of the responsibility as household translator. Her father, an intermittently heavy drinker, worked two or three jobs to survive financially. Mom, "a worrier," coped with anxieties by maintaining close ties to her church, often volunteering hours of her time. She had sought help for anxieties in the past but avoided the physician, who was not a Latino, and relied instead on her rosary beads and occasional visits to the neighborhood *curandera*.

A thorough history seemed to show that the onset of panic-attack symptoms was precipitated by a happy event: Milagra was accepted into the state university with a full-tuition scholarship. The family was at first ecstatic, very proud, and the envy of all their neighbors. However, as the late spring and early summer wore on, Milagra grew increasingly anxious: "How will I get to school? My car is too old. It will need many repairs. What about all my responsibilities at home? When will I have time to study? There are no buses or trains that travel reliably or conveniently to campus." After she accepted that she would have to visit the university, she planned a day to check out the campus and have an interview with university officials. On her way there, she experienced a full-blown panic attack, an experience that went well beyond the usual "nerves." Terrified, she pulled off the road and remained there with her heart racing, gasping for breath until a state police car pulled up to investigate. When she explained her situation, the policeman told her to move the vehicle off the bridge, or it would have to be towed. Feeling as if she were going to pass out, she calmed herself enough to travel down the highway, got off at the next exit at a gas station–convenience mart, and called home tearful, terrified and feeling defeated.

At home, her mother thought her daughter was going insane (because Milagra said as much), and took her to the parish priest. Father Reyes recognized the symptoms of a panic attack immediately (having ministered for years at the local psychiatric hospital), and referred her to a social worker. Milagra's mother called and set up the appointment, which was outside their immediate neighborhood, and they were transported there by Father Reyes. When she showed up for the first visit, Milagra expressed embarrassment at having to be brought by her mother and the parish priest.

Multidimensional/Functional Assessment: Defining Problems and Goals

A brief screening of Milagra's symptoms and concerns met many of the criteria for panic disorder with agoraphobia, including recurrent unexpected panic attacks characterized by heart palpitations, an accelerated heart rate, sweating, shaking, shortness of breath, nausea, and lightheadedness. She thought at times that she was losing her mind, and she began to dread the possibility of having another attack, which made her avoid going out even more, especially to public places where she might make a "fool of myself by fainting or running out" of the grocery store. She curtailed her chores alone and usually took her mother or one of her brothers "along for the ride." In addition to her anxiety symptoms, Milagra was becoming increasingly despondent (depressed?) about her college prospects. Although she had successfully put college out of her mind, she could no longer avoid it. Fortunately, she did not abuse alcohol or other drugs, but coped by burying herself in her books. She had no impulse-control problems of note, had a couple of good close friends, although no romantic liaison at this time, and was highly respected and depended upon by her family. Her dad was a little distant from her, but she was on good terms with him. Although he had always been a strict disciplinarian and had high standards for his children, he was never abusive in any way. She was in excellent health.

Her anxiety about leaving home was compounded by her sense of obligation to her family and by feelings that she was betraying her community. Her family was ostensibly proud of her and bragged to the neighbors and extended family, but quietly voiced anxieties about what they would do when Milagra "left us." In addition, many of her peers in school were not planning to go to college, and when word got around that she was accepted into school with a scholarship, she found it hard to endure accusations that she was going to become a "real gringa" and abandon her roots. These conflicted feelings added to her distress.

A functional analysis revealed a fairly straightforward correlation between symptoms and impending emancipation from home. After the initial excitement of having been accepted into the university, she became increasingly tense the more she thought about leaving home. Although she would avoid thinking about it much of the time, correspondence from the school began to arrive, and she realized she would have to go there soon to confer with university personnel and register for courses as well as to make arrangements to move and live on campus. She had only four months before classes were to begin, and she knew she could not put off her trip any longer. When she thought about leaving, she would become increasingly panicked, and begin to find reasons to stay at home, or at least not leave the immediate neighborhood. The symptoms would worsen, and she would find herself in her room, crying and trembling. Panic attacks increased as did her avoidance of thinking about school until she received her letter to come to the university for a meeting. It was at that point that she had a full panic attack when she tried to force herself to drive out of town.

After this initial assessment and rapport building with Milagra, the practitioner and she decided that the goal of treatment was to get her to drive to the university and begin her new adventure. After a couple of visits, the social worker, Gloria, expressed her appreciation for the help her mother and the priest provided, but suggested that Milagra come alone. The clinic was only a couple of blocks past Milagra's usual "boundary line." Although the thought of driving to the university, which was about an hour away (and included crossing a half-mile-long bridge), frightened her, she felt a sense of confidence that the practitioner was knowledgeable and communicated an optimism about succeeding.

Selecting and Designing the Intervention: Defining Strategies and Objectives

Although there would be time to take a more in-depth history, top priority in the first session was understanding the recent events that led up to the panic attack, and engendering a collaborative working alliance. Although the client was encouraged to see a physician for a checkup and consultation, she did not fill the prescription because she was skeptical of traditional medicine and anxious about taking medication. Since the abuse of alcohol or other drugs was carefully ruled out, in-depth assessment focused on the psychosocial factors potentially exacerbating the anxiety and panic symptoms.

The second step was to provide psychoeducation concerning the prevalence, patterns, and contributing causes of panic (table 7.1). The mother tended to imbue her daughter's experience with religious overtones, and Gloria did not challenge these interpretations. Milagra, however, having read about this disorder in a woman's magazine, was more inclined to consider physiological predisposition and psychosocial stressors. Gloria met with Milagra alone to develop a treatment plan and to initiate coping-skills strategies that she could begin immediately on her own. Gloria showed her basic breathing and muscle-relaxation techniques and used psychoeducation to help her reinterpret her physiological symptoms. She also recommended a book. These preliminary efforts at psychoeducation and relaxation training provided Milagra some immediate symptom relief.

During the second visit (she got a ride from a friend and her mother came along), Milagra reported that she was still experiencing panic attacks, albeit a little less frequently, and was unable to go outside for more than a few minutes because of her dread of another attack. However, thoughts about being trapped staying at home and not being able to go to college upset her even more. Although Gloria empathized with her concerns, she did not give any false reassurance that Milagra was going to make it to college. In addition to educating Milagra about the physical aspects of anxiety and how the mind misinterprets these events, Gloria wanted to discuss her fears about leaving home. Milagra expressed a number of concerns: "What about my dad? He's not always there for my mom. What about my little brother and sister? I'm not sure mom can keep up with them, and she spends a lot of time at the church. What about my friends? They are already telling me I'm too good for them now, that I just want to be like the rich Anglo girls." Gloria responded that Milagra seemed to feel extraordinarily responsible for the welfare of a lot of people, and might also be afraid of losing their affection. Rather than challenge these beliefs directly, however, Milagra was encouraged to listen to herself say out loud her worst fears about what she really thought would happen to her and her relationships with others if she successfully pursued her dreams, and consider alternative interpretations and scenarios.

During the next four weekly sessions Milagra continued to practice her meditation, breathing, and reinterpretation of her cognitive cues, and through journal writing appeared to come to an accommodation about how she could still be responsive to her family (by living at home for now), and her community (by eventually becoming a doctor and volunteering some time in the barrio). However, she had only six weeks before classes began. Gloria explained that although she had a better understanding of the role of anxiety, some skills to control it, and a better understanding of the other contributing causes, these insights would not be enough to relieve her terror of driving to the university on her own. The only way to overcome this irrational fear of driving out of town would be to confront it. "There's no way I'm going to do that . . . that scares the heck out of me! And what if I can't get home this time, or what if I get arrested?"

Gloria agreed that this must be quite frightening. To make it a little easier, they discussed how Milagra would learn to use her imagination and relaxation exercises to create a step-by-step hierarchy that she could use repeatedly to approach her fears in her mind's eye and practice remaining calm while covertly "driving" out of town before attempting it in vivo. Since Milagra had already felt some relief from relaxation exercises, she was positively disposed toward trying this. Gloria asked Milagra to close her eyes and practice her breathing exercise for a minute or two while concentrating on a neutral image in her mind's eye. Gloria asked her to imagine herself at home, comfortable, at ease, and relatively free from anxiety. She then said, "I want you to tell me by raising your finger when it becomes a little frightening for you (raised a little), moderately frightening (a little higher), or extremely frightening (straight up). When you start feeling anxious, use your breathing and muscle-relaxation exercise to calm yourself as much as you can." Gloria began to walk Milagra through a "typical" day of getting up, getting ready for classes, preparing her lunch, going out to the car, driving down the street to the edge of town by way of the main avenue, onto the entrance ramp to the highway, to the exit for the university a half hour away, into the parking lot, and into her first class. After several trials she was able to complete the exercise with, at worst, a moderate degree of anxiety. She agreed to practice it daily at home by using a tape of the session.

For the next week, Milagra practiced this "mental walk-through" daily. Although it was quite frightening at first, she was determined not to allow these panicky feelings to keep her from something she really wanted. After a week of daily practice, she felt that she was ready to try driving, but did not think she would be able to make it all the way. During her meditations, however, she spontaneously conjured an internal image of a strong, older, courageous woman whom she felt she could rely on to help her through this trial. "Is there anyone you know like that?" queried Gloria. Milagra said there was an old woman in her neighborhood, a *curandera*, whom she often thought of as someone who was loving and strong and, like her, a bit on the mystical side. Gloria agreed that the *curandera* seemed to be a person whom others relied on in times of trouble. Perhaps Milagra could obtain a figurine in one of the local bodegas, and bring it along with her for the ride as a representation of this woman. She agreed that this might help. Gloria also helped Milagra sketch a map of the area, in order to plan some "bail-out points," in case she felt that she could not complete her momentous journey.

For the next several days, Milagra gradually increased her driving distance, first down the street doing errands, then down the main thoroughfare until she approached the highway entrance ramp. It began clear that she actually had desensitized herself to much of the anxiety associated with getting back into the car and driving locally; she was also not overwhelmed by her fears of panic anymore, feeling that this experience was transitory and probably would not be as bad as before. However, it also became clear that her terror rose precipitously when she approached the highway ramp, because once on it, she felt there was no turning back, no escape route for at least a couple of miles. For two more weeks she drove locally but could not approach the ramp. Comments such as "maybe college just isn't for me" and "maybe I could just put things off for a year" were expected and understandable. Gloria reflected that, yes, maybe she was right. "Perhaps a year off would do you good ... and what would staying at home for the next year or so be like for you?" As they both played out this scenario, it became clear that Milagra considered this an unacceptable alternative. She felt she was approaching an inevitable and critical moment in her life: "I'm terrified, but I won't be left behind and stuck at home for the rest of my life ... I have to do it now."

Realizing that time was closing in, it appeared that Milagra needed one additional incentive to make this final leap. Gloria suggested that she borrow a friend's hands-free cell phone and keep the line open during the in vivo driving session. Milagra agreed to the plan. When Milagra called, she was in town and was just about to begin her approach to the highway ramp. Gloria coached her through her breathing exercises and provided gentle encouragement. Milagra became noticeably more afraid as the ramp approached, but was well in control. It was also apparent that she found considerable comfort in the fact that she had a connection to someone who could confront this threshold with her and talk her through it. The practitioner reminded her of the strength and confidence of the *curandera* whom she wanted to emulate. As she drove out onto the highway, however, the cell-phone connection broke up, and Gloria could not communicate with Milagra. Ten minutes later (it seemed much longer), she received a call from the other side. "I've done it! And you know what? It wasn't half as bad as I thought it would be! I can't believe it! I've done it!" For the next three weeks, Milagra drove back and forth to school, wandered the campus, imagined herself going to class. She purchased her books and parking sticker, and met a staff person at the International Student Center who was also Latina. She thought, "Maybe this won't be so terrifying after all."

Selecting Scales and Creating Indexes to Monitor and Evaluate Client Progress

A combination of the Agoraphobia Scale (measuring both anxiety level and avoidance) coupled with the Hamilton Depression Inventory (HAM-D) provided a sound accompaniment to the qualitative assessment (table 7.1). In addition, a series of indexes, including frequency of panic attacks, time or distance driving, and the SUDS to gauge anxiety level, were indispensable to evaluating change over the course of the intervention.

TABLE 7.1   The Client Service Plan for Milagra

Problems	Goals	Sample Objectives	Interventions	Assessment Tools
Long-term anxiety with recent onset of panic disorder	Leave home, enroll in school, and develop coping skills to eliminate panic disorder and avoidance behaviors (timetable: 4 months)	Become knowledgeable about panic disorder and agoraphobia through discussions, watching video, and reading a book from social worker (2 weeks)	Solid working alliance with client; examination of relationship of treatment expectations and impact of prospective outcomes on cultural beliefs	Agoraphobia Scale to gauge overall axiety and avoidance levels
Exacerbation of avoidance behavior brought on by the prospect of leaving home and community for college				HAM-D for co-occurring symptoms
Depression: sense of guilt, betrayal, and loss at the thought of leaving home	Reduce, eliminate depression; redefine the separation as normal moving on; find other ways to compensate to family and community	Examine and keep diary of anxiety-provoking thoughts, and challenge them based on discussion with social worker about "thinking errors" (daily)	Cognitive-behavioral coping skills, including psychoeducation regarding panic disorder and CBT; standard cognitive therapy techniques to examine dysfunctional thinking about leaving home, unrealistic fears regarding	Individual indexes: frequency of panic attacks; distance driven from home; amount of time away from home
				SUDS to measure subjective level of anxiety
		Practice anxiety-reduction methods: meditation and		

Problems	Goals	Sample Objectives	Interventions	Assessment Tools
		breathing exercises (10 minutes twice daily); gradually (as introduced by social worker) incorporate covert exposure to "car trip" hierarchy	panic symptoms, normative feelings of depression, and betrayal of family and culture	
		Begin daily in vivo graduated exposure (unaccompanied) by driving and parking as prescribed by "trip map" designed with social worker according to hierarchy of objectives. Use relaxation exercises and challenge cognitive errors until anxiety subsides to below 5 on SUDS	Imaginal desensitization techniques in combination with in vivo exposure to reduce her fear of driving out of town and going to public places alone.	
		2 months before school begins, drive over the bridge and to the university; biweekly trips after that to "hang around" campus and get comfortable	Case management: physical and psychiatric evaluation; work with community members (church personnel) to assist family as needed; later, contact and confer with university counseling to facilitate follow-up treatment as needed (e.g., making adjustments to school, dealing with social anxiety, depression, sense of loss, if necessary)	
		Make contacts with Hispanic-American club members during summer, and plan to meet a representative if possible		
		Examine cognitive errors regarding "betrayal and guilt"; focus on alternative ways to "give back" to family and culture as a college grad, future professional; delegate household jobs to brothers; work with church group to organize help for mother		

ASSESSMENT OF OBSESSIVE-COMPULSIVE DISORDER

Background Data

OCD and panic disorder with agoraphobia can both be addressed by some of the same assessment and intervention methods. Some clients may experience both conditions at different points in their lives, or symptoms of both may co-occur. Both are marked by severe and debilitating anxiety related to dysfunctional thinking, physiological symptoms, and attempts to ward off anxiety through avoidance: physically avoiding situations in agoraphobia, and in OCD, avoiding the anxiety caused by certain thoughts (obsessions) by engaging in compulsive rituals. In addition, both conditions can be effectively ameliorated through coping skills and exposure-based interventions, often combined with medication.

OCD is estimated to afflict about 2.5% of the population (Karno, Golding, Sorenson, & Burnam, 1988; Craske, 1999; *DSM-IV-TR*). Onset typically occurs in childhood or adolescence for males and young adulthood for women. Obsessions and compulsions are very common in the general population (Craske, 1999), but degree of impairment varies widely. Clients who meet the diagnostic criteria are at the severe end of the spectrum. OCD co-occurs with a number of other problems, especially other anxiety disorders and depression (Barlow, 1988; Craske, 1999; Steketee, 1993; *DSM-IV-TR*). Stress is a common precipitant to obsessional thinking and compulsions, and biological and psychological vulnerabilities are important predictors. Although cultural themes often color the nature of obsessions and compulsions, there appears to be little variation by gender or culture in treatment outcomes (Steketee & Shapiro, 1995).

Based on a review of the literature, Steketee (1997) reports that people with OCD are disproportionately unemployed, are less likely to be married (due to impaired social and sexual functioning), and often experience other problems in family functioning. Although most data on the family burden created by a member suffering from OCD are anecdotal, many family members seem to complain about the client's "manipulative behavior," which may include attempts to involve family members in the client's rituals. Clients may also demonstrate poor grooming and personal hygiene, among other behavioral problems. It appears that the majority of families suffer some degree of burden from caring for a family member with OCD, and most of the burden is carried by the principal caregiver. Family members suffer from feelings of frustration, anger, guilt, financial burden, and interrupted family activities. Although outcome data are largely limited to primary symptoms, Steketee (1997) recommends that more specific attention be given to understanding the social and occupational adjustment of the client and to including the family members in treatment to provide them with support and psychoeducation regarding the disorder and ways to manage it.

Theories

Psychodynamic explanations for the causes of obsessive-compulsive neurosis generally focus on the client's difficulties resolving love-hate feelings toward the love object, accompanied by defensive responses (e.g., isolation, undoing, reaction formation) to the perceived loss of mother's love. Aside from case-study analyses used to justify these theories, however, no developmentally sound research has ever provided substantive scientific support for them. Early conditioning theories (e.g., Mowrer, 1960) conceptualized obsessive-compulsive behaviors as a two-stage process in which some thought or image (obsession) was initially associated with a fear-inducing stimulus, and in response, an avoidance behavior (compulsive ritual) became reinforcing because it briefly reduced the anxiety. Early conditioning theories, however, came to be seen as insufficient to explain the *continuation* of obsessive-compulsive behaviors when the original stimulus is no longer active.

Contemporary theories regarding the cause and course of the disorder tend to focus on the interaction of genetic, developmental, cognitive, and behavioral factors (Barlow, 1988; Craske, 1999; Steketee, 1993; D. S. Riggs & Foa, 1993). Although the initial anxiety-producing thought may be trigged by some environmental event, perhaps during a period of stress, the obsessional thought is deemed very unacceptable and may be tied to an overwrought sense of responsibility. The person begins to engage in behavioral rituals in a vain attempt to neutralize the negative thought. Recent contributions of social-cognitive theory have been offered to illuminate the dynamics of obsessional thinking and role of compulsive rituals. Building on the foundation of Beck's cognitive model (1976), Salkovskis (1985) points out that negative automatic thoughts are usually distressing because of their plausible nature, whereas obsessions are not plausible (e.g., a client's fear that touching a doorknob will give him or her the AIDS virus), and the person experiencing them finds these thoughts irrational and unacceptable. He goes on to argue that although intrusive thoughts are common to many people, they become a source of considerable distress "only when they result in negative automatic thoughts through interaction between the unacceptable intrusions and the individual's belief system" (p. 573). These thoughts must be evaluated as "bad" by the individual in some way. Often they appear to be related to the idea that the individual is responsible for causing harm to himself or to another person. The person becomes distressed about the negative automatic thoughts that result from the intrusion, and may feel like a bad person merely for having had these bad thoughts. Often depression accompanies these negative self-evaluations. The compulsive thoughts or rituals then become futile efforts to neutralize the distressing obsession. Attempts to neutralize these disturbing thoughts through cognitive efforts alone are not likely to be successful. Salkovskis (1989) further hypothesizes that treatment must focus on helping the client realize that obsessional thoughts are irrelevant to prevent harm to oneself or others. That is, the intervention must focus on disengaging the cognitive linkage between obsessional thoughts and ritualistic protecting behaviors. Personal values embedded in cultural or religious thoughts and ritualistic influences may account for some of these fixed beliefs (Craske, 1999).

Key Elements of Multidimensional/ Functional Assessment

Essential features of OCD (Barlow, 1988; *DSM-IV-TR*) include recurrent obsessions or compulsions that a person typically has come to recognize as excessive or unreasonable and that are debilitating because they take up more than one hour per day and cause marked stress or impairment. Common obsessions include implausible thoughts about contamination by germs, persistent doubts (e.g., left the coffee pot on, therefore the house will burn down), excessive orderliness, and unacceptable thoughts of engaging in sexual or aggressive impulses. Compulsions are repetitive behaviors such as checking, ordering, counting, and hand washing and other behavioral or mental rituals meant to ward off anxiety or undo troubling thoughts. Clients typically recognize that engaging in the ritualized behavior cannot prevent the imagined negative consequences that they feel will result (e.g., my mother will become mortally ill if I don't fold my laundry in perfect piles).

Essential criteria for *DSM-IV-TR* diagnosis of OCD include the following:

Recurrent and persistent thoughts, impulses, or images are experienced as intrusive and inappropriate and cause marked anxiety or distress.

These obsessions are not simply excessive worries about real-life problems.

The person attempts to ignore or suppress such obsessions or to neutralize them with some other thought or action.

The person recognizes that the obsessions are a product of his or her own mind (not imposed from without, as in thought insertion).

Compulsions are repetitive behaviors or mental acts that the person feels driven to perform in response to an obsession, or according to rules that must be applied rigidly.

The compulsions are aimed at preventing or reducing distress or preventing some dreaded event or situation.

These compulsions either are not connected in any realistic way with what they are designed to neutralize or are clearly excessive.

At some point, adults recognize that these thoughts or behaviors are excessive (although children may not recognize them as such), and the obsessions or compulsions cause marked distress and interfere with interpersonal, occupational, or academic functioning. Practitioners should be aware that obsessions are fairly common, and that it is important to distinguish between obsessive rumination and excessive worrying associated with depression and anxiety. Obsessions associated with OCD tend to be unrealistic and are not seen as realistic by the client, whereas obsessions associated with other problems (e.g., ruminating over having actually caused an accident) may be congruent with the client's depressed mood. OCD can co-occur with other disorders, including other anxiety disorders, depression, substance abuse, and eating disorders, and many people with OCD also have a history of tic disorders. A careful analysis of the effects of the person's OCD on social well-being is also important. Clients may go to considerable lengths to hide their ritualistic behavior or obsessions. The practitioner should also closely assess family members to see if they engage in behaviors that inadvertently reinforce the client's obsessions and compulsions.

Functional assessment of OCD involves a more detailed account of the type, frequency, severity, and duration of both the obsessional thinking and the ritualistic behaviors. Determining what the nature of these obsessions and compulsions is, when they occur, and under what circumstances they occur is critical to helping the client monitor and track them. The social worker and client can then develop a hierarchy of obsessions as prelude to implementing graduated imaginal or in vivo exposure with response prevention (discussed below). Steketee (1993) recommends that assessment of obsessions include information about external sources of fear (tangible objects), internal triggers for fear (thoughts, images, impulses), and worries about the consequences of not engaging in the compulsive behaviors.

A variety of information-gathering methods should be employed, including self-report, behavioral tests, observation, reports of significant others, and standardized assessment. The assessment should follow a sequential plan. The first two sessions focus on psychoeducation about the nature of OCD and CBT (i.e., exposure with response prevention). A functional assessment identifies internal and external cues for obsessions, notes obsession-cuing situations, lists avoidance behaviors and mental rituals, and describes the involvement of significant others in rituals. Clients should report the information gathered in their self-monitoring diary/chart in the second session, and the practitioner should carefully confirm the diagnosis of OCD. In the third and fourth sessions, further review of self-monitoring is essential, and the practitioner should describe treatment in detail, help the client develop a hierarchy of obsessional situations, plan adjunctive activities such as homework and involvement of significant others, and schedule sessions (Steketee, 1993).

S. Taylor (1995) has summarized a number of different approaches to the assessment of OCD. These methods include behavioral avoidance tests in which the client is presented with the feared situation. For example, with a client who has an extreme fear of germs, test to see how close the client can approach touching a doorknob, or have the client touch a doorknob and see how long they can avoid washing their hands. Clients can report their SUDS level as described above in the assessment of panic disorder. An "in vivo" assessment can be compelling, but may be somewhat limited with respect to understanding other obsessional patterns or associated problems. Less obvious obsessions (e.g., privately counting or ritualistic thought patterns) may be more difficult to assess. Direct observation or use of diaries can be helpful for these more covert compulsions.

Instruments

A review of the literature suggests that the Yale-Brown Obsessive-Compulsive Scale (YBOCS; W. Goodman et al., 1989) is considered a valid tool for assessment and evaluation of treatment outcomes. Most investigators use the ten "core" items, which measure five parameters of both obsessions and compulsions: duration/frequency, interference in social and occupational functioning, associated distress, degree of resistance, and perceived control over obsessions or compulsions. Each core item is rated by average severity over the past week by the interviewer on a five-point scale (0 = none, 4 = extreme). Separate subscales for obsessions and compulsions are summed, although the ten items are usually summed as a global score. S. Taylor (1995) in a review of the psychometric literature on the YBOCS states that the scale has excellent interrater reliability, acceptable to good internal consistency, and good test-retest reliability; distinguishes people with OCD from people with other anxiety disorders; and correlates well with other OCD-related scales. It does tend to correlate significantly with measures of anxiety and depression, however, suggesting some weakness in discriminant validity.

The Obsessive-Compulsive Inventory (OCI; Foa, Kozak, Salkovskis, Coles, & Amir, 1998) is an excellent alternative to the YBOCS. It is reprinted here (instrument 7.2). It was developed with three goals in mind: to be more comprehensive than existing instruments, to allow for a wider range of severity scores than other scales, and to be easily administered to clinical and nonclinical populations. An eighteen-item version of the OCI has been developed, which improves the utility of the original instrument, yet retains excellent psychometric properties (Foa et al., 2002). The short version of the OCI comprises six subscales with three items each: washing (5, 11, 17), obsessing (6, 12, 18), hoarding (1, 7, 13), ordering (3, 9, 15), checking (2, 8, 14), and neutralizing (4, 10, 16). Internal consistency for the total OCI is good, test-retest reliability is very good overall for subscales and total score, and the subscales of the short OCI correlate very well generally with those of the longer version. Factor analysis supports the internal structure of the scale, and correlational analysis supports both convergent and discriminant validity. The eighteen-item OCI is scored by simply summing all items, and a cutoff score of 21 is recommended for identifying people who are likely to meet *DSM-IV-TR* criteria for obsessive-compulsive disorder. Individual items and subscale scores should also be examined to gauge the client's unique symptom configuration as well as subclinical distress.

INSTRUMENT 7.2   Obsessive-Compulsive Inventory–Revised

The following statements refer to experiences that many people have in their everyday lives. Circle the number that best describes HOW MUCH that experience has DISTRESSED or BOTHERED you during the PAST MONTH. The numbers refer to the following verbal labels:

	Not at all	A little	Moderately	A lot	Extremely
	0	1	2	3	4
1. I have saved up so many things that they get in the way.	0	1	2	3	4
2. I check things more often than necessary.	0	1	2	3	4
3. I get upset if objects are not arranged properly.	0	1	2	3	4
4. I feel compelled to count while I am doing things.	0	1	2	3	4
5. I find it difficult to touch an object when I know it has been touched by strangers or certain people.	0	1	2	3	4
6. I find it difficult to control my own thoughts.	0	1	2	3	4
7. I collect things I don't need.	0	1	2	3	4
8. I repeatedly check doors, windows, drawers, etc.	0	1	2	3	4
9. I get upset if others change the way I have arranged things.	0	1	2	3	4
10. I feel I have to repeat certain numbers.	0	1	2	3	4
11. I sometimes have to wash or clean myself simply because I feel contaminated.	0	1	2	3	4
12. I am upset by unpleasant thoughts that come into my mind against my will.	0	1	2	3	4
13. I avoid throwing things away because I am afraid I might need them later.	0	1	2	3	4
14. I repeatedly check gas and water taps and light switches after turning them off.	0	1	2	3	4
15. I need things to be arranged in a particular order.	0	1	2	3	4
16. I feel that there are good and bad numbers.	0	1	2	3	4
17. I wash my hands more often and longer than necessary.	0	1	2	3	4
18. I frequently get nasty thoughts and have difficulty getting rid of them.	0	1	2	3	4

SELECTING EFFECTIVE INTERVENTIONS

Research has not supported the use of psychodynamic interventions for people with OCD. In addition, early behavioral treatments such as thought stopping and mild aversive procedures were not shown to have any long-term positive effects (D. S. Riggs & Foa, 1993; Foa & Kozak, 1996). A strong consensus, however, has emerged among leading clinician-researchers that a specific application of CBT, exposure with response prevention (EX/RP), implemented over long periods of time, is the most effective psychosocial intervention for OCD. From one-half to three-quarters of clients appear to obtain substantial relief from their obsessive-compulsive symptoms, and show good long-term maintenance of gains. Those who relapse can be successfully treated with follow-up booster sessions and relapse prevention methods (Emmelkamp, 1994; Zinbarg et al., 1992; D. S. Riggs

& Foa, 1993; Steketee, 1993; Foa & Kozak, 1996). Recent studies have even revealed changes in brain functioning that demonstrate the deep and lasting effects of CBT for OCD (J. Schwartz, 1998).

Many clients with OCD report obsessions without any overt compulsive behavior. To address this problem, an intervention has been developed so that these clients can engage in prolonged exposure sessions by listening to a self-recorded audiotape of their own obsessive thought, impulse, or image, and then focus on avoiding the psychological compulsion to neutralize it or to engage in avoidance responses. A randomized controlled study with fifteen clients and fourteen controls demonstrated that audiotape exposure resulted in clinically significant gains with good maintenance of progress at six-month follow-up for about two-thirds of the clients (Freeston et al., 1997). Brief self-directed treatments that include combinations of bibliotherapy and self-directed in vivo and imaginal exposure to a planned hierarchy have also shown promising results (Fritzler, Hecker, & Losee, 1997). This brief intervention may be cost-effective for less debilitated OCD clients.

Minority clients have been markedly underrepresented in studies of OCD. A case analysis of two African-American women diagnosed with OCD demonstrated that current behavior therapies for this disorder were well received and showed positive results (K. E. Williams, Chambless, & Steketee, 1998). EX/RP has also been successfully implemented in partial hospitalization programs where it was combined with medication and other psychosocial interventions. Long-term outcomes at eighteen months were very positive (Bystritsky et al., 1996).

Evidence for the effectiveness of interventions in which family members are included show results similar to findings reported above for panic disorder and agoraphobia. Without addressing relationship problems directly, it appears that the significant other can enhance treatment and improve outcomes by assisting the client in carrying out EX/RP (Baucom et al., 1998).

Exposure with Response Prevention versus Medication

SSRIs have been demonstrated to be reasonably effective in the treatment of OCDs (D. S. Riggs & Foa, 1993; Foa & Kozak, 1996; H. I. Kaplan & Saddock, 1998), although about half of clients with OCD do not respond adequately to SSRIs alone (McDonough & Kennedy, 2002). There may be an initial increase in anxiety during the first two to three weeks, but many clients obtain long-term relief after that (H. I. Kaplan & Saddock, 1998).

Comparisons of CBT with and without medication have been examined in recent years. Results of a meta-analytic study demonstrated that EX/RP had outcomes comparable to antidepressants, but some evidence suggested that combined treatments may be preferable (Kobak, Greist, Jefferson, Katzelnick, & Henk, 1998). Other controlled trials have not shown that a combination of drugs and CBT (EX/RP) is superior to CBT alone (Van Balkom et al., 1998). Other reviewers have concluded that while both interventions are effective, neither results in complete remission of symptoms. CBT results in better overall outcomes, particularly when relapse rates, dropouts, and treatment refusers are considered. Relapse rates for those treated with medication alone, however, are considerably higher (Stanley & Turner, 1995). Much remains to be learned regarding what constitutes "best practice" for OCD, including more exploration of optimal treatment matching to client characteristics. It is likely that social work practitioners who employ CBT approaches will collaborate with psychiatrists to find the right combination on a case-by-case basis. EX/RP in combination with medication is currently considered the standard of care for OCD (Barletta, Beamish, Patrick, Andersen, & Pappas, 1996).

Exemplar Study: The Efficacy and Effectiveness of Exposure with Response Prevention.   Qualitative researchers often contend that the controlled conditions under which outcome research is conducted are not reflective of real-world practice. In partial response to these critics, M. E. Franklin et al. (2000) conducted a study to compare the effectiveness of EX/RP in a "service as usual" environment to results from four previously conducted controlled experiments. Participants were fifty-eight men and fifty-two women treated on a fee-for-service basis in a university-affiliated outpatient clinic. They ranged from eighteen to seventy-four years of age, and were almost all white. Forty percent were not taking medication at the time of the study. Outcome measures included the YBOCS, the Hamilton Depression Rating Scale, and the Beck Depression Inventory. All clients received EX/RP, including three treatment-planning sessions (information gathering, developing exposure hierarchy, education about OCD, and rationale for EX/RP), and fifteen sessions of EX/RP (including exercises, review of homework, and involvement of family and support people as determined by clinical judgment). Each session lasted for two hours, and treatment was conducted over the course of four weeks. Exposure exercises were "designed to trigger the patient's specific obsessional concerns. Patients were encouraged to persist with each exposure until the distress decreased noticeably. Exposure exercises were arranged hierarchically, beginning with the most distressing ones. Exposure exercises gradually progressed toward the most distressing situation or object, which was typically confronted during exposure session 6" (M. E. Franklin et al., 2000, p. 596). Clients were also assigned exposure homework for two hours between each daily session. They were instructed to refrain from engaging in their rituals throughout the entire treatment period. They were taught self-monitoring to become more aware of situations that triggered the urge to ritualize. If clients "slipped," therapists reviewed coping strategies with them. Clients were encouraged to seek help from support people or family members to resist ritualizing, or to call their practitioner for support and assistance.

All practitioners received training in EX/RP, but level of experience among the practitioners varied considerably. To offset this disparity, inexperienced practitioners received more supervision. Cases were assigned nonrandomly to practitioners. Eighty-six percent of treatment completers (100/110) improved significantly on three main outcome measures. The mean progress was comparable to results obtained in previous controlled trials. The study illustrates that the treatment context of clinical research may indeed be comparable to that of "natural" treatment environments.

Descriptions of Effective Interventions

A number of clinician-researchers have provided clear evidence-based guidelines for conducing EX/RP (Steketee, 1993; D. S. Riggs & Foa, 1993; Foa & Kozak, 1996). Although there are minor variations among authors, key treatment elements are synthesized below.

General Considerations.   The practitioner explains basic rationale for EX/RP to the client and conducts a detailed functional assessment of the client's obsessions and ritualized thoughts or behaviors. Clients are exposed progressively from the least anxiety-provoking item on the hierarchy to the most, as they successfully reduce their anxiety level at each predetermined stage. At each level, they are prevented from responding with their compulsive rituals until the anxiety subsides to a planned minimal level as measured on the SUDS. Although the EX/RP components are discussed separately below, they are implemented simultaneously. After the client has "conquered" the most anxiety-provoking obsession in the hierarchy, maximum EX/RP to the most troubling item is maintained over the remaining sessions. If this process is conducted frequently and long enough for the anxiety to subside during each exposure, the client stands a very good chance of overcoming this debilitating disorder.

EX/RP may be conducted in the office, in the natural environment, with or without the help of others, and with or without medication, depending on circumstances and client needs. The EX/RP plan is developed collaboratively during a detailed assessment, is tailored for the individual client, and often requires considerable creativity and ingenuity in its implementation.

Practitioners explain to clients all the details of the procedure. Family members, physicians, and others may collaborate in the treatment. These people should be in regular contact with the practitioner.

Here is the general format for this intervention. The first two or three sessions (which can last four to six hours, as needed) are devoted to a detailed examination of the client's obsessions and compulsions. About fifteen sessions will be required to complete the active EX/RP. By the eighth or tenth visit, the client should be receiving maximum exposure to the most anxiety-provoking step on the hierarchy. The sessions may last two hours or longer, often with two or more hours for homework to carry out the intervention alone or with the assistance of a supportive partner or other family member. Although this format may vary somewhat, case analysis suggests that intensive frequent visits are more effective than less-frequent visits. A typical session starts with ten to fifteen minutes for discussing homework and progress, but the bulk of the session is devoted to engaging in EX/RP. The last few minutes are devoted to discussing the next homework assignment.

Assessment.   Assuming the practitioner has conducted a thorough multidimensional assessment and identified or ruled out other co-occurring problems, one or two visits may be devoted to a detailed functional assessment of the type, frequency, intensity, and duration of obsessions and compulsions, and under what circumstances they occur. Obsessions are listed hierarchically from the least troubling to the most troubling. In each subsequent intervention, practitioner and client work "up the list" toward more anxiety-provoking stimuli. Confronting each anxiety-provoking stimulus (covertly or in vivo) is done in turn until the anxiety level for each one is substantially diminished, before moving on to the next objective on the list.

The practitioner helps the client develop and keep a chart or diary of thoughts or situations that provoke obsessional thinking and the subsequent compulsive ritual, gauge the degree of discomfort provoked by the obsessional thought, and measure the amount of time spent engaging in the compulsive ritual. The nature of these obsessional thoughts may be internal ("bad thoughts" about sex, harming someone, or having done something that, unrealistically, they feel might have caused harm to someone), external (concerns about "germs" from touching doorknobs, toilet seats, other people's hands), or concerns about safety (worrying about leaving on a lightbulb or the coffeemaker at home). Common themes may characterize these internal and external cues for people with OCD, but they are often highly idiosyncratic in their detail and meaning.

Keeping a chart or diary of obsessional concerns during the initial assessment continues to serve an important self-monitoring and evaluative function as clients track their own progress. By taking on this collaborative role in treatment, clients also begin to develop some autonomy and sense of control over their distress. They use the self-monitoring tool to guide their homework assignments and to measure progress.

During the assessment, the practitioner teaches the client how to use the SUDS. The level of distress associated with the feared thought or situation is measured at frequent intervals when they initially develop the fear hierarchy and, subsequently, when they are practicing the actual EX/RP. In this way, clients can judge and indicate their subjective level of distress for themselves, the practitioner, and a supportive assistant, and gauge how much progress they are making during the procedure.

Exposure.   During exposure, clients engage in and focus on the feared situation and exaggerate other "dirty" behaviors. Clients must then refrain from exercising the compulsion to undo, avoid the anxiety, or neutralize the obsessional thought until their distress subsides substantially (using the self-reported

SUDS based on a predetermined objective, say a drop from 80 to 30). The client should continue to move along the hierarchy only after each objective has been successfully achieved. Every five or ten minutes, the practitioner (or assistant) should ask the client what the anxiety level is (0–100). Although the amount of time the client can hold the exposure may vary, *it is critical that the exposure be prolonged and that it be maintained long enough for the anxiety to decrease significantly.*

In vivo exposure begins with the least anxiety-provoking situation and progresses gradually to the most anxiety-provoking situation usually within six to eight sessions. The most anxiety-producing items continue to be practiced for the remainder of treatment. Flexibility is key, as clients may need more or less time. As with exposure treatment in agoraphobia, the practitioner should gently but firmly push the client to expose to moderately or highly anxiety-provoking thoughts or situations. If the thought or situation is not sufficiently anxiety-provoking, they should move up the hierarchy to the next objective.

During exposure, the client's anxiety level can be periodically gauged every five or ten minutes by querying the client, and then applying anxiety coping skills that may include a cognitive challenge to the realistic degree of danger associated with the obsession, breathing or relaxation exercises, or some form of paradoxical intention such as an absurd exaggeration of the danger.

Although in vivo exposure is generally considered the most effective method, some clients may also benefit from imaginal exposure with or without the additional use of EX/RP in vivo, or as a warm-up to in vivo exposure. Although some clients find it hard to hold images in their mind's eye, the practitioner can assist them by painting a mental picture with them to re-create the anxiety-inducing situation. This part of the procedure can be done during the assessment phase when the practitioner carefully examines the nature of the obsessions and compulsive rituals. As with in vivo exposure, more anxiety-provoking scenes are generated gradually for imaginal exposure. The intervention process is similar to in vivo: develop a hierarchy, construct the scenes, expose clients to the mental pictures, and monitor clients' efforts to use behavioral or mental neutralizing techniques as compulsions to reduce their anxiety. This procedure should last most of the two-hour session, and the SUDS should be used every five to ten minutes.

Response Prevention.   Response prevention requires that the practitioner and client devise a way to block the response, which may include compulsive thoughts and behaviors. Covert or subtle compulsions such as subvocalizations, ritualistic blinking, or magical hand gestures must be identified and neutralized so as to not undermine the effectiveness of the exposure. Of course, the compulsive behavior may also be quite overt, such as repeated hand washing, or tapping loudly in specific numerical patterns. Regardless of the type of compulsion, however, *it is critical that maximum response prevention be employed.* Although a graduated approach to response prevention may be necessary initially, allowing progressively less response, maximum response prevention is the ultimate goal. Partial response prevention may actually make the problem worse by reinforcing the compulsion. Response prevention is planned at the same time that the fear hierarchy is planned, and the practitioner should anticipate sabotage such as subtle or covert minirituals, teach the supportive assistant to watch out for these, and as the client progresses through the hierarchy, eventually fade the intervention out.

Practitioner and client should estimate how far they are likely to progress in the hierarchy for each session, although this can be adjusted as needed. New situations can be added as things progress. Clients should be encouraged gently but firmly to expose themselves to situations that are challenging for them, but practitioners should avoid being overly ambitious or impatient. In general, the more autonomy a client takes during treatment, the better. The point of intervention is for clients to take as much control of resolving this problem as they can, and maintain gains over time. In other words, expose the client, check the anxiety level, wait, and urge the client to go further.

The typical session involves a review of the homework assignment and a detailed report of the success of the response prevention (i.e., time spent on homework, exposures accomplished, anxiety responses to exposures). Were there any violations? If so, have the client describe them. What obstacles got in the way of successfully completing the EX/RP homework? Did the client take any shortcuts or sabotage the response prevention? Did the client use any subtle neutralizing thoughts or behaviors to reduce anxiety? Generally, in addition to the time spent conducting procedure with the practitioner, it is recommended that clients continue practicing EX/RP for an additional two hours on their own (or with an agreed-upon support person), for a total of at least four hours of exposure treatment per day. It is agreed from the start that clients are restricted from engaging in all compulsive rituals during treatment. For example, "washers" are not permitted to wash beyond a timed shower (say every two or three days), and only one check of lights and appliances is permitted for compulsive checkers when they leave the house.

Toward the end of the intervention, a home visit can be used to reinforce gains and to assess subtle attempts to avoid the full exposure. The practitioner should also note the behavior of other family members to see if they are helping or unwittingly hindering the client's progress. Active intervention (EX/RP) should be carried out to solidify gains in the client's home environment, often the site of compulsive ritualizing.

After clients have succeeded in reducing anxiety and eliminating ritual responses, the practitioner should gradually disengage from involvement with them. Clients gradually take control of the treatment by doing more on their own, and practitioner and client should develop a follow-up maintenance plan. Supportive sessions or occasional booster visits may help solidify gains for the long run. At that point, clients may turn their attention to other problems in their life. Since EX/RP was never offered as an intervention that would solve all their problems or forever inoculate them against other difficulties, other interventions such as interpersonal psychotherapy, couples therapy, or cognitive therapy may be required.

IMPLEMENTING AND EVALUATING THE EVIDENCE-BASED INTERVENTION PLAN

CASE STUDY: GEORGE

George, a thirty-four-year-old married white man, arrived at the local mental health clinic with his wife Jan, thirty-two. He decided to come in for a long-standing problem that had recently gotten worse. In the waiting room, George decided, after a brief discussion, to come in alone, and Jan suggested that she might join him later in some sessions if it would be helpful. In the first visit, George was quite forthcoming about his troubles. Although he discussed in a somewhat roundabout manner, he finally got to the point: "I've been having a lot of trouble with an old problem. It has been taking me a long time to get home from work. Although my job is only 20 minutes away from home, I've been taking almost an hour and a half, almost two hours sometimes. Whenever I hear a bump in the road in my pickup truck, I am fearful that I have hit someone, a pedestrian, and even though I know rationally I have not hit anyone, I have to stop the truck and get out and look around to make sure I did not. Sometimes I have to make myself leave even though I cannot be 100% certain that I did not hit someone. I lie awake at night worried that in the newspapers the next morning they will report that a body was found off the side of the road in that area. This would make me think that I had actually hit and killed

someone, but the body went flying and I could not find it during dusk." When the social worker, Ted, inquired how long this had been going on, George indicated that he had been all right for a few years, since his two little girls came along (they are four and six). "Since I am responsible for them and working hard to keep up, I have not had much time to think about this old problem."

The "old problem" apparently was a repeated obsession that he had been responsible for the death of a young boy who was hit and killed by the car George's father was driving when George was a young boy himself. The boy had come down a hill through a stop sign onto the main road near their home in the early evening. The child appeared without warning, and George's father could not avoid hitting him. He never even hit the brakes. George, eight years old at the time, always remembered that he and his father were talking and laughing when the accident occurred, and felt that he must have distracted his dad and was, therefore, at fault. He had overheard his father say when the police arrived, "I was just talking with my son, and turned my head and there was this kid on a bicycle right in front of us." George always thought his father secretly blamed him for this. His dad was depressed for some time after that, and drank more heavily than usual. He recalls that he would come downstairs, and his dad would be talking to himself, angrily sometimes, as though arguing with someone. George said his dad was never the same after that, and he died of a heart attack a few years later.

At his dad's funeral, someone said to George, who was then twelve, "You're the man now ... you've got to be responsible ... be good and help out your mother and sisters." The neighbors and parish priests tried to be helpful, but George always felt that he needed to "take care of things" in a way most of his friends didn't understand. His mother, "a religious fanatic ... made sure I went to church every Sunday, and made me go to confession every week. I never felt like I could confess everything adequately, and felt guilty for overlooking things. I was afraid of having thoughts about sex, and I couldn't talk to anyone about it. As I got older I worked hard in school, but knew I had to get a job to help myself if I wanted to have a car or get money for college. My friends thought I was too serious, and I usually felt like I didn't fit in with them. I kind of forgot the incident as I got older, I guess, because I kept myself pretty busy. I drank a lot in college, but a couple of years after I got out, I stopped for a while. In the last few years I've started having a few again on the weekends. If I get drunk once in a while, it seems to quiet the noise in my head. I didn't think it would be any harm. I am captain of my bowling team, and we like to knock back a few during the games. I get on their case when they don't show up for practices on time or don't do their part with the equipment and so forth. They tell me to lighten up and don't take it so seriously. I got the job in the post office when I was twenty-five. It seemed like a steady thing, a secure job. It's boring sometimes, and the people in my location don't work too hard, but there's not much I can do about it."

"A few months ago, I heard that a guy in another post office got drunk and hit a kid and sent him to the hospital. For some reason I've started thinking about the old incident again, and my concern that I've hit something or someone when I'm driving just started up, like some kind of trigger was switched on. The problem I'm having is that I can't stop these thoughts, and I can't stop myself from stopping the truck and getting out to look and see it someone is lying in the road. I know these thoughts are crazy, but I can't make myself believe it. Sometimes I just go home, and go down in the basement to hide from my wife and kids and cry. I can't stand the stress it's causing me. I worry about every report in the morning paper, every accident or body they found, and I have to find out exactly where it was, and whether it could possibly have been me. I can't take this anymore. It's making me think about killing myself. It takes the fun out of everything I'm doing. I have a great wife and two beautiful little girls and I'm miserable most of the time. I can't stop thinking about this. I can't sleep. You gotta help me."

Multidimensional-Functional Assessment: Defining Problems and Goals

Although the content of George's obsessional thinking seemed triggered by a past event, a thorough assessment of the functional patterns of the obsession and compulsive checking was done. George appeared to meet the criteria for an OCD diagnosis, but his depressive symptoms and episodic binge drinking were significant as well. He seemed very tense much of the time. He reported trouble sleeping, and was irritable with coworkers. He also discussed "responsibility" as a recurrent theme in several areas of his life, and was often characterized by his friends as the "serious one" of the group.

Important relationships in his life appeared to be satisfying and going well. He and his wife loved each other, and their two children were doing well. At times he was overbearing at home, however, making sure "rules" about cleaning up and so forth were adhered to. When he was feeling particularly edgy and obsessing a lot, he was hard to approach and critical of those around him, sometimes alienating his wife for the day, and being a little harsh asking his daughters to behave themselves. His job was steady, and he had no immediate financial concerns. He was in good health.

He described his upbringing as "strict," although he felt that his parents had loved him. He had always had a hard time letting himself "off the hook" from relatively minor mistakes. His recent experience with obsessive-compulsive symptoms was not altogether new. Upon further examination, it became evident that he had, off and on, experienced an array of compulsive behaviors since he was young: compulsive blinking or ritualistic praying under his breath to ward off guilty feelings about "bad thoughts" as a young teenager (the old priest had told him not to think about sex or to masturbate unless he was ready to spend eternity in the fires of hell). This new twist on an already overwrought sense of responsibility was enough to cause additional compulsions to ward off guilt. These symptoms were exacerbated during times of stress in his life, and further marginalized him from ordinary social experiences such as dating, dances, proms, and other normative social activities.

A careful functional analysis of his presenting symptoms and reemergence of his compulsions seemed to connect several things: an increase in stress at work as a result of "efficiency" changes, an increase in drinking on weekends, and the report that one of his coworkers in another location (who was apparently driving under the influence of alcohol) had hit a child in a car accident. The child later died. Upon hearing this report, George was filled with anxiety and felt as though he were going to pass out. He took a break, and went out and sat in his truck for a few minutes, going over and over in his mind the last time he drove home on Saturday evening after having four or five beers over a two-hour period after a bowling-league tournament game. He felt flushed and panicky trying to remember if he had heard any "bumps" on the way home. Since the tournament was over two weeks ago with no adverse reports of accidents since then in that area of town, he was able to calm himself down to a point where he could go back inside to work. But the feeling lingered. His reaction to the news of his coworker's accident had been so acute that Ted began to think that George might also be suffering from post-traumatic stress.

On his way home from work, George began to think about the accident again, and started to observe every sound emanating from the suspension system in his old truck. It was dusk, and if he ever wanted to avoid feeling that sense of guilt again, he thought that he had better be exceptionally careful on the way home. Over the next couple of weeks, the sounds he heard, whether driving through the busy downtown area near work or on more rural road out of town, were enough to make him think something had happened. He began to stop the truck and look around "just to make sure" nothing had happened. This experience began to happen more often and took up considerable time on his way home. He didn't do this in the morning. He seemed to be able to shake off these thoughts in order to get to work on time. But at the end of the day, he found himself more keyed up on the way home.

Jan began to wonder what the problem was, but George made excuses and was not comfortable talking about it. After a couple of weeks, Jan became anxious about his evasiveness, began to think there was a problem, and confronted him about it. George responded angrily that "everybody needs to get off my back" and attacked her verbally, saying he was doing everything he could as a father and husband and she should just trust him. This outburst and the undisclosed reason for his lateness created a "cold war" atmosphere for about a week. George's struggles worsened. It seemed that the more he stopped his truck and looked around, the more obsessional he became, the more the thoughts bothered him, and relations with Jan were not getting better. One night he couldn't contain his feelings anymore and told her. He sobbed uncontrollably, saying he couldn't live like this anymore. Jan began to understand the problem. She thought he had left these problems behind long ago.

With the multidimensional assessment as backdrop, the practitioner and George developed a hypothetical summation of the problem: When under stress, George began to ruminate about being responsible for events beyond his control. Automatically he began to think, "What have I done, what could I have done differently?" His belief that he could undo or neutralize these troubling, anxiety-provoking thoughts by thoroughly checking every move he made was a long-standing problem. The argument for his guilt was unassailable: he could never completely disprove that he had harmed someone. However, the more he tried to prove that nothing happened while he was driving home, the harder it was for him to keep from stopping to look and double-check that he didn't hit anyone. He became increasingly anxious and despondent, began to drink more (which exacerbated his depression, anxiety level, and obsessional thinking), and became more alienated from those who could comfort and support him, especially his wife. This made him feel more isolated and guilty.

Ted and George decided that they had to address this problem directly. After a long discussion and examination of the developmental contributions to George's current difficulties, George knew he had to let go of this old way of dealing with his troubles and develop better ways of coping with his troubled feelings and daily stressors. He knew intellectually that the guilt was completely irrational and that the compulsive checking was futile. He could never resolve his anxieties by checking. He even laughed when he recounted the stories he made up to cover himself when one of his friends stopped to help him on the side of the road. "If they knew what I was really up to, they would think I was crazy."

After a couple of visits, George seemed a bit more at ease with himself and with the practitioner. Ted described to George how EX/RP works. He also suggested that George stop drinking for a while, at least until the obsessional symptoms and compulsive checking subsided. George agreed to try and felt that he probably would not have problem with abstaining, because he drank only on weekends. He also agreed to discuss these symptoms with a psychiatrist and at least consider taking medication if the physician thought it was indicated. George said that he understood the gist of the intervention and wanted to "get to work" as soon as possible. They then developed a hierarchy that gradually detailed the types of sounds that would trigger George's anxiety-ridden obsessive thoughts and his need to check out what happened. It seemed to occur only when was driving alone in his old pickup truck. The strength of the compulsion to check would depend on the type and force of the sound that heard. In general, the sounds ranged from minor sounds that he could sometimes overlook (like the sound of a small stone banging under the wheel well), to a louder "clunk," such as a branch hitting the bottom of the truck, or a loud bang like the sound an old suspension makes when you hit a pothole at a fairly good rate of speed. His anxious responses to these various sounds were rated on the SUDS. To hit a maximum of 100, there would have to be a loud bang and several people in the vicinity, say on a busy downtown street. It also became apparent that the sound did not have to emanate directly (he assumed) from the truck, but could be a loud noise produced nearby. In George's way of thinking, he could not *guarantee* that it did not come from his truck; therefore, he had to confirm it. His goal was to reduce his SUDS score to below 20; at that point, he felt he could "shake them off" and not have to check out each noise.

Selecting and Designing the Intervention: Defining Strategies and Objectives

The implementation of the EX/RP plan began right away (table 7.2). In order for George to implement it, however, he agreed to have his wife accompany him a few times, at least in the beginning. After a couples session, where the procedure was described and Jan's role explained, they were ready to start.

However, since George could not systematically and progressively control the loudness of the sounds that would occur, he would have to be prepared to pull off the road and maintain his exposure (tolerating the fact that he had heard the noise) without responding to it by getting out of the truck and checking

TABLE 7.2   The Client Service Plan for George

Problems	Goals	Sample Objectives	Interventions	Assessment Tools
Anxiety, guilty obsessional thinking about having struck pedestrians with his truck	Reduce, eliminate anxiety regarding the dysfunctional thinking	Read short manual and watch brief film on what OCD is and how EX/RP works	Relationship building: develop an atmosphere of openness and trust so he can commit to the treatment plan	SUDS to gauge progress with level of fear
Compulsive checking to confirm whether he had actually struck any one; moderately debilitating, spending up to 2 hours daily struggling with the compulsion	Eliminate obsessional thoughts and checking behaviors	Practice imaginal exposure daily at home for at least half an hour	Psychoeducation regarding the nature of OCD and how EX/RP works; include his wife in the discussions and implementation as a supportive assistant	Periodic assessment with OCI Other indicators of quality of life
Depression: trouble sleeping, thoughts of hopelessness, suicidal thoughts	Reduce depressive symptoms; further assessment needed	Practice in vivo EX/RP daily for 2–4 hours. First week accompanied by wife; second week alone	Incorporate SUDS in the functional assessment during the development of the hierarchy of fears (i.e., loudness of sounds while driving)	
Interpersonal trouble: irritability with wife and others at work; possibly related to his struggles with guilt-ridden obsessional thinking	Improve his ability to readily express his feelings to his wife and children; ask wife for support when he is troubled	Keep diary of progress daily for both imaginal and in vivo exposure	Teach imaginal exposure and relaxation exercises as preparation for in vivo exposure	
Episodic excessive alcohol use, mostly on weekends; reports drinking to cope with anxious obsessional thinking	Abstinence for now, pending further assessment after OCD symptoms have abated	Talk to wife daily about progress he is making with his difficulties	Daily (2–4 hours) in vivo exposure while driving Referral for psychiatric evaluation for possible antidepressants Lifestyle changes: increase aerobic exercise to reduce generalized anxiety and depression	

what happened. For two prolonged two-hour sessions, George agreed to "warm up" with imaginal exposure sessions to prepare for in vivo exposure. The social worker prepared George by teaching him relaxation exercises accompanied by deep breathing. He also learned to use a mantra, "Nothing happened, everyone is fine," to challenge the obsessional thought that he had struck someone with his truck. Gradually, Ted presented the obsession-inducing stimuli in ascending order of intensity, and when George indicated that he had the image in mind, Ted directed him to imagine sitting in his truck as if traffic had come to a stop. In his mind's eye he would have to remain sitting in his truck looking forward (not checking in his mirrors) and practice his deep breathing and his mantra. As they traveled up the hierarchy, George became increasingly anxious (after the sound of a large "bang" was inserted into the image). He shifted uncomfortably in his chair and was not breathing in a slow, relaxed way. The practitioner asked him his level of SUDS, which was 80. At that point, the social worker directed George to breathe deeply, focus on his mantra, and maintain the image in his mind. They sat for at least thirty minutes, and Ted occasionally requested a reading of George's SUDS. Gradually, the rating declined to 30. Ted directed George to practice this imaginal exercise daily at home an hour each night, with extra practice on the weekends (for at least two hours). After a week of covert desensitization, they decided to begin in vivo EX/RP.

Jan agreed to meet George at work every day for the next week and drive home with him in the truck. To get the process rolling, after that, George would be on his own, but they would go out together after he got home and on weekends for extra practice. Ted explained that the EX/RP would have to be done intensely and in a prolonged way in order to work. Jan and George met after work daily, and Jan (who was trained by Ted to be the coach) was prepared to assist George by sitting with him as he pulled to the side of the road after he heard a "40 or better" sounds. She would guide him in practicing his relaxation without getting out of the truck to check on what happened. He found this very difficult at first and, sobbing, begged Jan to tell him if anything had happened. Of course, Jan had been instructed not to reassure him, since she would be reinforcing the compulsive need to check. Jan, upset, called the practitioner one night and told him it was hard to see George suffer, and she didn't know if she could continue. Ted encouraged her not to give up and said that if she stuck with it for a few more days, George would begin to get some relief from his suffering and she would see some positive results.

The exposure sessions continued, and after a few days, George was breathing better during EX/RP even after some of the loudest bangs. He felt that he was ready to try it alone. The following week he was able to maintain exposure without checking, although he did find himself peeking in the mirror now and then, but eventually he curtailed that too. (Later on, when he had full control after even the loudest noises, he resumed checking "one time" as would be considered normal for responsible driving.) After one week of covert exposure and three weeks of daily in vivo exposure for about two hours a day (plus weekends), George felt as though he was over the worst of it. In addition to the in vivo exposure, George had eliminated his drinking during this time, was sleeping better, and was taking an antidepressant, which he felt may have begun to work. Ted agreed that this was an excellent beginning, but some follow-up was in order to prevent backsliding. In addition to continuing his self-guided EX/RP on the way home from work for an hour each day, George wanted to work on becoming a more relaxed and fun person with his wife and kids, and "not so serious all the time."They agreed to meet weekly in couples sessions, since George agreed that his marriage would be a good vehicle for addressing some of his interpersonal concerns. Other lifestyle changes included one or two beers on the weekends only after he discontinued his medication, and only if his OCD symptoms were well under control. He would avoid the use of alcohol to "quiet the noise" again. In addition (since he agreed that bowling could not be considered serious exercise) he decided to start running again, three times a week, to reduce generalized anxiety symptoms. Overall, his long-term prospects looked good, and he knew that he could always return for a booster session if he felt that his obsessions were coming back to haunt him.

Selecting Scales and Creating Indexes to Monitor and Evaluate Client Progress

To gauge his progress, George, Jan, and Ted relied primarily on George's self-anchored subjective level of distress (table 7.2). Later, he relied on the number of days that went by when he felt relatively trouble-free. Scores on the OCI were also checked periodically with the practitioner. As George improved, however, qualitative indicators began to tell the broader benefits of the relief he began to feel: his ability to laugh and have fun again with his kids and his friends, his general feeling of ease and lightness in his life, his lack of preoccupation with depressing thoughts, and, best of all, a renewed sense of intimacy with his wife, who didn't give up on him during treatment.

SUMMARY

Helping clients with serious anxiety disorders is very challenging and very gratifying. These disorders cause enormous suffering for millions of people. Social workers who learn exposure-based interventions for these and other anxiety disorders will find that their clinical skills are used to the maximum. Clients often suffer from other co-occurring problems as well. However, clients with anxiety disorders will not take the necessary risks to get better unless they feel the practitioner is competent and confident. The practitioner must give the client hope when dealing with what are often long-standing problems. Case management skills are often required to coordinate interventions that sometimes include collaborations with physicians, paraprofessionals, and social supports in the family and community.

CHAPTER 8

POST-TRAUMATIC STRESS DISORDER

Participation in combat, enduring torture, witnessing a killing, victimization by crime, escaping an attack on one's life, experiencing a terrorist bombing, surviving a natural disaster, suffering domestic violence, and victimization by sexual assault are all horrific events. Any one of them can have serious long-term negative effects on the psychological and social well-being of an adult or a child. These events are generally understood to be extreme psychological experiences, and many people have experienced at least one such traumatic event in their lives. Although many resilient people rebound from such experiences by virtue of innate temperament, ongoing social supports, or other protective factors, many people suffer from the residual effects of these stressful events for years. The cluster of anxiety-related symptoms and behaviors that include arousal, reexperiencing the traumatic event, and avoiding stimuli that remind the person of the event is referred to as post-traumatic stress disorder (PTSD).

Much of what was learned about assessment and treatment of anxiety disorders is directly applicable to evidence-based practice with traumatized people. Due to the nature of traumatic events and their effects, however, assessment and intervention with PTSD have unique aspects. Assessment of PTSD demands the standard multidimensional overview of a client's well-being as well as a thorough functional analysis linking key antecedents in everyday life to the worsening or improvement in the client's symptoms. Although working with people who suffer from PTSD is challenging, this condition has a good chance of responding favorably to CBT that includes some form of prolonged exposure to the thoughts or situations that provoke disabling anxiety.

ASSESSMENT

Background Data

Four major studies have provided PTSD researchers with a base for estimating the prevalence, consequences, and costs of PTSD. These include the National Comorbidity Survey (Kessler et al., 1995); F. H. Norris' survey (1990) of 1,000 persons in the southeastern United States; Resnick, Kilpatrick, Dansky, Saunders, and Best's telephone survey (1993) with a national sample of 4,008 women; and

190

Breslau, Davis, Andreski, & Peterson's survey (1991) of 1,007 adults. Although data-collection methods and measures varied, results demonstrated that 60–70% of people surveyed reported having experienced at least one traumatic event in their lifetime. However, the fact that someone has experienced a traumatic event does not doom them to develop PTSD. Factors that mediate whether someone develops the disorder include the nature and severity of the stressful event, its cognitive appraisal and interpretation, the inherent resiliency or vulnerability of the person, and the responsiveness and quality of social supports post-trauma. Lifetime prevalence of PTSD has been estimated to be 7.8% in the population, with 10.4% in women and 5.0% in men (Kessler et al.). Thus, large proportions of the population are exposed to traumatic events, and many of them demonstrate signs and symptoms associated with PTSD (Kilpatrick, Resnick, Saunders, & Best, 1998; Kilpatrick, Saunders, Veronen, Best, & Von, 1987). Costs associated with the effects of traumatic events have been estimated in the hundreds of billions of dollars (S. D. Solomon & Davidson, 1997).

In the twentieth century, war-related trauma (shell shock) encountered during World War I focused attention on the psychological effects of exposure to intense bombardment and associated death and dismemberment, and brought this condition into the realm of medical interest. This work continued after World War II and set the stage for a more formal recognition of PTSD as a psychiatric disorder (Keane, 1998). The National Vietnam Veterans Readjustment Study (NVVRS) was initiated in the mid-1980s to compensate for the methodological limitations of previous efforts to determine the effects of combat-related service in Vietnam. Its strategy was to measure premilitary-service, military-service, and postmilitary-service factors and their relationship to the psychosocial well-being of veterans years after service. The goals of the study (Kulka et al., 1988), which was funded by the Department of Veterans Affairs, were to determine the prevalence of PTSD and other psychological disorders that might have occurred as a result of participation in the Vietnam War, to examine the current life adjustment of individuals who participated in the war, and to study factors related to the development of PTSD (Keane, 1998).

The study revealed that veterans who served in the Vietnam theater were estimated to have rates of PTSD about six times as great (15.2% for men, 8.5% for women) as other veterans who served during the Vietnam era (2.5% for men, 1.1% for women), compared with rates for the civilian population at 1.2% for men, and 0.3% for women. Lifetime prevalence rates for Vietnam-theater veterans were 30.9% for men and 26.9% for women. PTSD rates for those who experienced low to moderate stress were 8.5% for men, 2.5% women, and for high war-zone stress, 35.8% for men and 17.5% for women. These differences were significant even after controlling for a wide range of demographic and other psychiatric and psychosocial measures. A range of other psychosocial disorders also accompanied a diagnosis of PTSD. These included substance abuse, marital and family adjustment problems, unemployment, and homelessness. Clearly, the data revealed that symptoms were directly related to the severity of the stressor.

It is important to remember that combat veterans were not the only victims of war. A fairly extensive literature has been compiled on the effects of war-related trauma and atrocities on civilians in Southeast Asia. The effects of war, imprisonment, loss of homeland, torture, traumatic emigration experiences, and dislocation resulted in a higher than expected range of psychiatric disorders, including PTSD, depression, and substance abuse. Many immigrants from Southeast Asia continue to suffer from mental health disturbances related to wartime trauma (e.g., B. E. Carlson & Russer-Hogan, 1991; O' Hare & Tran, 1998).

PTSD symptoms are generally more prevalent and more severe in women (J. Wolfe & Kimerling, 1997). F. H. Norris (1992) examined traumatic exposure in a large sample (*n* = 1,000) of men and women, and revealed that women were more likely to have suffered sexual assault, but men were more likely to have suffered from automobile accidents, physical assault, and combat exposure. Although men experienced higher rates of exposure to traumatic events in general, women suffered more severe symptoms overall, much of it associated with having been sexually assaulted. Among those who were victims of crime, women suffered more symptoms than men. Resnick et al. (1993) interviewed a random sample of over 4,000 Americans by phone, and found that 69% of women reported exposure to traumatic events, and 36% reported exposure to sexual or aggravated assault or the homicide of a close friend or family member. The overall sample showed a prevalence for lifetime PTSD of 12.3%, and rates were much higher for those who had been victimized by crime (26.0%) as compared to non-crime events (9.0%). Although rates of PTSD appear to be very high following a completed rape (greater than 90%), almost half of the victims show considerable remission of symptoms three months after the event (Rothbaum, Foa, Riggs, Murdock, & Walsh, 1992). Women with preexisting psychiatric difficulties were also more likely to develop PTSD symptoms after the traumatic event.

Rape as Traumatic Event

Rape is generally underreported because respondents do not respond in the affirmative when asked if they have been raped even though the event may meet the legal definition. In addition, victims often know the perpetrators and are reluctant to identify them and press charges. Rates of rape across studies vary because of inconsistencies in definitions of rape as well as the varying sensitivity of screening questions for identifying rape (Koss, 1993). Rape is one of the more frequent risk factors for PTSD in women because it often involves additional physical injury or even threat to life, and some women have been raped multiple times. As traumatic as rape is for a woman, however, the event does not inevitably result in long-term emotional disability. Rothbaum et al. (1992) studied the course of PTSD symptoms in ninety-five women assessed several days after they had been sexually assaulted. Although most met PTSD criteria soon after the event, about half gradually showed reduction in symptoms to subdiagnostic levels. Those who did not improve by the first month (postrape), showed little improvement afterward. Symptoms of rape-related distress included intrusive thoughts and images, anxiety, and depression. The authors demonstrated that those less likely to improve were identified soon after the sexual assault, based on scores on the Rape Aftermath Symptom Test and the Impact of Events Scale (IES). A host of factors will mediate the likelihood of developing PTSD, including early childhood neglect and abuse (including sexual abuse), substance abuse, history of other psychopathology, history of multiple violent events, and a history of inordinate physical and social risk taking (i.e., sensation seeking).

In addition to rape, other crimes have been shown to be a precipitant for the development of PTSD (Kilpatrick & Resnick, 1993). Criminal victimization is a relatively common occurrence, and rates of victimization are generally higher than those reflected in government statistics. Rates of PTSD are higher for those who have been raped as compared with other crimes. Substantial proportions of Americans are subjected to crimes against their persons, including rape and other physical assaults (Bisson & Shepherd, 1995). Psychological reactions to having been victimized by a crime are often similar to those of people who experience PTSD symptoms, and victims of crime are more likely than accident victims to manifest these symptoms three months after the event. Kilpatrick et al. (1987) interviewed 391 adult females from South Carolina about lifetime criminal victimization experiences, crime-reporting behavior, and psychological impact. More than 75% of the women reported having been victimized by a crime. Of all 547 crimes reported, almost half (49%) were sexual assaults, and 38.6% were burglaries. Over half of these crimes were not reported to the police. A subsequent analysis of the same sample (Kilpatrick et al., 1989) demonstrated that the development of crime-related PTSD (in about 20% of the crime victims) was predicted by age (younger women were more likely to develop symptoms), number of years since the crime occurred, having sustained a physical injury, having perceived threat of serious harm or death when the crime was being committed, and having been a victim of a completed rape. As with other traumatic events, the effects of having been victimized by a crime depended on a host of factors, particularly the degree to which one feared for one's life.

PTSD and Co-occurring Disorders

Most people with PTSD also have at least one other psychiatric disorder, and the prevalence of co-occurring disorders is similar for men and women (Kessler et al., 1995) Many problems co-occur with PTSD, including depression, anxiety, substance abuse, and somatization disorders as well as other functional psychosocial impairments that affect life at home and work. PTSD symptoms are also related to medical problems, particularly for women who have been sexually assaulted. Determining the time line for sequencing the development of these symptoms is more difficult, although it appears that a history of anxiety and depressive disorders may signal an increased risk of PTSD. Risks for direct personal exposure to traumatic events are increased for people who have a prior history of depression and substance abuse (Breslau, Davis, Andreski, Federman, & Anthony, 1998).

Recently, more attention has been given to the relatively common co-occur-rence of PTSD and substance abuse. Although it appears intuitively appealing that substance abuse develops as a way of coping with the physiological arousal that accompanies PTSD (the self-medication hypothesis), the relationship is actu-ally more complex (Hoffman & Sasaki, 1997; Stewart, 1996). Despite methodol-ogy limitations in the research, evidence is emerging that

- traumatic events and PTSD symptoms correlate directly with substance abuse;
- PTSD symptoms tend to precede a substance-abuse problem;
- those who drink following a traumatic event are more likely to do so episodically;
- symptom severity may be directly related to substance abuse;
- substance abuse may not only enhance the readiness of a person to expe-rience a traumatic event (e.g., have a car accident in which the drinker's passenger dies), but also physiologically prime the person to develop PTSD as a result of the event;
- PTSD symptoms may exacerbate existing substance abuse or precipitate the development of substance abuse;
- both disorders may share common causal factors (genetic or environmen-tal);
- the person's response to trauma may be more related to alcohol abuse than to exposure to the trauma itself; and
- although PTSD symptoms appear to precede the onset of problem drink-ing, the interrelationship is so complex and reciprocal in that withdrawal symptoms from abuse tend to exacerbate anxiety, depression, and other related symptoms serving to maintain the cycle of alcohol abuse and PTSD symptoms.

To quote Stewart (1996, p. 102): "It appears that a single unidirectional pathway to explain the overlap between PTSD and alcohol abuse is unlikely to be found. Instead, it seems possible that both self-medication and alcohol intoxication or withdrawal-induced intensification of PTSD symptoms contribute to the high degree of co-morbidity between alcohol abuse and PTSD diagnoses."

Theories

At the turn of the nineteenth century, psychoanalytic theories paved the way for the exploration of psychological trauma and its effects. "Hysterical neuroses" (S. Freud, 1966; J. Herman, 1992) were generally attributed to the failure of the indi-vidual to successfully repress infantile sexual impulses. However, psychoanalytic theorists have argued over the years whether hysterical neurosis is the result of actual childhood sexual seduction or unconscious fantasy on the part of the patient (J. Herman, 1992; Horowitz, 1997). These debates were accompanied by a lack of empirical evidence, which contributed to decades of confusion about the validity of a causal link between childhood sexual abuse and the development of future psychopathology. Nevertheless, some continue to opine that the causes of the development of future psychopathology of various kinds lie predominantly in the lack of "secure attachment" or other failures of parental nurturance during early childhood that would otherwise have provided a buffer, presumably, against future mental illnesses, including PTSD (Finkelhor & Browne, 1985; J. Herman, 1992; Van der Kolk, Weisaeth, & Van der Hart, 1996). It is asserted that traumatic events appear to interfere with a child's ability to regulate arousal level (through adequate functioning of the ego and its defenses), which may lead to problems in learning, mood regulation, aggression, and other interpersonal difficulties. Most of these theories, however, have often been based on post hoc analysis of case studies and correlational data between childhood experiences and adult psychopathology. More recently, longitudinal studies have looked for a causal connection between early childhood trauma and adult psychopathology, but these studies either do not consider the relative predictive power of childhood experiences within the context of other psychosocial influences over time, or they make unsubstantiated inferences regarding factors and causal links that could be explained more parsimoniously.

Although childhood victimization such as physical and sexual abuse or related forms of neglect appears to increase the risk for adult psychopathology (including PTSD), retrospective diagnosis is fraught with complexity, ambiguity, and reliability problems. Cathy Spatz Widom (1998, p. 81) is articulate about the complexities inherent in drawing cause-effect inferences about adult psychopathology from childhood data.

> Childhood experiences such as physical and sexual abuse and neglect are adverse events with immediate and long-term consequences. However, in considering child abuse and neglect as examples of adverse life events that have the potential to affect development and subsequent psychopathology, the assumption of well-being in the child's life prior to the victimization experience may not be a reasonable one. Although certain forms of childhood victimization may indeed be viewed as acute stressors, child abuse and neglect often occur against a background of more chronic adversity in multi-problem homes. Child abuse and neglect may be only one of the family's problems. Thus, the general effects of other family characteristics, such as poverty, unemployment, parental alcoholism or drug problems, or other inadequate social and family functioning, must be recognized and disentangled from the specific effects of childhood abuse and neglect.

Sorting out the effects of child abuse from other past and current contributing factors is difficult for clinicians and researchers alike. Clinicians should be cautious about attributing all adolescent or adult clients' complaints to their child-abuse history lest they overlook important contributing factors and co-occurring problems that may be more amenable to effective intervention.

Long-term outcomes of child abuse may also depend largely on other contextual factors, that is, how others respond to it at the time, including the response of the criminal justice and social service systems. Those surrounding the child can buffer or exacerbate the effects of the traumatic event itself. Much more needs to be established regarding the long-term effects of childhood victimization. It is likely, as with most of the problems addressed in this text, that the long-term consequences are the result of multiple interacting biological, psychosocial, and environmental factors that take a variety of developmental pathways.

Stress-environment theories are much needed to provide a "horizontal" complement to the "vertical" view of developmental pathology as a predictive model of PTSD. Multivariate theories now provide a more complete framework for understanding the complex linkages between traumatic events and PTSD symptoms. It has been well-established that a range of life stressors predispose people to greater health and mental health risks (see Dohrenwend, 1998, for relevant reviews). Although one should not underestimate the potential consequences of childhood abuse or other past traumas, chronic daily stressors may even be more predictive of adult disorders (Wheaton, 1994).

Problems abound with the developmental-diagnostic view as applied to PTSD. First, what constitutes traumatic versus nontraumatic is highly variable (Shalev, 1996). Second, the vast majority of people exposed to extreme stressors do not develop PTSD (A. C. McFarlane & Yehuda, 1996; Resnick et al., 1993; Shalev, 1996). Most acute trauma symptoms remit soon after the event, thus making acute symptoms poor predictors of who will manifest PTSD symptoms later. Conversely, PTSD symptoms can result from distressing but relatively common occurrences such as a nonfatal automobile accident. Third, symptoms associated with PTSD are generally not unique to this disorder (D. W. King, Leskin, King, & Weathers, 1998; A. C. McFarlane & Girolamo, 1996). The symptoms overlap considerably with depression, anxiety, somatization, and personality disorders, and co-occur with medical illnesses as well (M. Friedman, 1997). Fourth, factors that predict the development of the disorder may have less to do with traumatic events themselves and more to do with individual differences in appraisal of traumatic events, differences such as personality (e.g., negative worrying style) and gender (women are more likely to be diagnosed with PTSD despite lower exposure to traumatic events; Bowman, 1999). Perhaps the traumatic events acted as a precipitating trigger for other psychological vulnerabilities related to various other causes. This variability in the link between traumatic events and the development of PTSD may account, in part, for some of the inconsistent findings in the effectiveness of exposure-based treatments.

It has been suggested that research on PTSD has been too narrow or truncated. Shalev (1996) notes a disconnect between psychiatric research on PTSD and stress-coping theory (Holahan & Moos, 1994; R. S. Lazarus & Folkman, 1984). She outlines a number of factors that should be considered in a more complete multivariate model: pretrauma vulnerability (e.g., biological temperament, family history, social stressors), the severity of the stressor, preparedness for the event, acute responses, and coping resources that may provide a sense of control. She emphasizes that a distinction should be made between post-traumatic pathological symptoms and normative responses to a stressful event. The overlap in symptoms between PTSD and other anxiety disorders suggests that the interaction of developmental and stress-coping theories might provide a broader and more valid context within which to understand PTSD symptoms, rather than reifying PTSD as a disease.

Stressful events occur throughout the life span. Although the emphasis for assessment is on current functioning and adaptation (Holahan & Moos, 1994), how these events are appraised and whether a person's coping capacities are overtaxed will depend on a number of cognitive mediating factors that vary considerably from one individual to the next (R. S. Lazarus & Folkman, 1984; Bandura, 1986). Current psychological theories emphasize traumatic events as an assault on an individual's formerly stable cognitive model of the world, followed by either a relatively rapid psychological accommodation to the new related stimuli without further undue distress, or a long-term struggle, vacillating between confrontation and avoidance. The person must then reconcile these events by incrementally confronting them with gradually lessening psychophysiological distress (Rachman, 1980; Horowitz, 1997). Other psychological theories, such as conditioning and learned helplessness, may also provide partial and somewhat overlapping explanations for this psychological reconciliation process. Joseph, Williams, and Yule (1997) point out that dealing with traumatic events requires a balancing act of gradual exposure to frightening stimuli with time out for intermittent respite from the emotional stress caused by thinking about the traumatic event. Over time, this cognitive processing allows the individual to psychologically confront the event with a tolerable degree of discomfort. Although these theories vary somewhat in content and emphasis, they share a common theoretical core that points to the need for some level of covert exposure to the event and psychological reconciliation between the traumatic event and one's schema (sense of self and the world).

Psychological resolution, however, should not be understood as a process that takes place in a social vacuum. Social supports, both the emotional support of others and instrumental supports (meeting basic needs), can significantly moderate the effects of stress (Sarason et al., 1994). The quality of social supports before and after the trauma may be an important determinant for the manner in which people respond to a traumatic event and how speedily they recover from it. For example, research supports the buffering effects of family relationships for individuals exposed to community violence (Gorman-Smith & Tolan, 1998). The presence or absence of social supports may be the determining factor in long-term outcomes for someone who has suffered a severe traumatic event.

Although it should be understood that cultural factors will color the appraisal of and response to traumatic events, there is relatively little research on the effects of culture on the development, course, and treatment of PTSD (Marsella, Friedman, & Spain, 1996). One of the major problems in determining the role of race, ethnicity, and culture in relation to PTSD is the lack of good measures for these constructs. A review of racial differences among veterans with combat-related PTSD suggests strongly that veterans from different races are probably more alike than they are different with respect to symptoms and treatment response (Frueh, Brady, & de Arellano, 1998). Based on the NVVRS, however, Hispanics were shown to have higher rates of PTSD even after controlling for combat exposure and other background variables (Ruef, Litz, & Schlenger, 2000). Differences in treatment outcomes, however, may have less to do with inherent differences in response to traumatic events, and more to do with access to the treatment system (Rosenheck & Fontana, 1996).

Key Elements of Multidimensional/ Functional Assessment

The *DSM-IV-TR* provides guidelines that define and diagnose PTSD. In summary, clients meet the criteria for PTSD if they have been exposed to a traumatic event that involved actual or threatened death or serious injury, or a threat to the physical integrity of self or others, and their response involved intense fear, helplessness, or horror (or demonstrated disorganized or agitated behavior in the case of a child). The client must also manifest three categories of symptoms for a period of at least one month. First, the client persistently *reexperiences* the traumatic event through distressing recollections, dreams, "reliving" the experience, living with illusions, hallucinations, or dissociative flashbacks. The client may also experience intense psychological distress when exposed to internal or external cues that symbolize or resemble an aspect of the traumatic event. Second, the client must also demonstrate persistent *avoidance* of stimuli associated with the trauma and numbing of general responsiveness through efforts to avoid thoughts, feelings, conversations, or activities (including people and places) associated with the trauma; having trouble recalling important aspects of the traumatic event; significantly diminished interest or participation in familiar activities; a feeling of detachment from others; and a restricted range of expressing emotions and feelings toward others. The client may also experience a sense of a foreshortened future. Third, the client must experience persistent symptoms of increased *arousal* that were not present before the traumatic event, as indicated by two of the following symptoms: difficulty falling or staying asleep, irritability or outbursts of anger, difficulty concentrating, hypervigilance, or an exaggerated startle response. The practitioner should also examine to what extent the symptoms cause significant distress or impairment in social, occupational, and other important areas of functioning.

Given the heterogeneity of the causes and problems associated with PTSD, practitioners should go beyond diagnostic labeling of clients, and see the client's response to a traumatic event in a broader psychosocial context that takes into account both distal and proximate contributing factors (Naugle & Follette, 1998; Follette, Ruzek, & Abueg, 1998). A recent traumatic event such as rape can directly affect all domains of a client's psychosocial well-being, including mental status (e.g., depression, anxiety, dissociation), substance abuse, the quality of family and other interpersonal relationships, and community functioning (e.g., as a student or on the job). Nevertheless, the clinician should also be attuned to problems that existed prior to the traumatic event, and recognize that these problems may have been compounded by the recent trauma. For the client with a preexisting depression, substance-abuse problem, or poor interpersonal relationships, a rape may exacerbate these existing problems with additional psychosocial effects, including shame, humiliation, anger, interpersonal conflict, decreased functioning at work, and anxiety over health risks (e.g., HIV testing). It is reasonable to expect that a client with preexisting psychological difficulties and a lack of social supports will have a more difficult time recovering and dealing with a traumatic event such as rape than someone with a better pretrauma history. Although a number of preexisting problems may worsen a person's response to trauma, they may have to be addressed before progress can be made on reducing symptoms of PTSD.

Once major areas of well-being are reviewed, a detailed functional analysis of day-to-day coping is necessary to identify psychological distress and situational triggers that affect the client's symptoms and associated problems. The functional analysis provides a focused assessment to tentatively identify causal relationships among factors relevant to the target problem. Specifically, these may include automatic negative thoughts and images associated with the traumatic event, psychological arousal in the form of startle or chronic anxiety, and avoidance of specific people, places, or things that may remind one of the traumatic event. Linking these troubling thoughts, feelings, and behaviors with social and situational antecedents that trigger them can provide a useful and accurate working model to explain what psychosocial factors affect the client's symptoms and overall sense of well-being. Problems that add to client's difficulties may include living with an addicted person or being in a violent relationship, dealing with immediate financial stressors that might involve losing one's home or being evicted, and dealing with serious health problems and having no health insurance. By combining the MDF aspects of the assessment, the practitioner and client work together to identify the traumatic event that appears to be the primary precipitant of the client's distress, other contributing problems, any daily sequential patterning of psychosocial stressors that are exacerbating the client's symptoms, and linkages among distressing thoughts, feelings, behaviors, and situations that appear to alleviate or worsen the client's distress. Clients can collaborate in this ongoing assessment by using a chart or diary and by identifying their thoughts, feelings, and circumstances when they are feeling most vulnerable or most resilient.

Instruments

Two classes of instruments are related to trauma in general: those that measure the types, frequency, or severity of traumatic events, and those that measure the respondent's reaction to traumatic events (PTSD symptoms). A well-reviewed example of the first type is the Traumatic Stress Schedule (TSS; F. H. Norris, 1990; F. H. Norris & Riad, 1997). Traumatic events measured by this scale include being a victim of a crime such as robbery, assault, or rape; loss through homicide, suicide, or accident; personal injury; natural disaster; serving in combat; and serious automobile accident. The scale is available in English and Spanish versions, and has shown very good test-retest reliability. Rates of trauma measured with the TSS have been shown to be relatively stable across several samples, and, with ten items, the scale can be easily incorporated into routine screening and assessment protocol.

The emphasis in this section is on the second type of scale, however, measuring symptoms associated with post-traumatic stress. Several scales have been developed. The Mississippi Scale for Combat-Related PTSD (Keane, Caddell, & Taylor, 1988) contains thirty-five items that collectively measure reexperiencing, avoidance and numbing, arousal, and guilt/suicidal feelings. A civilian form of this scale uses an alternate instruction ("in the past" rather than "since I was in the military"). Different response categories are used depending on the question, but all are scored on a five-point scale. With a sample of 451 male and 217 female nonveterans, Vreven, Gudanowski, King, & King (1995) demonstrated very good internal consistency (.86), a multidimensional factor structure, but relatively weak relationships with other indicators of PTSD, suggesting that the Civilian Mississippi Scale may be a more general indicator of psychological distress. Vreven et al. concluded that evidence for the Civilian Mississippi Scale is somewhat mixed.

The Clinician Administered PTSD Scale (CAPS-1) was developed at the National Center for PTSD (Blake et al., 1990; Blake et al., 1995). It covers the seventeen PTSD symptoms in the *DSM-IV* diagnostic criteria, but includes others such as the impact of symptoms on social and occupational functioning, improvement in symptoms since previous CAPS–1 assessment, overall response validity, and global PTSD severity. Frequency and severity for each item are measured separately, and responses to each question are behaviorally anchored. The rating scheme allows for dichotomous scoring for diagnostic purposes, and continuous measures for evaluation. The CAPS-1 shows good evidence of test-retest reliability (.77 to .98), good internal consistency (.85 to .87 for major symptom clusters and .94 for all seventeen PTSD items), good sensitivity (.84) and specificity (.95), and good convergent validity in that the scale correlates well with other known measures of PTSD. A confirmatory factor analysis revealed a four-factor solution of moderately to highly intercorrelated subscales, suggesting that PTSD is more a collection of related symptoms and behaviors than a unified construct, and that most of the symptoms are not unique to PTSD (D. W. King et al., 1998). An alternative version (CAPS-2) is designed to assess current symptoms over a one-week period rather than the one-month criterion used with the CAPS-1. The CAPS-2 may be more sensitive to change, and may better lend itself to treatment evaluation. The CAPS instrument does require interviewers to be experienced in diagnostic interviewing, especially with PTSD diagnosis, and requires some degree of training in its use. It takes about forty-five minutes to complete.

The PTSD Symptom Scale (PSS), developed with female rape victims (Foa, Riggs, Dancu, & Rothbaum, 1993), comprises seventeen items that correspond to *DSM* criteria for PTSD. It comes in both client self-report form (PSS-SR) and practitioner structured interview form (PSS-I). Coffey, Dansky, Falsetti, Saladin, and Brady (1998) tested the PSS-SR against measures of stressful life events and psychiatric symptoms with a sample of 118 persons admitted for chemical dependency who reported at least one traumatic event in their lives. Internal consistency of the PSS-SR was excellent at .95 and .94 for the severity and frequency subscales, respectively. Total score was significantly correlated with the Symptom Checklist (SCL-90) PTSD scale and moderately correlated with the IES subscales that measure avoidance and intrusion. It also showed good sensitivity (89%) and specificity (65%) using a structured PTSD symptom interview as criteria. The PSS-SR shows good utility as well, in that it takes about ten to fifteen minutes to complete.

The PSS-I (instrument 8.1) provides a total score as well as subscale scores for reexperiencing, avoidance, and arousal. Items are measured on a four-point (0–3) frequency scale. The PSS-I shows good evidence of concurrent validity, given significant correlations with measures of PTSD symptoms and measures of anxiety and depression, and it has demonstrated excellent sensitivity and specificity with the *DSM* structured interview schedule (SCID; F. H. Norris & Riad, 1997). The PSS-I was shown to compare favorably to the CAPS-1 when administered with thirty-nine persons (combined clinical and community sample), all of whom met PTSD criteria and experienced traumatic events, including sexual assault, other violent assaults, or another traumatic event. Results showed good reliability and validity for the PSS-I as demonstrated by good internal consistency (.86 for all seventeen items; .70 reexperiencing, .74 avoidance, and .65 arousal subscales), excellent interrater reliability (all subscales well above 90%), and moderate to high subscale correlations with the CAPS-1 (Foa & Tolin, 2000). The practitioner should first identify the client's "target trauma" and second use all available information to make judgments about the severity of each item.

SELECTING EFFECTIVE INTERVENTIONS

Due to the lack of controlled studies, little evidence exists regarding the effectiveness of psychodynamic therapies for PTSD (Foa & Rothbaum, 1998; Foa & Meadows, 1997; Shalev, Bonne, & Eth, 1996; Kudler, Blank, & Krupnick, 2000). Part of the difficulty in assessing the efficacy of psychodynamic treatments is that hypotheses about the relationship between the intervention and the outcomes are not stated in ways that can be tested. Although descriptions of psychodynamic interventions for PTSD include generic aspects of effective interventions (e.g., the working alliance, establishing a sense of safety, recounting the events and mourning losses associated with them, regaining coping skills and a sense of connectedness to others), there does not appear to be any

INSTRUMENT 8.1   The PTSD Symptom Scale Interview (PSS-I)

Ask "In the past two weeks" (if < 2 weeks since trauma, ask "Since the trauma").
Probe all positive responses (e.g., "How often has this been happening?").

Not at all	Once per week or less/a little	2 to 4 times per week/somewhat	5 or more times per week/very much
0	1	2	3

Re-experiencing (need one for DSM criteria) (probe, then quantify)

____ 1. Have you had recurrent or intrusive distressing thoughts or recollections about the trauma?

____ 2. Have you been having recurrent bad dreams or nightmares about the trauma?

____ 3. Have you had the experience of suddenly reliving the trauma, flashbacks of it, acting or feeling as if it were re-occurring?

____ 4. Have you been intensely EMOTIONALLY upset when reminded of the trauma (includes anniversary reactions)?

____ 5. Have you been having intense PHYSICAL reactions (e.g., sweaty, heart palpitations) when reminded of the trauma?

Avoidance (need three for DSM criteria) (probe, then quantify)

____ 6. Have you persistently been making efforts to avoid thoughts or feelings associated with the trauma?

____ 7. Have you persistently been making efforts to avoid activities, situations, or places that remind you of the trauma?

____ 8. Are there any important aspects about the trauma that you still cannot recall?

____ 9. Have you markedly lost interest in free-time activities since the trauma?

____ 10. Have you felt detached or cut off from others around you since the trauma?

____ 11. Have you felt that your ability to experience the whole range of emotions is impaired (e.g., unable to have loving feelings)?

____ 12. Have you felt that any future plans or hopes have changed because of the trauma (e.g., no career, marriage, children, or long life)?

Increased Arousal (need two for DSM criteria) (probe, then quantify)

____ 13. Have you had persistent difficulty falling or staying asleep?

____ 14. Have you been continuously irritable or had outbursts of anger?

____ 15. Have you had persistent difficulty concentrating?

____ 16. Are you overly alert (e.g., check to see who is around you, etc.) since the trauma?

____ 17. Have you been jumpier, more easily startled, since the trauma?

PTSD severity is determined by totaling the 17 PSS-I item ratings. Scores range from **0–51**.

PTSD diagnosis is determined by counting the number of symptoms endorsed (a rating of 1 or greater) per symptom cluster—1 Re-experiencing, 3 Avoidance, and 2 Arousal symptoms are needed to meet diagnostic criteria.

A PTSD diagnosis also requires **symptom duration of more than one month** (criterion E) and **clinically significant distress or impairment** (criterion F). A manual is available from Nora Feeney and Edna Foa.

demonstrated elements of these interventions that are unique or specific to psychoanalytic theory. Other commonly employed interventions such as family or group methods have produced insufficient data from which to draw even marginally affirmative conclusions about their efficacy.

Overall, the most effective treatments for PTSD (tested mostly with combat and rape-related trauma) appear to include prolonged exposure (PE), eye-movement desensitization and reprocessing (EMDR), and other cognitive-behavioral coping skills such as stress inoculation training (Emmelkamp, 1994; Foa & Meadows, 1997; Rothbaum et al, 2000; Van Etten & Taylor, 1998). Although some form of imaginal exposure appears indicated for PTSD, no intervention has demonstrated great success in reducing all the associated symptoms, particularly physiological arousal. In addition, sensitivity to clients' ability to tolerate intense reimagining of traumatic events must be exercised through careful measuring of their subjective distress as these memories are broached. Some clients, such as people with serious co-occurring mental illnesses, may find the arousal induced through exposure overwhelming, and intervention can focus instead on developing better coping skills. For many traumatized clients, however, results are generally positive for reducing physiological arousal, intrusive traumatic thoughts, sleep disturbance, anxiety, and fear. Positive effects may be enhanced with supplementary hospitalization, medication, and additional psychosocial interventions (Blake & Sonnenberg, 1998).

Rothbaum et al. (2000, p. 67) reviewed twelve studies that employed exposure therapy, "all of which found positive results for this treatment with PTSD." Most of these studies met the methodological gold standard outlined in Foa and Meadows (1997). These standards include clearly defined target symptoms, sound measures, evaluators who are blind to the treatment conditions, trained assessors, well-defined intervention programs, random assignment to treatment and control groups, and good fidelity to the intervention model. Four studies investigated exposure therapies with Vietnam veterans, two with sexual-assault survivors (examined in detail below), and four with a variety of other trauma-related conditions. The authors concluded that "compelling evidence from many well-controlled trials with a mixed variety of trauma survivors indicates that exposure therapy is quite effective. In fact, no other treatment modality has evidence this strong indicating its efficacy" (Rothbaum et al., p. 75). Generally, exposure therapies have gained the most evidence of effectiveness and ease of use (by practitioners and clients), and appear to be the most cost-effective methods. However, practitioners should be flexible and ready to use combinations of in vivo exposure, imaginal exposure, and other stress-management techniques (similar to those examined in chapter 7) to help the client reduce symptoms, especially in the early stages of the intervention (Foa & Rothbaum, 1998).

Stress inoculation training (SIT; Meichenbaum, 1974) has also been employed as one component of a successful intervention for PTSD (as well as for the other anxiety disorders for both adults and children). This intervention includes an array of well-established behavioral techniques, including psychoeducation, relaxation training (e.g., muscle relaxation, breathing retraining, meditation), covert modeling, and role-playing. With regard to studies employing SIT with PTSD, only two met the methodological gold standard (Foa, Rothbaum, Riggs, & Murdock, 1991; Foa et al., 1999), and while both showed good results for SIT, it has not been demonstrated to be effective with clients other than rape-trauma survivors. Overall, exposure treatments have garnered the most evidence of effectiveness in controlled trials, have been shown to be effective with a wide array of trauma populations, and are typically as effective alone as when combined with other treatments such as SIT (Rothbaum et al., 2000).

The efficacy of EMDR is also supported by a growing number of controlled studies, and is considered "probably efficacious" for non–war-related PTSD along with exposure therapy and SIT. It has earned a sound degree of credibility, and should be considered a viable option for effective intervention with clients suffering from PTSD (Shapiro, 1996, 2002; Davidson & Parker, 2001; Edmond, Rubin, & Wambach, 1999; Van Etten & Taylor, 1998). Evidence supports the conclusion that EMDR is at least as effective as cognitive-behavioral interventions, and some studies have suggested that it may even require fewer sessions and related activities. However, more direct comparisons of EMDR and CBT are required before definitive conclusions can be drawn about their relative efficacy.

Although it has been debated whether EMDR is simply another variant on exposure therapy, the science to date has not supported the necessity of the dual attention (e.g., eye movements) component of the intervention. A recent meta-analysis of thirty-four controlled studies of EMDR (Davidson & Parker, 2001) revealed that (1) EMDR is an effective intervention (better that nonspecific therapies) for noncombatants with PTSD, but it is not superior to other exposure-based therapies; (2) the eye movement, or other alternating techniques, do not account for the effectiveness of the intervention; (3) when training was conducted by EMDR institute-trained practitioners, the interventions were no more effective than when other practitioners conducted the interventions; and (4) EMDR is no more or less effective with one treatment population than with another. Nevertheless, in another meta-analysis of twelve controlled studies, methodologically more rigorous studies of EMDR demonstrated robust effects (Maxfield & Hyer, 2002). However, serious criticisms have been brought to bear on methodologies employed (Foa & Meadows, 1997, e.g., lack of standardized measures, blind evaluations, measures of treatment adherence), and little evidence provides compelling support for the specific efficacy of the signature eye-movement component (Chemtob, Tolin, Van der Kolk, & Pitman, 2000; Shapiro, 1996; Foa & Rothbaum, 1998; Blake & Sonnenberg, 1998; Davidson & Parker, 2001; Lohr, Lilienfeld, Tolin, & Herbert, 1999).

An increasing number of comparisons of PE and EMDR have been conducted and have shown mixed results. Ironson, Freund, Strauss, and Williams (2002), treating rape and crime victims ($n = 22$), and S. Rogers et al. (1999), treating veterans ($n = 12$), both demonstrated superior results overall for EMDR in very brief, randomly controlled trials after three-session and single-session interventions, respectively. Ironson et al. (2002) also showed a significantly lower dropout rate from treatment for EMDR. However, both studies used relatively small samples and no follow-up measures. Lee, Gauvriel, Drummond, Richards, and Greenwald (2002) compared a combination of SIT and PE to EMDR. At three-month follow-up, the twenty-four completers all showed clinically significant gains, but those who received EMDR had made significantly greater gains. Contrary to these findings, Devilly and Spence (1999) showed that a combination of PE and CBT coping skills yielded superior outcomes when compared to EMDR in a randomized controlled trial with twenty-three participants who had experienced a traumatic event within four weeks of the study and who met PTSD criteria. After both groups received eight weeks of treatment, improvements for the CBT protocol were substantially greater for PTSD symptoms at posttreatment and three-month follow-up. S. Taylor et al. (2003) compared PE, EMDR, and relaxation therapy in a randomized controlled trial with sixty clients (forty-five treatment completers; dropouts did not differ across treatments) who met PTSD criteria, suffered for a mean duration of almost nine years, and had experienced a variety of traumas, including sexual assault, motor-vehicle accidents, and witnessing a homicide. Co-occurring disorders included depression (42%), panic disorder (31%), and social-anxiety disorder (12%). Although all three interventions showed positive results in reducing PTSD symptoms, PE showed significantly greater reduction in both reexperiencing and avoidance symptoms, demonstrated a more rapid reduction of avoidance symptoms, and showed a greater reduction in number of clients who met the criteria for PTSD. The authors added that their study met Foa and Meadow's gold standard (1997), and that, to the best of their knowledge, it was the first study using EMDR to meet that standard.

Overall, these studies met standards of sound experimental design and used standardized measures of good reliability and utility. Although lively debate and further research is likely to continue in comparing matters of theory, change process, and cost-effectiveness of PE and EMDR, evidence-based practitioners can take comfort in the fact that there are at least two interventions available that are likely to provide clinically significant relief for clients suffering from PTSD. As research continues, some optimal integration or client-treatment matching protocol may emerge.

Change Processes in Exposure Interventions

Social-cognitive theory accounts for the effectiveness of exposure therapies in the following way: Imaginal or in vivo exposure promotes symptom reduction by allowing patients to realize that, contrary to their mistaken beliefs, being in objectively safe situations that remind one of the trauma is not dangerous; remembering the trauma is not equivalent to experiencing it again; anxiety does not remain indefinitely in the presence of feared situations or memories, but rather decreases even without avoidance or escape; and experiencing anxiety/PTSD symptoms does not lead to loss of control (Foa & Meadows, 1997; Foa & Rothbaum, 1998; Rothbaum et al., 2000). Cognitive change occurs, not by direct cognitive intervention alone, but also as a result of behavior change.

Beck and associates (Beck, 1976; Beck et al., 1979; Oei & Shuttlewood, 1996) have theorized that it is the client's interpretation of events that causes the emotional response (cognition is primary), and, in turn, client's negative schemata, negative automatic thoughts, and information-processing errors contribute to the persistence of negative emotional states, including both depression and anxiety. Subsequent dysfunctional behaviors are also likely to become part of this problematic interplay of thoughts, feelings, and emotions. The theoretical change process of cognitive restructuring involves targeting these dysfunctional thoughts and changing them through disconfirmatory experiences, behavioral experiences that will successfully challenge negative or dysfunctional beliefs. These disconfirmatory experiences may work through exposure, habituation/extinction, increased self-efficacy, reduction in automatic negative thoughts, or some combination of these processes.

Emotional processing models also reflect the increasingly cognitive emphasis in contemporary behavioral theories. Fear responses are conceptualized in emotional processing theories as neural structures that contain memories and other cognitive components related to the anxiety, and they engender emotional, physiological, and behavioral responses (Rachman, 1980; Foa & Kozak, 1998; S. Rogers & Silver, 2002). The goal of treatment within the context of the emotional processing theory is to activate the fear structure, provide alternative corrective information, and attempt to disconnect stimuli from responses—in a sense, to dismantle the fear structure and change-related cognitions, physiological responses, and behaviors. In the long run, the client needs to learn and practice coping skills to maintain adaptive cognitive structures to prevent the reemergence of the original fear structure. The core intervention theoretically posited to cause changes in these fear structures is exposure to the feared mental images, preferably PE, until habituation, extinction, and dismantling of the fear structure occur.

Key findings in research on exposure therapies support the view that the exposure must be directly focused on an unwavering elicitation of the feared image in the mind (or, as with other problems, in vivo) without letting the client use mental or behavioral avoidance mechanisms. In EMDR, however, exposure to the feared stimulus is not constant and prolonged, but intermittent with periods of attention to other matters. Despite this key difference, results appear, more or less, to be comparable to more classic exposure-based therapies. S. Rogers and Silver (2002) support the view that, despite some incongruities with current emotional processing theories, EMDR is more akin to an emotional reprocessing intervention than to a simple exposure treatment. Critical review of specific and nonspecific effects of EMDR strongly suggests that EMDR may be effective for the reasons that other CBTs are—exposure to the feared mental images. Although the change processes for EMDR may be different than those purported for PE, some maintain that there is no evidence to substantiate any unique or specific effect to the eye-movement (or similar) alternating techniques (Lohr et al., 1999). Obviously, there are unanswered theoretical questions and competing explanations concerning why exposure therapies work, and it is unclear why EMDR is effective as well (Cahill, Carrigan, & Frueh, 1999). Thus, conclusions regarding the identification and nature of specific change processes for these effective interventions must remain tentative at this time (Tarrier et al., 2000).

Exemplar Study: Comparing Interventions Specifically Applied to Rape-Related PTSD.   Two Key studies (Foa et al., 1991; Foa et al., 1999) illustrate the supporting controlled research on exposure treatments and other cognitive behavioral methods for PTSD, and focus specifically on the treatment of rape-related trauma. Foa et al. (1991) compared the effectiveness of three interventions—prolonged imaginal exposure (PE), SIT, and supportive counseling (SC)—for PTSD with a wait-list control group. The researchers designed the interventions so there would be a minimum of overlap, and they expected that both PE and SIT would result in better outcomes than SC and the control. Forty-five women who had been raped more than three months before the study were randomly assigned to the four groups, and measures were taken at assessment, posttreatment, and follow-up (approximately three months). Treatment was provided by female therapists in nine ninety-minute sessions, biweekly for four and one-half weeks. In addition to a thorough assessment and evaluation of PTSD symptoms, additional valid self-report measures were included to measure symptoms associated with the aftermath of rape, depression, and anxiety. Interventions were performed by a combination of psychologists and clinical social workers hired and trained for the project. Interventions were monitored through supervision to enhance fidelity to the respective intervention models. In all three active treatments, the first two sessions included assessment and explanation of the rationale for the treatment. For the PE group, the additional seventh session included imaginal exposure (i.e. reliving the rape scene in the mind's eye of the client) as vividly as possible and describing it aloud in the present tense. The client would repeat this scene several times over the course of sixty minutes. The client took a recording of the session home to listen to it once daily. Additional in vivo exposure to feared situations (judged to be safe) were added based on client-therapist discussions. The SIT group employed an array of standard cognitive-behavioral coping skills, including breathing exercises, muscle relaxation, thought stopping to counter obsessional thinking, self-talk, imaginal modeling, and role-playing. Practitioners in the SC group provided standard unconditional support and facilitated general problem-solving techniques. The wait-list clients were contacted periodically for five weeks and then randomly assigned to either the PE or SIT group. Of the sixty-six original victims offered services, eleven refused treatment and ten dropped out, but attrition was comparable across treatment groups. Results demonstrated that both PE and SIT were effective interventions in the short run, and PE showed superior results at three-month follow-up. Both the SC and the control groups showed some reduction only in arousal symptoms. The investigators suggested that coping-skills approaches in SIT provided more immediate relief from symptoms, but PE (which produces high levels of arousal initially as clients imaginally enact the rape experience) showed more durable gains at follow-up. Practitioners suggested that the data supported an eclectic blend of both approaches.

In a later study, Foa et al. (1999) examined whether combining PE and SIT would be more effective than each treatment alone. Sixty-nine women who had been sexually assaulted and twenty-seven who were victims of nonsexual assault all met PTSD criteria. Extensive assessment included diagnostic interview and ratings of PTSD symptoms and social adjustment. Self-report measures included standardized anxiety and depression scales. Clients were randomly assigned to the following groups: combined PE and SIT, PE alone, SIT alone, and a wait-list group (ten clients). Measures were taken at assessment and at three, six, and twelve months. Interventions were conducted by seven doctoral-level female psychologists supervised by Foa and Dancu. The intervention consisted of nine twice-weekly sessions over five weeks, the first two sessions of which were 120 minutes long. Interventions provided were very similar to those described in Foa et al. 1991. Although all active treatments showed good results, PE was clearly the superior treatment. The investigators suggested that because of lower demand on the client to engage in simpler intervention (PE), fewer clients who received PE dropped out of treatment.

Descriptions of Effective Interventions

What follows is a brief overview of the essential components of both EMDR and CBT for victims of rape trauma. Notwithstanding debates about the essential nature of the eye-movement (and similar) alternating techniques, EMDR is considered a viable treatment for PTSD. The intervention requires that the client identify a number of details related to the traumatic memory, identify affective and physiological response elements, define the negative self-representation triggered by the traumatic experience, and identify an alternate positive self-representation (Shapiro, 2002; Chemtob et al., 2000). To implement the basic elements of EMDR, one should develop a sound working relationship with the client; provide psychoeducation about trauma and the rationale for the treatment; focus on trauma-specific memories and associated reminders; and teach coping skills to deal with trauma-related material as it emerges. The practitioner conducts a focused assessment of the trauma-related memory, including all associated negative and positive cognitions, associated emotions, and physical sensations along with self-anchored scales to rate the validity of the positive cognition (VOC scale), and to measure the client's distress at regular intervals with the SUDS. The practitioner instructs the client to hold the upsetting image in mind along with associated negative thoughts and bodily images connected with the traumatic memory. Then the client visually tracks the therapist's finger, which moves side to side about one foot in front of the client's face. After twenty or so repetitions, the client is requested to release the memory, take a deep breath, and report any cognitive, physical, or emotional changes. The practitioner may adjust the verbal instructions depending on the client's response. After subjective distress has been reduced to an acceptable level, the exercise begins again; however, this time the client works with the practitioner to install the positive image (using the VOC scale), and additional coping skills may be rehearsed to deal with future situations. After each session, care is taken to help the client recover from experiencing the traumatic images. The intervention is repeated and continuous reevaluation is conducted until the client meets the objectives.

Shapiro (2002) points out that dual stimulation (of which the eye-movement component of treatment is one form) is only one of several techniques that make up EMDR. She claims that the intervention is not merely a desensitization method but also "includes the elicitation of positive affects, evoked insights, belief alterations, and behavioral shifts" (p.1). The core of the technique, however, does not focus on behavior indexes, but rather is the "reprocessing of maladaptive information upon which experientially forged psychopathology is assumed to be based" (p.2).

PE protocol for sexual-assault victims has been clearly delineated as well. A more thorough, detailed examination is available in Foa and Rothbaum (1998). Although it is understood that a fair amount of judgment is required in choice of respective technique, Foa and Rothbaum recommend three basic treatment configurations based on their work and exhaustive reviews of the available controlled research: (1) PE alone, given its relative ease of use and lower demand characteristics on both client and practitioner; (2) PE and cognitive restructuring in combination for clients who have persistent ruminative or obsessive thoughts associated with disabling anger, shame, or guilt; and (3) PE and SIT for clients who need more work to deal with disabling anxiety symptoms before they can benefit more fully from PE. It is understood, regardless of the treatment regimen, that a thorough diagnostic and MDF assessment is required before the intervention can commence. Practitioners should spend a good amount of time connecting with the client, gaining the client's trust, providing some initial psychoeducation about the nature of the problem and the intervention, and (as with all evidence-based practices) projecting expertise and confidence that they can help the client. Practitioners should be empathetic and as active as necessary, and intervention should be relatively brief, with adjustments to length of stay made as needed. In general, these treatments share some common elements: a thorough assessment, psychoeducation, and clients' use of taped treatment sessions at home.

Specific components are described below (see Foa & Rothbaum, 1998). Modifications to the intervention plan depend on what the client is willing to try, how debilitated they are (do they need covert exposure as a "warm-up" prior to engaging in vivo?), and detection of co-occurring problems.

In *cognitive restructuring*, the practitioner identifies the source of the emotional distress, the specific emotional reaction, the troubling thought that preceded it, and the underlying beliefs (through the use of Socratic questioning). The practitioner helps the client challenge a belief by examining evidence to support of refute it. The client learns about the dysfunctional or irrational nature of the belief, and with help, changes it. Thought-stopping techniques may also be helpful. Clients may say "stop" aloud when the thought intrudes, say "stop" and simultaneously use some image to distract their thoughts, or say "stop" silently to themselves. At home, the client practices these techniques.

Progressive muscle relaxation works on all muscle groups. The client selects a verbal cue to instill relaxation as needed during the day, such as "calm," "easy does it," "I'm doing fine." The practitioner teaches the client cue-controlled relaxation by identifying a source of physical tension and using it as a stimulus to relax (breathe deeply, let it out slowly).

In *imaginal exposure*, clients close their eyes and narrate the traumatic event vividly in the present tense. They gradually increase the intensity of the imaginal event (with the practitioner's direct questioning and encouragement after one or two visits). The SUDS is used every ten minutes or so. The end of the session is a time for the client to "come down" and talk about the experience of reliving the traumatic event. The practitioner should be available by phone between visits.

Role-playing gives clients the opportunity to practice a new skill or improve on one (e.g., being more assertive at work). Clients and practitioners collaboratively develop a troubling scenario for the client that they want to work on, then act it out with both client and practitioner changing roles. The practitioner gives encouragement, feedback, and constructive suggestions for improvement as needed. Through covert modeling, clients can rehearse similar activities by practicing in their "mind's eye" at home and, by doing so, can prepare to engage in live exposure experiences by seeing themselves coping with troubling situations successfully.

In vivo exposure includes a thorough explanation of the procedure and use of the SUDS. A hierarchy of feared situations is constructed using the SUDS for each situation. Homework assignments are developed based on the hierarchy. The client places herself in a moderately anxiety-producing situation until anxiety drops by at least half. The client records SUDS ratings before and after each exposure.

The design of exposure-based therapies can be as creative as the situation warrants. Clients typically provide their own narrative accounts in the development of hierarchal scenarios, and the therapist may embellish them to increase therapeutic effect. Treatments may vary in duration of exposure per treatment event, and length of stay may vary. Clients can practice these techniques at home, and they can be facilitated by significant others who have been trained to collaborate in the intervention.

Interventions for Clients with Post-traumatic Stress Disorder and Co-occurring Substance Abuse

Given that CBT methods have been shown to be effective for both PTSD and substance abuse, combinations of skills can be used to address both problems

(Najavits, Weiss, & Liese, 1996). An evidence-based eclectic approach could include, for example, establishing a working relationship; psychoeducation regarding the reciprocal links between substance abuse and PTSD symptoms; brief medical intervention, perhaps including detoxification; self-monitoring of substance-using triggers (which may be related to trauma symptoms); teaching coping skills to avoid relapse related to reexperiencing trauma symptoms or substance abuse; graduated covert exposure treatments to reduce trauma-related distress; and facilitating increased social supports for long-term maintenance of gains. These methods can be readily incorporated into a comprehensive intervention plan for co-occurring PTSD and substance abuse.

Medication for Post-traumatic Stress Disorder

Foa and Rothbaum (1998) suggest that controlled studies support the usefulness of several types of antidepressants in providing some relief from PTSD symptoms. However, Shalev et al. (1996) assert that although common pharmacological agents such as SSRIs (antidepressants such as fluoxetine) and benzodiazepines (e.g., diazepam) may provide some relief for clients from acute symptoms, they are generally not sufficient to provide long-term relief or resolution.

IMPLEMENTING AND EVALUATING THE EVIDENCE-BASED INTERVENTION PLAN

CASE STUDY: JULIA

Julia was an eighteen-year-old college freshman who left home to attend a medium-sized university out of state. She had always been an excellent student, but was somewhat anxious socially, and was looking forward to "meeting people right off . . . I want to get out of my shell a bit." She met other young women in her dormitory and seemed to hit it off with them immediately. She was feeling right at home in no time. She called her parents, with whom she had always been close (she was the only child in the family), and told them how happy she was that she had decided to attend that university.

Her first semester passed uneventfully, and she continued to do well in school and enjoyed the company of her women companions. She was enthusiastic about picking up where she left off after returning to school for the spring semester. About halfway through the semester, just before spring break, she attended a party at a local fraternity house. There was considerable drinking and rumored use of some illicit drugs going on, but aside from a drink or two, Julia had little experience abusing alcohol or other drugs. Her best friend had attended the party because her boyfriend was one of the fraternity members. At one point, they became separated, and her friend was not to be found. "Oh well," she thought, "I need to work on getting over my shyness anyway. Here's my chance." She found herself in a room with three young men who seemed like they were having a good time. They invited her to stay, and seemed to have a lot in common. One of them was from her home state. They talked for some time, and Julia agreed to have some of the fruit punch they were serving.

With the loud music, talking, and the unexpectedly strong "punch" going to her head, she did not notice the time pass, or the fact that almost everyone had left the party. One of the guys got up, put a video on the TV, and closed the door. They invited Julia over to sit on a big couch positioned in front of the set. At that point, Julia assumed they were going to watch a movie, and since she was having such a good time, figured "why not?" It became apparent in a hurry that the movie was adult pornography with little plot and lots of graphic sex scenes. The guys laughed and cheered. Julia, although surprised at first, was pretty intoxicated and intrigued at this point. It did not become apparent to her that the young men in the room were going to try to encourage her to participate in sexual activity until one of them reached over and kissed her full on the mouth, and cupped his hands around her breast. After that, things spun out of control.

In recounting the following events, Julia was somewhat vague, only recalling images and feelings as she recollected what had happened that night several months past. She recalled being pushed down on the couch, and her clothes being pulled off by one of the young men. Before she could even

react, one of the males was on top of her with his fingers inside her vagina. Another had his mouth on her breasts. She was then quickly pulled up by her legs, and the first young man forced his penis into her. She recalled the penetration being somewhat painful, but then simply remembered being terrified and feeling completely out of control. She was raped again by the other male. In hindsight she remembered the two young men who raped her, and vaguely recalled the name of the young man who had been in the room earlier. She remembered crying, and the two men sitting her up at one point, and giving her another drink of punch. She was completely confused, since they now seemed to be acting very nice to her.

The next thing Julia remembered was waking up on a couch in the front of her own dormitory in rain. Her clothes were disheveled and felt like they didn't fit right. She went into her dorm, and found her girlfriend. She started crying, and when she was able to communicate some of what had happened, her girlfriend took her to the infirmary. She was checked out medically, and referred to the university counseling department for an appointment later that day. She reported the incident to the campus police, and later gave a statement to the state police as well. The third male at the scene was also contacted during the investigation. Although he later reported that he thought things might get out of hand, he was not actually there when the rape occurred. The two others were later suspended from the university on the basis of Julia's complaint and the police investigation, but the criminal trial would not take place for some time. The two men and their parents retained an attorney who maintained that Julia had been a willing participant in the sexual activity. She became additionally distressed because of that assertion.

With rape crisis counseling and the support of her family and friends, Julia was able to finish the semester, but felt like she was on "automatic pilot." She felt some vindication that two of the men had been suspended, but felt somewhat humiliated, depressed, and guilty about what had occurred. She left for home that summer with the hope that she would be able to put it behind her. During the summer, however, she became increasingly depressed and withdrawn, thought about the event in frightening images in her waking hours and, sometimes, in her dreams. At her waitress job at a local restaurant, she was having trouble keeping her mind on her work, sometimes mixing up customers' orders. The manager of the restaurant had to talk to her on a number of occasions. She was asked out on dates by some of the male patrons, but automatically refused. She often felt angry, bordering on hostile, in response to these inquiries. Although she kept busy reading during the day and working in the evenings, her social life was minimal. Her parents queried about her spending so much time alone, but they didn't push—they were happy that she seemed to be content to spend much of her time at home. Occasionally, her parents would hear her

sobbing in her room, sometimes late at night, but when they queried her, she said she was all right. When her dad asked if the assault was still bothering her, she responded that she thought about it sometimes, but that she would be all right. Her parents did not press her further to discuss it, and she did not bring it up.

As September approached, she seemed to her parents to be very anxious and irritable. They queried some more, and Julia began to say that she wasn't sure this was the right school for her anymore. As her annual medical exam for school was overdue anyway, she saw her physician, who noticed that she seemed depressed and anxious. She told Julia that she might still not be over the effects of the rape, and for the first time, Julia heard the words "traumatic stress" used in the context of her own experience. Her doctor told her that she would call the university and talk to a social worker who was on the staff of the university counseling center. The physician encouraged her not to avoid school, but to go back (it would start in a few weeks), and said that she could see someone to help her deal with her fears, anger, and depression. She prescribed an antidepressant to help "take the edge off some of the symptoms," but she insisted that Julia must follow through, and perhaps should talk to the social worker on the phone as soon as possible. After the initial phone call, Julia felt somewhat better. She was not alone in harboring these feelings, and she had a name to put to what she was experiencing: post-traumatic stress disorder.

Multidimensional/Functional Assessment: Defining Problems and Goals

Although Julia had spoken to the social worker, Amy, at length over the phone, Amy conducted a full assessment with Julia during the first visit. Some of the sleep disturbance had abated, but her mental-status exam revealed a young woman who was considerably depressed, had some suicidal ideation during the summer, avoided social situations, and found herself very frightened (i.e., light-headed, heart pounding) at times, for example, when she found herself in a corner in the library as a group of male students approached. She often jumped if someone quietly walked up behind her, or if she suddenly encountered someone coming around the corner in the laundry room. She ruminated that she must have done something to "set myself up . . . I mean, how could I have been so stupid?" Although her parents were very supportive to her, she thought she sensed her dad's disapproval at having put herself in that situation. She wondered if he blamed her, too. As she wondered about these things, Julia found it hard to concentrate on her work. Her mind wandered, and she found herself reliving the experience (or what she recalled of it) in her mind's eye, as if watching the same movie over and over again. She also found herself getting impatient with her new roommate, and became testy over things that normally didn't bother her. She felt more possessive about her things and "her space" in her room, and felt the need to have more control over her surroundings. She was afraid she would alienate her new roommate, too, and end up feeling even more isolated.

Her relationship with her friend who had taken her to the fraternity party became somewhat strained. Although they discussed the rape, Julia could not shake the feeling that her friend also blamed her. Although Julia was struggling through the day preoccupied and with low energy, she pushed herself to keep up with her work, but had little time for socializing. She was in good health, and avoided any use of alcohol because she was taking medication. As she discussed with her social worker, the medication was not going to make her problems go away. She was going to have to cope with these feelings better, deal with what happened to her once and for all. She felt angry that those young men had taken away her joy of living and were "keeping me from enjoying my time at college."

The social worker suggested they take a more focused or functional view to capture how these troubling thoughts, feelings, and behaviors were affecting her in different situations. Julia seemed to be mostly concerned about her feelings of depression and feeling detached from people, but also wanting to feel comfortable and not afraid of talking with men again. The social worker agreed that these three specific areas were not only all related, but also a good place to begin. On a daily basis, it appeared that one problem affected another. Julia awakened every day feeling somewhat pessimistic, and dreaded her work and dealing with people. She thought about how stupid others must think she was to have been taken advantage of. Perhaps some people who knew about the incident even blamed her for what happened because those two guys still had friends around campus.

These thoughts added to her negative mood, and seemed to precipitate a need to avoid others and "just stick to my work," since that, at least, was something she felt she had some control over and could feel good about. However, her avoidance of other people seemed to cause further rumination, and she had become increasingly withdrawn even from her good friend (who was also feeling guilty and somewhat responsible for leaving her alone the night of the party).

Amy and Julia decided that these three problems—feelings of guilt and harsh criticism of herself, her depression, and her anxious avoidance of other people—seemed to be interrelated, and stuck in a self-defeating cycle that made her feel helpless and more isolated. The seemingly automatic negative thoughts she had about herself added to her depression, and exacerbated her anxiety in social situations. The more she avoided them, the more anxious and demoralized she became, saying, "I feel more afraid of people now than before I came to college. I thought I'd be over this by now!" Her frustration at continuing to feel out of control enhanced her motivation to work on her problems. She wanted to feel better and to stop being afraid of people, particularly men. Her social worker, whom she now felt she could trust and who understood her, agreed that these were good treatment goals.

Selecting and Designing the Intervention: Defining Strategies and Objectives

After an extensive assessment, Amy outlined a tentative intervention plan to discuss with Julia (table 8.1). It included psychoeducation, cognitive restructuring, imaginal exposure, and role-playing and in vivo practice for social anxiety.

Psychoeducation.   Amy explained to Julia that much of the distress she was experiencing looked very much like the problems and symptoms associated with PTSD. Although the social worker didn't like using these labels, her depression, anxiety, guilt, startle reaction, and avoidance, among other problems, often occurred in people after they had experienced a horrible event, such as rape. Julia even had trouble admitting that she had been raped or saying "I was raped."

Amy explained that these feelings could linger for months or even years in people, and interrupt their lives in many ways. She explained that Julia's feelings were quite common and normal in someone who was raped, but that, because she had a supportive family and some real psychological strengths, she had a very good chance of learning to deal with these feelings and gaining some control over her life again. When she said "control," Julia began to cry and said, "That's what they did to me . . . they took my life away from me . . . my fun . . . my hopes in college . . . for meeting people . . . and I want it back."

Cognitive Restructuring.   Together they examined Julia's negative thinking about the event and about everyday events as well. She did feel somewhat to blame, and asked herself repeatedly, "Why did I go to that party? What was I doing alone in a frat house with those boys? Why was I drinking? Why did they pick me?" As they both examined her thoughts, feelings, and behaviors, Amy asked in response: Well, why shouldn't you have gone? What's wrong with going to a party? What was wrong with staying and talking with two or three male students? They seemed to be nice, didn't they? How could you have known that two of them were going to rape you? How were you supposed to have known? Should you never be alone with men again? Did you know how much alcohol they had snuck into your drink? Were there any other drugs in your drink? How do you know? As they collaboratively explored the situation, it became clear to Julia that she had been focusing mostly on blaming herself these past few months, rather than examining the culpability of those two men. She and Amy began to catalogue challenges to these intrusive and troubling thoughts. The more Julia discussed them aloud, the clearer she saw how hard she had been on herself since the incident, and how many factors related to the event had been out of her control.

As this line of inquiry proceeded, Amy and Julia began to develop a daily diary (in chart form), so that she could note some of these more troubling thoughts and her challenges to them. She was also to note the time of day and any important situational details. She said she found this easy to do, because she was able to create one on her portable computer, which she had with her most of the time anyway. She discovered that the rape had hurt her deeply, because she really thought that those guys had been interested in her, not just in using her. She discussed these thoughts and feelings with her social worker, who encouraged her to continue to explore this on her own as she kept her diary. She continued to note her challenges to these negative automatic thoughts for the next few weeks, although she sometimes felt like giving up, since the thoughts were often very distressing. Specific treatment objectives began to emerge: identify daily self-critical thoughts, feelings, and situations; then identify a counterargument to them.

Imaginal Exposure with Anxiety-Management Skills and Use of the SUDS. It became evident that, although they were discussing the events of the night Julia was raped, she had not really confronted the rape and examined the details. Although there was some ambiguity about the event, she was remembering more as time passed. The social worker explained to Julia the rationale for imaginal exposure, a graduated process by which she could learn to recount the rape experience in detail and, at the same time, learn to control and diminish her anxiety. She would have to reexperience some of the intense thoughts and feelings that had occurred in order to develop some sense of mastery over her feelings, and diminish the negative influence they were having on her life. Additional intervention objectives would be to learn controlled breathing, practice the SUDS, and engage in daily imaginal exposure until she reduced her anxiety to a score of 30 or less.

After Julia agreed, Amy explained to her how to develop and use the SUDS, and to signal when she was becoming too anxious (if she reached a score of 70). Together they discussed a detailed hierarchy of events that transpired before, during, and after the rape. During the discussion, it became clear that Julia was becoming increasingly anxious, and Amy was careful to gauge the anxiety to help her client get a feel for how the process worked. Amy also taught her some deep breathing methods, and encouraged her to breathe deeply and steadily, hold the image of what was occurring during the particular scene in her mind, and not mentally turn away from it. If she wanted to, Julia could stop the exposure intervention any time she wanted. She was in control of the pacing of events, and Amy was there to guide her through it.

Over the next few visits, they worked their way up the hierarchy, and Julia became increasingly composed and less emotionally distressed and anxious as she slowly recounted each detail of the rape. She also conducted the exposure in private every day for at least half an hour as agreed with the therapist. Over the next three weeks, she was beginning to feel "stronger," that the rape no longer "had a hold over me."

Role-Play and In Vivo Practice for Social Anxiety.   As they talked, it became clearer to Julia that what she really wanted to work on directly was talking to other people, including guys, and eventually to be comfortable alone with men. As she had already learned anxiety-management techniques (breath control and gauging her anxiety) when using imaginal exposure for the sexual assault, she could readily apply them when meeting people and engaging them in conversation. The social worker reviewed the deep-breathing exercises and encouraged Julia to couple deep breathing with her cognitive challenges to her "old tapes" that people were not going to like her or would reject her outright. Julia also took it upon herself to begin charting (i.e., self-monitoring) thoughts about initiating conversations with others, particularly men, to examine what she had been thinking and what was making her afraid. She discovered that she had always been shy because she was afraid that they would not want to talk to her, or would give her the brush-off.

Together Julia and Amy discussed social situations in which Julia would want to approach another person, and they arranged these situations hierarchically. First a young woman about her age in the college quad, the cafeteria, then at a party (increasingly personal settings). Then she would use the same hierarchy with young male students. A series of opening questions or topics of conversation were added to the proposed in vivo scenarios. Her objective was to make at least one social overture every day. She continued to keep her chart-diary, and reported successes in initiating conversations over the next two weeks. She was beginning to feel relaxed, and reported that much of the depression that had been burdening her for months was beginning to lift. She was beginning to have fun again, and was finally beginning to feel engaged in college life.

Although one might want to attribute the good results to the intervention itself, other events can also contribute to clinical improvement. One evening when Julia was working in the library, she went downstairs to get a soda and a snack from the vending machines. When she turned the corner, she encountered the third young man who had been at the scene just prior to the rape. They had not spoken together since the incident. He became very flustered. But, Julia took a deep breath as she saw he was becoming very anxious and said, "Hello, Todd, how are you?" Todd immediately began to apologize for not contacting Julia since the incident. He said that he had felt horrible about it, could not think what to say to her, and that he was very sorry. As Julia spoke with him, she felt a mixture of anger and compassion for him. He had not hurt her, but he had walked away when he felt things were becoming uncomfortable. At one point during the conversation, she suggested to him that perhaps he should talk to someone about what happened . . . but that he should not blame himself. At that point, his eyes welled up, and he wiped his face with his shirtsleeve. He said that he did blame himself, and that he had felt like a coward since the rape. He had cut off relations with his fraternity mates, who wouldn't have anything to do with him anymore. She later recounted in her diary how confident she felt speaking with him, and how she wished she could have done more to comfort him.

Selecting Scales and Creating Indexes to Monitor and Evaluate Client Progress

Fortunately, Julia was quite comfortable keeping a chart-diary, and her willingness to engage in self-monitoring provided an ideal opportunity for idiographic evaluation. Self-anchored indexes were used to measure depression, the number of times she initiated conversations, and her level of anxiety when thinking about the rape incident (table 8.1). The seventeen-item PTSD scale provided an ideal overall composite measure of PTSD-related distress symptoms.

SUMMARY

People suffering from the effects of traumatic events present serious clinical challenges to even the most experienced clinical social workers. There are a number of valid assessment instruments to accompany a thorough qualitative assessment. Cognitive-behavioral skills combined with exposure-based therapies are the most thoroughly researched approaches, and have been shown to be effective with PTSD. EMDR is also considered a viable option for treating PTSD. Although medication can be helpful to ameliorate some of the more troubling symptoms, it is not considered optimal care when applied without effective psychosocial methods. Although combinations of medication and psychosocial interventions can effectively ameliorate the symptoms and behaviors of PTSD, long-term positive outcomes remain a challenge.

TABLE 8.1   The client service plan for Julia

Problems	Goals	Sample Objectives	Interventions	Assessment Tools
Problems and symptoms associated with PTSD as a result of sexual assault	Reduce symptoms to a minimum	Use chart-diary to self-monitor situational-specific negative thoughts and response to them	Combined prolonged exposure and cognitive-behavioral coping skills	PTSD 17-item scale for overall symptoms
Depression: guilt, self-blame, crying, harsh self-criticism, trouble concentrating, some suicidal ideation	Reduce depression and related symptoms to pretrauma level		Psychoeducation, cognitive restructuring, anxiety-management skills, imaginal and in vivo exposure	Consider use of standardized depression scale Self-anchored indexes to examine degree of suicidal ideation
Anxiety, edginess, startles easily; troubled by mental images of the rape	Reduce excessive anxiety; increase control over images; develop anxiety-management skills	Learn breath control, use SUDS, and practice daily; develop hierarchy of rape-incident details; practice imaginal exposure daily for half an hour	Cognitive therapy/restructuring to examine negative critical thoughts and develop refutations Anxiety-management skills in conjunction with imaginal exposure to gain control over arousal associated with mental images of rape	Chart to monitor and examine patterns of thoughts, feelings, behaviors, and situations related to daily episodes of distress SUDS to measure anxiety level during imaginal or in vivo exposure exercises when coping with symptoms related to recollections of the rape or when dealing with social anxiety
Social anxiety, avoidance of social situations, especially encountering men alone	Improve social assertiveness and confidence in social situations	Develop hierarchy of social encounters; practice in vivo exposure daily	Anxiety-management skills in conjunction with in vivo exposure to practice social skills and reduce social anxiety with men and women in social encounters Case management: consultation with MD regarding antidepressant medication; referral to student organization dealing with rape on campus; peer consultation	

CHAPTER 9

DEPRESSION

Depression is one of the most common and debilitating psychosocial conditions in our society. As with most mental health disorders, the causes, course, and consequences of depression are multifaceted. Depression also co-occurs with a wide range of other mental health disorders, substance abuse, and health problems. Although biological and cognitive theories have dominated research on the causes of depression in recent decades, social scientists have become increasingly attuned to the deleterious effects of stressful social and environmental factors such as poverty, homelessness, interpersonal and community violence, and discrimination. The diagnosis and assessment of depression has been well-validated, and a number of effective pharmacological and psychosocial interventions are available to alleviate the symptoms of depression and improve social functioning. Pharmacological, psychotherapeutic, and clinical case management may be successfully combined for even the most depressed clients. This chapter reviews major aspects of assessment and intervention for depression in adults, and elderly depressed clients are given special emphasis.

ASSESSMENT

Background Data

General population estimates from the National Comorbidity Survey (Kessler et al., 1994) revealed that lifetime prevalence of major depressive disorder (MDD) was 12.7%, and 7.7% of people were diagnosed with the disorder within the previous twelve months. Another 4.8% and 2.1% were diagnosed with dysthymia for lifetime and previous twelve months, respectively. Women are more likely than men to have met the criteria for major depression in their lifetime (21.3% versus 17.1%) and within the previous twelve months (8% versus 6.4%). Other estimates of rates of depression (*DSM-IV-TR*; Kaplan & Saddock, 1998) in community samples vary from 10% to 25% for women and from 5% to 12% for men, suggesting that rates of depression among women may be twice that of men (Blumenthal, 1994; Sprock & Yoder, 1997; P. F. Sullivan, Neale, & Kendler, 2000; L. Chen, Eaton, Gallo, Nestadt, & Crum, 2000). Point prevalence (people diagnosed at any give time) has varied in studies from 5% to 9% for women and from 2% to 3% for men.

Rates of depression are higher in medical patients and people who do not have close interpersonal relationships. Major depressive episode is also associated with high mortality. Up to 15% of individuals diagnosed with depression will die by suicide. In addition, there is a fourfold increase in death rates of individuals with MDD after age fifty-five. First-degree biological relatives of people with MDD are one and one-half to three times as likely to be diagnosed with this disorder as are people in the general population (*DSM-IV-TR*; H.I. Kaplan & Saddock, 1998). International studies show that although rates of depression vary across cultures, women consistently show higher rates of depression and appear to experience longer episodes. In the United States, rates of depression may be increasing more rapidly among women than among men (Weissman et al., 2000). Depression is a heterogeneous disorder, but there appears to be little clinical utility for subtypes such as "melancholic" or "seasonal" depression.

Adolescence may be an especially critical time for the development of depression. In a longitudinal study of university students, several measures taken over a ten-year span revealed an upsurge in rates of depression between ages fifteen and eighteen, but the female rate rises to twice that of males (Hankin et al., 1998). Reviews of the research concerning women and depression (Blumenthal, 1994; Sprock & Yoder, 1997) have revealed evidence strongly suggesting that these differences are probably due to interacting causes, including biological factors (e.g., hormonal differences emerging during puberty), psychosocial stressors (e.g., multiple competing roles at home and work, sexual and physical abuse, sensitivity to losses, insufficient social supports, discrimination), and difference in socialization factors (e.g., favoring of boy children over girls and the subsequent cultivation of the self-effacing personality in young women). How these factors interact and change over time requires further investigation.

Although multiple factors appear to be at work in the increased risk of depression among women, a recent investigation of a clinical population demonstrated that women were more likely to have experienced a severe negative stressful event before the onset of their depressive episode (Spangler, Simons, Monroe, & Thase, 1996). Adult women's increased risk factors for depression include longer episodes that are more likely to develop into chronic and recurrent depression; a greater likelihood of depression's being triggered by negative life events, seasonal sensitivity, hormonal differences related to menstrual cycle, pregnancy, birth (postpartum depression), and menopause; and increased comorbidity with other disorders such as anxiety disorders and bulimia. Women are also likely to experience differential responses to medication, although evidence is sparse because women are not well represented in controlled clinical trials (Kornstein, 1997).

As with other mental disorders, depression is likely to co-occur with alcohol abuse and dependence. The NLAES (Grant & Harford, 1995) demonstrated that not only is the co-occurrence of depression and substance-abuse disorders prevalent in society, but it is even higher among women, African Americans, and middle-age-to-older Americans. A recent Australian survey of people ranging in age from eighteen to eighty (Rodgers et al., 2000) revealed that, although there is a strong association between people who drink heavily and symptoms of anxiety and depression, the relationship may be U-shaped. That is, those who do not drink at all and those who use alcohol heavily are more likely to experience symptoms of anxiety and depression. This relationship appears to be similar for both men and women. Given the substantial co-occurrence of depression and alcohol abuse, however, there is promising evidence that adding CBT for depression to standard substance-abuse intervention can help improve overall outcomes (R. A. Brown, Evans, Miller, Burgess, & Mueller, 1997).

Cultural differences regarding treatment and research on depression have been explored in qualitative investigations. For example, Koss-Chioino (1999) pointed out that although rates of depression among Puerto Rican women are comparable to women in the United States, the causes of depression may be somewhat culturally determined. She cites evidence that "traditional sex-role socialization encourages inhibition of assertiveness, which in turn leads to psychological problems, such as depression and psychosomatic symptoms" (p. 335). Depressive episodes may also be triggered by negative life events or role strains in family relations that may be somewhat distinct from other cultural contexts. Women's depression in primary health-care settings is likely to go undetected, and minority women appear unlikely to seek help from mental health or social service workers (Van Hook, 1999).

Older persons of color, in addition to being subjected to the other challenges of old age, are also more likely to have suffered from discrimination and other forms of oppression, given that they grew up before the civil rights movement brought many of these issues to a head (Beckett & Dungee-Anderson, 2000). Even more so than their white counterparts, African Americans, Native Americans, Hispanics, and Asian Americans are likely to have experienced poverty, fewer insurance benefits because of employment discrimination, poorer housing, and more health problems due to lack of access to health care. Socioeconomic problems are disproportionately incurred by racial minorities, and these factors appear to increase depression.

Over the past few decades, a growing number of immigrants from Southeast Asia have come to the United States, many of them traumatized by decades of war, and many having experienced imprisonment or torture. Most arrived as political refugees and, as a result of these stressors, have shown disproportionate signs of psychological strain, including symptoms of depression. Many of the continued symptoms of stress are associated with poverty, poor English-language proficiency, lack of social supports, and lower self-esteem (Kinzie et al., 1982; Nicassio, 1983; Tran, 1993). For many, there appears to be a direct dose-response relationship between the extent of traumatic stress and psychological and health-related consequences (Mollica, Poole, & Tor, 1998). However, premigration stressors may be moderated by level of acculturation. Immigrants who become more acculturated in their new host country are likely to suffer less stress and depression resulting from their premigration trauma experiences

(Ngo, Tran, Gibbons, & Oliver, 2001). These symptoms of stress and strain may be co-occurring with an increase in substance abuse (O'Hare & Tran, 1998). People from Southeast Asia, including those who have experienced war-related trauma, seem to experience depression and stress symptoms, in part, as somatic distress, an important factor that should be included in conceptualizations and measurement of depression (Kinzie et al., 1982; K. Uehara, Morelli, & Abe-Kim, 2001).

Depression and the Elderly

As the population of elderly people in the United States continues to grow, so will the demand and costs for interdisciplinary health and social work services. Increasing political, technological, ethical, and service-delivery challenges await the future of social work with the elderly (Feit & Cuevas-Feit, 1996). Although the rate of depression in older adults may be comparable to that of the general population, high-risk groups include older women and those with moderate to severe illnesses. In addition, older adults tend to be underdiagnosed for depression, in part because of minimization by the client, underdetection by professionals, or confounding psychiatric and medical symptoms (Dick & Gallagher-Thompson, 1996). The *DSM* criteria for depression may also lack sensitivity for detecting depression in the elderly. Underdetection for depression can increase risk of suicide, so practitioners should always screen for such risks. Caution should be taken with differential diagnosis as well. Sorting out depression from cognitive impairments and other medical complaints, bereavement reactions, substance abuse, and the side effects of medication can be challenging. Relying on multiple sources of data and focusing on the course of the disorder and the duration and progression of symptoms can help sort out the right diagnoses and causes of psychosocial distress.

Depression is a common ailment in older people with Alzheimer's disease (AD; Teri, 1996). Given that the likelihood of developing dementia increases with age, clinicians must be vigilant for its possible onset. Memory problems may be related to a number of disorders, including depression and dementia. In turn, dementia may be related to a number of medical conditions (such as substance abuse or cerebral-vascular disease). AD, which accounts for half or more of all cases of dementia, is the fourth leading cause of death in the United States and may last from three to twenty years from onset to the end of life. The prevalence of dementia in the community is estimated at about 3%, with rates climbing from about 1.5% for individuals in their late sixties to 16–25% for persons eighty-five years or older (*DSM-IV-TR*; H. I. Kaplan & Saddock, 1998; Callaway, 1998).

The primary cognitive deficits associated with AD include aphasia (deterioration in the use of meaningful language), apraxia (inability to perform ordinary motor activities such as brushing one's teeth), and agnosia (inability to recognize and name common objects such as a chair). These disturbances must be severe enough to indicate impairment and a decline in social or occupational functioning. Deterioration in cortical functioning may be manifested by difficulty or inability in planning and carrying out task-oriented behaviors that involve several sequential steps, such as preparing a meal, or difficulty coping with novel situations. AD generally has a progressive and irreversible course. Early-stage AD is marked by short-term memory loss, disorientation, personality changes, impaired judgment and information processing, and compromised problem-solving skills. The middle stage is characterized by difficulties in both short- and long-term memory, language, social skills, abstract reasoning, and activities of adult daily living. Late stage, which lasts less than two years, includes problems with getting around, speech deficits, greater disorientation and self-care difficulties, incontinence, and disinterest in eating. As memory deterioration may be one of the early signs of AD, it is important that clinicians make note of it and pursue further clinical diagnostic investigation rather than assuming it is related to depression. As a result of memory deterioration, orientation to time, place, and person may also be affected. Over time, personality changes may become apparent, changes that may be particularly disturbing to the client's family members (*DSM-IV-TR*; H. I. Kaplan & Saddock, 1998; Callaway, 1998). Thus, given the complex diagnostic concerns regarding depression and related psychiatric and other medical conditions, clinical social workers who serve the elderly should collaborate closely with medical specialists on assessment and intervention planning.

Anxiety disorders also commonly co-occur with depression (S. L. Smith, Sherrill, & Colenda, 1995). One study, conducted in the Netherlands (Beekman et al., 2000), examined the co-occurrence and risk-factor patterns for both anxiety and depression in a random sample of older people (ages 55–85) as part of a ten-year longitudinal study. Using well-validated standardized measures, they found that almost 48% of those who met the criteria for depressive disorder also met the criteria for anxiety disorder. Conversely, about 26% of those with anxiety disorder were also depressed. The only risk factor these two conditions shared, however, was a psychological marker "external locus of control" (a general sense that one's life is controlled by external forces more so than by one's own behavior). Anxiety disorders were particularly associated with a range of vulnerability and stress-related factors. Again, social workers should be acutely aware that psychopathology is highly variable and highly interactive with current stressors in their clients' lives, including the lives of their elderly clients. There are multiple possible sources of anxiety for the elderly person: stressors associated with retirement and the loss of friends and loved ones accompanied by subsequent feelings of loneliness, uselessness, and hopelessness. Medical problems, including the loss of normal functions such as eyesight and hearing, may add to fears of dying or becoming incapacitated. Other financial and situational stressors can exacerbate anxiety as well (S. L. Smith et al.).

Alcohol abuse is a serious problem among older Americans and often co-occurs with depression and other related psychosocial disorders. Liberto, Oslin, and Ruskin (1996) report that estimates of daily drinking among older people range from 10% to 22%, and estimates of heavier drinking from 3% to 9%. They also report that about half of these people would likely meet *DSM* criteria for abuse or dependence. Drinking rates among the elderly are higher for men, and consumption levels appear to be comparable among older African-American, Hispanic, and white men. Older persons who drink are also more likely to experience co-occurring anxiety disorder, drug abuse (especially prescription drugs), and other psychosocial stressors such as caretaker burden, poverty, and loneliness associated with grief and loss (Sanjuan & Langenbucher, 1999). The elderly are more vulnerable to negative health effects from consuming alcohol, even if they drink proportionately less than younger adults. Such problems include alcoholic liver disease, organic brain syndrome, obstructive pulmonary disease, strokes, gastritis, pancreatitis, and sleep disorders. Detoxification of the elderly also carries greater risks and is associated with a higher rate of mortality. Alcohol abuse can cloud the diagnostic picture and distort the clinical presentation of other disorders such as dementia and other organic illnesses associated with old age.

Theories

A range of biological, psychological, interpersonal, and stress-diathesis theories have been posited to explain the causes and maintenance of depression, but it has become increasingly clear that depression is more likely to be understood within an interdisciplinary matrix of interacting biopsychosocial processes. The role of biological processes in the predisposition for some people toward depression has been appreciated for some time now. Based on studies comparing monozygotic and dizygotic twins, twins separated at birth and raised by adoptive parents, and studies of first-degree relatives, evidence strongly suggests that biological factors predispose some people to depression. Estimates for increased risk due to inheritance are substantial, and the genetic component for bipolar disorder appears to be even higher (A. Schwartz & Schwartz, 1993; H. I. Kaplan & Saddock, 1998; *DSM-IV-TR*; P. F. Sullivan et al., 2000). A recent meta-analysis (with results based mostly on twin studies) revealed that familial genetic influence increases the risk of developing depression by a factor of almost three (P. F. Sullivan et al.). These researchers estimated the inheritability of depression at between 31% and 42% (as compared to schizophrenia and bipolar disorder, which may be as high as 70%). A survey that followed up about 2,000 subjects from the Epidemiological Catchment Area survey also demonstrated that inheritance factors were strong for depression (L. Chen et al., 2000).

As with a number of mental disorders, depression appears to be related to dysregulation of neurotransmitters (A. Schwartz & Schwartz, 1993; H. I. Kaplan & Saddock, 1998). Depletion of serotonin may precipitate depression, and dopamine activity may also be reduced in depression. Recently, research on animals (including primates) and preliminary findings in studies of humans have demonstrated that depression appears to be associated with hypersecretion of corticotropin-releasing hormone and subsequent overactivation of the hypothalamic-adrenal-pituitary axis, glands directly involved in hormone regulation and mood. There is suggestive evidence that these hormonal oversecretions may be influenced by genetic factors as well as environmental stressors (O'Keane, 2000). Nevertheless, to date no laboratory findings have been found to confirm a diagnosis of major depression. These various physiological processes may be related, and further research is needed to delineate their relationship to the various symptoms of depression and their degree of severity.

Cognitive and social-cognitive theories have dominated the psychological literature regarding depression over the past few decades. A number of theories have contributed to the understanding of depression (Dobson & Jackman-Cram, 1996), including learned helplessness theory (M. E. Seligman, 1975; Abramson, Seligman, & Teasdale, 1978), behavioral theory (Lewisohn, 1974), and perhaps most prominently, Beck's cognitive theory of depression (Beck, 1976; Beck et al., 1979; D. A. Clark & Beck, 1999). Learned-helplessness theory posits that depressed individuals are more likely to have stable, global, and internal attributions in response to negative life events (versus external attributions, or seeing problems caused by situational factors beyond their immediate control). These negative internal attributions can lead to hopelessness, helplessness, and depression. Lewisohn's behavioral theory focuses on the role of reinforcement contingencies inherent in interpersonal skills, and the interpretation of social reinforcers. According to Persons and Fresco (1998), Lewisohn's model posits that one's depression or happiness is in part contingent on the amount of positive reinforcement in one's life, the number and range or stimuli that one finds reinforcing, the availability of reinforcers, and one's skill in obtaining reinforcers.

Cognitive Theory.   Perhaps the most empirically developed theory of depression is that of Beck and colleagues (Beck, 1976; Beck et al., 1979; D. A. Clark & Beck, 1999). Cognitive theory of depression is an important development because it has shed light on psychological processes relevant to problems other than depression, including anxiety disorders. Beck's cognitive theory has evolved since the 1960s. The earlier formulation (Beck 1976; Beck et al., 1979) laid down the fundamental components that remain relevant to the current, albeit more complex, model. Although no assertions are made in cognitive theory regarding the ultimate cause of depression, priority or primacy is given to cognitive events within the interactions of physiological, behavioral, and environmental factors.

Three concepts constitute the major building blocks of the theory: the cognitive triad, schemata, and faulty information processing. The *cognitive triad* consists of three major cognitive patterns: first, the negative view of the self, that is, seeing oneself as defective some way, worthless, the cause of bad things happening, and so forth; second, a negative view of the world, that is, seeing the world as placing major obstacles in one's path to happiness; and third, holding a negative view of the future, that is, being pessimistic, expecting poor outcomes for one's efforts. These negative expectations of the self, the world, and the future are likely to negatively affect motivation, resulting in a sense of helplessness, hopelessness, and dependency, and may promote physiological symptoms of depression (e.g., low energy).

Negative schemata, the second major component of the cognitive theory of depression, are relatively stable cognitive patterns by which a person interprets life's experiences. Schemata may not always be active but, when activated by some external event, are likely to determine how the person will respond. If these schemata result in a distortion of life's events, they may lead to faulty information processing and misinterpretations that result in less than optimal or even maladaptive responses. The more distorted the interpretations, the more likely the negative schemata will affect behavior in a negative way. The more severe the distortions in reality, the less likely the person is to consider that negative interpretations are erroneous. These negative schemata appear to have their origins in one's social learning experience, including early life experiences.

The third major component of the cognitive theory of depression is *faulty information processing*, in which illogical or distorted thinking reinforces the negative view of self, the world, and the future. These faulty thinking processes may include arbitrary inference (drawing conclusions with little or no evidence to support the belief), selective abstraction (giving disproportionate weight to a small sample of evidence, perhaps viewed out of context), overgeneralization (erroneously applying conclusions based on small amounts of observational data), magnification or minimization (grossly over- or underestimating the significance of a particular event), personalization (erroneously relating external events to oneself), and absolutistic or dichotomous thinking (seeing events in polar extremes rather than on a continuum).

Recent developments in cognitive theory modify and add detail to the key concepts (D.A. Clark & Beck, 1999). A superordinate framework subsumes most of the prior theoretical developments within three categories: cognitive structures, information processing, and the products of cognitive structures.

Cognitive structures subsume the earlier concepts of cognitive schemata, and delineate various types, including cognitive-conceptual, affective, physiological, behavioral, and motivation schemata. The content of schemata (when activated in a depressed person) is constituted with elements of the cognitive triad as defined above. A more recently developed concept of *modes* (Beck, 1996; D.A. Clark & Beck, 1999) refers to hypothesized clusters of cognitive-conceptual, affective, physiological, behavioral, and motivational schemata organized in response to the particular demands on a person. These modes may be primal (emphasizing self-preservation), constructive (relationships and work), or minor modes (mundane and routine activities of daily living). *Personality* is understood as a relatively stable organization of various schemata and is most likely genetically predisposed. *Orienting schemata* guide the activation of modes in response to environmental stimuli.

Information processing may vary by different levels of activation by which environmental input is matched to relevant schemata and modes, accessibility by which information can be transferred from long- to short-term memory, levels of attention, and consciousness of information processing. Faulty information processes produce cognitive errors, which become even more pronounced when the client is affected by high emotional states such as depression and anxiety.

Products of cognitive structures constitute those thoughts, feelings, and behaviors that interact with cognitive structures in adaptive or maladaptive ways. Key cognitive products relevant to pathological conditions such as depression are the negative automatic thoughts presumably related to the client's problems. Cognitive constructions are ultimately the conceptual constructions (e.g., people, experiences, events) that provide meaning.

The above interacting cognitive structures, processes, and products are subject to self-referent activity that results in self-schemata. The interaction of depression-causing schemata and continuation of cognitive errors can become self-perpetuating. In the depressed person, this process may be expressed as "pervasive negativity toward the self" (D. A. Clark & Beck, 1999, p. 109).

Social-Cognitive Theory. Social-cognitive theory evolved empirically from early behavioral models (Bandura, 1977, 1986), and although cognitive processes are emphasized, social-cognitive theory more explicitly emphasizes the reciprocal interaction of psychological, physiological, and environmental factors. Social-learning theory (Bandura, 1977) engendered a "revolution" (Mahoney, 1977) in behaviorism by demonstrating the necessity of cognitive mediating factors to account for some of the limitations in reinforcement theory. Immediate, observable reinforcement in human behavior may be facilitative for behavior change, but social-learning theorists demonstrated that observable reinforcement was not necessary for behavior change. Social-cognitive theory emphasizes the role of cognitive processes that mediate external stimuli and behavioral responses. These cognitive processes include attention, retention, motor reproduction, and motivational processes. People essentially learn through information gathering, vicarious learning through observation of others' modeling behavior, and experience. Social-cognitive theorists see the development of psychosocial disorders as primarily the result of learning dysfunctional and maladaptive behaviors. As such, changing dysfunctional patterns of thinking, feeling, and behaving within the context of an individual's unique circumstances generally becomes a process of learning more adaptive ways of thinking and improving behavioral coping skills.

Cognitive-Behavioral Treatment. Cognitive-behavioral interventions are informed by cognitive theory, social-cognitive theory, and traditional (stimulus-response) behavioral theories. Currently, cognitive-behavioral treatment clearly emphasizes changing cognitions through direct cognitive means and behavioral-change techniques to disconfirm dysfunctional beliefs. This disconfirmatory experience is likely to increase self-efficacy by improving coping skills across different situations (Bandura, 1986). These success experiences can be highly reinforcing for the client.

Cognitive factors related to depression are best understood when seen within the context of social and environmental influences, which may provide a degree of competing risk and protective factors to precipitate or buffer an individual against the development of serious depression. Beck and associates (e.g., D. A. Clark & Beck, 1999) have begun to pay more attention, for example, to the appraisal of environmental factors in the causes of depression, and have incorporated stress-environment theoretical concepts into a more interactive model of cognitive theory (e.g., R. S. Lazarus & Folkman, 1984). Evidence for the relationship between depression and social-environmental conditions, stressful life events including losses (Stueve, Dohrenwend, & Skodol, 1998; G. W. Brown, 1998), has been known for some time. Other social-environmental stressors such as racism and discrimination have been linked to stress and symptoms of depression (Utsey & Ponterotto, 1996). However, in the Epidemiological Catchment Area study noted earlier (L. Chen et al., 2000), stressful life events were shown to be associated only with mild and episodic forms of depression rather than with major depression. Nevertheless, the addition of environmental stressors may increase overall vulnerability, and the environmental influences are likely to be unique to an individual and to the way those stressors are cognitively appraised. Although cognitive processes play a critical role, changing depression-causing cognitions may be initiated or precipitated through other routes such as biological interventions or environmental changes. Despite the lack of consensus among theoreticians regarding the specific causal pathways of depression, evidence suggests that facilitating environmental supports can have some preventive value. For example, a three-year follow-up survey with almost 2,000 elderly persons in Amsterdam demonstrated that social supports (including marriage) provided significant buffering effects against depression (Shoevers et al., 2000).

Key Elements of Multidimensional/ Functional Assessment

A considerable amount of research has informed the diagnostic criteria for the depressive disorders (*DSM-IV-TR*), and the data currently reflect a multidimensional view that includes physiological and psychosocial indicators of distress. Criteria for MDD include the presence of a major depressive episode defined by experiencing five relevant symptoms during the same two-week period. The symptoms represent a change from previous functioning (at least one of the symptoms is either depressed mood or a loss of interest or pleasure). The relevant symptoms include a consistently depressed mood; markedly diminished interest or pleasure in almost all activities; significant (unintended) weight loss or consistent decrease or increase in appetite; insomnia or hypersomnia nearly every day; psychomotor agitation or retardation nearly every day;

fatigue or loss of energy nearly every day; feelings of worthlessness or excessive or inappropriate guilt (which may be delusional); difficulty concentrating; recurrent thoughts of death (not just fear of dying), which may include recurrent suicidal ideation (without a specific plan), or a suicide attempt or a specific plan for committing suicide. As with other psychosocial conditions, the assessment is strengthened if data are collected from both the client and collateral observers.

MDF assessment requires going beyond merely enumerating the psychophysiological symptoms of depression; it demands an examination of the reciprocal nature of these symptoms with people in the client's social context. Depression is largely experienced as an interpersonal problem, as suggested in the discussion of cognitive and environmental theories above. Depression can be brought on or exacerbated by interpersonal conflict and problems, and, conversely, living with a person suffering with depression can put considerable strain on those around him or her. A depressed person may be relatively inactive (lying around the house brooding in silence for hours or glued to the television), relatively uncommunicative with others in the household (leaving partners to wonder what is wrong, or children, what they have done wrong). The depressed person may be irritable, argumentative, and uncooperative at work; actively avoid social gatherings; show little enthusiasm for leisure time on the weekends or planning vacations; or generally apathetic about making future plans. A seriously depressed person can cast a gloom over a household for months or years, and conflict may often erupt as, over time, empathy from loved ones erodes as the person's relative inactivity and apparent apathy is increasingly resented. Over time, the lack of cooperation, aloofness, and sparse communication or argumentativeness can lead to disaffection from family, friends, and workmates. Understanding depression in a broader psychosocial context can help in planning an intervention that goes beyond symptom reduction, but provides the family with an opportunity to better understand what is happening to their loved one, take their behavior less "personally," and speed the client's recovery by providing important social and emotional support.

Functional assessment should focus on how the depressed client's symptoms vary day-to-day in their social context (Persons & Fresco, 1998). Depressed clients may experience their depression more acutely at different times of the day, or at different times of the week (weekends may be particularly acute, removed from the distraction of work, and withdrawn from social contacts). The type, frequency, and severity of the client's signs and symptoms should be examined over time and across different social contexts: work, friends, family, and so on. The practitioner should also help the client track the occurrence of other emotional disturbances, behavioral problems, and interpersonal difficulties, all of which may be related to depression.

Screening for Suicide.   Client suicide may be one of the more worrisome concerns for practitioners. Although no social worker can offer 100% certainty of predicting and preventing client suicide, well-researched guidelines can heighten awareness of potential suicide and help the clinician know when to take preventative action. Based on a range of demographic and clinical data, guidelines for the assessment of suicide risk include both general indicators and specific risk factors for suicide (Peruzzi & Bongar, 1999). General indicators include being male, having a serious mental disorder (e.g., schizophrenia, alcoholism, depression); a history of suicide attempts; a history of suicide attempts in the family; being unemployed or experiencing other job-related problems; being unmarried or socially isolated; communicating suicidal intent, having made previous suicide attempts; possessing the lethal means to complete a suicide; communicating a sense of hopelessness (possibly an even better predictor than depression itself); having experienced chronic and stressful life events (including traumatic events); having aggressive or angry feelings; and suffering from serious physical illness.

In addition to general indicators, Peruzzi and Bongar (1999) suggest the following as predictors for clients diagnosed with major depression: attraction to death (fantasizing about it), experiencing anhedonia, suffering from psychic anxiety, having acute suicidal ideation, engaging in acute alcohol abuse, and experiencing interpersonal stress, especially losses and separations. These items should be assessed in all clients, with an increasingly detailed focus on any item that the client positively indicates. As a rule of thumb, all these risk factors should be gauged individually on a continuum from mild to severe, and they should be seen as additive, that is, suicide risk increases as the number of risk factors increases. When risk factors are identified, practitioners should follow them up over the course of treatment until it becomes clear that clients have improved, some of the acute problems are resolved, and they appear to be no longer at significant risk. Inpatient hospitalization should be seriously considered for clients who appear to be suicidal. If a client is treated on an outpatient basis, the practitioner should increase supervision of the client by being more available to the client (e.g., more frequent visits, phone contacts) as well as informing and recruiting significant others to monitor the client.

Practitioners have control over conducting and documenting a valid and thorough suicide assessment. They do not have control over whether a client ultimately completes a suicide. Nevertheless, there are some pitfalls to avoid in conducting suicide assessments. Bongar, Maris, Berman, and Litman (1992) examined malpractice data and clinical literature to identify common practice failures that can be avoided. They point out that prediction of suicide, given that it is a relatively rare event, is difficult. It also constitutes a troubling legal burden for practitioners because they are asked, essentially, to assume responsibility for another person's behavior. Nevertheless, social workers are expected to provide a reasonable degree of protection for clients against their suicidal actions. Bongar et al. itemized a number of procedural failures that practitioners can avoid in outpatient care. These include the practitioner's failure to

provide a diagnosis;

conduct a thorough mental-status exam;

complete a formal treatment plan;

provide a safe outpatient treatment environment;

document their clinical rationale, judgment, and significant observations;

refer a client for a medication evaluation;

specify criteria for hospitalization and/or implement hospitalization;

provide adequate supervision (if the social worker is a supervisor);

evaluate for suicide at intake and at other intervention transitions; and

secure prior records for medical/mental health history.

Although there are no guarantees that even the most thorough and skilled practitioner can prevent every potential suicide over years of practice, social workers can exercise prudence by providing thorough and well-documented assessments, keeping the client's interests paramount, and documenting their efforts to provide competent care. Conducting evidence-based assessment improves risk-management practices for social workers and their employers, and assures clients that they will receive the best care possible.

Special Considerations When Evaluating Depression in the Elderly. When conducting an assessment for depression with an elderly person, practitioners often have to consider related problems: cognitive impairment, functional capacity, decision-making ability, whether to bring in outside caretakers, and whether to place the client in a nursing home (Edelstein, Staats, Kalish, & Northrop, 1996). As with MDF assessment in general, gerontology researchers stress the need for a biopsychosocial framework, and emphasize that practitioners should avail themselves of multiple sources of data, observe the environment firsthand, use reliable and valid measurement instruments, observe interaction of the individual with significant others in their environment, take note of the consequences of the elderly client's behaviors on others, and test out their assessment hypotheses. Practitioners should also be mindful of their own biases about the elderly, such as, they are unproductive and disengaged from society, old folks get "set in their ways," and senility is inevitable. Performance decrements (related to depression and other forms of psychopathology) may manifest themselves differently than in younger adults; for example, the elderly may have more performance fears, lower expectations, memory problems, poor concentration, and fatigue. Other physical problems may also affect the elderly client's presentation and symptoms; for example, visual and auditory senses may be compromised, clients may suffer loss of physical flexibility and strength, and they may experience problems (such as pain) related to chronic illnesses and the effect of medications.

Depression and symptoms of physical illnesses can be intertwined in complex ways. Physical illness and depression can be reciprocally exacerbating, symptoms of both illnesses may be similar, medications can cause or exacerbate depression, and alcohol abuse may negatively affect medications, physical symptoms, and depression. The institutionalized elderly person and those undergoing medical treatment are more likely to be depressed. Practitioners should be alert to stressful negative events, health problems, losses, changes in social roles, lower income, late-life caregiving role, and other acute and chronic stressors as possible risk factors for depression (R. Wolfe, Morrow, & Fredrickson, 1996).

One of the most important assessment tasks may be to distinguish depressive symptoms from dementia (R. Wolfe et al., 1996; Safford, 1997). Cognitive, affective, and behavioral symptoms of dementia and depression overlap, but depression is generally more treatable than are symptoms of dementia. The depressed client is more likely not to be confused or have significant problems with everyday tasks than people with Alzheimer's disease, more likely to be anxious, and more likely to manifest the other classic symptoms of depression, such as early morning wakening. Depressed clients also appear to show more rapid onset and progression, have more problems with social skills, complain more about forgetfulness, underestimate their cognitive performance more, and display more negative memories. Clients with dementia have slower onset and progression, minimize or overlook performance deficits, show fewer classic symptoms of depression, show a decline in short-term memory, do worse on formal tests of cognitive performance, tend to show more confusion and confabulation, and demonstrate cognitive performance that is more consistently and pervasively impaired.

Most of what was discussed earlier regarding assessment of suicide risk in adult populations generally applies to the elderly as well. However, there may be some special considerations. Suicide appears to be more common among the elderly than among younger adult populations (R. Wolfe et al., 1996; Kennedy, Metz, & Lowinger, 1996). Up to 70% of late-life suicides are related to serious illness, and attempts are often made after having consulted a physician. Although the illness may play a central role, degree of hopelessness about whether their illness can be treated may be an even stronger predictor. Research on prevention and intervention with elderly suicide is very sparse.

Instruments

The Beck Depression Inventory (BDI; Beck, Ward, Mendelson, Mock, & Erbaugh, 1961) has become one of the most well-known scales for assessment of depression, and the psychometric properties of the BDI have been thoroughly documented. The item pool for the BDI was derived from observations of clinically depressed and other psychiatric patients, and compiled as a twenty-one item self-report scale that measures mood, pessimism, sense of failure, lack of satisfaction, guilt, sense of punishment, self-dislike, self-accusation, suicidal wishes, crying, irritability, social withdrawal, indecisiveness, distortion of body image, work inhibition, sleep disturbance, fatigability, loss of appetite, weight loss, somatic preoccupations, and loss of libido. These items are scored on a 0–3 scale, with cutoff scores 0–9 for none or minimal depression, 10–18 for mild to moderate, 19–29 for moderate to severe, and 30–63 for severe depression. Reviews of the psychometric properties have revealed that the BDI has very good internal consistency (mid-.80s on average) for both clinical and nonclinical populations, good test-retest reliability, and good factorial validity (measuring negative attitudes toward self and behavioral and somatic disturbances related to depression. Factor structures in various studies varied somewhat by study sample (Beck, Steer, & Garbin, 1988). Recently, the BDI-II was developed, with some modifications in item content and formatting covering a two-week (versus one week) reporting time to make it more congruent with *DSM-IV* criteria (Dozois, Dobson, & Ahnberg, 1998). Overall, however, the new version is quite similar to the original BDI. The BDI is a proprietary instrument, and agencies must incur some cost to use it.

Although scale developers often claim that their instrument measures unique features of a construct, these nuanced differences often have little clinical significance. Depression scales, including the BDI and the Hamilton Depression Rating Scale (HAM-D; Hamilton, 1960), tend to correlate highly (e.g., Hotopf, Sharp, & Lewis, 1998). The HAM-D has also been shown to be valid for detecting depression in demented patients for whom a cutoff score of ten is recommended (rather than the usual seventeen; Kertzman, Treves, Treves, Vainder, & Korczyn, 2002). The HAM-D is one of the most extensively used and well-validated scales in clinical research. It requires that the practitioner have a competent grasp of assessment for depression. There are no specific prompts, as such, and the interviewer must probe and examine each symptom category in a face-to-face semistructured interview. The HAM-D is in the public domain and may be used without cost (instrument 9.1).

Brief depression screens can improve detection and assessment of depression in the elderly (Dorfman et al., 1995). The Geriatric Depression Scale (GDS; Yesavage et al., 1983) was designed specifically to detect depression in elderly clients. It is a screening tool, and as such, a positive score (from 11 to 14) should prompt a more in-depth assessment and diagnosis for depression. The GDS was developed from a pool of one hundred items suggested by practitioners and researchers. It was administered to a sample of nondepressed elderly people (more than fifty-five years of age), some of whom were hospitalized. The thirty items that correlated best with a diagnosis of depression were retained for the scale. Items that emphasized somatic symptoms were not included because they also correlated with physical symptoms experienced by nondepressed older adults. The yes/no format allows for easy administration. The GDS was shown to have both high internal consistency and split-half reliability. Edelstein et al. (1996) reviewed the literature regarding the GDS, and cited evidence that supports good sensitivity and specificity but, as might be expected, suggested that the GDS may not be as accurate for seriously cognitively impaired adults. The GDS appears to be more sensitive to detecting depression in the elderly than the HAM-D, the BDI, or the Zung Depression Scale (Dick & Gallagher-Thompson, 1996).

INSTRUMENT 9.1   Hamilton Depression Rating Scale (HAM-D)

The total Hamilton Depression (HAM-D) Rating Scale provides an indication of depression and, over time, provides a valuable guide to progress.

Classification of symptoms which may be difficult to obtain can be scored as:
0 - absent; 1 - doubtful or trivial; 2 - present.
Classification of symptoms where more detail can be obtained can be expanded to:
0 - absent; 1 - mild; 2 - moderate; 3 - severe; 4 - incapacitating.

In general the higher the total score the more severe the depression.
HAM-D score level of depression:
10-13 mild; 14-17 mild to moderate; >17 moderate to severe.

Assessment is recommended at two-week intervals.

Symptoms

1.	Depressed mood	0 1 2 3 4
2.	Guilt feelings	0 1 2 3 4
3.	Suicide	0 1 2 3 4
4.	Insomnia—early	0 1 2
5.	Insomnia—middle	0 1 2
6.	Insomnia—late	0 1 2
7.	Work and activities	0 1 2 3 4
8.	Retardation—psychomotor	0 1 2 3 4
9.	Agitation	0 1 2 3 4
10.	Anxiety—psychological	0 1 2 3 4
11.	Anxiety—somatic	0 1 2 3 4
12.	Somatic symptoms—GI	0 1 2
13.	Somatic symptoms—general	0 1 2
14.	Sexual dysfunction—menstrual disturbance	0 1 2
15.	Hypochondrias	0 1 2 3 4
16.	Weight loss—by history	0 1 2
	—by scales	0 1 2
17.	Insight	0 1 2

Total Score _____

A comprehensive review of the GDS (Stiles & McGarrahan, 1998) summarized the psychometric data and administrative recommendations. Although there are briefer versions of the GDS, the original thirty-item version of the scale is recommended, given that it is the most researched version. It can be used as a self-report instrument, but is probably better administered by clinical staff. Recommended cutoff scores range from 11 to 14 as an indicator of depression (using 11 might increase false positives; 14 will reduce false positives). Based on the original scoring (with individual items rated yes = 1 and no = 0), 0–10 is generally considered normal, 11–19 mildly depressed, and 20–30 severely depressed. Research on the GDS shows relatively consistent support for it relia-bility and validity, including good internal consistency, test-retest reliability, and good sensitivity and specificity in discriminating between depressed and non-depressed individuals. Using the GDS with seriously demented clients is proba-bly of questionable validity, although it should be considered valid for those who show only mild to moderate symptoms of dementia. Most studies have shown moderate to high correlations between the GDS and other standardized depres-sion scales, thus arguing for its concurrent validity. The GDS has been translated into many languages, although data regarding reliability and validity with other cultures and races are mixed. More cross-cultural research with the GDS is needed. The GDS is in the public domain, and reprinted here (instrument 9.2).

Because depression scales do not target common co-occurring symptoms in the very old, scales that measure cognitive impairment may also need to be included in assessment and implemented by practitioners trained specifically in conducting thorough mental-status exams. One of the better-validated and most commonly used scales for measuring cognitive impairments is the Mini-Mental State Examination (Folstein, Folstein, & McHugh, 1975), considered perhaps the best all-around screen for cognitive impairment including dementia. It takes five to ten minutes to administer, and a score of 23 or less is the cutoff for cognitive impairment with high sensitivity. The twenty-item screen for cognitive function-ing measures orientation, attention, and concentration, recall memory, ability to follow a three-step command, and other gross indicators of problems with cog-nitive functioning.

SELECTING EFFECTIVE INTERVENTIONS

Research evidence has consistently demonstrated that depression can be suc-cessfully treated in most cases with psychosocial interventions, medication, or a combination of both. Most of the controlled research on psychosocial interven-tion for depression over the past fifteen years has focused on two approaches: cognitive therapy, which will be referred to here (for the sake of consistency) as cognitive-behavioral therapy (CBT; Beck et al., 1979; Shelton, Hollon, & Davis, 1993; D.A. Clark & Beck, 1999), and interpersonal psychotherapy (IPT; Klerman, Weissman, Rounsaville, & Chevron, 1984; Elkin et al., 1989; Klerman & Weissman, 1993; Weissman et al., 2000). Both approaches have been endorsed by leading professional organizations as effective forms of psychotherapy for depression, although evidence specifying the effective mechanisms of change has not been clearly demonstrated (Hollon & Carter, 1994; Oei & Shuttlewood, 1996).

Although some of the outcome data have been mixed with regard to the effectiveness of CBT for severe depression or its relative effectiveness when compared to antidepressant medication, CBT has accumulated a solid record of effectiveness when compared to control and comparison groups treated with other psychotherapies (Hollon et al., 1993; D.A. Clark & Beck, 1999). However, findings from the landmark NIMH Treatment of Depression Collaborative

INSTRUMENT 9.2   Geriatric Depression Scale (GDS)

Choose the best answer for how you felt this past week.

*1. Are you basically satisfied with your life?	yes	NO
2. Have you dropped many of your activities and interests?	YES	no
3. Do you feel that your life is empty?	YES	no
4. Do you often get bored?	YES	no
*5. Are you hopeful about the future?	yes	NO
6. Are you bothered by thoughts you can't get out of your head?	YES	no
*7. Are you in good spirits most of the time?	yes	NO
8. Are you afraid that something bad is going to happen to you?	YES	no
*9. Do you feel happy most of the time?	yes	NO
10. Do you often feel helpless?	YES	no
11. Do you often get restless and fidgety?	YES	no
12. Do you prefer to stay at home, rather than going out and doing new things?	YES	no
13. Do you frequently worry about the future?	YES	no
14. Do you feel you have more problems with memory than most?	YES	no
*15. Do you think it is wonderful to be alive now?	yes	NO
16. Do you often feel downhearted and blue?	YES	no
17. Do you feel pretty worthless the way you are now?	YES	no
18. Do you worry a lot about the past?	YES	no
*19. Do you find life very exciting?	yes	NO
20. Is it hard for you to get started on new projects?	YES	no
*21. Do you feel full of energy?	yes	NO
22. Do you feel that your situation is hopeless?	YES	no
23. Do you think that most people are better off than you are?	YES	no
24. Do you frequently get upset over little things?	YES	no
25. Do you frequently feel like crying?	YES	no
26. Do you have trouble concentrating?	YES	no
*27. Do you enjoy getting up in the morning?	yes	NO
28. Do you prefer to avoid social gatherings?	YES	no
*29. Is it easy for you to make decisions?	yes	NO
*30. Is your mind as clear as it used to be?	yes	NO

*Nondepressed answers = yes; all others = no.

To score the GDS, count the number of capitalized (depressed) answers.

Score: _____ (Number of "depressed" answers)

Research Program (Elkin, Parloff, Hadley, & Autry, 1985; Elkin et al., 1989; Elkin, 1994) revealed a relatively poor showing for CBT. The study compared the efficacy of CBT, IPT, and tricyclic antidepressant pharmacotherapy (TCA) with a placebo condition that included minimal supportive therapy. It was considered the most ambitious test to date comparing CBT to pharmacotherapy. Conducting the study simultaneously at three different sites, the investigators randomly assigned 250 nonpsychotic, unipolar depressed outpatient clients to sixteen weeks of treatment in one of these four conditions. Results indicated little difference among the three treatment conditions, and relatively little difference in outcomes between CBT and IPT in symptoms or levels of functioning. For the more severely depressed clients, pharmacotherapy was superior to placebo controls, and IPT seemed to fare better than CBT. However, according to Hollon, Shelton, and Loosen (1991), CBT outperformed the placebo group on some measures, and follow-up at eighteen months showed the long-term effects of CBT to be somewhat better than the other treatments (Shea et al., 1992). These results echoed previous findings (Kovacs, Rush, Beck, & Hollon, 1981), although long-term outcomes for all of the interventions were unimpressive overall. More recent evidence has also provided modest support for the relapse-prevention potential of cognitive-behavioral treatment when applied after a trial of antidepressant medication (G. A. Fava, Rafanelli, Grandi, Canestrari, & Morphy, 1998).

In the first comprehensive meta-analytic review of CBT using a common outcome measure (the BDI), Dobson (1989) examined twenty-eight controlled studies from which thirty-nine contrasts could be made between CBT and non-CBT, pharmacotherapy, and other psychotherapies. Ten studies demonstrated that clients receiving CBT improved significantly more than 98% of those who received no treatment (including wait-list control clients). Nine studies showed that those receiving CBT had better outcomes than 67% of those receiving behavior therapy. Eight studies demonstrated that CBT clients fared better than 70% of clients receiving pharmacotherapy, and seven studies showed that clients receiving CBT obtained significantly better results than 70% of those receiving other forms of psychotherapies. Although Dobson's finding were generally favorable toward CBT versus medications, Hollon et al. (1991) noted methodological weakness in some of the core studies Dobson (1989) had reviewed.

Because previous data comparing cognitive and pharmacological therapies had been flawed for a number of reasons, Hollon et al. (1992) conducted a controlled trial to offset some of these weaknesses. One hundred and seven depressed clients who met strict diagnostic criteria and cutoff scores on the HAM-D and the BDI were assigned randomly to four conditions: pharmacotherapy with discontinuation of medications after twelve weeks, pharmacotherapy with continuation of medications for one year, CBT, and combined cognitive and pharmacotherapy. Randomization continued until sixteen clients completed each protocol, yielding a final complete sample of sixty-four. Data showed no difference in attrition among the four groups. Clients were assessed at intake, six weeks, and twelve weeks (posttreatment) by evaluators blind to treatment condition. Data showed no difference in outcomes between CBT and imipramine treatments, and no advantage to combining these treatments over implementing them alone.

Noting the mixed findings resulting from comparisons of CBT and TCA medications, Thase et al. (2000) conducted the first comparison of CBT with the newer generation of antidepressants, the SSRIs. Their sequential comparison of two groups of male clients demonstrated that SSRI medications outperformed

CBT on four out of six outcome measures, including the HAM-D, the Automatic Thoughts Questionnaire, the Dysfunctional Attitudes Scale, and the Affects Balance Scale. They attributed some of the apparent advantage of the SSRIs to better treatment compliance, given what they surmised to be fewer and less severe side effects of the newer medications. Additional studies are needed to replicate comparison between SSRIs, CBT, and other therapies.

Some researchers have cited the "heterogeneity hypothesis" to account for the inconsistency in outcomes for CBT; that is, differential outcomes may be a function of various interactions between dysfunctional thinking and different degrees of life stress. A. D. Simons, Gordon, Monroe, and Thase (1995) conducted a study in which fifty-three clients, who completed the treatment protocol, provided data on several valid measures of depression, electroencephalograph readings, and two environmental-stressor scales. Results demonstrated that severe negative life events lessened the expected impact of treatment on dysfunctional attitudes. In a follow-up study, Spangler, Simons, Monroe, and Thase (1997) tested whether the interaction of cognitive dysfunction and negative stress predicted the client's response to CBT. As in the initial study, clients generally showed good improvement as a result of treatment, but findings indicated that CBT was effective regardless of the client's degree of cognitive dysfunction or occurrence of recent and severe stressful life events. The authors concluded that CBT is usually effective regardless of interactions between specific cognitive dysfunctions and stressful events.

Since the NIMH collaborative study, evidence that IPT is a viable intervention for depression has continued to accumulate (Klerman & Weissman, 1993; Weissman et al., 2000). In a brief review of IPT, Markowitz (1999) concluded that the results of IPT were often comparable to those achieved with a trial of imipramine, clients developed new social skills up to one year after the termination of treatment, and IPT provided more benefits for some clients than CBT. IPT apparently has shown substantial benefits across all age groups, including adolescents, adults, and the elderly. Combining IPT and TCAs has been shown to yield good long-term outcomes for elderly patients with depression. In a randomized controlled study of older clients (C. F. Reynolds et al., 1999), elderly depressed clients were assigned to four treatment groups: medication (nortriptyline) and IPT, medication and medication-clinic visits, placebo pill and IPT, and placebo pill and medication clinic. Those receiving IPT plus medication were least likely to relapse.

Change-Process Theory: Explaining How and Why Psychosocial Interventions for Depression Work

Although cognitively based theories have provided productive models for examining the psychological processes associated with specific problems such as depression and anxiety, it is less clear how these theories inform therapeutic change processes or account for the effectiveness of various psychosocial interventions. Comparable outcomes among different interventions for depression (e.g., CBT and IPT) make it difficult to establish the efficacy of specific and unique theory-based methods. Common or different therapeutic mechanisms may be at work among different approaches. Despite the relative effectiveness of CBT, no change processes have been shown to be specifically or uniquely related to positive outcomes with depressed clients. "The pattern of findings for cognitive therapy has paralleled other findings for other therapies; clear superiority over no treatment conditions, but little difference in comparison with other forms of therapy . . . Taken as a whole . . . meta-analyses do not provide strong evidence for specific action in cognitive therapy for depression" (Oei & Shuttlewood, 1996, p. 95).

In cognitively oriented interventions, the task in therapy is to change schematic models from dysfunctional (e.g., negative, pessimistic) ones to more adaptive ones (Teasdale, 1995), but there may be multiple ways to accomplish that, not just cognitive. Behavioral approaches emphasize that, although the process that maintains the problem may be cognitive, effective interventions often focus on behavior change where corrective learning experiences may have multiple impacts on cognitive, emotional, and behavioral functioning (G. T. Wilson, 1995). Behavioral homework activities in CBT ("testing out" dysfunctional thoughts) may account in large part for the effectiveness of cognitive therapy (Robins & Hayes, 1993). Medication and other interventions (e.g., regular vigorous exercise; see Salmon, 2001) can also cause clinically significant changes in mood, cognition, physiological function, and behavior. Given that clients' depressive concerns are often manifested in the context of interpersonal problems, it is quite possible that CBT, IPT, and some experiential therapies, although ostensibly different in technique, operate effectively through a combination of change processes that focus on interpersonal distortions, associated negative moods, and behavior changes that actively alter these processes (S. M. Johnson & Greenberg, 1995; Jensen, 1994; Ablon & Jones, 2002; Watson, Gordon, Stermac, Kalogerokos, & Steckley, 2003). Perhaps variations in both intervention techniques and change processes among these different approaches will have to be accounted for, at least in part, by client differences.

Exemplar Study: Testing Change Processes in Cognitive Therapy. A recent controlled investigation (Jacobson et al., 1996) compared key intervention components of CBT to the complete CBT model to examine whether all the components of CBT are necessary to achieve the desired therapeutic effect. According to Beck et al.'s theory (1979), the key active ingredient in CBT is the targeting of core cognitive structures (schemata) for change. Jacobson et al. compared "Behavioral Activation" (engaging in semistructured activities) and identifying and modifying automatic thoughts with the full CBT package (which also includes identifying and modifying core dysfunctional cognitive schemata). One hundred and fifty-two participants (110 women, 42 men) who met *DSM* criteria and scored above the conventional cutoffs of the BDI and the HAM-D were randomly assigned to the three treatment conditions, and measures were taken at intake, termination, and 6-, 12-, 18-, and 24-week follow-ups. Data were analyzed based on 137 clients (an 8% attrition rate) who completed between twelve and the maximum twenty sessions. Experienced cognitive therapists provided all the services. Fidelity checks were conducted randomly on 20% of the sessions to ensure that each treatment protocol was adhered to.

Treatment conditions were as follows: *Behavioral activation* (BA) included monitoring daily activities, assessment of pleasure and mastery associated with those activities, engaging in increasingly more challenging tasks that engendered pleasure and mastery, cognitive rehearsal of engaging in these activities and identifying obstacles in the process, identifying behavioral techniques to use to overcome these obstacles, and enhancement of social skills to overcome obstacles. *Activation and modification of dysfunctional thought* (AT) included identifying cognitive distortions and identifying thoughts that preceded mood shifts during sessions, using a diary as a self-monitoring tool to identify negative thoughts and the circumstances, challenging the rationality of these thoughts, developing more functional responses to them, examining clients' cause-effect reasoning about attributions regarding successes or failures in their lives, and use of homework to evaluate their negative interpretations. In this treatment condition, all BA activities could be incorporated as well. *CBT* (complete form) emphasized the identification and modification of more stable core beliefs (schemata) that underlie the negative automatic thoughts and distortions in reasoning, through a careful deductive analysis of underlying assumptions and challenges to them through homework assignments. In addition to the full CBT condition, which incorporated both BA and AT, eight sessions had to be specifically targeted toward core assumptions.

Results showed that a complete regimen of CBT was no more effective than either BA or AT. In fact, BA was as effective as the full CBT protocol. A follow-up study (Gortner, Gollan, Dobson, Jacobson, 1998) examined data at 6, 12, 18, and 24 months after active treatment. One hundred and thirty-seven clients were followed up with measures used in the original study. At two-year follow-up, there were no significant differences among the three treatment groups with regard to relapse indicators. The authors summarized: "The three treatment conditions were virtually identical on every criterion measure, including recovery and relapse rates, number of well weeks, and survival time to relapse" (Gortner et al., pp. 380–381). This study is but one that challenges a major tenet of CBT and practice: that core negative schemata must be addressed directly to cause stable improvement in depressed mood. Since behavioral activation is a relatively straightforward intervention method, it is possible that either core cognitive schemata can be changed through behavior changes alone, or that other change processes alone or in combination result in a reduction of depression.

Clinical Case Management for Depression in the Elderly

Given that depression in the elderly is often linked to losses, loneliness, withdrawal, and social deficits, improving clients' instrumental and social supports may be essential for maintaining therapeutic improvements. Naleppa and Reid

(1998) conduced preliminary research to integrate a short-term task-oriented intervention into a long-term case management model. Sowers-Hoag (1997) also emphasizes the need for multiple "traditional" case management services for the elderly, including case finding, multidimensional assessment, comprehensive care planning, coordination of services, and monitoring and evaluation of services. Although a number of interventions (including medication and psychotherapy) are effective for treating depression in elderly people, these interventions are of little use if clients, especially those who lack social and instrumental supports, do not have the means to obtain treatment, or cannot be monitored effectively in the community. One innovative program (Morrow-Howell, Becker-Kemppainen, & Lee, 1998) uses frequent phone contacts to increase socialization and maximize autonomy in the elderly. The intervention (called Link-Plus) combines supportive therapy with case management services to provide meals, transportation, opportunities for socialization, and psychiatric services. In addition to accessing these services, case managers help the client overcome environmental and psychological barriers to using the services, and ensure service quality and continuity through monitoring and evaluation. Initial evaluation of this model was promising.

Supportive, psychoeducational and problem-solving intervention can be readily incorporated into an eclectic model that includes psychotherapeutic and case management components. For example, a brief eight-week psychoeducational program for helping grandparents who are raising their grandchildren was evaluated (D. Burnette, 1998). The eclectic intervention included enhancement of social supports, stress-management skills, dealing with family/interpersonal problems, parenting skills for a "new" generation of children, examining availability of legal and social services, addressing neighborhood and community problems, and accessing available services. The evaluation demonstrated significant improvement in client depression scores. Rife and Belcher (1994) developed an innovative job-finding service (Job Club) for elderly unemployed workers. The service instructs participants in areas such as job interviewing, writing résumés, completing applications, and facilitated social support and the sharing of job leads among the members. Results demonstrated significantly better outcomes for finding employment compared to traditional job-finding services, and participants had significantly lower scores of the GDS at posttest. Cummings (2003) demonstrated in an uncontrolled evaluation that brief motivational enhancement therapy for elders in an assisted-living residence improved psychological well-being and social supports. The program emphasized social interaction of participants with hands-on participation in gardening-related activities. Such program can be a cost-effective addition to comprehensive strategies to improve quality of life for the elderly.

Descriptions of Effective Interventions

Cognitive Behavior Therapy.   CBT for depression is a set of integrated cognitive and behavioral techniques used to identify, assess, and change negative and dysfunctional beliefs and associated problem behaviors (Beck, 1976; Beck et al., 1979; Hollon & Carter, 1994; R. E. Clark et al., 1999). Clients are helped to modify dysfunctional thinking through rational discussion and behavioral disconfirmation in the form of "homework" assignments. These assignments may also include one or more standard behavioral interventions (e.g., coping skills, problem-solving and communication skills, stress management). In actual practice, considerable latitude is employed in crafting a CBT plan for the individual client.

Cognitive-behavioral therapists are expected to be actively engaged with the client in testing dysfunctional beliefs. It is understood that practitioners will cultivate a sound therapeutic alliance based upon a foundation of the "core ingredients" of the helping relationship (warmth, genuineness, positive regard, basic trust) (Beck, 1976; Orlinsky et al., 1994; Klosko & Sanderson, 1999). The process of CBT for depression generally follows a sequence.

1. A thorough biopsychosocial assessment is conducted.

2. Suicide assessment is carefully carried out.

3. A therapeutic structure is established and respective roles delineated.

4. Tasks are planned to jump start the client's level of activity (e.g., spend an hour per day organizing work at home, or begin a long-neglected task); seemingly complex tasks are broken down into manageable steps.

5. The cognitive model of depression is explained (i.e., schemata, negative automatic thoughts, and dysfunctional information processing); the CBT practitioner avoids judging or labeling the client, but accepts the client's initial construction of the problem.

6. The practitioner actively engages the client in a Socratic exploration of the problem and discovers where some of the sources of the problem may be.

7. The client is taught how to self-monitor and record automatic thoughts and associated moods. Examination of the client's negative automatic thoughts may lead to an exploration of underlying assumptions, perhaps themes that seem to permeate different areas of the client's life and recur over time.

8. The client is taught how to examine evidence of these troubling thoughts, consider alternative explanations, and identify the real implications of the belief if it is true.

9. The client learns how to identify cognitive distortions and perform collaboratively planned homework assignments to test hypotheses regarding these negative assumptions or negative automatic thoughts.

10. The client is encouraged to participate in active self-monitoring of these thoughts and record responses to them. The client may use diaries, logs, or charts to record these experiences. Significant others may assist as needed in the assessment or may carry out homework assignments with the client. With repeated homework experiences and associated tasks, dysfunctional beliefs are likely to be disconfirmed.

11. The practitioner helps the client identify underlying assumptions (schemata) that maintain the negative automatic thoughts.

12. The practitioner works with the client on developing a plan to cope with the possibility of relapse, and focuses on how the client will implement new coping strategies in the face of future stressors and disappointments that may reactivate negative automatic thoughts.

The practitioner may be relatively active in the beginning stage of the intervention, becoming gradually less active as the client takes more initiative in questioning and testing negative or depressing thinking, associated feelings, and behaviors. During each session, an agenda is set, homework reviewed, new homework assigned, and feedback obtained about each visit. In addition to the homework tasks assigned for testing dysfunctional beliefs, other behavioral treatments may include assertiveness training, anger management, relaxation techniques, improving productivity (e.g., time management, getting organized), managing panic attacks, and guided imagery for covert rehearsal.

Cognitive Therapy for Late-Life Depression.   A meta-analysis of interventions with the elderly demonstrated considerable promise for a number of interventions, particularly cognitive and reminiscence therapy (Scogin & McElreath, 1994). Case-study research has also provided some support for cognitive therapy for depression in the elderly (e.g., Gupta, 2000). Thompson (1996) outlined recommendations for adapting CBT for older clients, given that they may be experiencing some degree of cognitive impairment. He recommends the use of the GDS and a thorough mental-status exam as part of a comprehensive assessment. Brief CBT should be used in combination with medication for maximum therapeutic benefit. Although CBT for depression is usually provided in sixteen to twenty sessions, practitioners should be prepared to be flexible with treatment duration. In addition, presenting material more slowly and using memory aids (e.g., writing down homework assignments, using a notebook, presenting information on a whiteboard or projector screen) are all modifications that can be helpful for the older client.

Thompson (1996) suggests a three-phase approach. In the early phase (sessions 1–3) a good working alliance is established, and clients are instructed in the basic principles of cognitive theory and CBT. Clients are also instructed how to self-monitor dysfunctional thoughts that occur between sessions. In the middle phase (sessions 4–12), clients are taught core cognitive and behavioral skills for identifying dysfunctional thoughts, and practitioners then gently challenge these beliefs through rational examination and behavioral hypothesis testing. Clients are also encouraged to identify and increase pleasurable activities in their lives. In the final phase (sessions 13–16), clients focus on honing their skills for dealing with stressful situations to prevent relapse. Some clients may also be referred for follow-up interventions such as continued medication or electroconvulsive therapy.

Thompson (1996) recommends that individual sessions be structured this way: present the agenda; conduct assessment (including the use of measures); identify and discuss problem assumptions or dysfunctional beliefs; review homework assignments; address areas of apparent resistance; present a new or continued topic as needed; and summarize the session and give a new homework assignment. A similar application of CBT for anxiety in the elderly has also been shown to be effective, with results showing clinically substantive reductions in co-occurring depression (Stanley et al., 2003). Since many depressed elderly clients also suffer from anxiety disorders, it may be fruitful to incorporate anxiety-management skills into CBT for older clients.

Description of Interpersonal Psychotherapy.   Although Weissman et al. (2000) refer to a number of theoretical influences in the development of IPT, they explicitly endorse a firm commitment to the basic principles of evidence-based practice: "We are convinced . . . that all theories and schools require evidence from testing, and that the most powerful evidence comes from carefully designed, well-controlled investigative trials" (p. 4). IPT emphasizes three main component processes: symptom function (main physiological symptoms such as disturbances in sleep, appetite, and energy), social and interpersonal relations (based on learning experiences, current social supports, personal coping skills, and competence), and personality and character problems (more enduring dysfunctional traits including poor self-esteem and chronic difficulties relating to others). The IPT practitioner intervenes in the first of these two processes: physiological symptoms of depression and problems of interpersonal relations. Although IPT does not focus on character change, improved coping skills may compensate for problems in those areas as well. Although IPT shares generic psychotherapeutic skills such as basic counseling techniques, improving interpersonal problem solving, and communication, the authors assert that it is more than merely "supportive" therapy.

> IPT . . . intervenes with symptom formation, social adjustment and interpersonal relations, working predominantly on current problems and at conscious and preconscious levels. Although the IPT therapist may recognize unconscious factors, they are not directly addressed. The emphasis is on current disputes, frustrations, anxieties, and wishes as defined in the interpersonal context. IPT aims to help clients *change* rather than to understand and simply accept their current life situation. The influence of early childhood experience is recognized as significant but not emphasized in the therapy. Rather, the work focuses on the "here and now." Overall treatment goals are to encourage mastery of current social roles and adaptation to interpersonal situations. (p. 9)

IPT is to be understood within the broader framework of the medical model, and its adherents actively endorse the notion that the client adopts the "sick" role. IPT practitioners recognize that other interventions may be preferable for some clients, and its developers do not claim that IPT is universally effective for all depressed clients. IPT is a goal-focused intervention, and is relatively short term. The main techniques used include exploration, encouragement of affect, clarification, communication analysis, use of the therapeutic relationship, behavior-change techniques, and other adjunctive techniques. Although past relationships are recognized as potentially important in understanding the genesis of the client's main problem, the therapeutic focus is on current relationships. Since IPT is rooted somewhat in a neo-Freudian tradition, practitioners of IPT may recognize the importance of defense mechanisms, but the focus is squarely on improving current interpersonal relations. However, IPT practitioners part company with their CBT counterparts in at least one significant way: although distorted thinking may be acknowledged along the way in therapy, no systematic effort is made to analyze the content of these thoughts other than to better understand them within the context of the client's interpersonal functioning. The IPT practitioner is active, not neutral or passive, and puts emphasis on the core ingredients of basic helping. Transference (the displacement of clients' unconscious thoughts, wishes, fantasies, etc. on the practitioner), although recognized as a legitimate construct by IPT practitioners, does not become a focus of treatment. Positive transference is left untouched; negative interpersonal interactions with the therapist are dealt with openly in an effort to resolve them. Above all, client autonomy (not dependency) is encouraged.

Based on the writings of the leading developers and proponents of IPT (Weissman et al., 2000; Markowitz, 1999), the basic approach is outlined below.

In the initial sessions, practitioners conduct a thorough review of depressive symptoms, characterize the depression as an illness, and evaluate the client for medication.

Both past and present relationships are examined for quality and satisfaction, significant problems, met and unmet expectations, and changes the client would like to see in their relationships.

The problem is defined as a relationship-based formulation, and the practitioner and client plan the intervention goals together.

The client is provided with a basic introduction to the philosophy and procedures of IPT.

In the intermediate sessions, the practitioner and client focus on one of three major problem areas: grief, interpersonal role disputes, or role transitions.

If the problem is grief, the practitioner should facilitate the mourning process, examine the loss and attending symptoms, and help the client reconnect with other social supports to help alleviate the depressive symptoms associated with loss.

If the focus in an interpersonal role dispute, the conflict should be identified, and problem-solving strategies reviewed to help ameliorate the conflict.

If the focus is a role transition, the practitioner might assist the client in mourning the old role by examining thoughts and facilitating the expression of feelings about the loss. They can then address the new role in a more positive light with an emphasis on attaining mastery of the new role and accessing support systems that may facilitate the new role.

If the client has interpersonal deficits, the practitioner should help the client reduce their isolation and encourage the formation of new relationships.

If the client's interpersonal problems seem to recapitulate within the context of the therapeutic relationship, the practitioner should use that opportunity to help the client resolve their interpersonal dispute. In other words, the therapeutic context becomes a laboratory for helping the client better understand and manage interpersonal problems.

Termination focuses on helping the client plan to maintain their gains in the future.

IPT for Treating Depression in Elderly People.   Weissman et al. (2000) note that mood disorders are common among the elderly population, and are often accompanied by disproportionately high suicide rates. Effective psychosocial interventions for the elderly are important, given the higher risks associated with taking medication (e.g., side effects, drug interactions). In addition, losses and role transitions experienced by the elderly lend themselves to goals of IPT (Klerman & Weissman, 1993). Controlled trials of IPT with elderly clients have demonstrated that IPT can be effective when administered in much the same way as it would be for younger clients, although a variation on the original IPT model geared toward maintenance of late-life depression (IPT-LLM) has also been developed. In addition to balancing dependency needs with the need to maintain independence, practitioners should expect to remain active in the treatment, and encourage small gains, be flexible in scheduling meetings, and help clients tolerate some of their interpersonal difficulties if making major changes is impractical or unwanted by the client (Klerman & Weissman, 1993).

Medications

Overall, data support the effectiveness of SSRIs for the treatment of mild to moderate depression. Higher doses may be helpful for more severe depression, although alternative therapies may be superior (H. I. Kaplan & Saddock, 1998). The most common side effects in the central nervous system involve headache, sexual dysfunction, nervousness, insomnia, drowsiness, and anxiety. Fluoxetine, as well as other SSRIs, may cause sleep interruption as well, prompting physicians to add a more sedative drug to the medication regimen. SSRIs have been considered generally safer than other antidepressants should the client overdose (H. I. Kaplan & Saddock, 1998). Although SSRIs are frequently prescribed for the elderly with good results (Dick & Gallagher-Thompson, 1996), less research on SSRIs has been conducted with the elderly than with younger adults (R. Wolfe et al., 1996).

Although not as frequently prescribed for depression anymore as are the SSRIs, TCAs are still considered a viable option for some depressed clients (H. I. Kaplan & Saddock, 1998). TCAs have a clinical reputation for more serious anticholinergic side effects and greater potential toxicity than the newer SSRIs. These side effects, which are shared with SSRIs, include blurred vision, dry mouth, constipation, and urinary retention. TCAs also have a reputation of being more sedating than SSRIs. Social work practitioners should be aware that overdoses through error or in a suicide attempt are not uncommon, and overdoses of TCAs can be fatal, particularly in the physically compromised elderly person. Physicians generally begin by prescribing lower doses of TCAs (25 mg to 50 mg), gradually increasing them to a therapeutic dose (e.g., 150 mg) over the course of a couple of weeks. Therapeutic benefits are likely to begin within two to four weeks (H. I. Kaplan & Saddock, 1998; Dzieglielewski & Leon, 1998).

More recently, however, research has seriously challenged the broad claim of superiority of SSRIs over TCAs for either their therapeutic effect or less severe side effects (I. M. Anderson, 2000). In some cases, amitriptyline (a TCA) may have superior effectiveness, and the tolerability of these drugs appears to vary from patient to patient. Direct comparisons of these drugs in controlled trials are warranted.

Monoamine oxidase inhibitors (MAOIs) have come to be considered a third option for an antidepressant (Dzieglielewski & Leon, 1998; H. I. Kaplan & Saddock, 1998). These drugs work by increasing amine neurotransmitter levels. Therapeutic effects are usually noticed within two to four weeks with the dosage gradually increased from 15 mg to 90 mg. MAOIs, although considered to be as effective as newer antidepressants (and possibly effective with atypical depression), carry a high risk of causing hypertensive crisis due to potential interactions with ingredients in common foods. MAOIs also tend to interrupt normal sleep, and may cause insomnia and daytime drowsiness. Other side effects include edema, weight gain, and sexual dysfunction. Overdose of MAOIs may induce coma, and an overdose of these drugs with other antidepressants may be fatal.

Dzieglielewski and Leon (1998) offer prudent suggestions for social workers providing interventions for clients who are taking antidepressant medication. Clients usually need to take these medications for several months to achieve their full benefit. As a client prepares to discontinue their use, social workers can help plan for this transition by increasing clients' awareness about the possible recurrence of symptoms, ensuring that clients have good social supports, encouraging them to consider the continuation of psychosocial intervention after discontinuing medications, preparing them with an action plan if the depressive symptoms seem to be recurring, and involving significant others in a relapse-prevention plan.

Electroconvulsive therapy (ECT) is also a viable option for treating severe depression in the elderly. The safety and efficacy of ECT has been well documented (Dick & Gallagher-Thompson, 1996), but some researchers note potential complications associated with ECT, including hypoxia, arrhythmias, delirium, transient hypertension, and memory disturbances (R. Wolfe et al., 1996). Nevertheless, many elderly people who do not respond well to medications or other therapies obtain substantial relief from their depression with ECT, and suffer few if any adverse side effects.

IMPLEMENTING AND EVALUATING THE EVIDENCE-BASED INTERVENTION PLAN

CASE STUDY: GRANDMA LONG

Grandma Long came into the social worker's office led by her daughter An. She was obviously quite depressed, stared down at the floor, refused to look at the social worker, and, except for occasionally sighing and crying softly to herself, said very little throughout the interview. An recounted the story and the reasons she had reluctantly come into the clinic.

About a month before, Grandma Long's sixteen-year-old grandson Thu (a nephew of An, her brother's son) was shot and killed during a robbery outside of the family restaurant after closing hours. The funeral was a few days later, and the extended family was greatly distraught. He had been a hard worker in the restaurant and a good student in school. The extended family had worked hard to keep their sons and daughters out of the growing gang culture that had evolved over the past few years in the nearby neighborhoods. It was not clear who committed the crime, and no arrests had been made.

Prior to the killing, Grandma Long had been increasingly despondent. Her son-in-law, Hung, had recently purchased the Asian restaurant that he, Grandma Long, and Hung's wife, An, had all worked in for the past few years. Hung, now the boss (after many years of working over eighty hours per week), wanted to make it clear that he was in charge. He asked that Grandma Long no longer be allowed in the kitchen. Grandma Long had for many years been manager and head chef in a number of Asian restaurants both in Vietnam and in the United States. She and Hung had often butted heads, but the former owner had a way of keeping them focused on different tasks. For the past few months Grandma Long had been pushed out altogether and was feeling, in her words, "used up, worthless, no longer needed." After the killing, she became incapacitated with depression, refused to eat, was losing weight, and expressed a desire to die as soon as possible. Other family members were coming by often to offer her tea and conversation, and to keep an eye on her.

Grandma Long left Vietnam just before the fall of Saigon. She was in her late forties then, had witnessed many years of war, lost several extended family members, and felt she had left such violence behind when she came to the United States. She brought her daughter An, who was twenty-one at the time, with her. They lived in Vietnamese neighborhoods in a midwestern American city for a number of years, working in restaurants. After An met Hung and got married, they moved east so Hung could take a new job. They had a daughter, and since then have been living and working in the same neighborhood. They lived near the restaurant in a three-story house with Grandma Long and other family members. Everyone worked hard, and child care and other domestic duties were shared along tra-ditional lines. Grandma Long (whose name means "the dragon") lived up to her name as the one in charge (the children called her "dragon lady" behind her back). Grandma Long often opined that the old ways were fading, that children did not respect their elders in the United States. She tried to exercise her authority over the children in the household, but feared that they were being pulled too easily into the fast and seductive American culture outside the extended family enclave. When Thu, her favorite grandson, was killed, it was the validation of the worst of her lifelong fears. War and more killing, she felt, had followed her to America.

Multidimensional/Functional Assessment: Defining Problems and Goals

Just before the killing, Grandma Long had been somewhat despondent and more irritable than usual. She seemed less assertive around the house, less inclined to orchestrate domestic duties, and less inclined to exercise her authority since she had been "demoted" at the restaurant by her son-in-law. She seemed distracted, staring out the window for long periods of time, and often was forgetful, once leaving the tea kettle on and falling asleep in her easy chair. The smell of the burning empty kettle brought one of the other family members downstairs. When Hung found out, he was angry and said if it happened again, Grandma Long would have to move out and go to an "old folks' home."

At other times, Grandma Long seemed fidgety and nervous, would sigh a lot and sometimes cry. She did not sleep well at night, often getting out of bed early in the morning to sit in her chair in the main room. Often she repeated the refrain, "I'm no use to anyone. I should just die soon. It would make things a lot easier for everyone." She seemed to feel a great sense of shame due to her lower status in the family. She often complained of pains and feeling ill, and had visited the neighborhood herbalist. She was taking various concoctions in her tea, and felt that these admixtures ameliorated her physical symptoms. Still, her mood had not improved. She also visited the doctor at the local clinic. She suggested that Grandma Long was depressed, ruled out any incipient dementia, and offered medication (an SSRI), which was declined. Grandma Long had little faith in standard American medical practices. Other than her somatic complaints, her health was deemed to be very good.

Although she was feeling that everyone had abandoned her and pushed her aside, Grandma Long actually had many social supports and was still respected in the family. Some members still felt that she was the "go to" person on cooking and other domestic matters. Younger members of the community would often come by to see her and ask her about the "old days" in Vietnam or try to get her recipes. At these times she seemed a little more animated and (her daughter related) demonstrated some of the "old spark." But when her visitors left, she would lapse back into a sense of despair. Nevertheless, she had considerable family and community support despite her depressed state, shame, and sense of worthlessness. After the news of the killing reached her, she become incapacitated. Her day-to-day functioning declined even further, and she no longer accepted visitors. She stopped eating. She lay in bed and said she just wanted to die.

Selecting and Designing the Intervention: Defining Strategies and Objectives

During the week after the killing, neighbors and friends came and went in the household, helping with meals and cleaning, and keeping an eye on Grandma Long. There was not much else they could do at the time. A week after the funeral, household routines and restaurant duties resumed despite a lingering cloud of sadness and anger. Grandma Long seemed to be fading away, and the family knew they had to take action. After An conferred with the clinical social worker, Jen, on the phone in the local mental health clinic, Grandma Long was admitted to a general hospital that had a special geriatric psychiatric unit. Grandma Long remained there for a few days, as she was losing weight and somewhat dehydrated. After a number of examinations and tests, the psychiatrist in charge said she needed to be discharged as the insurance would not cover an extended stay. Medication was recommended again. Jen would continue to follow the case on an outpatient basis. The social worker met with the family and established a plan for individual grief counseling for Grandma Long, but also encouraged An, her husband, and other members of the family to participate in family sessions for grief counseling and, eventually, to work out some of the interpersonal conflicts that emerged in the initial assessment with Grandma Long. Eventually, Jen set up a case management plan to make occasional home visits with the family to see that improvements were maintained (table 9.1).

The social work practitioner was well versed in evidence-based approaches to working with depression in the elderly. She was also attuned to the local Southeast Asian culture, and had considerable experience working with families and indigenous community helpers such as the Asian apothecary and the Vietnamese Catholic priest. Jen met with Grandma Long, An, and Hung, and decided that Grandma Long needed, at least initially, some individual attention to grieve the loss of her favorite nephew. She made it clear that she also wanted to include An and Hung at some point in the family sessions but felt that it was premature to deal with family conflicts at the time. She also recognized the family's grief over the loss of their nephew, and invited An, Hung, and other family members to attend a group session that included other Vietnamese community members who had also lost loved ones.

Jen concluded that IPT would be helpful for Grandma Long. Initially, the emphasis on addressing her grief seemed to be in order. The grandmother spoke long and glowingly of Thu, and how he would stop by often to see her. She was obviously very proud of him, and brought in pictures of him and documents that attested to his academic prowess and other accomplishments. He had won second prize for a story he had written about his grandmother and her experiences in Vietnam before coming to America. Over the course of two to three months, Grandma Long began to brighten. She was sleeping better (which may have been because of the antidepressant medication that she finally agreed to try along with her herbal mixtures), and she had gained a significant amount of weight. She was not talking about suicide anymore, and some of her attention was now refocused on domestic duties. Nevertheless, she continued to feel that her status in the family had seriously diminished.

At some point into the third month, Jen asked Grandma Long if she would like to have her daughter and son-in-law return for a few visits to see if some of their differences could be worked out. Grandma Long's belief that she was "useless" seemed intractable. The practitioner felt that these negative beliefs could be resolved, but not without resolving some of the family role conflicts. The grandmother was still in good health and could certainly contribute more to the family at home and perhaps in the restaurant. It seemed that IPT could be used to resolve the role conflict in a family intervention and, at the same time, that elements of CBT could be applied to help Grandma Long examine and (through behavior changes) disconfirm her negative view of herself as "used up, worthless."

Jen had developed a strong alliance with her client, and felt that it was time for Grandma Long, An, and Hung to meet. During the week, however, Jen began to think that she had miscalculated by scheduling both the grandmother and the couple together. She felt that she should see the couple first to report on Grandma Long's progress, but also to test the possibility that the son-in-law would relent somewhat about banishing Grandma Long from the restaurant altogether. When they all met in the waiting room, Jen asked Grandma Long if it would be OK to meet with her daughter and son-in-law alone for a few minutes. Grandma Long seemed pleased to be deferred to in this decision, and she agreed. During the couple's visit, Jen explained that Grandma Long had become a bit less depressed, although she would probably always grieve the loss of her grandson on some level. Jen then posed the problem of the long-standing conflict between Hung and Grandma Long. As Hung spoke, it became clear that he had worked incredibly long and hard under an abusive boss. When he finally had his "own place," he felt he had to establish complete control over the business to ensure its success. Nothing, in his eyes, could be worse than if his business failed. He did not feel that he could expend the energy or the stress of fighting with his mother-in-law in the kitchen, run his business, and maintain his marriage. The social worker acknowledged that these seemed to be reasonable concerns. But, as the business was going very well and Hung had a sense that things were well under his command, perhaps they could discuss the possibility of some important role that could be delegated to Grandma Long—not make-work, but some important place where she could make a real contribution to the business. Would Hung be willing to discuss this with her?

The social worker met with Grandma Long and suggested that all three of them could meet the following week to discuss some things about the home and the business. The grandmother agreed. In that discussion, they all agreed that the business was going well and that there was considerably more help in the kitchen than before. Many of the employees were young people engaged in preparatory cooking work and other ancillary jobs (e.g., running the dishwasher). Hung agreed that, at times, things were getting out of hand in the restaurant. He had also discussed with other restaurant owners at his social club that his employees lacked training, a task for which Hung had neither time nor patience.

It occurred to Hung in conversations with his wife that he had been disrespectful to Grandma Long, and that she might be the ideal person to train the younger employees and to keep them "in line." (She was, after all, the "dragon lady.") Hung had become frustrated in dealing with them, and felt the need to delegate more responsibility to his head chef, spend some time talking to his customers, get out of the restaurant once in a while, and deal more directly with his suppliers. It might also give him more time to look into opening up another restaurant on the other side of town. Hung realized he had been somewhat abrupt in the past with Grandma Long. Jen motioned to him to talk with Grandma Long directly. He picked up the cue and (after apologizing to her for showing disrespect) asked if she would be willing to take over the training and supervision of the kitchen help. Grandma Long (after saying "I told you so") agreed. Jen made follow-up visits to the home and the restaurant, when invited. Grandma Long appeared to be doing well and was once again energetic in the kitchen, attending to her new charges. Soon after Grandma Long discontinued her antidepressant medication (it had been about sixteen weeks), An reported that her serious symptoms of depression had not returned. Grandma Long seemed to have "adopted" some of the young people who worked for her, which seemed to please her very much. But pinned up over the calendar at the far end of the kitchen was a photo of Grandma Long and her grandson Thu, always in view.

Selecting Scales and Creating Indexes to Monitor and Evaluate Client Progress

Instruments useful in this case included the Mini-Mental State Examination (Folstein et al., 1975), which was used during Grandma Long's hospital stay, and the GDS used by the social worker for both assessment and periodic monitoring (table 9.1). Individual indexes included her level of activity around the house (how often she engaged in domestic duties), hours sleeping, and number of meals she took daily. Other important indexes included suicide risk factors, particularly indications of helplessness or suicidal ideation.

TABLE 9.1   The client service plan for Grandma Long

Problems	Goals	Sample Objectives	Interventions	Assessment Tools
Symptoms of major depression that appear to be exacerbated by an acute grief reaction (favorite grandson killed during a robbery)	Alleviate acute symptoms related to grief; sort out assessment of prior depression from grief reaction	Allow for expressions of grief during weekly visits; review and reminisce about her relationship with her grandson; review mementos and pictures; help her express grief over other losses in her family	Eclectic use of both IPT and CBT	Mini-Mental State Examination
			Short-term IPT to initiate resolution of acute grief symptoms	GDS for depression
				Other functional indexes: hours of sleep; meals eaten; hours of activity at home, and (later) at the restaurant; suicidal indicators
			IPT to address grief and role conflicts with family members that appear to be related to her sense of "worthlessness"	
Suicidal thinking, feelings of shame, guilt, worthlessness; lowered activity level, sleep disturbance, loss of appetite, and loss of pleasure in life. Other somatic complaints: vague references to aches and pains	Ameliorate symptoms related to major depression; return to normal level of functioning	When she begins to show some increase in energy, activate daily routine gradually over time; plan domestic activities one at a time; increase as needed	CBT to examine cognitions regarding her sense of "worthlessness"; disconfirm these beliefs by improving role performance	
			Family session(s) to clarify communications and assist in resolving role conflicts that involve her	
Problem in family relations: conflict with son-in-law over authority, respective roles	Resolve family dispute; ideally, adjust respective family roles to the reasonable satisfaction of all members	As depression abates and energy increases, plan to reintroduce her to the business; incorporate her role as trainer initially for 2 hours 1–2 days per week; increase as needed and required	Case management activities: coordinate monitoring and evaluation with psychiatrist regarding medication compliance; confer with local community helpers as needed	

SUMMARY

Depression is among the most common and debilitating disorders in the nation, and co-occurs with the full range of psychosocial disorders. Contemporary theories now emphasize the interaction of biological, cognitive, behavioral, and situational factors in the etiology and continuation of depression. Following a thorough assessment, social workers can avail themselves of at least two psychosocial interventions that have been shown to be effective with depression: CBT and IPT. Given that social and instrumental supports are critical to long-term maintenance of gains, particularly for the elderly client, case management provides a coherent framework for coordination of psychosocial and medical interventions.

CHAPTER 10

ANTISOCIAL AND BORDERLINE
PERSONALITY DISORDERS

Among the most challenging, intriguing, and often frustrating clients encountered by social work practitioners are the "personality disordered." Often enduring from childhood or adolescence, the problems of these clients can confound even the most attentive and skilled practitioners. The causes of these chronic disorders of thinking, affect, behavior, and relating to others range from inherited temperament, childhood abuse, the role modeling of significant adults, maladaptive coping within pathogenic environments, and combinations of these factors. Psychoanalytic theories, based primarily on correlational studies and case analyses, have not provided explanations that stand up to longitudinal research. Aside from research on psychopathy, personality "trait" theories (e.g., Millon & Davis, 1995; Cattell, 1965; Eysenck, 1960; Goldberg, 1993) have found relatively little utility in mainstream mental health services. Practitioners, by necessity, usually refer to *DSM-IV-TR* diagnostic descriptions, where *personality disorder* is defined as "an enduring pattern of inner experience and behavior that deviates markedly from the expectations of the individual's culture, is pervasive and inflexible, has an onset in adolescence or early adulthood, is stable over time, and leads to distress or impairment" (p. 685). Nevertheless, there remains considerable controversy regarding the reliability and essential validity of diagnostic categories for personality disorders (Crits-Christoph, 1998; Tryer, 1995; Widiger & Corbitt, 1995; Hare & Hart, 1995; C. W. Johnston & Alozie, 2001).

Although not all clients who are "personality disordered" run afoul of the law, many do and are sometimes treated within an informal framework referred to as "forensic social work" (A. R. Roberts & Brownell; 1999; Odiah & Wright, 2000), an offshoot of forensic psychiatry (Jager, 1999). Within this professional context, social workers may be involved in writing reports or providing expert testimony regarding the determination of a self-mutilating and drug-addicted young woman's fitness to stand trial, a violent husband's likelihood of repeating domestic violence, or an adolescent sex offender's chances of relapsing in the community. Social workers are also required to be knowledgeable about informed consent, confidentiality, and what constitutes professional malpractice, they may be called upon to advocate for clients involved in the criminal justice system and often provide primary interventions for these clients as well.

Personality disorders tend to co-occur with other psychosocial problems, including anxiety, depression, severe mental illnesses, interpersonal and community problems, and substance-use disorders. Some have argued that two of the more common personality disorders, antisocial and borderline personality disorders (APD and BPD), may share common etiology and behavioral characteristics (e.g., manipulativeness, suicidal thoughts, substance abuse) and may be variations on the same disorder, with males and females disproportionately diagnosed APD and BPD, respectively (Paris, 1997a). Despite the challenge in caring for these clients, a body of outcome research for treating APD and BPD has begun to emerge. Given that APD and BPD are two of the more commonly treated personality disorders in human service environments, they are the focus of this chapter.

ASSESSMENT OF ANTISOCIAL PERSONALITY DISORDER

Background Data

There are two somewhat overlapping approaches to defining people as antisocial: the *DSM* diagnostic description (APD) and a personality type described as psychopathic. The *DSM-IV-TR* criteria for a diagnosis of APD emphasizes a pervasive pattern of disregard for, and violation of the rights and safety of others (e.g., unlawful acts, chronic deceitfulness, impulsiveness, violence), chronic irresponsibility with regard to work or financial commitments, and lack of remorse for hurting others or otherwise infringing on others' rights. Although not synonymous with criminality, many of the people, mostly male, who run afoul of the law also meet the criteria for APD. The concept of psychopathy, originating with Cleckley's classic book *The Mask of Sanity(1941),* has been operationalized as the Psychopathy Check List (PCL-r; Hare, Harpur, Hakstian, Forth, & Hart, 1990). Psychopathy emphasizes two major factors: selfishness, callousness, and remorseless use of others; and a chronically unstable and antisocial lifestyle. These elements overlap with a diagnosis of APD. Thus, psychopathy constitutes a broader construct and should be considered along with a diagnosis of APD.

Prevalence rates for APD are estimated to be about 1–3% in the general population, 3% in males and 1% in females, and rates in clinical samples have ranged from 3% to 30%. Kessler et al. (1994) estimated lifetime *DSM-III-R* diagnoses of APD at 5.8% for men, 1.2% for women, and about 3.5% for the general adult population. Although people diagnosed APD are not always criminally involved, about three-quarters of people in prison are considered to be antisocial personalities. Over time, from the teens until around age forty, the criminal activities of people later diagnosed with APD are relatively constant, but begin to decline after age forty and virtually cease beyond age fifty (Robins, 1966; Hare, McPherson, &

Forth, 1988; Kessler et al.). Those diagnosed with APD are less likely to have completed high school and show much lower incomes overall than the general population (Kessler et al.) When such people are criminally active, they tend to be generalists, not specialists, and engage in a variety of criminal activities, including drug use, domestic violence, robbery, and rape (L. U. Simon, 1997).

APD often co-occurs with substance abuse. About 70% of people diagnosed as APD abuse alcohol, and a third or more abuse other drugs (Regier et al., 1990). Sexual excesses, substance abuse, child abuse and neglect, and domestic violence are often part of their behavioral repertoire. APD may co-occur with a range of other disorders, including those related to anxiety, depression, somatization, gambling, and borderline, narcissistic, and other personality disorders.

People who fit the criteria for APD should be carefully screened for perpetrating domestic violence. A sizeable proportion of domestic batterers are sociopathic and/or antisocial (Gleason, 1997). As will be reviewed more thoroughly in chapter 11, Bograd and Mederos (1999) note a number of risk factors for domestic violence that mirror characteristic behaviors of people with APD, including unresolved substance abuse, a history of two or more acts of domestic violence or sexual assault, and a history of violent criminal acts. The latter may include violation of restraining order, use of weapons, ongoing threats of violence, and obsessional behaviors toward a partner, such as intense jealousy, stalking, harassing, and bizarre forms of violence marked by sadism or an attempt to depersonalize the victim.

Given the high rates of co-occurring disorders among APD, practitioners are likely to confront these problems in a variety of combinations (Hotaling & Sugarman, 1986). For example, T. G. Brown, Werk, Caplan, and Seraganian (1999) found that almost two-thirds of fifty-three adult males (ages 23–61) from three domestic-violence treatment facilities had a current substance-use disorder and almost all of them met the criteria for a lifetime diagnosis of a substance-use disorder. More than half had a problem with polysubstance use as well. Severity of substance abuse was directly related to severity of psychiatric symptoms, including acts of verbal and physical violence. Although a small clinical sample, this group was screened for their willingness to participate in treatment and take responsibility for their actions. One might infer that they probably represent a less psychopathic and antisocial sample than other groups. Dutton, Bodnarchuk, Kropp, Hart, & Ogloff (1997) demonstrated in a combined group of both mandated and voluntary male participants in domestic-violence treatment (three-quarters of whom had a substance-use disorder) that those with personality disorders (including both BPD and APD) were more likely to perpetrate violent acts after treatment. Male batterers have also been found to show greater levels of personality-disordered traits commensurate with APD and BPD (Gleason, 1997; Dutton, Starzomski, & Ryan, 1996), and their level of abusiveness seems to be exacerbated by excessive drinking (Hastings & Hamberger, 1988;

Hamberger & Hastings, 1991). Although all batterers do not meet the criteria for psychopathy, APD, or other personality disorders, there is likely to be a subgroup of batterers who do, and these are more likely to be less responsive to treatment and to repeat their offenses (Huss & Langhinrichsen-Rohling, 2000).

The co-occurrence of conduct disorder, APD, and substance abuse has also been shown among people diagnosed with severe mental illnesses such as schizophrenia and major affective disorders (Mueser et al. 1999) and among depressed outpatients (J. D. Carter, Joyce, Mulder, Sullivan, & Luty, 1999). Those with co-occurring substance-use disorders and APD are also more likely to engage in HIV-risky behaviors: unprotected sex and intravenous drug use (Kelly & Petry, 2000). Forty-four percent of substance-abusing clients admitted to a midwestern drug treatment facility were diagnosed with APD, showing no significant differences between white and black clients, and rates of APD among men significantly exceeded the rate for women, as would be expected in the general population as well (W. M. Compton et al., 2000). Surveys of incarcerated individuals (a group that contains a disproportionately high rate of people with APD) also show higher rates of people with drinking problems (Wright, 1993). Among alcoholic incarcerated offenders, men show greater degrees of psychopathy than women (Walsh, 1997).

Theories

Both genetic and environmental factors appear to increase the risks of developing APD and substance abuse among offspring of people with APD. Having a first-degree relative with APD may increase the likelihood of manifesting these signs and symptoms by a factor of five (H. I. Kaplan & Saddock, 1998). Daghestani, Dinwiddie, and Hardy (2001) note a range of theories that may collectively account for APD, including the influences of heritability (as demonstrated by genetic twin and adoption studies) and other biological factors such as neurological impairments. Children with a history of abuse and neglect, conduct disorder, and ADHD appear to have an increased likelihood of later being diagnosed with APD. Although male offspring of a person with APD are more likely to develop both APD and a substance-use disorder, females are more likely to develop a somatization disorder (*DSM-IV-TR*). Studies of adoptees have demonstrated that, for both men and women, genetic predisposition for petty criminality is well established, but these risks are moderated by gender relative to social status, institutionalization during childhood, and being raised in an urban setting, among other social influences (Sigvardsson, Cloninger, Bohman, & von Knorring, 1982). Biological research on the causes of aggressiveness and impulsivity often associated with antisocial and criminal behavior has demonstrated a negative correlation between serotonin levels and aggressive behavior. Although these influences may be genetic in origin, they can be exacerbated or mitigated through environmental influences (Lane & Cherek, 2000).

APD and substance abuse and dependence are both, in part, genetically transmitted, and there appears to be some interaction between these two sources of genetic influence in some people (van den Bree, Svikis, & Pickens, 2000). A child born of at least one mentally ill parent and placed in an adoptive home soon after birth was more likely to show an increased risk of antisocial behavior if that child had a biological parent who was alcoholic or antisocial, or if the child experienced adverse environmental stressors (Cadoret & Cain, 1980). Electroencephalograms and neuropsychological testing with young males have shown greater frontal-lobe activity in people with childhood conduct problems and antisocial-personality indicators (Deckel, Hesselbrock, & Bauer, 1996). Such findings suggest a common biological substrate among antisocial personality, substance abuse, and biological reinforcement processes.

Biological processes, however, probably interact with environmental liabilities and risks to cause a disorder that is determined by multiple factors interacting over time (Martens, 2000). The preponderance of evidence suggests that those diagnosed with APD come from the lower socioeconomic strata (Kessler et al., 1994; Kohn et al., 1998). This fact suggests at least some role of environmental factors in the development of antisocial behavior. The interactive and reciprocally reinforcing effects of biological and environmental factors may result in cognitive structures (i.e., negative schemata, dysfunctional beliefs, expectancies, thought processes) related to problems with self-regulation, impulsivity, emotional dysregulation, and aggression. However, although childhood risk factors in general have been known for some time to be good predictors of APD in adulthood, genetic and environmental influences are difficult to disentangle (Rutter, 1997).

One longitudinal study begun in south London in the early 1960s (Farrington, 2000) examined white boys from ages eight to ten, sampled from primary schools. Response rates to the survey taken in (roughly) ten-year intervals over thirty years remained high at each measurement point (>90%). Results revealed that males identified to be APD at age eighteen were over three times as likely to be arrested between ages twenty-one and forty. The most important predictive factors for future diagnosis of APD and criminal convictions included having a parent who was convicted of a crime, large family size, low intelligence, disrupted family life, and having been raised by a young single mother. Another longitudinal study of a representative population in New Zealand (Moffitt, Caspi, Dickson, Silva, & Stanton, 1996) followed boys from ages three to eighteen. A battery of measures was taken every two years for more than 1,000 subjects. Although it was the rare boy who did not engage in some kind of antisocial behavior at some point (<6%), those children manifesting behavioral disorders by age three were much more likely to develop long-term patterns of conduct-disordered and, later, antisocial behavior. Late-onset problems, usually precipitated around puberty, were more transitory and less likely to persist. The problems associated with early-onset type were primarily associated with a range of early learning and neurological problems, including "cognitive, language and motor deficits, comorbid attention deficit and hyperactivity, extreme aggressiveness, reading difficulties, impulsivity, adverse family social contexts, and poor parenting" (Moffitt et al., p. 419). Similar conclusions have been found in populations of adult offenders (e.g., Vitelli, 1997). When adults with APD are followed up, long-term outcomes appear to be best predicted by initial severity of their APD symptoms (D. W. Black, Monahan, Baumgard, & Bell, 1997). Given the proclivity for early-onset conduct-disordered children to engage in violence, as one would expect, adults with APD are also more likely to engage in a range of violent acts, especially those with higher indicated levels of psychopathy, a personality trait marked by "callousness, impulsivity, egocentricity, grandiosity, irresponsibility, lack of empathy, guilt, or remorse" (Hare, 1999, p. 185). These traits are especially dangerous and troubling when identified in violent sex offenders, people who are virtually nonresponsive to treatment (Hare, 1999).

Fishbein (2000) notes a lack of interdisciplinary research on antisocial personality, and this lack of communication among various disciplines has hindered understanding the interactions among biological, psychological, social, and criminal-justice processes.

> Studies indicate that vulnerability to antisocial behavior is partially a function of genetic and biological make-up that manifests during childhood as particular behavioral, cognitive, and psychological traits (e.g., impulsivity, attention deficits, or conduct disorder) and are measurable in physiological and biochemical responses . . . Instead of viewing evidence from these various disciplines as independent sources of biological and social dysfunction, these sources of evidence should be seen as a continuous, developmental sequence of interacting factors. That is, basic genetic or acquired biological traits contribute to measurable biochemical and physiological conditions that predispose individuals to a constellation of particular behavioral and temperamental outcomes . . . Biological vulnerabilities are, in turn, influenced by socio-environmental factors that act as triggers, offering one explanation for the disproportionate number of residents prone to antisocial behavior in lower income neighborhoods where triggers are more prevalent. Put simply, abnormalities in certain neurobiological mechanisms heighten sensitivity to adverse environmental circumstances, increasing the risk for an antisocial outcome. (pp. 1–3)

Widom and Toch (2000) describe a transactional view that incorporates the contributions of temperament, early attachment and loss, parental guidance and modeling (e.g., the influence of parenting skills, proper disciplining, adequate nurturance, the parents' own modeling of self-control and prosocial behaviors), and environmental contingencies (e.g., intermittent rewards and punishments for committing crimes). All of these influences can theoretically be examined within a transactional and ecological framework where cognitive, behavioral, physiological, interpersonal, and environmental factors interact over time and across situations to either increase or decrease the likelihood of antisocial behavior (Rutter, 1997; Martens, 2000). An interdisciplinary view of the causes, course, and consequences of APD would likely lead to more integrated understanding and more effective interventions and policies rather than approaches that are largely driven by political ideology.

Key Elements of Multidimensional/ Functional Assessment

The *DSM-IV-TR* diagnosis of APD includes four basic criteria. The first is evidence of a pervasive pattern of disregard and violation of the rights of others occurring since the age of fifteen as indicated by at least three of the following: repeated unlawful acts, chronic deceitfulness, impulsiveness, hyperaggressiveness (e.g., fights, assaults), reckless disregard for the safety of self or others, consistent irresponsibility with regard to work or financial commitments, and lack of remorse when having hurt or otherwise infringed on others' rights. The other three criteria are that the individual should be at least eighteen (although the diagnosis as indicated above can be applied to minors), there is evidence of onset of conduct disorder prior to age fifteen, and antisocial behavior did not occur exclusively during a period of major mental illness. Again, practitioners should be aware of problems with reliability in applying this diagnosis, and of a high rate of co-occurrence with other problems and diagnoses (M. D. Cunningham & Reidy, 1998). A more complete diagnostic picture should include elements that emphasize psychopathy in addition to criminal behavior.

Social workers are likely to encounter many clients who demonstrate some of the behaviors described in the current diagnostic criteria. Key considerations include the chronicity and pervasiveness of antisocial behaviors, psychopathic attitudes regarding the rights of others, and the context within which these behaviors occur. A multidimensional assessment should draw heavily on a historical time line to substantiate these facts across various domains of living (work, relationships, etc), and practitioners should avoid diagnosing in response to a client's recent presentation in one particular situation. Regardless of whether the client clearly meets the criteria for APD, it is important to examine potential co-occurring problems and disorders. Given the predictive value of childhood and adolescent risk factors, a thorough history is in order, particularly evidence of behavioral problems (e.g., school disruption, truancy, fighting, stealing, run-ins with the law, substance abuse) from childhood through adolescence (Daghestani et al., 2001). Practitioners should look for consistency and congruence with current problems in interpersonal relations, job disruption, and evidence of dangerousness to others.

Assessing risk for violent behavior is one of the more challenging and critical goals of an MDF assessment of people diagnosed with APD. Research findings support a range of risk factors that contribute to an assessment of violent behaviors and the reasons for it. These factors include temperament, childhood history of abuse and neglect, history of conduct disorder, hyperactivity, family conflict, witnessing or being a victim of domestic violence, growing up in a violent community, previous involvement with alcohol and other drugs, and criminal involvement. Given the heterogeneity of risk factors and the unique combination of factors that contribute to the proclivity toward violence, Howells and Day (2002) emphasized the critical importance of conducting a functional analysis of factors that may precipitate aggressive or violent behavior. This detailed sequential analysis of proximate factors that maintain the cycle of violence in the individual's life is essential for focusing intervention planning. Gendreau (1996a) argues for the benefits of combining population risk data (i.e., actuarial and risk-assessment data) with a client-specific functional analysis of day-to-day behavior. This assessment needs to be linked to intervention planning that targets specific problems and needs of the client, such as criminal and antisocial attitudes, impulse control, substance abuse, use of leisure time, social relationships, and work.

Notwithstanding the insufferable insights of clinical Monday-morning quarterbacks, risk-assessment research strongly suggests that *predicting* violent behavior in an individual client is a difficult task for even the most seasoned and scrupulous practitioner. It is not an activity that lends itself to "clinical intuition." There is a difference between correlational prediction based on general risk-assessment data and predicting if, when, and under what circumstances an individual is likely to become violent. Nevertheless, practitioners are called upon in clinical and legal settings to make their best estimates of risk. In recent years, some progress has been made in this regard. A study conducted with 799 violent offenders discharged from a maximum-security therapeutic community (M. Rice & Harris, 1995) demonstrated that the following factors (measured with the Violence Risk Appraisal Guide) were predictive of further violence: a positive score on the PCL-r, separation from parents before age sixteen, having never been married, behavior problems in elementary school, having failed on prior conditional release, a property-offense history, an alcohol-abuse history, and a diagnosis of APD. Those with a diagnosis of schizophrenia and older clients were less likely to be violent. Based on these factors, the investigators accurately predicted 75% of the cases that failed (which were 43% of those released). M. D. Cunningham and Reidy (1999) suggest that practitioners improve their estimates by using a number of evidence-based strategies, including referencing population base rates and clinical sample base rates, clearly defining the severity of the behavior in question, and considering contextual factors such as drug use at the time of the violent event. They also recommend that practitioners avoid the following practices: relying on illusory correlations, putting much confidence in one's own clinical impressions (which tend to disproportionately focus on previous "correct" guesses while forgetting "wrong" guesses), use of projective testing for diagnostic purposes, and an overemphasis on *DSM* diagnosis of APD. Monahan (1996), a well-known authority on the challenges of predicting violence, suggests that, future research should do the following: (1) disaggregate dangerousness into risk factors including the type and degree of harm, and likelihood of its occurrence; (2) employ a multidimensional approach to assessment and risk evaluation; (3) measure harm on a severity continuum, and employ multiple measures; (4) estimate risk over time and across different contexts; (5) use known statistical data to predict harm from known risk factors; and (6) use representative samples in research and include research goals that both assess and manage risk. There may be serious consequences to the use of well-intended treatments not supported by evidence-based assessment of violence risk. For example, M. Rice (1997) notes that early enthusiastic efforts to treat psychopathic violent offenders demonstrated not only failure, but an actual increase in the chances of future violence. She concludes that there are currently no psychological treatments that significantly reduce risk of repeat offenses.

Practitioners must also be aware of the pernicious influence of racial stereotypes when making evidence-based assessments. In addition to the tendency to give harsher sentences to people of color for drug offenses, African Americans are also likely to be sentenced more harshly, based on the perception that they are less likely than whites to reduce criminal behavior with age. Given the evidence that antisocial behavior tends to remit during middle age, it is reasonable to hypothesize that criminal sentencing for older citizens should be less severe for many drug-related crimes. C. W. Johnston and Alozie (2001) conducted a multivariate analysis of about 5,700 arrested people in Arizona and found that while non-Hispanic white defendants began to receive more lenient sentences at around age fifty-two, these diminished sentences were not extended as often to blacks and Hispanics. Not only are many people of color more likely to be sentenced and sentenced more harshly, but this bias continues even when these offenders have reached the declining years of their criminal careers.

Instruments

Given the risk of violence by clients diagnosed with APD, the predictive validity of assessment for the purpose of making decisions regarding court-ordered interventions or conditional release to the community is of critical importance. Thus, an instrument that would reduce the likelihood of making the wrong decision about releasing criminals into the community would be particularly valuable. Evidence consistently supports the use of the PCL-r (Hare, Harpur, Hakstian, Forth, & Harts, 1990; Hare, 1991) as a valuable aid in making these decisions. Bodholdt, Richards, and Gacono (2000) discuss the historical and conceptual roots of the PCL-r, and note that the items are similar to the profile of the psychopathic personality conceptualized by Cleckley (1941). These traits include superficial charm, absence of thought disorders, lack of anxiety, untruthfulness, lack of remorse, failure to learn by experience, lack of insight, and lack of any life plan. In contrast, the current criteria of the *DSM-IV-TR* focuses almost exclusively on criminal behavior, and is understood to be based more on a model of social deviance (Bodholdt et al.). Other items on the PCL-r overlap with some of these indicators as well.

A series of studies with several forensic samples have supported the reliability and validity of the PCL-r. Hart, Kropp, and Hare (1988) used the PCL-r with a cutoff of 34 (to identify the high-risk group) with over 200 inmates who were released to the community. The data clearly demonstrated that the PCL-r improved predictive ability of practitioners beyond the statistical contributions of inmates' age, criminal history, and release type. Those who scored high performed very poorly following conditional release from prison, by participating in more frequent and more serious criminal activities and by failing to develop a stable noncriminal lifestyle.

Although earlier factor analyses of the PCL showed several factors measuring psychopathy, many of the samples were of inadequate size, and there were other problems in interpretation of the analyses. Harpur, Hakstian, and Hare (1988) examined the factor structure of the PCL, using exploratory factor analysis from five samples of male prison inmates (mostly white), and found good congruence of factor structure across different samples with good to excellent interrater reliabilities and internal consistencies. The best solution appeared to contain two factors: factor 1, selfishness, callousness, and remorseless exploitation of others; factor 2, chronically unstable and antisocial lifestyle. In multiple samples of prison and forensic inmates Harpur, Hare, and Hakstian (1989) demonstrated very good internal consistencies (mid-.80s) for both factors 1 and 2. The PCL-r also demonstrated good concurrent and discriminant validity in that factor 1, as expected, correlated significantly and more highly than factor 2 with standardized measures of anxiety (-.20 and -.26) and narcissism (.45), whereas factor 2 correlated with a diagnosis of APD (.55, .61, .66) in three separate samples. In a similar study with eighty forensic patients, Hart and Hare (1989) showed good concurrent validity between the PCL and APD, but good discrimination between the PCL and Axis I diagnoses. Studies with similar populations provided equally strong support (Forth, Hart, & Hare, 1990). A study of a Swedish forensic population (violent offenders with schizophrenia) demonstrated that the PCL-r was the strongest predictor of recidivism (using a cutoff score of 26) compared to several other factors over the course of a follow-up period of more than four years (Tengstrom, Grann, Langstrom, & Kulgren, 2000). The PCL-r has also been shown to be reliable and valid for adolescents, including black youths (Brandt, Kennedy, Patrick, & Curtin, 1997), and both black and white adult inmates (Cooke & Michie, 1997). A recent rigorous validation of the PCL-r using item response theory showed strong support for the factor structure, reliability, and validity of the subscales (Cooke & Michie). Item response theory focuses on the performance of each individual item as it relates to the overall factor that it is theoretically expected to measure.

The PCL-r (Hare et al., 1990) is a twenty-item instrument. Each item is scaled to indicate the degree to which the trait or behavior applies to the respondent: 0 = definitely does not apply, 1 = may or may not apply, 2 = definitely applies. The PCL-r is a proprietary instrument. It cannot be used without purchasing the instrument and the training materials, and requires expertise in forensic evaluations. Nevertheless, the items of the PCL-r may be a helpful guide for detecting psychopathy in nonforensic settings as well. The twenty items (Hare et al. 1990) are

1. glibness/superficial charm
2. grandiose sense of self-worth
3. need for stimulation
4. pathological lying
5. conning/manipulation
6. lack of remorse or guilt
7. shallow affect
8. callousness/lack of empathy
9. parasitic lifestyle
10. poor behavioral controls
11. promiscuous sexual behavior
12. early behavior problems
13. lack of realistic goals
14. impulsivity
15. irresponsibility
16. failure to accept responsibility
17. many short-term relationships
18. juvenile delinquency
19. revocation of conditional release
20. criminal versatility

Factor 1 (selfishness, callousness, and remorseless use of others) is scored by summing items 1, 2, 4, 5, 6, 7, 8, and 16. Factor 2 (chronically unstable and antisocial lifestyle) is scored by summing items 3, 9, 10, 12, 13, 14, 15, 18, and 19.

In summary, reviews of the PCL-r (Bodholdt et al., 2000; M. D. Cunningham & Reidy, 1998) have demonstrated that it has very good internal consistency, interrater and test-retest reliability, and good construct and criterion validity, and has been normed with prison inmates and forensic psychiatric patients. The PCL-r is also highly intercorrelated with the brief PCL screening version, but the screening version is not intended to be substituted for the full PCL-r when used as part of a comprehensive assessment. Again, these items can provide a basis for raising concern about the presence of psychopathy in a client, but the PCL-r should be administered by people with special training and experience in working with correctional or forensic populations. Despite the strengths of the PCL-r, it has limitations and should be used within the context of a broad MDF assessment that includes known base rates for recidivism (Freedman, 2001; Serin & Brown, 2000).

SELECTING EFFECTIVE INTERVENTIONS

People who meet the criteria for APD may be encountered in any number of treatment environments, including outpatient or inpatient mental health and substance-abuse treatment settings, court-ordered treatment, specialized forensic settings and prison-connected therapeutic communities (Daghestani et al., 2001). L. M. Simon (1998) points out that 70% of inmates meet the criteria for APD, but most individuals under correctional supervision are not in prison. Many of these people on probation or parole are not adequately supervised in the community. Reviewers of the current research literature generally agree on the importance of employing well-controlled studies to justify the use of interventions with offenders, given the risks to the community. They also agree that the evidence supports structured programs for cognitive-behavioral skills combined with contingency management, and that psychodynamic and similar psychotherapies are of little value with these populations (Daghestani et al.; L. M. Simon, 1998; Lipsey & Wilson, 1993; Gendreau, 1996a, 1966b). Community-reinforcement approaches that include contingency management for people who abuse alcohol and other drugs (see review in chapter 6) are also relevant to treatment of the forensic population. Nevertheless, despite the promising results from emerging behavioral programs, practitioners must be cautious about participants who may fake compliance with interventions until they are completed, to obtain reduced sentences or to put the best face on at a parole hearing. Long-term interventions and close monitoring of clients by mental health, substance-abuse, and criminal justice professionals are essential.

The conclusions from reviews of the literature regarding what is effective for offending adults parallels approaches shown to be effective with adolescent juveniles (Palmer 1996; see chapter 13). Outcome studies of adult- and juvenile-offender programs have demonstrated effect sizes from .17 to .77 in meta-analytic reviews (Lipsey & Wilson, 1993). However, the primary focus in this chapter is on adults treated in forensic programs.

Prison-based therapeutic communities (TCs) have become increasingly accepted by the criminal justice system and the public, particularly for nonviolent drug offenders. This trend is supported by promising evidence of outcomes showing a reduction in drug use, crime, and recidivism and an increase in prosocial behaviors (H. K. Wexler, 1995). The TC movement began with Synanon in the late 1950s as an alternative to AA and conventional therapeutic treatments geared toward middle-class patients. The Synanon movement has evolved, but the basic concept lives on in well-known residential programs such as Daytop Village and Phoenix House. According to H. K. Wexler (1995), TC's core ingredients include the overarching principles of self-help, a hierarchical structure and strict rules of conduct within the residence, use of emotionally charged group encounters, and educational seminars. Lengths of stay of at least one year are strongly recommended. Implementing TCs in prison has become increasingly popular, and H. K. Wexler (1995, p.63) recommends that they be developed with the following "central features": a clear and consistent treatment philosophy, an empathic and safe environment, recruitment of committed staff, clear rules of conduct, employment of ex-offenders and ex-addicts, use of peer role models and peer pressure, use of relapse-prevention strategies, continuity of care from residential to aftercare in the community, and "maintenance of treatment program integrity, autonomy, flexibility, and openness." Attention to TC programming has increasingly focused on problems that co-occur with substance abuse.

Although drug-court treatment diversionary programs have shown some positive gains, most evaluation studies have suffered from methodological weaknesses, including high attrition rates from the original sample (and possibly "creaming" the less dysfunctional and more motivated inmates), lack of random assignment, and lack of long-term follow-up. In one nonrandomized quasi-experimental evaluation, Vito and Tewksbury (1998) compared drug-court graduates of a diversionary program in Kentucky to those who chose not to participate in the program. Both African-American and white participants who successfully completed the one-year treatment program showed substantively lower reconviction rates than those who chose not to participate. They speculated that the reasons for the apparent success were good mutual support between the criminal justice and treatment communities, adequate screening of potential candidates for the program, implementation of evaluation technologies, and reliable drug-abuse monitoring systems (e.g., urine testing).

In evaluating three similar prison-based drug rehabilitation programs in Delaware, New York, and Texas, K. Knight, Hiller, and Simpson (1999) noted that all three demonstrated that prisoners who received the standard prison drug program plus an aftercare follow-up program showed less relapse than those who received just the standard prison program. The latter, in turn, showed less recidivism than those who received no treatment. Nevertheless, even the best-performing groups showed, overall, considerable rates of recidivism. However, the authors point out that one of the key problems in making comparisons across studies is the lack of consistency in measuring relapse (how to detect and measure drug use), and recidivism (rearrest or reincarceration), and a lack of broad-based psychosocial measures to account for other outcomes.

Exemplar Study: Staged Approaches to Prison Aftercare Programs. The trend in the offender literature has begun to support the emphasis of staged long-term approaches to intervention with inmates in drug TC's while in prison and after release. One noted program in Delaware (S. S. Martin, Butzin, & Inciardi, 1995; Inciardi, Martin, Butzin, Hooper, & Harrison, 1997) evaluated combinations of a three-stage model against a comparison group (who received no TC in-prison treatment, but managed to obtain some treatment after release). Stage 1 included an in-prison TC intervention (focused on reducing criminal attitudes, engendering prosocial attitudes, and planning a drug-free life). In stage 2, inmates worked at real jobs in the community during the day but returned to prison or an associated facility at night. In stage 3, work release was completed, and the offender was on parole. Offenders attended counseling sessions, periodically returned to the prison TC for booster sessions, and kept in touch with their counselor. Of the 448 mostly male African-American study participants (out of 1,002 originally interviewed), 77% of those who completed the three-stage program were not arrested at eighteen month follow-up as compared to 57% of those who received the two-stage program, 43% for those who had received TC only, and 46% for the comparison group. A similar pattern of results was found for clean urine analysis (47% for three-stage intervention, 31% for two-stage, 22% for prison TC only, and 16% for the comparison group). Generally, the more treatment received, the better the results.

Although in-prison TCs with aftercare are a positive development in the field of correctional rehabilitation, confidence in the outcome research must be tempered with caution, given the methodological weaknesses in the evaluation designs. In addition to sample attrition and a lack of random assignment to treatment conditions, there is also the overarching problem of how and why many of these people come to be imprisoned in the first place. The "war on drugs" has resulted in disproportionately imprisoning blacks and Hispanics, and has resulted in their receiving longer sentences. The best psychosocial interventions will not mitigate the essential injustice of disproportionately imprisoning people because they are poor and members of racial minorities.

Sex Offender Outcome Studies

Sex offenders may be considered a subset of people who otherwise fit the criteria for APD. Their calculated exploitation of children and lack of remorse, at a minimum, qualify them as criminally antisocial and psychopathic. Although practitioners should not be optimistic about treatment success with sex-offending clients, cognitive-behavioral interventions have been shown to result in some modest improvements. Maletzky and Steinhauser (2002) reported on the treatments of over 7,000 clients treated over twenty-five years. A variety of cognitive-behavioral methods were employed, but the elements of these treatment packages were not consistent. Nevertheless, with *less severe clients* (exhibitionists and child molesters rather than homosexual pedophiles and rapists) modest gains were demonstrated. Although 62% of clients were followed up to five years, those who dropped out must be conservatively considered treatment failures. Overall, it is reasonable to cautiously conclude that CBT may have a modest positive effect with less severe sex offenders.

W. L. Marshall (1996) reviewed results from group treatment that included empathy training, respectful confrontation to reduce denial and minimization of the offense, masturbatory reconditioning to reduce deviant sexual fantasies and increase "normal" fantasies, and relapse-prevention strategies. He concluded that these cognitive-behavioral programs have been encouraging, particularly for youthful offenders, but that these approaches have not yet been subjected to a sufficient amount of controlled research to justify placing a high degree of confidence in these methods. Hall (1995) reviewed ninety-two studies and found twelve in which treatment groups were compared to alternative treatment or control conditions. Although the clients across studies had been convicted of heterogeneous offenses, ten of the twelve studies included adult male sex offenders who committed their crimes against children. Results showed some modest success for CBT and hormonal treatments. Quinsey, Harris, Rice, and Lalumiere (1993) carefully examined the methodological shortcomings of many of the studies reviewed by others. The major limitations in sex-offender research include lack of random assignment and control groups, inadequacy in dealing with attrition and dropouts in calculating the results, and the use of comparison data from other populations to estimate the significance of recidivism in treatment groups. The authors argue that when more rigorous methodological criteria are employed, there is little evidence to conclude that interventions for sex offenders are effective. Although some cognitive-behavioral programs with close external (law-enforcement) supervision appear promising for some, outcomes do not reach levels that are sufficient to put children in the community at risk. Furby, Weinrott, and Blackshaw (1989) concluded in their review that clients deemed to be sexually aggressive should be considered intractable and nonresponsive to treatment. Considering all the current evidence, the priority for dealing with sex offenders must be confinement of the offender and protection of potential child victims. Some flexibility in this position may be justified for less severe adolescent offenders.

Descriptions of Effective Intervention Methods

After thoroughly reviewing the extant empirical literature, several reviewers have concluded that behavioral programs conducted within the context of community-reinforcement or contingency management approaches are currently the most effective psychosocial interventions (Gendreau, 1996a, 1996b; McGuire & Hatcher, 2001; Prendergast, Anglin, & Wellisch, 1995). Recommendations based on their reviews include the following:

Develop a sound and sensitive working relationship with each client.

Conduct an individual MDF assessment of each client's deficits, needs, and strengths and readiness to change.

Use Standardized measures such as the PCL-r and scales for common co-occurring problems such as the Addiction Severity Index (see chapter 6).

Use cognitive-behavioral coping skills to help clients challenge negative criminogenic attitudes, learn self-monitoring to detect at-risk situations, avoid triggers for crime-related activities (e.g., using drugs), and learn self-regulation skills, which aim to control impulses and anger, manage stress, improve poor motivation, and cope more effectively with negative moods. These coping skills are also commensurate with the goals of relapse prevention (see chapter 6) for those offenders who abuse drugs.

Have clients observe the modeling behavior of others to learn alternative ways of dealing with situations that can provoke criminal acts.

Help clients develop better social problem-solving methods to deal better with social isolation and improve interpersonal skills.

Implement community-reinforcement strategies.

Use contingency management methods, such as giving or withholding rewards for prosocial activities. This strategy includes the possible reinstatement of punishment, if necessary.

Monitor interventions for treatment fidelity.

Provide long-term interventions with follow-up and good coordination with adjunctive services as needed.

Within these basic intervention principles, practitioners and program managers must also make an effort to match the intervention plan to the interests and needs of each individual client. Reinforcers and contingencies must be provided and enforced consistently. Positive reinforcers should be used in much greater proportion than the use of punishment, if punishment is to be used at all (it is the least preferred technique). Traditional case management is also necessary to coordinate the community resources necessary to help clients avoid relapse and achieve their prosocial rehabilitative goals. These community contacts may include drug testing and related service agencies (e.g., methadone maintenance), psychiatric services, job-site supervisors, probation or parole officers, spouses, and other family members.

Collaboration between Social Work and the Criminal Justice System: Therapeutic Justice and Therapeutic Jurisprudence.

People are ultimately responsible for their own decisions and actions. If social workers believe in "empowering" people, then they must simultaneously advocate for their clients' rights and communicate an expectation that they respect the rights of others. When a client does something positive for himself or for another person, social workers consider the act an expression of the client's free will. When a client performs a criminal act, social workers must, likewise, hold him accountable and responsible for that decision. Although there are mitigating psychological and environmental factors to consider (e.g., florid psychosis at the time of the act, being in a life-threatening situation), a balanced approach to assessing client responsibility is needed to effectively apply therapeutic and criminal justice strategies for the common goals of improving the psychosocial well-being of clients and protecting innocent people in the community.

Nygaard (2000) has noted a disconnection between the criminal justice system and the behavioral sciences that tends to result in a reactionary and polarized approach to criminal behavior (i.e., punishment versus treatment). An alternative to these extremes is a growing appreciation and understanding of two related concepts: therapeutic justice and therapeutic jurisprudence. Nygaard explains that *therapeutic justice* employs the criminal justice system not just as a means to confine and punish, but as an opportunity to engender change in the client, using the leverage of the penal system and a range of existing social forces including professional therapeutic means. These efforts go beyond the prison walls, and use a continuum of efforts in the community to enhance change and prevent recidivism. Such an effort must be interdisciplinary in both research and practice. According to his view, therapeutic justice is all about change, about creating a clinical and penal climate in which transgressors are encouraged to change and, for the offenders who sincerely want to change, about assisting them in their endeavors. Nonetheless, people who are correctable or have treatable conditions bear the ultimate moral responsibility both for the change resulting from treatment and their condition afterwards; this applies whether one has a physical ailment, an addiction disease, a more complex emotional problem, or has committed a crime. The system can help one do what one cannot do for, or by, himself. It can restore hope where despair exists. It can coordinate individual and component efforts. It can intervene. But it cannot rehabilitate. We have learned that lesson. Change is tough. Therapeutic justice is not a soft, easy remedy. (p. 23-14)

Therapeutic jurisprudence is a focused effort to use court proceedings to advance therapeutic outcomes (D. B. Wexler, 1991). An example of therapeutic jurisprudence within the broader context of therapeutic justice would be the civil commitment of a substance-abusing mentally ill man who was guilty of committing assault. Sentencing might include close monitoring and continued compliance with medical and psychosocial intervention. The mentally ill man is not exonerated from his criminal behavior, but, rather than institutionalizing him indefinitely, he is simultaneously treated and held accountable for his actions. *Holding the client accountable for his behavior must be understood to be a therapeutic process* in order for client progress to be tied inextricably to community safety. Social workers have an ethical duty to enhance the psychosocial well-being of both clients and the larger community around them.

Social workers have long been ambivalent about their relationship with law enforcement and the criminal justice system. This ambivalence is perhaps justifiable, given some of the inherent biases and discriminatory policies. However, such excesses do not obviate the potential for collaboration when therapeutic and criminal justice goals are commensurate. Unfortunately, the practice of "remanding a client for counseling" from the bench has often been a dubious practice at best. As O'Hare (1996a, p. 421) has noted, social workers risk "participating in a muddled enterprise where clinicians pretend to treat and clients pretend to comply at the behest of the criminal justice system." A clarification of the goals and responsibilities of the therapeutic community and the criminal justice system, however, can help reduce this ambiguity of goals and responsibilities and result in clearer accountability standards for clients. Current examples of potentially effective collaborations between social workers and the criminal justice system include outpatient civil commitment for treatment of the mentally ill who have committed crimes, diversionary treatment programs for nonviolent drug offenders, and advocacy for substance-abusing mothers (contingent on treatment compliance and sobriety) to regain custody of children in the child welfare system. Rather than loose or informal arrangements, such collaboration between various social services and criminal justice requires more clearly defined integrative programs, including clearer mandates for the use of evidence-based practices, clearly defined intervention goals, adequate supervision and evaluation of client outcomes, and more rigorously designed program evaluation and research.

Rooney and Bibus (2001) provide the following guidelines for an ethical and legal framework for working with involuntary clients: assure informed consent and protection of their legal rights (due process); exercise beneficence and paternalism with judgment; intervene when necessary and within legal limits for the good of the client and/or to protect others in society; empower clients to the extent one can in order to affirm their worth and dignity, enhance their strengths, and prompt them to take initiative in problem solving; keep clients informed of their legal requirements as well as choices and options they may have; communicate openly and honestly with clients and avoid deceptive methods; and advocate for the protection of clients' rights and fair treatment under the law.

IMPLEMENTING AND EVALUATING THE EVIDENCE-BASED INTERVENTION PLAN

CASE STUDY: TIM

Tim was a twenty-six-year-old white male who had recently been arrested for being drunk and disorderly. At his arrest, he was carrying a small amount of methamphetamine. He was seen by a social worker, George, in a combined mental health/substance-abuse treatment agency as part of a contracted diversionary program for first-time drug offenders. This was not, however, the first time that Tim had broken the law.

Tim had been in trouble off and on since adolescence. Raised in an economically disadvantaged mixed-race working-class neighborhood, Tim vaguely recalls his father coming in and out of the picture during his childhood and adolescence. He clearly recalls the violent beatings his father gave to his mother in their narrow galley kitchen, as well as the beatings he received himself. His father was often drunk, intermittently provided financial support, and occasionally would be around for months while he was "on the wagon." Tim recalls these periods of sobriety as almost worse than when his father was drinking, because his father would become unbearably strict in an effort to "rehabilitate himself and everyone around him." As his father relapsed and spent more time out of the picture, Tim began to skip school, started hanging out on the streets, began to shoplift, and engaged in other forms of criminal activity. Later, he "graduated" to stealing objects out of cars and snatching purses. During this time he also began to drink, sniff glue and other inhalants, and occasionally smoke pot when he could afford it or steal it. Occasionally he was paid in drugs to act as courier for local drug dealers. Tim was remarkably adept at not getting caught, and maintained a reputation among the adults in the community of being a "nice boy." Eventually he was sent to foster homes because of his chronic truancy during early adolescence. His mom could not control his behavior, and his age virtually precluded adoption. At that point, his father was absent from his life.

After a few stays in foster homes, Tim eventually moved back home with his mother. Tim decided that moving from one place to another was not preferable to staying home. He remained there until he was eighteen, and worked sporadically. After eighteen (having failed to finish high school) he moved out, and began working in phone sales for a variety of companies selling a range of speculative products (e.g., vacation timeshares, stocks and bonds, other investment schemes, etc). He was quite adept at these endeavors and was able to make a decent living, maintained an apartment, and drove a late-model car. He successfully lied about his age and qualifications on numerous occasions to obtain better-paying work, and his employers did not delve too deeply into his more grandiose claims, given his sales track record. As he moved into more sophisticated sales jobs, he was able to afford better clothes and the desirable accoutrements of the "high-powered" salesperson. He was charming, and engaging, could converse well on any number of subjects, and had a first-rate reputation in his product area. Tim also had to keep moving around because of his ques-

tionable sales methods. He showed little compunction for misrepresenting the truth to older people and the infirm when selling insurance policies. He came across as quite sincere, very credible, and very persuasive in person. He was also accused on more than one occasion of sexual assault. In one case, the young woman was fifteen years old, but charges were dropped for lack of evidence. In another case, the woman was an adult, but charges were dropped by her for unknown reasons.

None of Tim's brushes with the law ever amounted to a conviction. He was arrested just prior to his intake at the clinic. He had been drinking heavily and snorting methamphetamine all day, celebrating yet another "big score" in his current sales job, and got involved in a bar fight with someone who was also intoxicated. The bartender (with the help of other patrons) pushed them into the street where the fight ensued, and police were called. When he emptied his pockets in the local police station, the methamphetamines were discovered, and Tim was arrested. He presented himself before the judge as suitably contrite, and was mandated to outpatient substance-abuse treatment at the local mental health center, an agency that had a contract with the state drug-court diversionary program.

Multidimensional/Functional Assessment: Defining Problems and Goals

George, the social worker, obtained Tim's previous criminal and social service records. It appeared from these data that he would easily have met the diagnostic criteria for conduct disorder and, now, APD. Risk factors were congruent with Tim's increasing antisocial behavior: his father's alcoholism, Tim's impulsivity, having witnessed domestic violence and having been abused himself, feeling that he could trust few people in the world. His history and current presentation were of someone who clearly had developed the ability to be deceitful, lie, and otherwise take advantage of people while showing little remorse. His brushes with the law, which involved stealing, allegations of rape, chronic drug abuse, and other problem behaviors, represented a long history of criminal activity from youth into adulthood. George was inclined to think that Tim played down these details, and took little responsibility for the accusations. At times George observed that Tim would disproportionately focus on one relatively innocuous event in great detail with considerable affect, while avoiding or glossing over other more egregious facts concerning his alleged illegal activities. He would admit as little as possible about crimes for which he had been charged or arrested, and volunteered information for little else. His arrest for drug possession was his first time being charged as an adult for a serious crime. His day-to-day coping skills were generally good. He complained about being bored often, had few friends outside of work acquaintances, and aside from moving from one job to another (not all that unusual in sales), worked consistently. He had no steady romantic relationship, but prided himself on "having an easy time getting any woman I want." He reported his health as excellent (despite neglect and poor health habits). Although he owned up to the possibility that he possibly drank a bit too much at times, he generally denied drug abuse ("aside from an occasional joint"), and even suggested that the drugs found on him at his arrest were not really his, but someone else's that he was just holding for them.

Overall, it appeared to the social worker that Tim was downplaying his drug use and other illegal activities, and his sincerity about "getting better and improving myself" was somewhat affected. The tip-off seemed to come when he began to use psychotherapeutic clichés about "getting myself together and really . . . I mean, really dealing with my issues." Nevertheless, George realized that, at this point, there was little point in confronting him with his apparent deceitfulness; he would continue to gather more data and move forward with a detailed functional assessment.

In examining the details of Tim's everyday life, it appeared that he was not uniformly conning people, abusing drugs, or attempting to otherwise exploit people. Although these themes appeared to be somewhat consistent overall, he was not unlikable or without the ability to develop acquaintances, even a friendly relationship with another man or a romantic relationship with a woman. These relationships, appeared to be somewhat short-lived, however, and were usually terminated by him. Although he did not present his work or his relationships as exploitive, there appeared to be a pattern of increasing his "conning" behaviors when he was feeling threatened in them. A sense of "I'll get them before they get me" clearly came through as the social worker discussed Tim's "survival strategies" at work or in his dealings with women. He tended to see perceived slights or not getting his way as a very serious matter and a provocation that he would not stand for. Compromise equaled capitulation, and "giving in is for losers." His drinking and drug use appeared to increase during times of stress, and simultaneously it seemed that his other problematic behaviors tended to increase. These included more quick sexual liaisons with women and increased conflict at work, often leading to a change of employment. At other times, he suggested that he actually felt quite good, but "it never lasts." When queried about what those times were like, Tim suggested that once, when he was twenty, he had a relationship with someone and, during that time, felt better than he had ever felt in his life. But "she left me for someone else . . . I'll never let that happen again." Whether it was work, his relationships, or something else, the pattern seemed to be that he experienced a sense of being threatened, he drank more or used drugs, he became more impulsive and somewhat exploitive to those around him with the consequences creating more conflict and consequential stress, and, at some point, a more serious problem would erupt, a problem that he would have to escape or retreat from.

Over the course of a few visits (he was mandated for weekly counseling for a year with monthly reports to his probation officer), Tim and George came to a tentative understanding regarding what the goals of their work together would be. They agreed that Tim would abstain from drug use for the time being (although he continued to downplay it, he agreed in principle); examine his relationships with other people, including his customers, workmates, and any romantic associations he might have; and reduce incidents of explosive anger and conflict that caused him more problems. The social worker, after a few visits, put it succinctly: "You tend to treat people in a way that suggests that you just want to get something from them, like a sale, a favor, or sex, but you don't want to give them anything of yourself in return. Is that about right?" Despite appearing very angry at this suggestion that "I'm just a user," Tim acknowledged that there "might be a little something to that."

For Tim, however, the most important consideration for being in treatment seemed to be to "comply with the courts and get this behind me." George made it clear that full reports regarding any illegal behavior would be going to the probation officer, and that he and the probation officer were working as a team. George was also realistic in his outcome expectations for Tim: there would be no personality reconstruction here, but a reduction, even an elimination, of illegal activities was possible. Tim might not cultivate deeper and genuine feelings, even empathy, for others, but he could reduce the threat that he posed to others in the community either through exploitation or his drug use. These latter goals would be much more difficult to monitor and hard to hold him accountable for. Regarding his taking advantage of people on the job, there appeared to be a fine line between his exploitive quasi-criminal behavior and what is often condoned in many work environments.

Selecting and Designing the Intervention: Defining Strategies and Objectives

Appealing to Tim's self-interest, George endeavored to find some motivation for working on his problems, other than simply "staying out of trouble." In using a motivational interviewing style, he was able to help Tim arrive at a sort of cost-benefit analysis (using the pros and cons approach one might use in sales) of what kind of trouble his conning others and use of illegal drugs (to the extent that he admitted it) had caused him. He was, after a time, willing to admit that his drug use didn't really "fill the void" all that well and that, at times, he got sick of it and wondered why he was often "bored with reading or exercise or other activities that people seem to enjoy." Although lots of his acquaintances in his line of work enjoyed golfing, he thought "golfing is stupid. Using sticks to hit little balls into holes . . . I don't get it." He didn't see that the companionship might be a big draw for some people aside from the nature of the activity itself. He clearly understood the drawbacks to getting arrested. That was an easy evaluation for him to make. He also felt bad when he had to leave a job that he liked because his sales tactics raised one too many eyebrows. As for his relationships with women, he seemed to be unaware that they might be interested in anything other than just being with him. When George asked him what he "brought to the table" for the woman who had his interest, he seemed to be stumped by the question, suggesting (as though it were obvious) "well, me of course." When asked, "What is it about you that makes a relationship such a good deal for the woman?" he became angry and sullen, and wanted to end the session early.

The first goal was to help Tim avoid or cope with the triggers associated with his "occasional" drug use (table 10.1). Since he was not willing to own up to much, they decided to discuss his drug use as a "hypothetical" based on his past experiences. Triggers included "when I'm bored, angry, frustrated, and lonely." Further exploration focused on these thoughts, feelings, behaviors, and situations, and they both came up with a useful list of realistic alternatives to drug use, ways he could assuage his negative feelings and avoid using substances. (He had not agreed to abstinence with alcohol, because since it is legal, but George helped him identify alcohol use as a trigger for drug use.) Cognitive exercises focused on his real fear of being arrested and going to prison (he had never been incarcerated except for a few hours once), and, conversely, he cognitively reviewed all the legal things he enjoyed about his freedom.

To cope with physiological tension, George showed Tim some basic relaxation exercises, and discovered that he had always had trouble sitting still "ever since I was a kid." Anger-control exercises were also planned and carried out using a combination of imagery to recreate specific circumstances that elicited his anger, role-playing, rehearsal, and practice for situations that arose at work or in the community. He had underperformed in school all his life, and never graduated high school or received an equivalency (although he had fake high school and college diplomas available and regularly lied on his résumé. They discussed the possibility of his getting a graduate equivalency degree from high school and, taking a business class in the local community college, but the suggestions just seemed to anger him.

George also helped Tim develop a behavioral map to identify those times and circumstances when he was most likely to feel the desire to drink heavily or use drugs, and reviewed the list of alternatives. To implement contingency management in the program, they also decided to meet bimonthly with the probation officer to reinforce the team approach, but George agreed to discuss only those matters directly salient to the charges, and not reveal anything that was unnecessary, although absolute confidentiality on these matters could not be guaranteed. Over time, Tim began to show more interest in examining his transitory relationships and the lack of intimacy he felt with others, but it was difficult for George to judge his level of sincerity on these matters. Nevertheless, Tim continued to show genuine interest in "staying out of trouble," the primary goal of the intervention.

Selecting Scales and Creating Indexes to Monitor and Evaluate Client Progress

George used the PCL-r primarily to screen Tim for his level of "psychopathy," although he was not expecting to detect substantive changes in scores at outcome (table 10.1). He also decided to use the ASI, although the extent to which he thought Tim would be honest about his use was questionable. Nevertheless, it served as a useful assessment and clinical tool over the course of the intervention. George and Tim also developed a series of one-item (0–10) self-anchored indexes to track his main objectives and goals. These included an "urge" scale to monitor thoughts, feelings, and situations where he felt particularly at risk to "hypothetically" drink or use drugs, or to lose his temper at work or other social circumstances, and he would use these situations to work on the communication skills that he practiced in sessions with George.

ASSESSMENT OF BORDERLINE PERSONALITY DISORDER

Background Data

People diagnosed with BPD demonstrate a selection of characteristic behaviors that may include some combination of: severe mood swings, short-lived psychotic episodes, unpredictable and often impulsive behaviors frequently associated with highly conflicted relationships, suicidal or pseudosuicidal gestures, and other risky or dangerous behaviors. The mood, ideals, and aspirations of people characterized as having BPD are often ephemeral as they fly from one commitment or set of plans to another, depending on how they are feeling at any given moment, particularly in regard to their own self-worth, self-confidence,

TABLE 10.1   The client service plan for Tim

Problems	Goals	Sample Objectives	Interventions	Assessment Tools
Illegal activities, specifically drug use	Reduce substance use and eventually abstain	Monitoring triggers (cognitive, emotions, behaviors, situations) that increase likelihood of drug use	Cognitive-behavioral skills employed with contingency management; service implementation conducted through a case management framework to integrate mental health, substance-abuse intervention with probationary requirements	PCL-r Possibly the ASI and other drug-use indexes or index of "urge to use" to assess/evaluate ability to resist the desire to use
Angry outbursts, desire to strike out, hurt others when he feels provoked	Reduce intensity of anger and increase time between provocation and his response; improve his ability to respond verbally rather than physically	Practice identifying provocation and practice nonaggressive responses twice weekly, and come to visits prepared to discuss examples	Cognitive appraisal of risks of use (imprisonment)	
Exploitive relationships; difficulty connecting with others on a genuine level; difficulty experiencing empathy	Define potential relationship problems, explore them, provide education regarding how these may be problematic; have client at least consider further discussion	No specific relationship objectives because client does not genuinely acknowledge a problem at this time	Relaxation exercises to reduce physiological tension	
			Contingency management plan: meeting with social worker and probation officer to discuss progress and reinforce consequences if drug use resumes	
			Cognitive appraisal of provoking situations, role-play and rehearsal during sessions, and homework practice	

and self-image. These alterations are often accompanied by wide swings of mood (e.g., crying, screaming, raging outbursts, threats of harm to self or others), often followed by a brief return to tranquility or euphoria. People with BPD often describe themselves as feeling empty, bored, or confused about who they are, and are often characterized as having an unstable self-image (identity diffusion). People diagnosed with BPD are often described as intolerant of being alone, although their relationships are often fraught with upset, drama, conflict, and sometimes violence. Moods and perceptions regarding those with whom they become involved tend to oscillate between two extremes of "all bad" or "all good." These emotional extremes often accompany the heightened drama of their tumultuous relationships. People categorized as "borderline" appear to be particularly sensitive to any apparent change in a relationship that may trigger fears of "abandonment" even when the separation is temporary. Their relationships tend to be marked by initial euphoric attachment and overidealization of the other person, but disappointment and conflict seem inevitable and often arrive swiftly as the client with BPD insists that their love "object" is less than they thought and cannot supply them with adequate attention. Perhaps the most troublesome behavior for clinicians is the tendency for the person with BPD to threaten suicide and engage in sometimes frequent self-mutilation and other self-destructive acts. Their acts of self-mutilation do not usually indicate an actual suicide attempt, although they are often seriously depressed, which puts them at increased risk for an actual suicide. People diagnosed with BPD may engage in activities that indirectly put themselves or others at risk of harm, such as promiscuous and unprotected sex, reckless driving, spending money impulsively, abusing drugs and alcohol, or engaging in outright aggressive acts (*DSM-IV-TR*; Linehan, Kanter, & Comtois, 1999; Linehan, 1993a). Needless to say, the distorted cognitions, erratic emotions, and impulsive and at times dangerous behaviors of the client with BPD are challenging treatment-management issues for even experienced practitioners.

Estimates of BPD range from 1% to 2%, in the United States, and women are more likely to get this diagnosis. As many as 10% of clients in outpatient mental health facilities and 20% of inpatients reportedly fit the diagnostic criteria for BPD. From one-third to more than one-half of clients diagnosed with any personality disorder are also likely to fit the criteria for BPD. The symptoms of BPD are more prevalent in adolescents and young adults, and tend to attenuate over time. Many clients diagnosed with BPD no longer meet the criteria for BPD as they move into their thirties and forties. BPD is likely to co-occur with a wide range of other diagnoses, including mood disorders and substance abuse, and clients may demonstrate symptoms of other personality disorders such as histrionic disorder, narcissistic disorder, and APD (H. I. Kaplan & Saddock, 1998; *DSM-IV-TR*).

Evidence suggests that people with BPD are likely to experience violence and sexual abuse both as children and as adults. In one recent study (Zanarini et al., 1999), 290 hospitalized patients with BPD (average age twenty-seven, 85% white) were compared with 72 controls who were diagnosed with another Axis II disorder. Both diagnostic groups were similar in age, marital status, and race. More of those in the BPD category were female. Results showed that violence was a fairly common experience among BPD patients, 33% experienced physical abuse at the hands of their partner, 31% had been raped as an adult, 21% reported they had been raped by a known perpetrator, and 11% reported multiple episodes of rape. About 50% of the female patients with BPD reported an adult history of physical assault and/or rape. Male patients with BPD were about half as likely as females (25%) to have been physically assaulted and/or raped. Violence against these BPD patients was significantly more common than among controls. These patients were also more likely than other Axis II clients to have had a substance-abuse problem prior to age eighteen and to have experienced abuse and neglect as a child, including physical neglect, any form of sexual abuse, sexual abuse by a noncaretaker, emotional withdrawal by a caretaker, and failure by the caretaker to provide physical protection.

Although correlations between BPD and substance abuse have been shown to be significant, the cause-effect linkages are complex and are potentially mediated by a number of important factors. After an extensive ten-year review of the research, Trull, Sher, Minks-Brown, Durbin, and Burr (2000) considered a number of possible explanations for the correlation between BPD and substance abuse. First, the overlap between BPD symptoms and substance abuse may be an artifact in that both problem areas are marked by impulsive behavior; second, they may both share a common (but noncausal) factor such as age of onset for the disorder (late teens, early twenties); third, both disorders may share a common risk factor such as childhood trauma; and, fourth, causes and/or exacerbates the other. Although these are reasonable hypotheses for further testing, the authors conclude, "It is not possible at this point in time to declare simply that BPD causes or leads to SUD or vice versa" (p. 244).

Although practitioners have observed that impulsivity is a common behavior among people diagnosed with BPD, Hochhausen, Lorenz, and Newman (2002) noted that little laboratory research has provided support for this contention. They used computer-based tests of impulse control to compare Caucasian and African-American female inmates who met criteria for BPD with a similar group of inmates who did not meet the criteria, and found that both African-American and Caucasian inmates with BPD showed significantly greater impulsivity than those without the diagnosis. Underscoring the heterogeneity of a diagnosis with BPD, they also found that BPD was correlated with APD, psychopathy as measured by the PCL-r, and established measures of depression and anxiety.

Theories

Perhaps because there were no competing alternatives, psychoanalytic conceptions of BPD and its treatment dominated the mental health field until recently. Current psychodynamic conceptualizations are derived from a combination of classical psychoanalytic theory (S. Freud, 1966, 1923, 1938; A. Freud, 1946; Strean, 1986) and its derivatives, including developmental ego psychology, attachment theory, and Kohut's self-psychology (e.g., Mahler, 1968; Bowlby, 1980; Baker & Baker, 1987). Classic psychoanalytic theories involve a number of interacting systems, including the "structural view" (id, ego, and superego), the dynamic point of view (regulation of sexual and aggressive drives), the topographic perspective (unconscious, preconscious, and conscious mind), the functions of the ego and defense mechanisms (e.g., repression, projection, denial, rationalization, intellectualization), and the genetic or developmental perspective (oral, anal, phallic— including the oedipal phase—and latency) continuing to puberty and adolescence, where psychosocial elements from earlier phases might be recapitulated.

Developmental ego psychology, based on S. Freud's later emphasis on the ego (see also A. Freud, 1946), was developed further by Mahler, Bowlby, and others into a more explicitly interpersonal developmental model. Healthful relationships were purported to have derived from the successful negotiation of psychosocial phases. Conversely, psychopathology resulted from serious failures to negotiate these important psychosocial developmental thresholds. The individual's internal mental representations of these relationships (i.e., object relations) developed sequentially as follows: the autistic phase, where basic physiological needs are met; the symbiotic phase, a blending of self with mother who satisfies or frustrates needs; and the subphases of the separation-individuation stage, where the toddler gradually moves toward a degree of separate identity while maintaining a constant internalized and integrated image of the maternal object. In a healthful situation, the toddler resolves the "splitting defense," and the internalized representation is integrated; in other words, it does not vacillate between extremes of "all good" and "all bad." Serious developmental failures in these stages may result in the vacillating moods, tumultuous relationships, and impulsive behaviors of a future "borderline" client.

The concept of the borderline personality was coined by A. Stern (1938) for patients who appeared to be on the borderline between psychosis and neurosis. This geographical metaphor reflects a theoretical developmental continuum of psychopathology (i.e., psychotic to borderline to neurotic) that mirrors the stages of developmental ego psychology: respectively, autism, symbiosis, separation-individuation. Failure in one stage theoretically will result in a corresponding degree of psychopathology. Clients with serious pathology, but less severe than psychosis, may be characterized as demonstrating "primitive" defensive functioning (denial, projection, splitting, failures in normal repression), which reflects disruption in ego development during the separation-individuation phase (Gunderson, 1984; Masterson, 1981; Kernberg, 1975). As Kernberg (1976) concisely puts it, "These patients' capacity for encompassing contradictory (good and bad) self- and object-images is impaired" (p. 146).

> Individualization includes the gradual replacement of primitive introjections and identifications with partial, sublimatory identifications fitting into the overall concept of the self. Emotional maturity is reflected in the capacity for discriminating subtle aspects of one's own self and of other people and in an increasing selectivity in accepting and internalizing the qualities of other people. Mature friendships are based on such selectivity and the capacity to combine love with independence and emotional objectivity. (p. 74)

Although Kernberg's concepts of the borderline-personality organization diverge somewhat from the more descriptive criteria for BPD in the *DSM*, the differences are more theoretical than practical for the average practitioner. The narcissistic personality suffers from some of the same presumed ego deficits, but is better organized, and more stable behaviorally and emotionally. This client is also markedly more grandiose, arrogant, and defensively difficult to influence or confront. Interpretation is employed to help clarify, explain, or gently confront clients on distortions related to communications in therapy or problems external to therapy (Kernberg, 1975; Baker & Baker, 1987).

These theoretical assertions, based primarily on correlational studies and uncontrolled case analyses, lead to the following treatment recommendations in psychoanalytic/psychodynamic practice: (1) identification and interpretation of emerging primitive part-objects within the context of the transference (unconscious projections on therapists that they are mean, hurtful, untrustworthy, etc); (2) helping clients understand how these self and object representations can oscillate or reverse (e.g., the client may start to act mean and see the therapist as a vulnerable, frightened victim); and (3) helping clients understand that both their positive and negative conceptualizations of the relationship with the therapist need to be reconciled into one whole and more complex relationship. "The successful integration of mutually dissociated or split-off, all-good and all-bad primitive object relations in the transference includes the integration not only of the corresponding self and object representations, but also of primitive affects, leading to affect modulation, to an increase in the capacity for affect control, to a heightened capacity for empathy with both self and others, and a corresponding deepening and maturing of all object relations" (Kernberg, 1999, p. 169). Stated concisely, the goal of treatment of the person with BPD is to resolve identity diffusion and primitive defensive operations, and help the client move toward a more integrated view of internalized self object (pp. 168–169).

Psychodynamic psychotherapy with borderline clients has been modified somewhat from long-term interpretive analytic work into a briefer, more supportive approach that emphasizes current functioning and gentle confrontation. Interpretations of unconscious material, typically employed with healthier "neurotic" clients in psychoanalytic treatment, is saved for a later stage of treatment when the client is more stable and is on the way to better integration of "good-bad" self and other object representation. Premature interpretations of unconscious conflict with its genesis in early childhood could confuse the patient's already unsteady grip on reality and possibly provoke "transference psychosis" (Kernberg, 1976). Interpretations are present-focused to help the client cope with more immediate problems. Limit-setting regarding session rules and reality clarification is dealt with more directly. Priorities in treatment include behaviors that are dangerous to self or others, behaviors that are potentially disruptive to the continuity of treatment, and communications that indicate a lack of honesty in treatment.

There have been efforts in recent years to empirically validate psychodynamic explanations of BPD. M. I. Stern, Herron, Primavera, and Kakuma (1997) conducted a correlational study comparing fifty-five hospitalized people with BPD and twenty-two with major depression. Using a series of measures including psychiatric functioning scales and scales designed specifically to measure perceptions of self and others, they found some expected differences. Patients with BPD were more hostile, emotionally labile, and unstable than people with major depression. However, a good proportion of the findings were mixed or did not support study hypotheses. For example, there were no differences in perceptions of control or nurturance from early caregivers, and other differences washed out when age and gender were controlled for.

De Bonis, De Boeck, Lida-Pulik, Hourtane, and Feline (1998) used a qualitative/quantitative grid method to capture clients' unique positive and negative affect valences for self and others (a key object-relations construct), and compared small samples of depressed patients with BPD, depressed patients without BPD, and people with no known psychiatric diagnosis. Results showed that self-descriptions of both depressed groups were more negative than the psychiatric controls. In addition, depressed patients with BPD had greater affect-valence discrepancy for others, but the depressed-only group showed no differences on negative view of the self. As with the prior study, these data provided mixed support for the object-relations theory.

Fonagy et al. (1996) compared eighty-two psychiatric inpatients with matched outpatient controls on psychiatric measures, attachment style, and capacity for self-reflection (ability to reflect on their own and another's mental state, a theoretically important factor in object-relations theory). As one would expect, inpatients showed significantly greater psychiatric problems and unresolved attachments than outpatients. With regard to patients with BPD, they were found to be more likely to have experienced childhood abuse, unresolved trauma or loss, were less likely to have experienced their parents as loving but neglectful; and were less able to reflect on their own or another's state of mind. This impaired ability to conceptualize the mind of the abusive caregiver may be related to unresolved attachment conflicts and a factor in the development of borderline pathology (Fonagy, Target, & Gergely, 2000).

S. J. Goldman, D'Angelo, and DeMaso (1993) compared forty-four children (about ten years of age) with BPD and one hundred without BPD and found greater rates of pathology in the parents in the families of the BPD group. Types of pathology in descending order of frequency included substance-abuse problems, depression, and antisocial personality. There was no evidence that the interviewers were blind to the diagnostic status of a child during the interview. The authors suggested that interacting environmental and biological risk factors of one or two parents with significant psychopathology may contribute to the development of BPD, although they suggested that causality cannot be inferred from this study.

Given that longitudinal designs would strengthen the cause-effect argument for the genesis of BPD resulting from poor parenting, Bezirganian, Cohen, and Brook (1993) examined data collected over three years in an attempt to causally connect maternal inconsistency and high maternal overinvolvement with the development of BPD in a random sample of 776 adolescents. Given that *DSM* criteria for BPD were not available at the time of the baseline interviews, diagnoses were made after the fact based on other personality-disorder related items. Logistic regression was employed to examine whether theoretically relevant factors predicted BPD status. Results showed that an interaction of maternal over-involvement and maternal inconsistency predicted BPD diagnostic status better than chance alone. However, most of the measures employed in the study, including those that measured maternal overinvolvement and maternal inconsistency, were below acceptable standards for internal consistency, and there was no indication how much of the variance of BPD was explained by maternal overinvolvement or inconsistency.

Although the investigators who made these long-overdue attempts to test the validity of psychodynamic theories of BPD should be applauded for their efforts, the studies suffer from fatal methodological flaws. Some are based primarily on clinical populations, and thus vulnerable to Berkson's bias (clinical populations tend to have more correlating problems). Some are correlational in nature, in which case they merely suggest that certain current self-reported thoughts, feelings, or behaviors are associated with other presumably pathogenic processes or events. Some are based on retrospective data and thus subject to the distortions of recall memory. Some have serious limitations in the measures employed. To date, the only substantive claim to be made is that chronic problems during childhood and adolescence act as risk factors for increased psychological and interpersonal problems in adolescence and adulthood. The theoretical processes that may account for *how* these past events cause BPD are not adequately addressed by these studies. Developmental cause-effect processes remain wide open to interpretation. Based on longitudinal data predictive of other disorders, it appears likely that a combination of factors including biological temperament, substantive child abuse/neglect, and a host of environmental stressors are needed to account for increased risk for serious psychopathology.

Many people subjected to abuse and other forms of trauma do not develop BPD, and many people who manifest borderline symptoms have never been abused (Paris, 1997b; Sabo, 1997). Indeed, there is little evidence that early childhood abuse as an individual factor is more important than other environmental assaults that occur later in life (see Rutter & Rutter, 1993). Evidence suggests that practitioners employ evidence-based multidimensional theories to support their assessment protocol. Childhood trauma, although not to be overlooked as a risk factor, is often not a sufficient explanation for adult psychopathology (Trull et al., 2000; Paris, 1997b; Sabo, 1997).

Cognitive-analytical theory (CAT; Ryle, 1997) emphasizes influences from both cognitive/phenomenological psychology and psychoanalytic theory. This model conceptualizes BPD as a dysfunction marked by alternating multiple self-states. Self-states are cognitive-affective-behavioral psychic structures that represent internalized models of interpersonal functioning (i.e., repertoire of reciprocal roles) that develop over time. In a reasonably well-functioning person, these roles are adequate for giving and receiving what is necessary for healthy interpersonal relations. People with BPD seem to be "prone to abrupt and discomforting shifts between markedly contrasting states . . . accompanied by depersonalization-derealization experiences . . . understood in the proposed model to be the effect of switches between partially dissociated self states" (Ryle, 1997, p. 83). Commonly encountered self-states reflect some of the key symptoms of BPD in character: idealization, emotional blankness, loss of control, rage. Ryle differentiates his model from psychoanalytic theory by emphasizing dissociation of these self-states rather than emphasizing the failure of repression and the reliance on splitting and projection as main defenses. The application of this theory to treatment emphasizes assisting the client in recognizing, understanding, modifying, and integrating these self-states with commensurate improvement in cognitive and interpersonal functioning. Although the research is in its early stages, Ryle recommends the use of controlled trials to compare the efficacy of treatment with other extant models. Uncontrolled evaluation suggests that about half the clients studied benefited from CAT, but those with more severe symptoms tended to respond poorly to the intervention (Ryle & Golynkina, 2000).

The theoretical foundation for dialectical behavior therapy (DBT; Linehan et al., 1999; Linehan, 1993a) is built on a range of theories and conceptual frameworks. It is suggested that BPD is partly caused by a deficiency in the ability to regulate emotions, a deficiency that has its roots in genetic predisposition, prenatal trauma, or other early trauma. This temperamental vulnerability may include a high sensitivity to emotional stimuli, a tendency toward intense emotional reactions, difficulty in calming down, and poor modulation of emotional responses. This dysregulation in a child may be exacerbated by what Linehan calls an "invalidating" environment, that is, circumstances in which emotional dysregulation and poor coping skills are reinforced through confusing and disconfirmatory communications in the home or by punishment of otherwise normal emotional expression. As a result, children may begin to consistently doubt the veracity or genuineness of what they think and feel. In such an environment, painful emotions may be ignored or disregarded, and emotional expression discouraged in general. People in the environment may simply refuse to accept the accuracy of the child's labeling of her own emotions, or they may be generally unresponsive to children's emotional needs. Theoretically, the consequences of such interactions may impair children's ability to accurately identify and regulate their own feelings, a problem that may negatively affect identity development and future ability to cope with emotional distress, regulate behavior, and maintain stable interpersonal relations. As with similar theories that place the causes of psychopathology in family relations (e.g., dysfunctional family communications, the schizophrenogenic mother), more developmental research is needed to account for these specific processes.

Key Elements of Multidimensional/ Functional Assessment

BPD (*DSM-IV-TR*) is marked by a pervasive pattern of instability of interpersonal relationships, self-image, and affects, and marked impulsivity beginning by early adulthood and present in a variety of contexts, as indicated by five or more of the following: (1) frantic efforts to avoid real or imagined abandonment; (2) a pattern of unstable and intense relationships marked by extremes of idealization and devaluation; (3) unstable self-image or sense of self; (4) impulsivity in areas that may cause harm to the client (e.g., substance abuse, risky sexual behavior); (5) recurrent suicidal gestures, threats, or self-mutilating behavior (e.g., scratching one's arm with a broken piece of glass to the extent that significant bleeding occurs); (6) affective instability or mood lasting a few hours or days; (7) chronic feelings of emptiness; (8) problems controlling anger; (9) transient paranoid or dissociative symptoms.

In a thorough review of the literature regarding the reliability and validity of the *DSM-IV* criteria for BPD, Gunderson, Zanarini, and Kisiel (1995) concluded that BPD was rarely diagnosed alone, that there is considerable overlap with other personality disorders (e.g., histrionic, avoidant), and that many criteria are based on theoretical inferences versus observable behaviors. Although some scientific work has been done on the reliability and validity of the disorder, these empirical developments have not "altogether mirrored the disorder's clinical base" (Gunderson et al., p. 154), an assertion that may be interpreted to mean that the diagnostic criteria as conceptualized by psychodynamic clinicians are not congruent with *DSM* criteria. (However, the construct validity of the psychodynamic "clinical" conceptualization has never been validated either.) BPD also overlaps with Axis I diagnoses such as mood disorders and PTSD, and although there is adequate reliability in identifying many of these signs and symptoms, there is a lack of construct and predictive validity (Dahl, 1995).

Initially, a thorough examination of the client's presenting problems is in order, to determine if they are commensurate with the *DSM-IV* diagnosis for BPD, particularly with regard to impulsive behaviors, highly conflicted relationships, self-harm and suicide risks, and emotional dysregulation. Fears regarding "abandonment" or problems with a stable self-image are more subject to inference and hence less reliable. It is important to carefully examine the historical consistency and duration of these behaviors as well as to examine factors in the current environment that may partly account for the client's emotional and behavioral instability. Ongoing threats by an abusive partner, a history of domestic violence, sexual assault, and involvement in criminal activity, among other situational factors, may account for "borderline" symptoms and behaviors. Practitioners should also carefully consider co-occurring disorders such as substance abuse, depression, major mental illness, anxiety disorders, and eating disorders. These problems may be primary problems, not merely other manifestations of borderline personality. Given the variety of symptoms associated with a diagnosis of BPD, thorough history taking carefully considers cause-effect linkages between significant past events (e.g., traumatic events including sudden losses, physical or sexual abuse, victimization as result of a crime) and current co-occurring problems. A family history should note the presence of parental mental illnesses, substance abuse, domestic violence, criminal behavior, and other significant pathology and disruption in the client's childhood and adolescence. The fact that BPD symptoms overlap with a range of other disorders should make practitioners conservative about applying this label before other explanations are ruled out.

A careful functional analysis of clients' daily encounters with stressful situations and their pattern of coping emotionally and behaviorally is essential. Circumstances that clearly appear to precipitate clients' more egregious and potentially harmful behaviors should be highlighted (e.g., the client burning her forearm with a cigarette after a domestic dispute). One might also expect periods of inactivity and low energy due to depression associated with disappointments or precipitated by what would otherwise be seen as normative stressors (e.g., an argument with someone at work). Given the likelihood of distortion, lying, or malingering, one should also make the attempt to engage significant others in the assessment, and possibly include them in the intervention at some point. Obtaining collateral assessment data can go a long way to clarifying incongruities in the client's self-report and gets the perspective of others who see the client across a wider array of circumstances. The client's presentation in the consulting room or hospital can be quite different than at home or at work. A thorough MDF assessment that collates multiple points of view can provide a solid base for intervention planning.

Instruments

A number of scales have been developed to identify BPD. The revised Personality Diagnostic Questionnaire (PDQ-R; Hyler, Skodol, Kellman, Oldham, & Rosnick, 1990; Patrick, Links, Reekum, & Mitton, 1995) is a 152-item self-administered, true-false instrument that includes subscales for eleven personality disorders, including BPD. It takes twenty minutes to complete. Patrick et al. examined three cutoff scores with inpatient and outpatient populations to determine the ideal cutoff scores for the BPD subscale that would provide the best sensitivity and specificity for psychiatrist-determined diagnosis of BPD. Overall, sensitivity and specificity ratings were inadequate and relatively inconsistent across three clinical samples. The PDQ-R was shown to have fairly high false positive ratings with an inpatient sample (n = 87; Hyder et al.).

The Borderline Syndrome Index (H. R. Conte, Plutchik, Karasu, & Jerrett, 1980) comprises fifty-two dichotomous items for detecting the presence of BPD. Until recently, little psychometric evaluation was conducted on this instrument. Marlowe, O'Neill-Byrne, Lowe-Ponsford, and Watson (1996) found modest correlations between the Borderline Syndrome Index, the BDI, and a general index of psychopathology. However, the instrument performed poorly overall as a screening device for detecting BPD.

One BPD screening instrument has been developed on a theoretical base that reflects Kernberg's theories (1975) on borderline-personality organization. The Borderline Personality Inventory (BPI) is a short (fifty-three-item, yes-no) self-report instrument (Leichsenring, 1999). A four-part study was devised to test the factor structure, reliability, discriminant validity, and sensitivity and specificity cutoff scores. An initial 100-item version of the scale was administered to a small sample of clients diagnosed with BPD to establish interrater reliability (.90). In addition, fifty-three items correlated significantly with diagnostic criteria for BPD, and the twenty items with the highest correlations were scaled to determine a diagnosis of BPD. Based on additional samples of clients with and without BPD ($n = 484$), factor analysis was conducted, and four subscales were identified: identity diffusion, primitive defense mechanisms, impaired reality testing, and fear of fusion. On the twenty-item subscale, the BPI demonstrated very good sensitivity (85–89%) for accurately identifying people diagnosed with BPD, and very good specificity (82–90%) for identifying those who did not meet BPD criteria ("neurotic" or diagnosed with schizophrenia). Internal-consistency reliability for the four subscales ranged from acceptable to good, and test-retest reliabilities were good overall. Intercorrelations among the four subscales were moderate, as would be expected, and the subscales were invariant across sex and age. Thus, overall psychometric characteristics suggest the BPI could be used as a self-administered screening tool for BPD in mental health treatment environments.

The Borderline Personality Disorder Severity Index (BPDSI; Arntz et al., 2003; see 10.1), a semistructured instrument that mirrors *DSM-IV* criteria for BPD, was developed and refined in a two-part study with a relatively small but mixed population from a mental health clinic. The original interview format (Weaver & Clum, 1993; instrument 10.1) showed very good psychometric characteristics overall. The BPDSI is currently undergoing further psychometric evaluation, and factor structure, reliability, and validity appear strong. In addition, a score of 19 or more appears at this time to be an indication of borderline psychopathology (J. Giesen-Bloo, personal communication, March, 2005).

INSTRUMENT 10.1   Borderline Personality Disorder Severity Index (BPDSI)

This interview is about a number of things people can experience. You decide whether you feel you have experienced the particular item within the last three months and how often it has happened. All questions are asked in the same way, but if you don't understand them completely you can easily ask for some explanation. Do you have any questions about this so far?

Because we will only talk about the past three months, it's important to determine which period that was. Today is (date), three months ago it was (date). That was around (important event/day in general and/or specific for the patient).

<u>Notes preceding each question are meant for the interviewer and are not meant to be read out loud to the patient.</u>

The following scale is used to provide a frequency score for all items except "Identity," which has an alternate scale. Record the scores for each item on the SCORING FORM (see appendix F).

0 Never
1 1x in 3 months
2 2x in 3 months
3 3x in 3 months/1x a month
4 4 to 5x in 3 months/1x in 3 weeks
5 6 to 7x in 3 months/1x in 2 weeks

6 8 to 10x in 3 months/2x in 3 weeks
7 1x week/11 to 15x in 3 months
8 several times a week but less than half of the week
9 More than half of the week/almost daily
10 Daily

1. Abandonment: These items refer to frantic efforts attempted by the interviewee with the goal to prevent someone with whom interviewee has a relationship, is bonded with or is dependent on from abandoning him/her. Examples are, among other things, begging someone not to leave or physically trying to prevent someone from leaving.

1.1 Did you, in the last three months, ever become desperate when you thought that someone you care about was going to abandon you?
(when scoring positive, clear examples are required)

1.2 Did you, in the last three months, try to keep someone who's important to you and who wanted to avoid you (or whom you thought wanted to avoid you) with you in a fanatical way?
(e.g. continuous ringing up, checking, seducing . . . only exaggerated, forced, frenetic ways are scored)
(This item is about real and imagined abandonment; when scoring positive, clear examples of attempts are required) (Also scoring of examples/incidents that return at items 1.3, 1.4 and 1.5)

1.3 Did you, in the last three months, ever beg or cry for someone not to leave you?

1.4 Did you, in the last three months, ever threaten to do something to make sure that someone wouldn't leave you? (e.g. blackmail, lies, murder, suicide)

1.5 Did you, in the last three months, ever try to keep someone from leaving you in a physical way? (e.g. by standing in front of a door, holding on to someone)

1.6 How often did you, in the last three months, have a strong desire to hear someone tell you he/she loves you, cares about you, is not abandoning you, finds you attractive, et cetera.
(this can happen with partners, family and friends)

1.7 How often did you, in the last three months, ask other people for affirmation, whereas the aim of the affirmation was reassurance that someone will not abandon you?

2. Interpersonal relationships: There are three characteristics for this criterion. First of all, there must be a pattern of instable relationships, which can be characterized by regular conflicts and imminent or actual break-up. Secondly, these relationships must be intense, meaning that strong emotions are involved (e.g. euphoria, aversion, anger, resentment, despair). Thirdly, the interviewee must at some moments devaluate the other person (e.g., "he's really very mean"). At other moments the interviewee could idealize the other person (e.g. "my boyfriend is the most wonderful, attentive and strongest person I ever met"). These persons use, in psychoanalytic terms, splitting as a defense mechanism.

Partner relationship

2.1 Were there moments, in the last three months, when you thought that your partner was everything you wanted and other moments at which you thought he/she was awful?
(the conviction is essential i.e. intra-psychological, so it's not necessarily about the actual relationship)

2.2 How often, in the last three months, did you have ups and downs in your partner relationship?
(the focus is on the actual relationship)

2.3 How often, in the last three months, did you break up your partner relationship and/or got together again?
(score both "on" and "off," so two times of breaking up and getting together again gives a score of 4 not 2)

2.4 How often, in the last three months, did you start one or more new partner relationship(s) and/or did you end these?
(score both "on" and "off" separately)

Other relationships

2.5 Were there moments, in the last three months, when you thought that your friends/family members/colleagues and/or other important persons were everything you wanted and other moments at which you thought that he/she was awful?
(the conviction is essential i.e. intra-psychological, so it's not necessarily about the actual relationship)

2.6 How often, in the last three months, did you have ups and downs in your relationships with friends/family members/colleagues and/or other important persons?
(the focus is on the actual relationships)

2.7 How often, in the last three months, did you break up your relationships with friends/family members/colleagues and/or other important persons and/or got together again?
(score both breaking up and getting together)

2.8 How often, in the last three months, did you start one or more new relationships with friends/family members/colleagues and/or important persons and/or did you end relationships?
(score both breaking up and getting together)

3. Identity: Self identity is a stable sense of self which provides unity of personality over time. The type of identity disturbance characteristic for borderline personality disorder exists as extreme shifts in the self-image of the person in question (who am I?). These shifts manifest themselves in sudden changes with respect to jobs, career goals, sexual orientation, personal values, friends and the fundamental feeling one has about oneself (e.g. good or bad). These items must only be scored if the identity disturbance doesn't fit the developmental age of the person in question (i.e. normal adult identity shifts are not taken into account).

3.1 Were you, in the last three months, in diverse situations or with various people so different that you didn't always behave as the same person and that you didn't know anymore who you truly were?
0 Absent
1 Questionable/some support
2 Probable not knowing who he/she is, but not very clearly defined
3 (Quite) clear not knowing who he/she is, but not very dominant
4 Dominant, clear and well-defined not knowing who he/she is

3.2 Did it happen, in the last three months, that the idea of who you are changed strongly?

0 Absent

1 Questionable/some support

2 Probable instability of self-image

3 (Quite) clear instability of self-image

4 Clear and dominant instability of self-image

3.3 Did it happen, in the last three months, that the feeling of your being a good or bad person changed strongly?

0 Absent

1 Questionable/some support

2 Probable instability of sense of self

3 (Quite) clear instability of sense of self

4 Clear and dominant instability of sense of self

3.4 What have been your long-term goals for life in the last three months? For example which education, job and/or career would you want or wish for? Have these goals changed in the last three months?

(clients in treatment often say their only goal is to get better and/or finish treatment well; this is scored as avoidance)

0 Absent

1 Questionable/some support

2 Probable instability of long-term goals/probable avoidance of dealing with long-term goals

3 (Quite) clear instability of long-term goals, but not very dominant/(quite) clear avoidance of dealing with long-term goals, but not very dominant

4 Clear and dominant instability of long-term goals/clear and dominant avoidance of dealing with long term goals

3.5 Have you changed, in the last three months, in your view of what is morally right or wrong? (. . . in your view about your standards and values/what you can and what you can't do/what's good and bad)

(question intensity/direction/frequency of changes)

0 Absent

1 Questionable/some support

2 Probable instability of moral values

3 (Quite) clear instability of moral values, but not very dominant

4 Clear and dominant instability of moral values

3.6 Have you had trouble, in the last three months, to determine what is important in your life? Has this changed in the last three months?

0 Absent

1 Questionable/some support

2 Probable instability of personal values/probable avoidance

3 (Quite) clear instability of personal values, but not very dominant/probable avoidance but not very dominant

4 Clear and dominant instability of moral values/clear and dominant avoidance

3.7 Have you had trouble, in the last three months, to determine what sort of friends you would like to have? Does the sort of friends you have change often?

(some people say they don't have friends; this is scored as avoidance)

0 Absent
1 Questionable/some support
2 Probable instability with regard to friends/probable avoidance with regard to friends
3 (Quite) clear instability with regard to friends, but not very dominant/probable avoidance with regard to friends but not very dominant
4 Clear and dominant instability with regard to friends/clear and dominant avoidance with regard to friends

3.8 Did you, in the last three months, ever doubt if you wanted a sexual relationship with men or women? [After the interviewee's reply:] How often has this changed in the last three months?
(stable heterosexual/bisexual/homosexual orientation is scored 0)
0 Absent
1 Rarely
2 Has probable doubts with regard to sexual orientation
3 Has (quite) clear doubts with regard to sexual orientation
4 Has serious doubts with regard to sexual orientation

4. Impulsivity: Next are a few examples of things people can act on impulsively. Things of which you later thought that you should not have done or things that caused or could have caused problems for you or your environment. (Behavior with the primary goal of eliminating negative feelings and/or inducing positive feelings is essential; <u>not</u> the behavior with the primary goal to damage oneself or others.) The core characteristic of this criterion is the inability of the person to control his/her impulses, through which he/she gets involved in behavior that is satisfactory in the short term but can be damaging in the long term. The behaviors mentioned below are examples; they don't cover the full spectrum of impulsive behaviors.

4.1 How often, in the last three months, did you irresponsibly spend money and/or spend more money than you actually can spend? (e.g. gambling, impulsive buying, making many and long phone calls)

4.2 How often, in the last three months, did you have sex with people you didn't or hardly know?

4.3 How often, in the last three months, did you have unsafe sex? (sex without considering the possible self-damaging consequences and/or pregnancy)

4.4 How often, in the last three months, did you have too much alcohol and/or did you use alcohol at the wrong moments?
(with alcoholic people: note the standard use of alcohol at 4.4.A on the score form, everything on top of that is scored at 4.4)

4.5 How often, in the last three months, did you use too much soft drugs and/or did you use soft drugs at the wrong moments?
(with drug addicts: note the standard use of soft drugs at 4.5.A on the score form, everything on top of that is scored at 4.5)

4.6 How often, in the last three months, did you take pills? (not with the goal of suicide but with the goal to get high)

4.7 How often, in the last three months, did you use hard drugs?
(with drug addicts: note the standard use of hard drugs at 4.7.A on the score form, everything on top of that is scored at 4.7))

4.8 How often, in the last three months, did you have episodes of binge eating?
(all binge eating is scored, with or without loss of control, with or without planning etc.)

4.9 How often, in the last three months, were you reckless in traffic? (e.g. driving too fast or under the influence of alcohol)
(not caused by dissociation)

4.10 How often, in the last three months, have you committed thefts?
(with what intention? It's essential that it's done to get a good feeling or to push aside a bad feeling, it's not about enriching oneself)

4.11 How often, in the last three months, did you do things impulsively that could have gotten you in trouble or actually did get you in trouble? (e.g. cancel appointments, not keeping to agreements, subscribe to a course/education, book a vacation)
(not self-mutilation or suicidal behavior; note answers on score form)

5. Parasuicidal behavior: The next questions inquire if you tried to hurt or wound yourself in the last three months.

Self-mutilation with self-injury as immediate consequence, i.e. tissue damage or physical pain, without any suicidal intention

5.1 How often, in the last three months, did you deliberately hit yourself or did you hit your head, fist, knuckles or other body part into something? Or smash a window with your fist and/or other body part?

5.2 How often, in the last three months, did you scratch or pinch yourself?

5.3 How often, in the last three months, did you bite yourself? (what generally speaking hurts, so not nail biting)

5.4 How often, in the last three months, did you tear your hair? (can also be eyebrows or eyelashes)

5.5 How often, in the last three months, did you cut yourself? (also cutting relatively shallow, more or less resulting in scratches)

5.6 How often, in the last three months, did you burn yourself? (cigarette, clothes iron)

5.7 How often, in the last three months, did you stick needles and such in your body?

5.8 How often, in the last three months, did you harm yourself on purpose?
(e.g. swallow sharp objects, take dangerous substances, enter sharp/dangerous objects into body openings like the vagina, penis, ears etc.; note well on the score form)

Suicide (plans/attempts)

5.9 How often, in the last three months, did you want to kill yourself?

5.10 How often, in the last three months, did you tell other people that you wanted to kill yourself?
(not scored when it's about passive suicidal ideation, e.g. telling others "I wish I was dead")

5.11 How often, in the last three months, did you make plans to kill yourself? (when these plans led to particular steps, score at 5.12)

5.12 How often, in the last three months, did you take steps towards killing yourself? (when these steps led to an attempt, score at 5.13)

5.13 How often, in the last three months, did you attempt to take your own life?

6. Affective instability: Mood changes are striking changes with regard to a dejected/depressed, irritable, anxious, desperate and/or angry mood. Affective instability refers to the alternating, instable quality of mood of the interviewee. Even though the mood alteration is often abrupt, a sudden onset of the change in mood is not required. Instead, this criterion specifies frequent affective shifts that are indeed strong but of relative short endurance (hours rather than days or weeks).

6.1 Are you aware of such mood shifts towards a dejected (depressed) mood? How often, in the last three months, did this happen?
(not due to Axis I diagnoses)

6.2 And how often, in the last three months, towards an irritable and/or edgy mood?
(not because of Axis I)

6.3 And how often, in the last three months, towards an anxious mood?
(not because of Axis I)

6.4 And how often, in the last three months, towards a desperate mood?
(not because of Axis I)

6.5 And how often, in the last three months, towards an angry mood?
(not because of Axis I)

(when in doubt of the influence of Axis I diagnoses, score the items)

7. Emptiness: Chronic feelings of emptiness are often linked with feelings of boredom, loneliness, worthlessness or feelings "you can't define."

7.1 How often, in the last three months, did you feel bored or empty inside?
(This is about feelings of emptiness or boredom resulting in stress or inadequate behavior. Inadequate behavior also includes the negative influence of these feelings on normal or adequate behavior. For example not being able to do anything while it was desired or necessary to do something.)

7.2 How often, in the last three months, didn't you do anything as a consequence of these feelings of emptiness or boredom, while you actually did want to do something?
(e.g. stay in bed instead of doing shopping)

7.3 How often, in the last three months, did you do things as a consequence of these feelings of emptiness or boredom, while you actually did want to do something else?
(e.g. going out instead of working; alcohol and drug abuse can also belong to this criterion)

7.4 How often, in the last three months, did it happen that you couldn't take a moment to rest?
(e.g. cleaning or pacing up and down; this is interpreted as avoidance of rest to keep feelings of emptiness away)

8. Outbursts of anger: The next questions are about outbursts of anger or rage. Inappropriate anger refers to the intensity of anger of the person, which is not in proportion to the cause of the anger. Manifestations of extreme physical (violent) behavior, like hitting people or throwing things, can indicate a lack of anger control with regard to anger/rage. The rage is often expressed in the context of an actual or experienced lack of care/attention, loss or neglect.

8.1 Does it happen that you experience a bad temper and/or have a fit of rage? How often, in the last three months, did this happen?

8.2 How often, in the last three months, did you act cynical and/or sarcastic to other people?
(stinging, sneering, mocking)

8.3 How often, in the last three months, did you swear, scream and/or slam doors? (make noise)

8.4 How often, in the last three months, were you so mad that you weren't approachable anymore, that you couldn't be brought to reason anymore?
(outbursts of anger)

8.5 How often, in the last three months, did you throw things, break things, et cetera?

8.6 How often, in the last three months, did you attack others?
(physically)

9. Dissociation and paranoid ideation: Some people strongly react to stressful events. Some people with borderline personality disorder develop transitory paranoid or dissociative symptoms during periods of stress. These symptoms are rarely of such severity that an additional diagnosis can be made (i.e. psychotic disorders). The stressor often is an actual, supposed or anticipated absence of the care/attention of a caretaker (e.g. partner, parent, or therapist). In such situations can the actual or supposed return of care/attention result in remission of the symptoms? The dissociative symptoms consist of periods of dissociative amnesia (sometimes expressed through the person's feeling of "losing time"), depersonalization (i.e. the feeling of becoming estranged from yourself or moving away from yourself) or derealization (i.e. the feeling that the external world is unreal or unusual). These periods usually last a few minutes or hours.

Dissociation: depersonalization (9.1), derealization (9.2), consciousness (9.3), memory (9.4 and 9.5)

9.1 To what extent, in the last three months, did you feel not like yourself anymore, as if you stood outside yourself, or did you experience yourself as in a movie or dream?
(self is both body and mind) (not because of drugs)

9.2 To what extent, in the last three months, did you perceive the world around you entirely different, or experience it entirely different, so that this appears very strange or unreal to you?
(e.g. other people look unfamiliar or like robots) (not because of drugs)

9.3 To what extent, in the last three months, didn't you know anymore what you were doing or where you were?
(not because of drugs)

9.4 To what extent, in the last three months, did you, all of a sudden, not recognize people and/or objects familiar to you anymore ?
(not because of drugs)

9.5 To what extent, in the last three months, couldn't you quite remember important things anymore?
(not because of drugs; clinical judgment of the importance of something, so not always out of the interviewee's perception)

Paranoid ideation

9.6 To what extent, in the last three months, did you have trouble with being very suspicious or distrusting other people?
(not because of drugs) (the idea is essential)

9.7 To what extent, in the last three months, were you convinced that other people were out to get you, that you were being pursued?
(not because of drugs) (this item is about a temporary delusion)

9.8 To what extent, in the last three months, were you convinced that other people were unfairly treating you?
(not because of drugs) (this item is about a temporary delusion)

SELECTING EFFECTIVE INTERVENTIONS

There is little controlled intervention research with people suffering from personality disorders in general (Turkat, 1992; Crits-Christoph, 1998) including research on interventions for BPD. Based on a limited number of controlled studies, however, cognitive-behavioral methods are now considered a first-line approach. Dialectical behavior therapy (Linehan, 1993a; Linehan et al., 1999) is a cognitive-behavioral intervention intended to help people with BPD learn to self-regulate their dysfunctional thinking, problem behaviors, and emotions more effectively. The term *dialectic* implies that clients struggle to better tolerate extremes of emotion, and to change from rigid dichotomous thinking about themselves and others to seeing themselves and others in a more balanced and less extreme way. For the practitioner's part, the dialectic involves balancing the need to accept some of the clients' distress and troubling behaviors while, helping clients develop the skills to better regulate their emotions and control their problem behaviors.

There is very little evidence to support the effectiveness of psychodynamic therapies with clients diagnosed with BPD. However, some efforts have been made to test this approach. For example, Bateman and Fonagy (1999) compared psychoanalytically oriented partial hospitalization with standard outpatient care for thirty-eight borderline patients (nineteen completed treatment). The psychoanalytically oriented group consisted of combined individual and group therapy, weekly expressive therapy, weekly community meetings, and medication review. Therapy was provided by psychiatric nurses who "had no formal psychotherapy qualifications" (p. 1565). Control patients received outpatient services that included medication review, problem-solving therapy, community follow-up visits, and no formal psychotherapy of any kind. Results were measured over eighteen months, and results showed superior outcomes for the experimental group on several measures, including depression, suicidal acts, self-harm, improved social functioning, and inpatient days. Interpretation of the results, however, is problematic. The experimental group received substantially more treatment overall. Thus, the study appears to be more a comparison of the structure, intensity, and amount of treatment rather than a test of psychoanalytic intervention. Given that the nurses providing the treatment had no formal psychotherapeutic credentials, the study does little more than point out that severely troubled clients may require more structured and intensive services.

Linehan and associates have formulated a successful cognitive-behavioral approach DBT to help BPD clients cope with negative affect while reducing self-destructive and other maladaptive behaviors. Results demonstrated better treatment compliance and fewer days in the hospital than those receiving alternative psychotherapy. Components of the approach were employed in a problem-solving framework and included cognitive modification, behavioral-skills training, contingency management, and exposure to behavioral cues. Given the relative paucity of evidence, a series of related investigations conducted by Linehan and associates will serve as our exemplar study.

Exemplar Study: The First Controlled Trial of Dialectical Behavior Therapy.   A study by Linehan, Armstrong, Suarez, Allmon, and Heard (1991) is one of the few controlled trials conducted with people diagnosed with BPD. Forty-four women (twenty-two in each group) matched on diagnosis, number of parasuicidal behaviors, age, hospitalizations, and prognosis were randomly assigned to either DBT or treatment as usual (TAU) in the community. Individual therapists in this study used behavioral management skills, contingency management, cognitive modification, and exposure to emotional cues. These techniques were balanced with standard supportive therapeutic methods, including empathy, reflection, and acceptance. Group sessions employed psychoeducation that included behavioral-skills training in three areas: interpersonal functioning, distress tolerance, and emotion regulation. Clients attended weekly one-hour individual and two-and-one-half-hour group sessions for a year. Assessment/evaluation measures were taken at baseline, 4, 8, and 12 months. A combination of standardized and unstandardized scales were used in the study to measure frequency of parasuicide episodes, suicide attempts, amount of psychiatric and medical treatment the client received, measures of depression, and hopelessness. There were significant pretreatment differences between the two groups on important clinical indicators. Results showed fewer (median of 1.5 versus 9) and less severe episodes of parasuicidal behavior and fewer days in the hospital compared to TAU clients, but no differences in depression, hopelessness, suicidal ideation, or reasons for living. Attrition rate for the DBT group was less than one-third than for the TAU group (16.7% versus 58.3%). DBT patients also spent less time in psychiatric hospitals (average 8.46 versus 38.86

days) and had fewer admissions. In the last four months of treatment, the TAU group engaged in suicidal behavior almost twice as often as did the DBT group. The authors suggested that the low attrition rate in the DBT group might be attributable to directly addressing therapy-interfering behaviors and development of a solid working relationship as an important component of the intervention.

Subsequent analyses of the same clients also revealed less parasuicidal behavior, less anger, and better adjustment with regard to social functioning, work, and global adjustment for DBT clients (Linehan, Heard, & Armstrong, 1993; Linehan, Tutek, Heard, & Armstrong, 1994). Gains, which were generally maintained over the course of one year's follow-up, did not appear to be an artifact of experimental treatment factors such as lower fee for DBT clients, more therapy or phone contacts, or the novelty of being involved in an experimental treatment. With other psychiatric indicators (e.g., depression, hopelessness, suicidal ideation), there were no significant differences. Limitations of the study include the fact that over one-quarter of the TAU clients never made it into treatment, and DBT therapists had more experience in treating clients diagnosed with BPD. Although generalizations from this one study of twenty-two women with BPD should be made cautiously, the differences with regard to reduction in parasuicidal behaviors were substantial. Other reports have offered positive narrative accounts of implementing DBT (Corwin, 1996; B. C. Miller, 1995), including in partial hospital settings (Simpson et al., 1998) and inpatient programs (C. R. Swenson, Sanderson, Dulit, & Linehan, 2001).

Additional controlled investigations of DBT for BPD are under way. Researchers in one controlled trial in the Netherlands (Verheul et al., 2003) randomly assigned fifty-eight women who met BPD criteria to DBT versus treatment as usual (mental health or substance-abuse treatment). The intervention began four weeks after random assignment, and clients were treated by psychologists and social workers for one year. The DBT group showed superior outcomes overall: almost three times as many patients were retained in the DBT group for the entire year, four times as many clients (eight versus two) attempted suicide in the TAU group (although the difference was not statistically significant), and DBT clients demonstrated significantly less self-mutilating behavior (35% versus 57%) than those in the TAU group.

DBT has provided a promising alternative to previous treatments for BPD. In addition to the lack of replication, however, other substantive questions regarding the change-process theory behind the techniques as well as the relative effectiveness of individual components of the overall approach remain to be addressed. From an evidence-based perspective, it is far from clear that many of the theoretical assumptions are either valid or necessary to account for the effectiveness of DBT. In addition, although one can extrapolate from the efficacy studies of CBT with other serious problems (PTSD, substance abuse, anxiety disorders, depression, antisocial behaviors), it seems quite reasonable that the core components of DBT are likely to hold up well in future research. They include a sound working alliance, core CBT coping skills, facilitating social support, and contingency management strategies. Although the theoretical concepts and practices of DBT may appear daunting, one study demonstrated that a diverse group of clinicians could, with adequate training, grasp the concepts (Hawkins & Sinha, 1998). However, as the authors pointed out, "Conceptual mastery does not guarantee adherence to a model, or even the ability to practice it adequately, and whether the knowledge acquired in this training initiative translates into practice approximate to Dr. Linehan's model remains to be determined" (p. 384).

Descriptions of Effective Intervention Methods

Although Linehan (1993a, 1993b) describes DBT as employing a wide range of standard CBT methods, she stresses that DBT is distinguished from CBT in the following ways: First, it emphasizes acceptance and validation of the client's behavior as it is experienced by the client in the moment. Second it intervenes in client behaviors that interfere with the process of therapy. Third, it emphasizes therapeutic relationship and dialectical processes. Although one could argue whether these factors truly diverge from standard CBT practice, they are given priority in the practice of DBT.

The now classic text and workbook (Linehan, 1993a, 1993b) describe DBT theory and intervention methods in great detail. In a nutshell, DBT, at its core, is an assertive combination of intensive social support for the client in the context of the practitioner-client relationship, a careful functional behavioral analysis, and teaching coping skills to decrease dysfunctional thoughts and behaviors, increase functional behaviors, and improve overall quality of life. Although the treatment may be applied somewhat flexibly, formal DBT employs several modalities, including individual therapy, supportive group, structured skill training, phone consultation, and other ancillary treatments such as hospitalization as needed. An important dimension of DBT is an early emphasis on contracting with the client regarding attendance at sessions, commitment to staying in treatment for a substantial time (e.g., at least one year), agreements to reduce suicidal and parasuicidal acts, and not engaging in behaviors that disrupt or interfere with treatment. The practitioner is also explicit about adhering to other fairly standard guidelines for ethical practice. The tone of DBT, while commensurate with CBT methods in general, is a model for most forms of psychosocial intervention: the client contracts to participate constructively for specific reasons, and the practitioner practices true informed consent by telling the client in clear terms what their work together is about and how it will be carried out.

The core goals of DBT are to help the client reduce dysfunctional thinking, develop a "dialectical" way of thinking (i.e., moderation, balanced, integrating or reconciling apparent contradictions), and reduce harmful behaviors by learning a range of coping skills. In addition to experiencing depression, emotional turmoil, and suicidal feelings, people diagnosed with BPD often struggle with tumultuous and often abusive relationships, other mental health disorders, substance abuse, problems with changing jobs, unstable housing, health problems that go untreated, criminal activity, risky sexual behaviors, and gambling. Cognitive-behavioral methods employed successfully with these other problems are congruent with the methods employed in DBT. The emphasis on reducing dysfunctional thinking is quite similar to the methods employed in standard cognitive therapy. Dysfunctional thinking includes absolutistic or dichotomous thinking, drawing conclusions from too little data, overgeneralizing from one occurrence, catastrophizing problems, etc. (see chapter 9 for a more extensive discussion). Reducing suicidal ideation, parasuicidal acts, and potentially genuine suicidal acts is a priority as well. In addition to cognitive therapy methods, there is a strong emphasis on employing behavioral analysis and standard behavioral problem-solving methods. Linehan (1993a, p. 100) summarizes: "In most cases, the behavioral analysis will show that there are skill deficits, problematic reinforcement contingencies, inhibitions resulting from fear and guilt, and faulty beliefs and assumptions. Thus, a treatment program integrating skill training, contingency management, exposure strategies, and cognitive modification is likely to be required. The behavioral target of each strategy, however, is dependent on the behavioral analysis." Clients also use problem-solving skills to move toward a more moderate approach to life, improving lifestyle functioning and overall psychosocial well-being.

The process of DBT has four stages (Linehan et al., 1999). In stage 1, the practitioner addresses some of the most immediate and troubling behavioral disturbances typically associated with BPD: suicidal threats, treatment compliance, co-occurring problems such as substance abuse or homelessness, problems with interpersonal functioning, emotional dysregulation, and difficulties tolerating stress. In stage 2, although the more dramatic behavioral problems have perhaps been brought under some control in stage 1, the client continues to suffer emotional pain in "quiet desperation," pain that may be related to PTSD. The goal of stage 2 is to help the client reduce emotional distress through the use of exposure methods (similar to those reviewed in chapters 7 and 8). In stages 3 and 4, the focus is on moderating distress or unhappiness, and moving toward more fulfilling engagement in life.

Linehan et al. (1999) discuss several general modes of service delivery. These include motivational enhancement of the client by reinforcing client progress; skill building (i.e., capability enhancement) to help clients learn to cope better with emotional distress through standard behavioral techniques; generalization through homework assignments, in vivo interventions, and phone consultations; increasing environmental supports in a positive therapeutic environment, family sessions if warranted, and positive social supports; and enhancing the practitioner's capabilities and motivation through support, consultation, and supervision.

Specific behavioral coping-skills methods are geared toward the particular problems experienced by clients diagnosed with BPD, and further specified for the individual client. The major behavioral skill categories include core mindfulness, distress tolerance, emotion regulation, interpersonal effectiveness, self-management, and exposure and cognitive modification.

Core mindfulness (influenced by Zen teaching) teaches the client to experience the moment through observation, reflecting on an event less emotionally, and fully participating in events with less self-consciousness. Clients are also taught to be less judgmental about the events, focus their concentration on one thing at a time, and emphasize being effective and achieving goals over getting caught up in emotion-driven contests to prove they're right.

Distress tolerance is taught to clients based on the amount of emotional pain they continue to deal with. Learning how to accept distress as a part of life is an important goal for clients who may typically avoid it through numbing themselves, cutting, themselves, drug abuse, promiscuity, or other unheathful behaviors.

Emotion regulation is taught to help clients to be less controlled by their emotions. This skill includes identification of the feeling, identifies the function of the emotion (often a form of communication), and emphasizes reducing their vulnerability to the "emotion mind" through increased self-efficacy and problem solving (e.g., mastery activities), engaging in activities that increase positive emotional events, acting in ways that are in opposition to the emotion evoked in a situation (e.g., respond in a pleasant way in an uncomfortable social situation), and increasing awareness and acceptance of emotions.

Interpersonal-effectiveness skills emphasize clear and effective expression in routine or novel interpersonal and social situations to cope effectively. Many of the skills are similar to those in standard assertiveness and interpersonal-skill training programs such as expressing thoughts and feelings clearly, being assertive, saying no, and asking for assistance.

Self-management skills include generic behavioral skills for solving problems and successfully getting things done. These skills include setting realistic goals, behavioral self-analysis, analysis and optimizing of the environment, learning self-reward techniques, and dealing realistically with relapses and partial successes.

Exposure and cognitive-modification strategies are likely to be used to help change a client's cognitive and emotional responses to trauma-related stimuli (graduated covert exposure is a core component of dealing with the effects of trauma). CBT methods for PTSD were covered in chapter 8, but the reader should refer to Linehan (1993a) for recommended application of these methods to clients with BPD. Once clients have achieved some level of emotional and behavioral stability, methods that help them recognize the continuing effects of trauma can be employed to deal with them more effectively.

A more detailed accounting of these cognitive-behavioral skills for addressing primary and secondary behavioral targets can be reviewed in Linehan's text and companion workbook (1993a, 1993b).

IMPLEMENTING AND EVALUATING THE EVIDENCE-BASED INTERVENTION PLAN

CASE STUDY: FRANCINE

Francine is a thirty-four-year-old white female who came to see a social worker, Gail, at the local mental health clinic at the urging of her husband. He was becoming increasingly concerned about her strange behavior. Francine and her husband, Geoff, live in a relatively isolated rural area with their twelve-year-old daughter, Tabatha. Francine came to the social worker very depressed, talking of "ending it all," although she had no specific plan. She said she had been depressed all her life, she had not held a job for some time, and she was having a terrible time with Tabatha, who virtually ignored Francine's attempts to set limits or get her to help around the house. She described her relationship with her husband as" "OK, not great," but they had no specific problems, although she'd lost interest in having sex with him over the past couple of years. Geoff was a maintenance person for the local township, worked hard, and was typically dirty and very tired when he came home in the evening. Francine said she did not find him appealing any more. Francine had worked as a receptionist in the past, but quit her job a few months ago, and had not worked since then. She said she could not get along with the peo-

ple at work, that they did not accept her. Upon further inspection, it seemed that in her first week on the job she found out that she had not been invited to a party. When she heard others discussing it around the lunch table, she became upset, and started screaming at them "Don't f—— with me. If you don't like me just say so!" Someone took her aside, apologized about the oversight, and tried to explain that the get-together was for a long-time employee who was leaving, and the party had been planned and people invited long before Francine started working there. No slight was intended. Francine then felt humiliated because of her behavior, left work, and did not return. She said she took off in her car to go home, sped out of the parking lot, and almost had an accident with a passing car. She pulled the car over to the side of the road and started gasping and crying, and was reaching for her tranquilizers when a police cruiser came by. He noticed the pills and the scratches and cuts on her arms, and transported her to the local hospital ER. It was revealed later that she may have experienced a panic attack, described by Francine as "freaking out . . . something that happens now and then."

Multidimension/Functional Assessment: Defining Problems and Goals

Recently, Francine found herself reminiscing about her mother, who died a few years ago. Her dad was still alive. She described him as always having treated her very special, because her mother was sick often (depressed, she thinks, and using lots of medication), and Francine had to "take over the house" now and then. She described her father as being somewhat flirtatious with her when she was a teenager, but does not recall it ever going beyond that. Her parents were never abusive, but she describes herself as often feeling alone. She had few friends because her parents discouraged it, and she characterized her home and family as "too weird to bring home any friends." Francine did attend a community college for a couple of years, during which time she struggled with a moderate drug problem (alcohol, marijuana, and cocaine). She described what sounded like a series of somewhat tumultuous and abusive relationships, and she had obtained counseling for a brief bout with bulimia during that time.

She sometimes described intense feelings of anger at herself, and often felt guilty for not being a better person, wife, daughter, and mother. She described how she would like to hurt the "little demon-girl inside her" for not being better. During these times, she would often hide in the attic (when no one else was at home) and cut up her arms with a hobby knife or broken pieces of glass. Although she usually hid her arms with long sleeves, she had recently exposed veins in her wrist during this process, which resulted in excessive bleeding that required emergency intervention at the hospital. Although her husband often worried about her depression off and on, he became alarmed when he saw the scratches and scarring on her arms. Further examination over the course of a few weeks revealed that Francine did have a friend who had been sharing some benzodiazepine medication with her to "help me with my nerves." Francine was taking them off and on when she wanted to "calm down." Her husband described intense emotional outbursts by Francine. He said he tried to help her, to calm her down, but she would not listen to him, and seemed to become more enraged at him the more he tried.

A detailed functional assessment revealed that Francine often awoke in the morning quite depressed, had a hard time getting out of bed, but after some struggle, helped get her husband and daughter ready for the day. She would then sit over her coffee for an hour, feeling "tired and empty." She would often brood for most of the morning, many of her thoughts focused on intense self-loathing and "how I want to kill that little girl inside of me." Sometimes she drew pictures of herself or what she saw as the bad girl inside of her, and marked up the picture with depictions of stab wounds. Over the last couple of months, she had become increasingly incapacitated and often would not leave the house for days. Sometimes she would go for three or four days without showering, and did increasingly little by way of housework, shopping, or meal preparation. In family meetings, her husband and daughter helped Gail get a more complete account of what their daily life was like. Apparently Geoff and Tabatha would offer to assist with household responsibilities, but Francine would frustrate these attempts with emotional outbursts and accusations that they didn't like the way she did things, and that they were trying to take over and push her out of the home altogether. Geoff tried patiently to assuage her anger, but Tabatha and Francine would end up in screaming matches. She did expect her daughter to pick up the slack with the housework, however, although Francine would take little initiative to teach her daughter how to do anything. She was not actively looking for a job either, which caused considerable tension with her husband. The couple was barely making it financially, and could be described as living just above the limits of rural poverty.

After these outbursts, Francine would become withdrawn, and sulky, and Tabatha would make attempts to reconcile with her, apologizing for upsetting her. Francine would be inconsolable, and alternate between blaming Tabatha for being a bad daughter and herself for being a bad mother, wife, and so forth. The family felt they could no longer cope with her. Geoff was, on the whole, one to "muddle through . . . my mom had problems, I'm kind of used to it." Tabatha appeared depressed during these sessions, but said she had friends, and was doing pretty well in school. "I just feel guilty when I leave the house, because I don't know what it's going to be like when I get home."

Francine presented signs and symptoms of BPD (self-loathing, distorted self-image, self-mutilating and parasuicidal behavior, chronic feelings of emptiness, difficulty connecting with others, intense anger, vacillating feelings that caused considerable conflict in her relationships), but also presented a number of co-occurring problems: serious depression, possible panic disorder, drug abuse, and parenting-skill deficits. On a daily basis, she appeared to be immobilized with depression from the first thing in the morning, had little structure to plan her day, avoided daily responsibilities, spent time ruminating about past regrets and problems, and used tranquilizers to manage her moods. This pattern had become more stable over the past two months or so, and her depression, anxiety, conflicts, and emotional outbursts with her family and self-harming behaviors appeared to have increased in intensity. Her own construction of the problem was put succinctly: "I need to die and come back as a new person. I hate myself. I need to be made new." Gail acknowledged Francine's self-loathing and recognized the pain that she had been in for some time. With Geoff present, she provided the couple with some psychoeducation regarding these co-occurring problems, and talked about how they might work together to help Francine learn to better cope with her distress and enjoy her family and her life more. Gail tried not to focus immediately on Francine's problems exclusively, so as not to further convince her that she was the "bad" one. But they did agree on tentative goals for the intervention: to eliminate the self-hatred and self-mutilation, alleviate and help her cope better with some of the depression and anxiety, help her sleep better, and improve relations at home with her husband and daughter (table 10.2).

Selecting and Designing the Intervention: Defining Strategies and Objectives

In response to Francine's query "So where do we start?" Gail suggested a psychiatric evaluation for the depression and panic attacks, and a medically supervised withdrawal from the tranquilizers in order to obtain a better assessment of these problems. In consultation with the psychiatrist, Gail agreed that Francine's self-mutilation did not appear to be suicidal in any way, but they would continue to monitor her for any intent to really harm herself. Geoff was provided with psychoeducation regarding suicidal risk factors, and was encouraged to observe and discuss these concerns with Francine on a regular basis. Francine agreed, and seemed to respond positively to the attention. Antidepressant medication was prescribed a few weeks later, and Geoff, was asked to monitor the dispensing of the medication to see that Francine took the prescribed amount on a regular basis. Little was said at this point about her self-harming behaviors.

After a few weeks of preliminary meetings, referral, and follow-up assessment, the social worker recommended and described to Francine the use of DBT. Francine agreed that it was time to get some help. Gail focused immediately on Francine's main concerns: her depression, panicky feelings, maintaining a drug-free lifestyle, improving her relations with her husband and daughter, and reducing or eliminating her self-mutilating behavior. Gail taught Francine core mindfulness skills and cognitive therapy to help Francine to avoid "freaking out" every time something moderately upsetting happened around the house. Rather than react, Francine was taught to focus on observing what was going on without making any immediate judgment about the event (e.g., her daughter would come home from school in a bad mood because one of her girlfriends or a boy she liked rebuffed her). Gail incorporated some basic cognitive therapy techniques to help Francine stop and consider what she herself was thinking and feeling, and to gauge whether her response was reasonable and measured, given the situation. They role-played Francine listening, not reacting based on her own feelings, but reaching out to her daughter with a query such as "Why don't you sit down with me and tell me what happened today." The phrase "it's not about me" seemed to come up spontaneously, and Francine (laughing for the first time) showed some awareness that others around her might be experiencing distress as well, and that not everything that happened was directed at Francine or was intended to upset her. Francine tersely characterized her self-absorption: "Perhaps it's time I pulled my head out of my ass, and paid attention to others."

After the next few visits, Francine began to direct some of her anger and suspicion toward the therapist: "I don't think you really like me; you think I'm a 'head case' don't you; why don't you just tell me I'm a f——ing a——hole, and get it over with." In each case, Gail expressed concern about Francine's anger, asked her to talk more about how she was feeling and what was going on at home (and, later, at work), and provided some honest feedback to Francine about how it felt to be attacked in that manner. She used these exchanges as opportunities to educate Francine about her inclination to assume that other people thought very poorly of her, despite there being no evidence that they intended to be negative toward her. After several encounters like this, Francine began to more realistically consider that perhaps these were distortions on her part. To the extent that people actually did respond to her negatively, it might have something to do with the way Francine was communicating to them, since she was often sarcastic, critical, or ignored others altogether when she was "in a mood." Over time, Francine began to see that, rather than reacting negatively "like everybody else," Gail made every attempt to use these exchanges as an opportunity to teach Francine something that could be helpful to her. This modeling behavior seemed to have a positive effect, as Francine commented on one occasion: "I wish I could not take things so personally like you. I have to get a grip when I think someone doesn't like me or doesn't like something I've said. I mean . . . so what if they don't? I can't freak out every time I think someone is angry at me or doesn't approve of me."

Having eliminated the use of tranquilizers and started taking her prescribed SSRI medication, Francine began to feel a little more energy in the morning. Self-management skills were discussed and used to focus on structuring her mornings, gradually taking on more and more productive activities. They agreed that after completing her chores she would reward herself with either a bath or a walk (depending on needs, the weather, etc.) at about midday. Over the next few weeks, these activities (basic housecleaning, shopping for groceries, preparing meals, etc.) were increased, and Francine became increasingly confident and less anxious going into town and accomplishing basic errands. She did have a tendency at times to "space out," and discovered during her sessions that she would become immobilized and begin ruminating at certain times. She struggled with the desire to go upstairs and cut herself, as the ruminating often led to negative, self-critical thoughts. Through negotiation, the social worker and she agreed that she could schedule a time to sit and "brood" for exactly twenty minutes late in the morning after she completed her chores, and then reward herself with a walk or a bath. Gail also showed her some simple relaxation and meditation exercises she could do for a few minutes when she felt some of her frustration and anger rising. Francine told her friend next door that they could walk together only if she did not talk about using drugs anymore. When Francine asked about cutting herself (which often followed her intense brooding periods), Gail told her that not cutting herself would be preferred, but that decision was up to her. The social worker chose to focus on helping Francine self-monitor her own mood and use positive alternatives when she was feeling angry, depressed, or desperate.

Over the course of a few weeks (with periodic brief visits that included her husband and daughter), she made considerable gains in being active during the morning, was more productive, was less depressed, and became more available to her daughter when she came home after school. She began to feel "like a real mom," as her daughter seemed happier to come home and looked forward to telling her mother all that was going on in school during the day. "Maybe I'm not as screwed up as my mother was," Francine quipped at one point. "I don't have to be a chronic 'nut-job' like her if I don't want to. I can be there for Tabatha. It doesn't even take much. I just have to put her needs ahead of mine for a few minutes a day. That's not really much to ask of someone."

Early afternoons seemed to be the toughest time for Francine. By then, her schedule was done and she found herself becoming bored and preoccupied. She would begin to feel like going upstairs and cutting herself, and it was still a struggle not to give in to it. She needed to find a way to "fill in the gap" before her daughter came home a couple hours later. Gail and she decided that this window of vulnerability had to be closed and dealt with directly. The depression had subsided somewhat, and Francine had developed enough confidence in her self-management skills so that Gail felt she could challenge Francine a bit more. For the next few weeks, Gail helped Francine improve her distress tolerance and emotion regulation by developing an imaginal hierarchy of things that caused her emotional pain. These included images of her mom being ill when Francine was a child, feelings of embarrassment when she could not invite friends over, and more contemporary stressors such as being in a group of people and having a conversation without becoming upset, jealous, anxious, or angry. With a combination of guided imagery and relaxation exercises, Gail helped Francine to list these covert stressors from most to least distressful. Starting with the least distressful image, Gail helped Francine develop these images in her mind's eye, tolerate them while maintaining her composure, and accept them (if they were past events that could not be changed). Francine imagined herself coping with current stressors more effectively. As they worked their way down the list, Francine began to feel more confident that her emotional reactions to events past or present could be controlled or at least tolerated. This possibility came as a relief to her, and she began to feel, over time, that perhaps she could venture out into the world again. Going out would provide more opportunities to fill up that troublesome part of the day.

Francine spontaneously asked the social worker for some advice on how to polish her résumé. Gail offered some pretty standard advice on how Francine could present her work experience, and how to present herself at her best in a job interview. Francine's desire to get a part-time job outside the home presented an excellent opportunity to work on helping her gain confidence and overcome her anxiety about dealing with people again. She could further work on integrating her distress tolerance, and emotional regulation, and improving her interpersonal-effectiveness skills in a stressful situation (a job interview where she felt she was being judged). A few different scenarios were drawn up, and Gail provided the role-playing environment for Francine to field tough questions and challenging situations by learning to relax, breathe, not take it personally, and respond calmly, knowing that her worth as a person was not "on the line" in every job interview. After a few sessions of role-playing and rehearsal, she felt she was ready to try again.

Over the following weeks, Francine found a part-time job as a receptionist in a physician's office, and although she felt somewhat overwhelmed by the task of dealing with people on a daily basis, decided to take the position. She talked with her husband and daughter (who insisted they had to reschedule their private time for after dinner), and they agreed it was a good move. Her husband was relieved, as they needed the extra income. Francine decided to attend sessions every other week instead of weekly. She continued to struggle with anxieties regarding work and feeling comfortable dealing with other people. Her progress was reviewed, and she and Gail developed a relapse-prevention plan. They focused on identifying those potential "potholes" that Francine had to look out for, and wrote down a menu of constructive coping responses. There were also daily routine skills she needed to continue to work on: identifying negative and self-destructive thoughts, practicing calm communication skills with her husband, spending undivided time with her daughter every day if only for five to ten minutes, and taking time out for herself daily to do something she found enjoyable. Since her job was about three-quarters of a mile from her home, she was able to walk and practice her relaxation skills to and from the job.

During follow-up several months later, she appeared to be less preoccupied with her past ruminations. Her daily anxieties seemed to be much more focused on realistic concerns. Her confidence in being able to cope with them had grown. She continued her medication, although she said she had talked with her physician about cutting down. She no longer used tranquilizers. Her daughter seemed more at ease, her husband more relaxed (although, as Francine agreed, "we need to work on us"). The scars on her wrists and forearms were still visible, but with time would gradually fade. Rather than provocatively displaying her wounds, she wanted increasingly to hide them, particularly at work. Her daughter, who had taken up making costume jewelry with a friend, gave her mom a collection of bracelets, which Francine would wear in multiples, and proudly show off to her new companions at work.

Selecting Scales and Creating Indexes to Monitor and Evaluate Client Progress

Any number of standardized and idiographic indexes would be helpful for both the initial assessment as well as for monitoring and evaluating client progress (table 10.2). The BPDSI would be useful for gauging the change in severity of

TABLE 10.2   The client service plan for Francine

Problems	Goals	Sample Objectives	Interventions	Assessment Tools
Depression: mood disturbance, cognitive distortions of self-image, self-loathing, sleep disturbance (early a.m. wakening), lack of self-care, withdrawal, low energy (poor personal hygiene, low activity level); feelings of emptiness	Alleviate most major symptoms of depression; improve sleep, increase structured activity level, improve hygiene, overall appearance, self-image	Identify specific cognitive distortions about self and others and test them at home and elsewhere as opportunities arise	Dialectical behavior therapy (coupled with family visits) Psychoeducation regarding anxiety/depressive symptoms and problems with emotional/behavioral regulation; discuss core aspects of DBT	Any one of an array of depression, anxiety scales to help client track her symptoms BPDSI to track core symptoms of BPD Self-anchored scales to help client self-monitor progress: on a scale of 1-10, degree of

Problems	Goals	Sample Objectives	Interventions	Assessment Tools
Anxiety: generalized anxiety, anxiety attacks (rule out substance-abuse withdrawal), interpersonal anxiety (very anxious in social settings, work settings, self-conscious, becomes easily upset, defensive)	Rule out panic attacks/substance-abuse withdrawals; improve anxiety-management skills in social/work situations	Increase daily household objectives as client improves	Cognitive therapy: a mindful consideration of distortions regarding herself and others; test distortions through role-play and practice in vivo Core mindfulness skills to help her cope with others' behaviors	self-loathing, desire to cut, desire to use drugs, level of depression, anxiety about a specific event Frequency scales: number of times scratched or cut, minutes spent in productive conversation with daughter or husband; number of conversations initiated at work with coworkers
Substance abuse: taking nonprescription benzodiazepines; history of drug abuse when younger	Eliminate use of alcohol and nonprescription drugs	Practice breathing, meditation skills daily for increasing amounts of time (initially 5 minutes, then 10, up to 20 minutes)	Structured daily activities with daily goals and rewards to increase activity level Cognitive therapy (as above) to interpret provocative stimuli	
Self-mutilation: scratches wrists, forearms with blade or glass fragment; no clear suicidal intent	Eliminate self-mutilation	Use relaxation skills when she thinks of drug seeking; take "stress breaks" doing something enjoyable; when opportunity arises, implement in vivo practice of interpersonal skills; initiate one conversation a week up to daily as she returns to work, has more social contacts	Stress-management skills: breathing and relaxation exercises to cope with symptoms Role-play to cope with interpersonal situations that cause anxiety, miscommunications Exposure therapy to approach anxiety-provoking situations socially/at work	
Parenting problems with adolescent daughter; difficulty dealing with her needs	Improve relations/parenting skills with daughter; improve attention to daughter's age-specific needs	Sit and talk (mostly listen) with daughter 5 minutes daily after school, longer as she becomes comfortable	Case management: coordinate medical/psychiatric review of medications and symptoms Planned brief structured time for daughter daily	
Minimal intimacy with husband; little affection; poor communication	Improve relationship with husband in taking care of daughter and household; improve communication and empathy	Later in evening, initiate conversation with husband; first half is to focus on daily responsibilities of home, then each other; plan one activity together each weekend; first for 1 hour (e.g., a walk), then longer if their enjoyment increases	Communication and problem solving with husband to improve relationship and intimacy once client's major symptoms abate	

symptoms over time, and the HAM-D (see chapter 9) would be useful for assessing changes in depression level. Individual indexes could be employed to measure severity of the urge to cut, use of tranquilizers, severity of anxiety, frequency of cutting, and duration of time spent with daughter or problem solving with husband.

SUMMARY

Social workers are likely to encounter clients who "fit the profile" of the personality disorder in both specialized and general practice environments. Acquiring multiple collateral reports is essential to conducting a thorough MDF assessment. Despite the overall lack of research on clients diagnosed with APD and BPD, cognitive-behavioral and contingency management approaches have been shown to be very promising, and are often provided in the context of a case management team. Despite the difficulties and frequent frustrations associated with working with these troubled clients, evidence-based practice can substantively help them improve their self-management skills, enjoy a better quality of life, and become less of a problem for their family and the community.

PART THREE

PSYCHOSOCIAL PROBLEMS OF COUPLES, CHILDREN, AND FAMILIES

CHAPTER 11

DISTRESSED COUPLES

Using evidence-based interventions with couples is important not only for improving intimate adult relationships, but also for enhancing work with children and families. Thus, this chapter serves both as a critical overview of assessment and intervention with distressed couples and as a prelude to the chapters on childhood and adolescent disorders. Although systems frameworks have helped practitioners expand their perspective from individual psychopathology to the family and community, many popular couples and family approaches remain relatively untested. Two major evidence-based couples approaches for which substantive bodies of outcome research do exist are emphasized in this chapter: behavioral couples therapy and emotion-focused therapy.

ASSESSMENT

Background Data

A range of psychosocial factors contribute to the problems and distress experienced by couples, and the resulting distress can have serious consequences on the individual mental health of both partners and their children (Gottman, 1998, 1993b; R. L. Weiss & Heyman, 1997). Although divorce rates in North America have seen some decline in recent years (S. M. Johnson, 2003), divorce rates still range from 40% to 50% for first-time marriages and are estimated to be even higher for second marriages. The consequences of couples conflict, separation, and divorce include increased automobile accidents and fatalities, physical illness, suicide, homicide, depression, anxiety, social withdrawal, and other behavioral problems. Dysfunctional couples are more likely to suffer stress-related health problems (e.g., compromised immune-system response, higher blood pressure) as a result of their conflicts (Gottman; R. L. Weiss & Heyman, S. M. Johnson).

Couples problems and their treatment have also been examined from the perspective of individual disorders. One or both partners may suffer from a serious mental health or substance-abuse problem that reciprocally interacts with marital distress. Recently, more attention has been paid to couples where one has a serious disorder such as depression (K. D. O'Leary & Beach, 1990; Beach & O'Leary, 1992), alcoholism (O'Farrell et al., 1993; O'Farrell & Fals-Stewart, 2003), or anxiety disorders (Craske & Zoeller, 1995). The relationship between individual psychopathology and couples problems, however, is complex. One must consider, at a minimum, the age of onset of the partner's disorder, whether it is recurrent, the impact of marital stress on the individual's disorder, the effects of the disorder as a stressor on the partner's psychological well-being, and quality of the couple's relationship. Theories that suggest that one partner is unconsciously gratifying dark unresolved needs via their partner's disorder, or that the disorder of the "identified patient" serves some form of regulatory function in the family system have given way to multivariate explanations for couples' distress. A more accurate picture of the relationship between individual psychological disorders and marital distress is that these two problems are likely to interact and exacerbate one another (Halford & Bouma, 1997; Gottman, 1998, R.L. Weiss & Heyman, 1997).

Violence between couples

Findings regarding the cause and correlates of domestic violence have begun to accumulate (Gelles & Cornell, 1990; Holtzworth-Munroe, Bates, Smutzler, & Sandin, 1997; Holtzworth-Munroe, Smutzler & Bates, 1997). Violence against women is all too common, and much of it goes unreported. About 25% of American women have been physically abused by a partner in their lifetime, about 8% of women have reportedly been raped by their husbands, and many of these women die at the hands of their batterers (U.S. Department of Justice, 2000; Pagelow, 1992). Almost five million women annually are raped or physically assaulted by partners (U.S. Department of Justice, 2000). Although men are also assaulted, twice as many women suffer injuries, and these injuries are generally more severe. Women who live with female partners are less likely to be abused than women who live with male partners. Males who live with male partners are more likely to suffer abuse than males who live with female partners. Fifteen percent of males living with a male partner reported being raped, assaulted, or stalked by their partner (U.S. Department of Justice, 2000).

Battering of women was barely recognized in the research literature until the 1980s (Holtzworth-Munroe, Bates et al., 1997), due, in part, to its low priority as a national civil rights or legal concern, and its tendency to be dismissed by therapists and emergency-room attendants as the result of the woman's psychological problems (Pagelow, 1992). Women are at high risk for a range of psychological consequences that result from battering, including PTSD, depression, and low self-esteem. These symptoms are related to the severity and chronicity of the violent behaviors. In response to the age-old query "Why do they stay?" researchers have concluded that "battered women have many understandable reasons for remaining with an abusive partner, including fear of further abuse, economic dependence, commitment to one's spouse, and the belief that the partner will change" (Holtzworth-Munroe, Smutzler, & Sandin, 1997, p. 197). However, they point out that many battered women do eventually leave their abusive husbands.

Violence has been reported by up to one-quarter of couples during courtship, and marital violence is more likely in newlyweds and those under thirty years of age. Aggressive behavior among newlyweds has been shown to correlate with marital dissatisfaction even when controlling for negative communication styles and stressful life events (Lawrence & Bradbury, 2001). In a longitudinal study of couples, K. D. O'Leary et al. (1989) revealed that 31% of men and 44% of women had engaged in aggression against their partner in the year before they were married. At eighteen months after marriage, the rates dropped to 27% and 36%, respectively, and at thirty months, 25% and 32%. Women's violence declined significantly from one time interval to the next, but not men's. The most common forms of aggression were pushing, grabbing. and shoving. Age appeared to be the most important determinant of rates of aggressive acts. In a follow-up investigation based on the same research sample, K. D. O'Leary, Malone, and Tyree (1994) examined predictive factors of aggression and concluded that men's violence appeared to be more strongly related to a history of domestic violence in their own family of origin, but women's violence in their early marriages appeared to be a continuation of previous violent behavior. Other factors such as personality characteristics and the influence of marital discord also contributed to what is a multivariate model of violent behavior. O'Leary et al. stressed, however, that pathways to violence as well as the consequences to the object of that violence are quite different for men and women. In addition, most of these violent acts are not severe and do not result in serious bodily harm. In their study, about 2% of the aggressive acts resulted in the victim being "beaten up."

Men who abuse their partners are generally more likely to score higher on various measures of psychopathology, including poor self-esteem, depression, aggressiveness, hostility and anger, personality disorders, dependency needs, and disturbed relationship patterns. Men who feel powerless (e.g., unemployed, underemployed and dissatisfied with their jobs) are also more likely to use violence. Other correlates of men's battering include having more children in the family, financial problems, living in poor housing conditions, having had a violent childhood, disparity in the partners' educational/occupational status, sexual difficulties, poorly balanced power-sharing in the relationship, social stressors, and social isolation. Minority rates of couples violence also appear to be related to socioeconomic factors. Although substance abuse is a significant correlate of couples violence, its causal relationship to the abuse is complex—either the result of disinhibiting effects or a ready excuse to be abusive. Regardless of its specific role, substance abuse appears to be a catalyst to couples violence (Gelles & Cornell, 1990; Holtzworth-Munroe, Bates et al., 1997; Pagelow, 1992).

Couples violence also appears to be related to negative communication patterns between the partners. For example, a husband's controlling behavior tends to drive a communication pattern that is marked by anger, contempt, and belligerence, a cycle that is difficult to terminate once initiated. One reason it is important to study violent couples is that there appears to be a strong direct relationship between marital distress and husband's violence (Holtzworth-Munroe, Smutzler, & Bates, 1997). In a comprehensive review of studies from 1970 to 1984, Hotaling and Sugarman (1986) found four key factors associated with men's violence toward their wife: use of violence toward children, sexual aggression toward their wife, alcohol abuse, and having witnessed violence between their parents as a child or adolescent. In two case-controlled studies comparing clinical and community samples (Hastings & Hamberger, 1988; Hamberger & Hastings, 1991), male batterers were found to show greater levels of personality-disordered traits commensurate with BPD and APD, and their abusiveness seems to be mediated by alcohol abuse. However, Marcus and Swett (2002) call for an emphasis on the violent couple's relationship to better understand couples violence, rather than overemphasizing individual psychopathology, because evidence has consistently shown that both partners are likely to be violent. These violent relationships tend to be associated with high-risk emotions: anger, rage related to rejection sensitivity, insecurity, jealousy, and negative affect. Likewise, as one would expect, nonviolent relationships are marked by empathy, intimacy, trust, love, and a sense of security.

In the legal arena, domestic violence has increasingly become recognized as a crime rather than a private family matter or personal problem. Nevertheless, law-enforcement protection of women from their violent partners often fails, with consequences that include further serious physical injury and often death at the hands of their abusers. Pagelow (1992, p. 103) makes a key point regarding the importance of using social science evidence as a tool in the pursuit of social justice: "None of the legislative changes benefiting women could have occurred without empirical research findings." Evidence-based practice is more than employing psychosocial interventions that work; it is using social science evidence to inform policy analysis and support social action.

Effects of Couple Distress on Children

Couples who navigate the sometimes difficult waters of marital and family stress and conflict may provide positive role modeling and engender psychosocial resilience in their children. Lindahl, Clements, and Markman (1998) demonstrated convincingly that the parents' ability to manage conflict in their marriage enhances their children's psychological well-being. However, raising children can introduce stress and strain on a couple's relationship. These stressors may be due to differences in parenting philosophies, the accumulated role strain of balancing careers with children's activities, rigid gender roles regarding parenting responsibilities, and dealing with a behaviorally disturbed, disabled, or seriously ill child (Sanders, Nicholson, & Floyd, 1997). Reciprocally, marital distress and conflict associated with divorce increases the likelihood of greater psychological, emotional, behavioral, and interpersonal adjustment problems for children (Sanders et al.; Grych & Fincham, 1990). Children who witness marital violence, particularly conflict that is open, frequent, intense, physically aggressive, and unresolved, are at much greater risk to suffer these negative psychosocial effects (Holtzworth-Munroe, Smutzler, & Sandin, 1997). Children of divorce also suffer mental health problems both as children and as adults. They are more likely to obtain less satisfaction from family life, are more anxious, and have more difficulty coping with life's stressors (Sanders et al.; Gottman, 1998). These problems may vary somewhat by age and gender, and long-term outcomes may be mitigated to some degree should consistent parenting resume postdivorce. The mechanisms by which these effects are processed may include modeling (e.g., overt hostility and violence), the direct stress caused by marital conflict, and the negative effects of marital conflict on parent-child relationships.

The implications of these findings are important for planning interventions with children and their families. As Sanders, Nicholson, & Floyd (1997) aptly point out, there has been very little overlap or integration between the literatures on interventions with couples and interventions with children. "When a couple presents with parenting difficulties, therapists are encouraged to, first, diagnose the problem as primarily a marital problem or a parenting issue, and then, second, implement the appropriate course of marital or parenting intervention. It is rarely acknowledged that these two components may be inextricably linked, or that therapists should be experienced in treating both types of problems simultaneously" (p. 234). There is little research addressing how to modify marital interventions to address adjustment problems in children. Although intervening with a couple during divorce to aid their children's adjustment has become popular, there is little research evaluating these programs. For some childhood and adolescent disorders, incorporating cognitive-behavioral interventions into a family therapy model has only recently received empirical attention, as will be seen in subsequent chapters.

Gay and Lesbian Relationships

Gay and lesbian couples share many of the same concerns and challenges as heterosexual couples. They face some unique psychosocial and political challenges as well, such as interstate recognition of gay marriages. As with heterosexual couples, gay and lesbian couples seek constancy and intimacy in relationships; experience similar problems over money, household duties, sexual relations, infidelity, and parenting differences; and are as likely to be satisfied in their relationships as their heterosexual counterparts (Ossana, 2000). Kurdek (1998) surveyed over 200 gay, lesbian, and heterosexual couples, and found many similarities in their overall affective appraisal of their relationships, problem solving, and relationship satisfaction over a five-year period. B. J. MacDonald (1998) found rates of interpersonal violence to be comparable, and found that these couples shared problems related to control, power and dominance, sexual dysfunction, and struggles for autonomy and independence. This investigator also found that balance and equality in relationships tended to be a sign of relationship health (as seems to be the case in heterosexual couples). A recent qualitative analysis of a small sample of gay people in relationships found that gay couples were similar to straight couples in their use of maintenance behaviors such as task sharing, communication, and spending time together (Haas & Stafford, 1998). Even with regard to concerns such as HIV/AIDS that at one time were perceived as uniquely "gay issues," there may be more similarity than otherwise. In a recent survey of gay and straight couples with mixed HIV status, Beckerman, Letteney, and Lorber (2000) found they were equally concerned about HIV transmission, effects of uncertainty on the relationship, and fluctuations in emotional closeness and distancing.

However, the different challenges faced by gay and lesbian couples should not be minimized. As predicted, Kurdek (1998) found that lesbian couples reported more intimacy than heterosexual couples, and both gay and lesbian couples reported more autonomy in their relationships than heterosexual couples. B. J. MacDonald (1998) highlighted unique challenges for gay and lesbian couples in a thoughtful review of the literature: discrimination, stigma and homophobia, lack of comparable economic and political parity, the threat of HIV/AIDS (which disproportionately affected the gay community), and alienation from their own families. As a result, gay and lesbian couples may be more inclined to remain closeted about sexual orientation, a dilemma that places the resolution of couples conflict in a somewhat different social context than that of straight couples. Gay and lesbian couples may engage in relational maintenance behaviors that focus on solidifying their bond as a way of coping with sociopolitical pressures in society, that is, as a buffer against social stigma (Haas & Stafford, 1998). Practitioners should also not overlook within-group differences. One should not expect that all gay, lesbian, or heterosexual couples operate on the same principles.

Ossana (2000) points out some unique considerations when working with gay and lesbian couples: different developmental challenges for each member of the couple, the lack of available role models for gay couples' relationships, and the different way of forming gender-role identity that each partner brings to the relationship. One partner may be "out" and the other quietly "in the closet." Barriers to living openly as a couple continue in this society, and gay couples continue to face public-policy barriers, family rejection, and difficulties fitting into nongay social rituals (Ossana, 2000). Any and all of these stressors, past or present, can inject psychological strain into the relationship.

The Importance of Cultural, Racial, and Ethnic Differences in Couples Relationships

Cultural, racial, and ethnic identity can be powerful forces in making or breaking a relationship. Cultivating a long-term relationship with someone can be greatly enhanced by a mutual identification with common cultural ancestry, including a desire to share it with one's children. Conversely, the joining of different racial, ethnic, or cultural heritages through marriage can also be exciting. Appreciating and blending customs, beliefs, mythologies, rituals, music, food, and other traditions into a new family can result in a unique cultural pastiche.

Although little research has been conducted on racially or culturally mixed couples, a number of clinical scholars have made thoughtful observations. A. C. Jones and Chao (1997) point out that couples should attempt to be consciously aware of cultural issues, see cultural differences as a potential enhancement to their relationship, and use their cultural mix to develop each one's cultural, ethnic, or racial identity further in a positive and affirming way. They also warn of potential pitfalls however, such as mismatched ethnic identity and acculturation conflict (as when a couple, both of Cantonese ancestry, have differences in negotiating American norms, given different levels of acculturation and assimilation); minimizing the potential impact of cultural, ethic, or racial differences (an Irish-Catholic man and reformed Jewish woman of Orthodox parents may face friction as they plan marriage and children); different strategies for coping with racial, ethnic, or cultural bias, discrimination, and oppression (e.g., one avoids it, one confronts it openly).

Evidence suggests that there are both similarities and differences among couples by race and culture. For example, German couples were shown to be more likely to engage in negative and coercive interactions than Australian couples (Halford, Hahlweg, & Dunne, 1990). Hispanic and non-Hispanic white couples in the southwestern United States appeared to be more similar than different in levels of marital distress after controlling for other demographic factors, and showed only a modest difference in the relationship between level of acculturation and marital distress among wives (Negy & Snyder, 1997). Oggins, Leber, and Veroff (1993) examined the sexual and marital satisfaction of both African-American and white couples, and showed that for both groups, men reported less of a contingency between sexual satisfaction and marital intimacy than women. However, lower-income black women (compared with white women) appeared to pay greater attention to sexual satisfaction in its own right. In a retrospective qualitative study of white, African-American, and Mexican-American couples who had been married for twenty years or more, conflict generally declined after the rearing of children, but African-American men reported a more confrontational style over the years, an opinion with which their wives generally concurred (Mackey & O'Brien, 1998).

Theories

There is a striking split in the literature on couples problems between theories based largely on speculation and those supported by empirical evidence. Pathological behavior within the context of psychodynamic couples assessment, for example, is seen largely as the result of poor ego development related to disturbances in early attachment or object relations. These disturbances lead to interpersonal (i.e., "relational") problems that affect choice of mate and later cause relationship dysfunction (Scharff, 1995; Bowlby, 1969; S. M. Johnson & Greenberg, 1995; Meissner, 1978). The goal of treatment is to help the couple clarify interpersonal distortions (i.e., displacements, projections), see each other more realistically, interact less defensively, and obtain a more mature level of intimacy. Although these theories continue to have some intuitive appeal, there is relatively little evidence that specifically links early mother-infant/toddler interactions with adult relationship problems. Confirmatory evidence of such a link would require, as Furman and Flanagan (1997, p. 189) point out, "a longitudinal demonstration that examines whether childhood attachment is predictive of adult romantic attachment and characteristics of the marital relationship. Unfortunately, such a study does not yet exist." Indeed, any model linking childhood experiences and subsequent adult relationships is likely to involve a combinations of factors that interact over time, such as innate temperament, early childhood experiences (nurturance versus abuse and neglect), peer influences, intimate experiences in adolescence and young adulthood, social and cultural context of early romantic relationships, and a host of other psychological risks and resiliencies. Theories that overemphasize the influence of early childhood also fail to account for sources of change and variability during the course of the marital relationship itself (Karney & Bradbury, 1995). A simple causal linkage between early "attachment" behaviors and adult relationships is likely to remain a theory in search of evidence.

Although multidimensional theories of relationship development await further investigation, current theories that attempt to explain couples' well-being and distress generally focus on the quality of interactional attributions and behaviors. Much of contemporary couples theory has its roots in social exchange theory (Thibaut & Kelly, 1959). Levinger (1976) applied these concepts to marriage and suggested that the success or failure of marriage depended on three main factors: each spouse's weighing the attractions of the relationship, barriers to leaving, and the availability of attractive alternatives. Behavioral exchange theory has provided the bedrock for contemporary marital theory. It emphasizes the importance of interacting rewards and punishments between partners and their correlation with overall marital satisfaction (R. B. Stuart, 1969, 1980; Jacobson & Margolin, 1979). Interventions developed in this tradition tend to focus on changing interactional behaviors to increase mutual satisfaction through improved communication and problem solving. P. L. Johnson and O'Leary (1996) tested this hypothesized relationship between behavior exchange and marital satisfaction and demonstrated that they do, indeed, correlate significantly. In addition, they demonstrated that an individualized approach to assessment whereby couples identified ten positive and ten negative behaviors in their relationship was as reliable and valid as using validated psychometric instruments that included over 100 items. Findings such as this illustrate the importance of using thoughtful idiographic assessment.

The increased emphasis on cognitive theory has also had its impact on behavioral approaches to couples theory and practice. Several practitioner-researchers have incorporated traditional cognitive concepts (Baucom, Epstein, & Rankin, 1995; Kayser, 1997) to account for the interpersonal distortions and misattributions that occur between partners as a result of social learning history or current situational stressors. For example, couples may use selective attention (focusing only on a partner's mistakes), arbitrary inference ("You're late . . . Are you seeing someone else?"), overgeneralization ("You *never* do anything nice for me!"), dichotomous thinking ("I take all the responsibility around here and you take none!"), and mind reading ("You've been quiet all night . . . You're angry at me, aren't you!"). Cognitive-behavioral intervention includes an examination of dysfunctional cognitive thinking about the relationship (without inferring unconscious motives), clarification through improved communications, and behavioral tasks to disconfirm these distorted beliefs or erroneous expectations. The partners' respective cognitive schemata, that is, their more enduring beliefs or expectancies about relationship and intimacy, may require more careful and probing examination. Beliefs and associated feelings and behaviors may need to be repeatedly challenged and disconfirmed over time in the relationship before they can change. For example, being suspicious or vigilant, despite much reassurance, because of a former lover's infidelities can have long-term effects on mutual trust. Such problems with "basic trust" need not be rooted in early childhood, but can be instilled as a result of a prior betrayal in adulthood. Other deeply hurtful experiences may require more "cognitive reconstruction" than just challenging distorted thinking. Only behavioral disconfirmation over time, in the form of constancy in a loving relationship, is likely to heal these psychological wounds.

Operating within the same general framework of social exchange, Gottman (1993b) developed an empirical model that examines interpersonal processes over the course of the relationship. He contends that his structural model supports a "*process cascade* in which criticism leads to contempt, which leads to defensiveness, which leads to stonewalling. The findings of his research suggest that these four processes are particularly corrosive to marital stability" (p. 62). Divorce may not be far off when these behaviors far outweigh positive interchanges. Gottman's research (1993a) led him to suggest five typologies of marriage (three stable: "validators," "volatiles," and "avoiders"; and two unstable: "hostile," and "hostile/detached") based on ability to balance positive and negative interactions. The stable marriages, in differing ways, demonstrated a five-to-one ratio of positive to negative interactions. Gottman (1993b) suggests that couples therapy should focus on interrupting the negative reciprocal cycle between the partners employing three main strategies: nondefensive and nonprovocative speaking, nondefensive listening and validation, and tactful editing (clarification of what was communicated). The process should be accompanied by efforts to calm heightened arousal during marital discussions. As the negative interactions ease, the couple can use repair mechanisms to ease tensions and improve communications overall.

Karney and Bradbury (1995) also emphasized the central place of behavioral theory and its focus on mutual attributions and interactional rewards. However, they suggested that the focus on behavioral theory has been overly narrow and lacks a sense of context, such as environmental stress, within which the behavioral changes are occurring. They also address another aspect of healthy relationships not addressed in contemporary couples theory, the role of social support. Pasch and Bradbury (1998) demonstrated the importance of both positive interactions during problem solving, and the need to provide social support to the other spouse when dealing with nonmarital problems as well. The provision of social support to one's spouse predicted positive marital outcomes over two years during early marriage, a critical time during which most divorce proceedings are initiated.

Despite the limitations in the research, a multidimensional social-cognitive framework for marital theory is emerging (Karney & Bradbury, 1995; Lindahl, Malik, & Bradbury, 1997). The vulnerability-stress-adaptation model suggests that marital outcomes emerge from the interaction of three domains: enduring vulnerabilities, adaptive processes, and stressful events. Enduring vulnerabilities include those intraindividual qualities each partner brings to the relationship. Adaptive processes refer to communication between partners, attributions partners make about each other, and partners' ability to provide support and understanding to each other (Karney & Bradbury, 1995). Adaptive processes are shaped by the personal strengths and weaknesses (or enduring vulnerabilities) that spouses bring to marriage, such as stable demographic, historical, personality, and experiential factors; and the stressful events, developmental transitions, and chronic or acute circumstances that spouses encounter. One implication of this theory is that even couples who are good problem solvers can succumb to marital failure if environmental stressors overwhelm them, and they lack the resources to deal with them (Lindahl et al.). Further research on the impact of social, environmental, and economic stressors on marriage is needed to enhance social-cognitive couples theory.

Current theories of couples well-being and dysfunction clearly owe a debt to social exchange in the behavioral tradition. Many of the data have focused on negative reciprocal interactional processes that, once they become negative, tend to spiral out of control. Couples who are adept at "short-circuiting" those negative patterns by self-editing, lowering their own level of criticism, reducing arousal during these exchanges, and sticking to the issue at hand, tend to have better communications (e.g., good listening without interrupting), which results in a more constructive and supportive climate (R. L. Weiss & Heyman, 1997; Gottman, 1998, 1993b). Couples who practice good "rules of engagement" during arguments may also store up a bank of goodwill or "positive sentiment override" (R. L. Weiss & Heyman) that can be tapped during more stressful periods. However, there are limitations to a theory built primarily on interactional processes. In addition to a host of methodological shortcomings, these theories tend to be *correlational rather than developmentally explanatory*; that is, they do not explain how relationships succeed or fail over time. Couples theory in the social-cognitive and social exchange arena would be enhanced by examining influences that develop in both individuals and couples over time within a broader social-environmental framework that includes a greater emphasis on cross-cultural factors as well (Halford, 1998; Gottman, 1993b; Karney & Bradbury, 1995).

Key Elements of Multidimensional/ Functional Assessment

Assessing distressed couples may be more challenging than assessing an individual. Couples assessment involves individual assessments of each partner and understanding the development of interactional patterns between them over time. Children may also be part of the assessment picture; more attention will be paid to the broader family assessment and that of children in subsequent chapters. A thorough assessment of each partner is important for several reasons. First, each partner may have different reasons for seeking help, different motivation level, different goals, and different understanding of the problems at hand. Second, one or both of the partners may be suffering from individual problems or a psychiatric disorder that may require special attention beyond that of understanding the couple's behavior. One partner may be seriously depressed, may refuse to travel outdoors due to panic attacks, may suffer from OCD, may have a substance-abuse problem, or may suffer from PTSD. It is a reasonable working assumption, however, that although individual problems may have their own developmental causes and trajectory, these problems are likely to strain the relationship, and, in turn, the couple's conflict may further exacerbate a partner's disorder. Third, one partner may not feel ready to disclose certain information in the presence of the other partner, and it may be critical for the practitioner to be informed of this matter.

A thorough examination of each partner's relationship history (beyond family of origin) may also reveal information salient to the current relationship. What does each partner bring to the relationship? Has either been married before? What were previous relationships like? Were they positive with pleasant memories or were they fraught with conflict? Was there any history of abuse? What expectations did they bring and do they still have about the current relationship and what they want from their partner? Are these expectations reasonable? Are their impressions, attributions, and cognitions congruent with regard to the other partner's actual behavior? This relationship history can then provide a foundation for a developmental time line. How long have they been together? At what point (in terms of major developmental milestones) are they in their relationship? Are they newlyweds struggling with young children, or a more experienced couple trying to keep up with more adventurous adolescent sons or daughters? Are they struggling to finance their young adult's college education? Practitioners should avoid superimposing the expectations of standard "stage theories" on couples. However, they should take note of common milestones (having children, children leaving home, approaching retirement), and examine the unique aspects of the relationship at these thresholds.

A functional assessment is necessary to capture the pattern and sequencing of a couple's positive and negative interactions over time (Fraenkel, 1997; Sayers & Sarwer, 1998; F. J. Floyd, Haynes, & Kelly, 1997). The functional analysis should include their unique developmental trajectory (i.e., courtship and marital life cycle) as well as their day-to-day interactions concerning key problems, such as parenting differences, money, sharing household responsibilities, fidelity, sexual problems, and difficulties with in-laws. Processes to be described should include distorted cognitions (misattributions) about the relationship and one another, emotional expression, negative and positive communication patterns and deficits, and other situational problems. Relationships with families of origin, social supports, work relationships, and other community relations (e.g., friends and acquaintances) should be examined as well. Work-related stress or financial problems can seriously strain a couple's relationship. More severe environmental barriers due to poverty, discrimination, poor living conditions, and other social stressors must also be considered.

It is important that the couple have an opportunity to discuss a moderately distressing problem within the session during the assessment phase, so that the practitioner can observe how they interact and what problem-solving methods and communication styles they employ. After a period of observation, the practitioner can use a stop-action method to interrupt the couple and help them examine important aspects of their own communication process, including cognitions (beliefs, expectations, attributions) regarding the relationship and their partner, emotional content associated with those cognitions, and specific behavioral interactions. Both partners are likely to have different views regarding their partner's behaviors, the quality of the relationship as a whole, and "what happened and when" in day-to-day interactions. Nevertheless, the practitioner should, at least initially, strive to keep the discussion purely descriptive, to keep the emotional timbre low and matter-of-fact, and to avoid making confirmatory judgments at the time. This "neutral" position can help establish an overall sense of fairness. The practitioner can then begin to tentatively formulate a hypothetical model of a key problem: "Let me see if I understand this . . . first, you do X, and then you say Y, and then Z happens. Do I have that right?"

Once the practitioner and couple generally agree on the problem content and a description of the problematic interaction, it is important to establish a problem hierarchy and decide on intervention goals. Goals of treatment (i.e., changes each partner wants in the other and in their relationship as a whole) should be mutually agreed upon. Which problem should be addressed first? Taking on the most challenging one may not be the best place to start. A more manageable and less contentious but important issue, perhaps balancing the budget may be a good starting point. Approaching problems gradually and achieving small successes along the way can help clients increase their self-efficacy in problem solving, improve their emotional response to one another, and increase optimism that "we can work it out." Individual problems should also be broken down into steps (again, hierarchically), so that the couple can begin with a more manageable part of the problem (e.g., making a list of household expenses, attend a free seminar on home budgeting at the local high school, review résumé-writing tips), and lead gradually up to more contentious challenges (e.g., moving or changing jobs). Indeed, not every problem needs to be solved. Couples can live quite happily together by "agreeing to disagree" about some problems for which the resolution is not critical at the moment. Sometimes, as other problems are resolved, the improvements in mutual goodwill, problem solving, and communication skills generalize to these other problems as well.

As discussed in chapter 2, the practitioner should be prepared to use a few different methods of reporting in order to compare the consistency of responses: the face-to-face interview; self-monitoring techniques that the couple can work on at home, such as keeping individual diaries or a joint chart to record times they worked constructively on the problem together; and brief, reliable, and valid couples assessment scales, a few of which are discussed below.

Given that violence between partners is not a rare event, and given the potential harm to both the partner and children, practitioners should always screen for domestic violence as a routine part of assessment for all adult clients, both individuals and couples. In the presence of domestic violence, couples work may not be feasible. Although some practitioners maintain that domestic violence should always preclude couples work, there is growing consensus that this policy may be overly broad, and may preclude effective work in cases where the violence is at a low to moderate level. Although there is an acute need for further research on the matter, assessment of couples battering and determining which couples may be amenable to successful intervention can be informed by what is currently known about risk factors.

Bograd and Mederos (1999) suggest three preconditions for assessment with male-on-female violence (which can be modified for gay couples): (1) the male must be a voluntary participant in the therapy; (2) modification in disclosing confidential information during individual assessment interviews must be an option (e.g., the woman may disclose that she has been victimized to the practitioner, but does not want the practitioner to disclose yet); and (3) the practitioner must "be frank and clear about the allocation of responsibility and the inappropriateness of abusive behavior regardless of circumstances" (p. 296). In addition to a couples assessment session that focuses primarily on interactional concerns in the marriage, the practitioner should also conduct individual meetings within which domestic violence is explored. Bograd and Mederos make it clear that the practitioner cannot mislead the victims into believing that their security can be guaranteed by the practitioner, and the client must be well-informed of the potential risks.

The goals of the individual assessment interview are to learn about the nature of any violence between partners and functional details (context, sequence of events leading up to it, the type, frequency, severity, consequences of the violence); understand the intended function of the violence and its effects; evaluate the degree of intimidation used and fear elicited in the victim; examine whether there is a broader pattern of violence and intimidation; consider the real possibility of serious injury or death; and arrive at an informed decision about the feasibility and wisdom of proceeding with couples work.

Bograd and Mederos (1999) further suggest that if any one of the following risk factors exists, practitioners should seriously considering forgoing couples therapy:

unresolved substance abuse;

a history of two or more acts of domestic violence (to wife or children), including rape;

history of violent criminal acts including violation of restraining order;

previous use of weapons;

ongoing threats of violence;

obsessional behaviors toward the partner such as intense jealousy, stalking, and harassing; and

bizarre forms of violence marked by sadism or an attempt to depersonalize the victim.

Conversely, couples intervention *may* be considered if

both partners agree to therapy;

the incidents of violence have been few or the incidents have been confined to less harmful forms of aggression such as pushing, shoving, or open-handed slaps that do not result in physical injury;

there is minimal psychological abuse;

there are no threats of lethality and the woman does not fear violent reprisals; and the abusive partner takes responsibility for his behavior and for controlling his anger without making excuses or blaming others.

A thorough review of Bograd and Mederos 1999 is recommended. The use of assessment instruments such as the Conflict Tactics Scale and the Danger Assessment Scale have been recommended as useful adjuncts to a thorough clinical interview (S. A. Anderson, 2001).

Social workers may not always be the first in line to assess domestic violence. Often medical professionals are in a position to determine whether violence has taken place. Such data can be instrumental in the successful prosecution of domestic-violence cases. Two key areas where medical professionals can improve assessment and provide solid evidence for court proceedings are in documenting medical injuries accurately (clear descriptions, photographs), and accurately recording the verbal reports of their clients (in quotes), rather than making interpretations or inferences about what they thought their clients meant. Recording the time of the interview and the time the injuries were said to have occurred also strengthens the evidence (U.S. Department of Justice, 2001). Social workers can also improve their recording of verbal reports from clients about the specific nature (who, what, where, and when) of the violence, and work closely with health-care professionals on a routine basis to gather solid physical evidence of physical abuse. Case management coordination of data gathering and, later, interventions may be invaluable to successful intervention with victims of domestic violence.

Instruments

A number of well-tested instruments have been widely used in practice and research with couples and can serve as useful adjuncts to an MDF assessment. The Marital Adjustment Test (MAT; Locke & Wallace, 1959; Fredman & Sherman, 1987) is one of the most widely used measures of marital satisfaction. The MAT is a fifteen-item scale that takes only a few minutes to complete and has weighted scores that sum to a potential total ranging from 0 to 60. It has one global measure of marital satisfaction, eight questions regarding specific areas of possible disagreement (e.g., finances, recreation, affection, friends, sex), and six questions measuring conflict resolution, communication, and cohesion (e.g., how disagreements are resolved, leisure preferences, willingness to confide in the other). It has excellent internal consistency reliability, and discriminates well between adjusted and maladjusted couples.

The Dyadic Adjustment Scale (DAS; Spanier, 1976) has been considered one of the more valid and useful scales for the assessment of marital adjustment. The original DAS is relatively brief (thirty-two items) and has been shown to discriminate between distressed and nondistressed couples. Although there has been some controversy regarding whether the DAS is unidimensional or multidimensional, it was originally designed to measure four areas of marital adjustment: consensus on important areas of marital functioning, dyadic satisfaction, marital cohesion, and the expression of affection. Recently, Busby, Christensen, Crane, and Larson (1995) undertook a reanalysis of the factor structure of the DAS with 242 couples, and demonstrated that, according to their data, the DAS is best conceptualized as a multidimensional instrument that measures three subscales corresponding to the following areas: consensus (in decisionmaking, leisure activities, values, affection), marital satisfaction (instability of the marriage, level of conflict), and cohesion (activities engaged in together, exchanging ideas of interest with one another). Their three-factor model resulted in a fourteen-item brief scale that demonstrated a high degree of construct and criterion validity as well as good to excellent internal consistency and split-half reliability for brief subscales. The fourteen-item revised DAS can be examined in Busby et al. The revised DAS has also been shown to correlate highly ($r = .78$) with the Kansas Marital Satisfaction scale, which appears to yield comparable results in distinguishing distressed from nondistressed couples (Crane, Middleton, & Bean,

2000). One of the limitations of these two scales, however, is that the samples overrepresent white couples. Validating these scales with minority couples is a potentially rich avenue for social work research.

Should the practitioner be primarily interested in measuring relationship satisfaction, a practical and brief alternative may be the Relationship Assessment Scale (RAS; Hendrick, 1981, 1988; Hendrick, Dicke, & Hendrick, 1998). The original version was based on research showing a correlation between self-disclosure and marital satisfaction with fifty-one couples (Hendrick, 1981). A more recent version of the RAS is a seven-item Likert-scale global measure of relationship satisfaction, with total scores ranging from 7 to 35. Reliability of the scale has been shown to be high, and the RAS correlates highly with the long version of the DAS (Hendrick, 1988; M. J. Vaughn & Matyastik Baier, 1999). The RAS also discriminates couples who stay together and couples who break up. It has been shown to have relatively consistent measurement properties by gender and ethnic background, and can be used with nonmarried people involved in a relationship (Hendrick et al.). This option is important, because practitioners can use this brief scale with "nontraditional" couples.

A more recent addition to the set of available instruments for assessing couples relationships is the Marital Disaffection Scale (Kersten, 1990; Kayser, 1996). This twenty-one item self-report scale measures the degree to which a person has lost their feelings of love and affection for their partner on a four-point scale: "very true" (4), "somewhat true" (3), "not very true" (2), and "not at all true" (1). Although the scale uses the term *marital*, the items do not preclude its use with any couple that has existed for a significant amount of time. Two studies support the reliability and criterion validity of the scale. Kayser (1996) administered the scale to seventy-six spouses recruited through community sources for the study. Mean age was about thirty-two, and couples had been married for a mean of eight years. In another study, 354 spouses were surveyed (mean age forty-six and mean length of marriage was twenty-one years). Internal consistency ratings were high (>.95), and the scale correlated with other related measures moderately to high in the expected direction (Kayser, 1996; Tuliatos, Perlmutter, & Holden, 2001). The scale also includes several reverse score items to measure intimacy. The entire scale is printed here (instrument 11.1).

SELECTING EFFECTIVE INTERVENTIONS

Although a tremendous amount of descriptive and theoretical literature has been written about couples therapy, surprisingly few formal interventions for couples have been tested in controlled trials. These include EFT and BCT. Since the early nineties, the pace of research on couples therapy has slowed, but theoretical developments with an eye toward integration and eclecticism have continued. What follows is a brief overview of interventions shown to be effective with distressed couples, followed by suggestions for incorporating the best of these approaches into flexible evidence-based guidelines.

INSTRUMENT 11.1 Marital Disaffection Scale

Please answer all questions using the following scale:

Very true	Somewhat true	Not very true	Not at all true
4	3	2	1

1. If I could never be with my spouse, I would feel miserable. 4 3 2 1
2. I find it difficult to confide in my spouse about a number of things. 4 3 2 1
3. I enjoy spending time alone with my spouse. 4 3 2 1
4. I often feel lonely even though I am with my spouse. 4 3 2 1
5. I miss my spouse when we're not together for a couple days. 4 3 2 1
6. Most of the time I feel very close to my spouse. 4 3 2 1
7. I seem to enjoy just being with my spouse. 4 3 2 1
8. I look forward to seeing my spouse at the end of the day. 4 3 2 1
9. My love for my spouse has increased more and more over time. 4 3 2 1
10. I find myself withdrawing more and more from my spouse. 4 3 2 1
11. When I have a personal problem, my spouse is the first person I turn to. 4 3 2 1
12. Apathy and indifference best describe my feelings toward my spouse. 4 3 2 1
13. I feel little, if any, desire to have sex with my spouse. 4 3 2 1
14. My spouse has always been there when I needed him or her. 4 3 2 1
15. I would prefer to spend less time with my spouse. 4 3 2 1
16. I have more positive than negative thoughts about my partner. 4 3 2 1
17. I have a lot of angry feelings toward my spouse. 4 3 2 1
18. I am not as concerned about fulfilling my obligations and responsibilities in my marriage as I was in the past. 4 3 2 1
19. I try to avoid spending time with my spouse. 4 3 2 1
20. There are times when I do not feel a great deal of love and affection for my mate. 4 3 2 1
21. I enjoy sharing my feelings with my spouse. 4 3 2 1

After reversing the scores on items 1, 3, 5, 6, 7, 8, 9, 11, 14, 16, 21, sum all items. The higher the score, the greater the level of disaffection.

BCT is clearly the most extensively researched of the couples interventions, and has accumulated a solid record of demonstrated effectiveness for reducing couples' distress in over thirty controlled trials (Hahlweg & Markman, 1988; Alexander, Holtzworth-Munroe, & Jameson, 1994; Gurman, Kniskern, & Pinsof, 1986; Baucom & Epstein, 1990; Jacobson & Addis, 1993; Lebow & Gurman, 1995; Lebow, 2000). Usually, BCT includes three main components in the intervention: behavioral exchange (quid pro quo contracting), communication training, and problem-solving skills. In almost all controlled trials, BCT has been shown to be more effective than no treatment in reducing harmful conflict, improving communications, improving interpersonal behaviors, and increasing relationship satisfaction (Halford, 1998; Hahlweg & Markman; Lebow & Gurman). Only about

70-75% of clients show improvement from BCT, however, and many clients relapse over time. Although BCT has accumulated the most evidence as an established treatment for marital distress, it has not been shown to be markedly superior to other nonbehavioral approaches such as insight-oriented couples therapy (IOCT) or EFT in direct comparisons (e.g., Snyder et al., 1991; S. M. Johnson, 2003) or in meta-analysis (Shadish et al., 1993). The addition of explicit cognitive elements has not markedly improved the outcomes of BCT (Baucom & Epstein, 1990; Jacobson & Addis, 1993; Halford, 1998), and (as with other approaches) the effective processes of BCT have not been clearly determined.

In the course of its evolution, BCT has incorporated modifications that go beyond behavior change as the only indication of success. Integrative behavioral couples therapy (IBCT; Christensen, Jacobson, & Babcock, 1995) was developed to enhance "acceptance" between partners when some problems seem intractable. IBCT is based on the assumption that, to be happy as a couple, not all problems need to be resolved. In fact, some couples can become more intimate by learning to accept some of their differences. To this end, the methods include empathic joining (trying to understand the partner's needs and feelings to reduce some of the pain felt mutually), detachment (developing mutual intellectual understanding and distance from the problem), developing some degree of tolerance for the problem (to diminish the ongoing struggle to change it), and cultivating self-care skills to reduce overreliance on the other person to satisfy all of one's particular needs. One preliminary randomized trial with twenty-one couples (treated for a mean of twenty-one sessions) demonstrated that IBCT resulted in greater satisfaction and more clinically significant gains than traditional BCT (Jacobson, Christensen, Prince, Cordova, & Eldridge, 2000). Halford has also embellished BCT by changing the focus from changing the partner to each partner's improving their own self-regulatory behaviors. "In the context of relationship problems, self-regulation involves focusing on each partner's attempts to change their own behavior, cognitions and affect to enhance their personal satisfaction with the relationship" (Halford, 1998, p. 621). Initial exploratory investigations appear to be promising. Investigators are hopeful that emphasizing self-regulatory mechanisms of change rather than changing the other person may lead to more lasting benefits of couples therapy.

The major alternatives to BCT include EFT (S. M. Johnson & Greenberg, 1985a, 1985b, 1988; James, 1991; A. Goldman & Greenberg, 1992) and IOCT (Snyder & Wills, 1989; Snyder et al., 1991). Based somewhat on variants of psychodynamic theory and practice, both EFT and IOCT emphasize changing partners' behaviors by increasing insight into their relationship through either direct interpretation (IOCT) or improved emotional expression (EFT). Both EFT and IOCT have been shown to be reasonably effective at improving relationship satisfaction (Halford, 1998), although these conclusions are based on a very limited number of trials and few direct comparisons to other approaches. In a study comparing BCT and EFT (S. M. Johnson & Greenberg, 1985a), EFT was shown to be superior when compared with one skill component of BCT (problem solving) in a sample of mildly distressed couples. In a comparison with BCT (Snyder & Wills, 1989; Snyder et al.), IOCT was shown to have better long-term outcomes, although it was alleged that the BCT method employed did not include relational aspects that are part of BCT as well (Jacobson, 1991). Given the limited evidence from direct comparisons and meta-analytic studies, it is difficult to argue that one approach is markedly superior to another.

A few key outcome studies of EFT have been conducted since the mid-1980s. In the initial study, S. M. Johnson and Greenberg (1985a) assigned forty-five couples (fifteen each) to eight one-hour sessions of EFT, problem-solving training (PS, a component of BCT), and a control group (wait list). Several measures were taken at pretreatment, posttreatment, and follow-up. Husbands in the EFT group reported significant improvement over the other two conditions, and wives in both EFT and PS reported improvements over the controls. Couples in both treatment groups improved compared to controls on measures of intellectual intimacy, consensus, reduction in target problems, and overall goal attainment. EFT couples, however, reported greater cohesion, intellectual intimacy, and reductions in target complaints, than couples receiving PS. Wives in the EFT condition also improved more in emotional expression and expression of affection. Two-month follow-up measures showed gains for the EFT couples consistent with those at posttest. The authors emphasized that EFT resulted in behavioral improvements (e.g., negotiations, other behavior changes) despite a lack of explicit focus on these skills. They suggested that "it may be that the increase in trust and responsiveness, which is the goal of the EF treatment, has an effect in these areas" (p. 181). In a follow-up study, S. M. Johnson and Greenberg (1985b) treated and evaluated those who had been in the wait-list control in the previous study, and showed that, although no substantive improvements had occurred during the waiting period, they improved after eight sessions of EFT in all outcomes and maintained their gains after two months.

James (1991) conducted a controlled trial in which EFT (twelve sessions) was compared to an intervention consisting of a combination of EFT and CT augmented by the addition of communication training (CT), that is, eight sessions of EFT and four sessions of CT. Forty-two couples (average length of partnership about ten years) were randomly assigned to three treatment conditions (including a wait-list control), and the interventions were measured for fidelity to their respective models. Both treatment groups had generally superior outcomes at posttest and follow-up. But aside from improved communications in the EFT plus CT group, there were few differences between them, suggesting that the addition of CT to EFT resulted in only marginal improvement. The results suggested that the goals of improving marital satisfaction and lessening target complaints were more responsive to treatment than improving emotional bonds, a goal that may require more lengthy intervention.

A. Goldman and Greenberg (1992) compared EFT with integrated systemic marital therapy (ISMT), where therapist consultants assisted a primary therapist in using systemic techniques such as reframing and prescribing the symptom. Forty-two couples were randomly assigned (fourteen each) to one of two treatment conditions (ten sessions), or a wait-list control group. Couples were all white and had been together for eleven years on average. Fourteen therapists (with masters in psychology, counseling, or social work) received twelve hours of instruction and additional supervision in their approach. Couples in the two treatment groups demonstrated more marital satisfaction, conflict resolution, reductions in target complaints, and goal attainment. Two-thirds of the treatment couples were rated in the nondistressed range after treatment, with no differences between the two treatment groups. The other 33% showed some clinical improvement, although they could not be considered treatment successes. Results for EFT couples deteriorated over time at follow-up, perhaps as a result of the persuasiveness of the team approach, or because these couples were more severely distressed than couples previously treated in studies of EFT. The ISMT approach was more explicit about changing couples behaviors, while the EFT was more focused on changing emotional perceptions and interactive experience within the couples.

Exemplar Study: Insight-Oriented Couples Therapy versus Behavioral Couples Therapy.   Given the key theoretical and practical debate generated by comparing IOCT and BCT, the investigation by Snyder and associates (Snyder & Wills, 1989; Snyder et al., 1991) will serve as this chapter's exemplar.

BCT was considered the only empirically demonstrated effective couples intervention until the mideighties. Snyder and Wills (1989) pointed out that although EFT (S. M. Johnson & Greenberg, 1985a) is also based on psychodynamic principles, implementation of EFT does not explicitly require identifying early, perhaps unconscious, causes of intrapsychic and interspousal difficulties. IOCT, on the other hand, was designed specifically to uncover and interpret unconscious conflict that presumably causes intrapsychic and interspousal conflict, in order to improve the couple's relationship. The investigators (Snyder & Wills) recruited seventy-nine predominantly white midwestern couples, who were randomly assigned to BCT (twenty-nine), IOCT (thirty), and wait-list control group (twenty). Therapists were four masters-level social workers and one psychiatric nurse. Pains were taken to examine treatment biases, and examination found that all practitioners were comfortable with "pluralistic practice." Considerable efforts were also taken to ensure treatment fidelity. IOCT, as described by Snyder and Wills (p. 41),

> emphasized the resolution of conflictual emotional processes that exist either within one or both spouses separately, between spouses interactively, or within the broader family system. This approach attempted to integrate individual, couple, and family functioning by addressing developmental issues, collusive interactions, incongruent contractual expectations, irrational role assign-

ments, and maladaptive relationship rules. Therapists used probes, clarification and interpretation in uncovering and explicating those feelings, beliefs, and expectations that spouses had toward themselves, their partners and their marriage, which were either totally or partially beyond awareness, so that these could be restructured or renegotiated at a conscious level. The emphasis was on the interpretation of underlying dynamics that contributed to the current, observable marital difficulties.

Both approaches were applied over an average of nineteen sessions each, and attrition rates were negligible. Results showed that both interventions performed comparably well at termination and at six-month follow-up on measures of psychological distress, and more so on couples satisfaction. The authors suggested that, despite the procedural differences in the two approaches, the comparable outcomes might be attributed to common core therapeutic processes.

Four years later, fifty-five couples were followed up and interviewed by phone. Results showed a striking difference in outcomes between the two groups. Those who had undergone BCT showed a divorce rate of 38%, whereas those who had received IOCT had a divorce rate of 3%. In addition, those in the IOCT group who were still married showed greater marital satisfaction. Results suggest that psychodynamically oriented methods may help modify underlying cognitive attributions about the interactional problems between the partners. Perhaps understanding the "underlying rules" of the relationship is necessary for couples to generalize the benefits of marital therapy across situations and maintain their behavior changes.

These studies provoked lively debate regarding the relative efficacy of BCT and IOCT. Jacobson (1991) argued that the type of IOCT used appeared to have much in common with clinically sensitive BCT, thus demonstrating that enhanced BCT was better than the older, more behaviorally focused BCT. Respective camps also argued over which approach was more likely to benefit from investigational bias. However, it was clear in the original study (Snyder & Wills, 1989) that the investigators went to considerable pains to examine the biases of the investigators (who generally expected BCT to be superior), and noted that they used BCT as explicated in Jacobson and Margolin 1979 (described in more detail below) without attention to later cognitive embellishments. Nevertheless, without further replication or additional efficacy and change-process studies, it is hard to determine which approach is superior or even what the essential components of each intervention are. Results from a single study can easily be anomalous. Further research might reveal reliable differences.

Couples Therapy for Specific Mental Health Problems

A recent comprehensive review of the literature on empirically supported couples and family interventions for marital distress and adult mental health problems supports the view that couples and family interventions can often augment results for an individual with a specific disorder (Baucom, Mueser, Shoham, Dainton, & Stickle, 1998). Using relatively strict methodological criteria for reviewing the literature, the authors noted that there are different purposes in applying couples and family interventions when one person is a primary target of that intervention. First, some interventions are seen as partner- or family-assisted treatments to help in the implementation of a treatment regimen (as when the partner or family helps a mother overcome agoraphobia). Second, a couple's or family's interactional behaviors may be the focus of treatment insofar as those behaviors have a negative impact on a family member with an individual disorder (as when helping family members not to reinforce a father's excuses for heavy drinking). Third, a couple or family may have difficulties that need to be addressed, and their collective behaviors may exacerbate the symptoms of a family member who may also be the focus of individual treatment (e.g., helping a family with a mentally ill son by reducing conflict, improving communications, and problem solving to improve overall family climate and reduce stress). What the evidence does not support are early family-therapy theories that assert that individual "identified patient's" symptoms or problems were caused by the family's behavior.

With regard to findings, Baucom et al. (1998) concluded that couples and family work may be as effective as individual interventions for OCD, agoraphobia, and alcohol-abuse disorders, and couples and family work may enhance the individual client's therapeutic success. Involving a partner or other family member in assisting in exposure treatments for people with OCD or agoraphobia, for example, can help the individual succeed. Engaging a partner or family member in helping the drinking spouse or other family member can boost therapeutic outcomes as well. That family psychoeducation with mentally ill people is effective has been supported by a wealth of evidence. Lastly, although it is not clear that couples interventions are superior to individual treatment when a partner is depressed, it appears that couples therapy "might be preferable to individual psychotherapy among maritally discordant couples with a depressed wife because it leads to improvement in both depression and marital discord" (Baucom et al., p. 68). However, if the partners are not distressed, individual treatment may be more effective in many cases.

BCT is prominently represented in research on applying couples work to individual disorders. It was shown to be effective for couples where the alcoholic spouse voluntarily participated in treatment, (e.g., O'Farrell et al., 1993; McCrady et al., 1986; O'Farrell & Fals-Stewart, 2003). This approach treats spouses together by focusing directly on reducing drinking and improving the relationship. BCT was also shown to be effective in reducing depressive symptoms in one spouse while improving marital functioning overall (Beach & O'Leary, 1992). In a controlled trial comparing couples therapy with medication, EFT was found to have superior results for the female spouse at six-month follow-up (Dessaulles, Johnson, & Denton, 2003). Few controlled trials have been conducted with other couples approaches when applied to an individual partner's disorder.

Interventions for Sexual Dysfunction in Couples

It is not uncommon for couples to experience some problems with sexual expression or for one or both partners to experience a diagnosable sexual dysfunction. The *DSM-IV-TR* categorizes them as disorders of *sexual desire* (hypoactive or sexual aversion disorder), *sexual arousal* (female arousal disorder or male erectile disorder), *orgasmic disorders* (difficulty achieving orgasm in females or males, and premature ejaculation in males), and *sexual pain disorders* (pain associated with intercourse; involuntary contraction of outer muscles of the vagina, causing marked distress). In addition to the fact that the validity of the current taxonomy for sexual disorder has been questioned (R. C. Rosen & Leiblum, 1995), it is also understood that the notion of sexual dysfunction is highly relative to cultural context. Reliable data on the prevalence of sexual dysfunctions is hard to come by, given the highly variable methods used in relevant surveys. However, recent estimates based on reviews of epidemiological data suggest that from one-quarter to one-half of all women and about 15% of men experience disorders of low sexual desire, about 20% of women and 10% of males experience inhibited sexual arousal, and from 5% to 15% of both men and women experience inhibited orgasm, although premature ejaculation is experienced as a problem by 30% to 40% of men. Sexual pain disorders are more common for women than for men (15% versus 3%; *DSM-IV-TR*; Dzieglielewski, Resncik, Nelson-Gardell, & Harrison, 1998).

Multidimensional assessment for sexual dysfunction is now widely recommended for couples (Dzieglielewski et al., 1998; Rosen & Leiblum, 1995). There is a greater emphasis on understanding sexual dysfunction within the context of the individual's interpersonal history and the quality of their current relationship. In addition, special consideration should be given to a thorough history of sexual behavior, especially to history of sexual abuse. Rape, incest, and sexual molestation, depending on type, severity, and relationship to the abuser, may have a profound effect on a person's ability to enjoy sexual intimacy as an adult (Barnes, 1995). In addition to a thorough history taking, assessment of current sexual functioning should focus on both the individual and the dyad. Individual factors that may impede sexual expression include depression, anxiety, distorted cognitions that may inhibit sexual enjoyment, substance abuse, overall fitness, and other specific medical concerns. A medical examination should be given high priority when sexual dysfunction is present.

As for the couple, practitioners and researchers have come to see the necessity of formulating the sexual assessment within the context of the couple's overall relationship (Rosen & Leiblum, 1995). Problems in couples' relationships can either contribute to sexual difficulties or become a barrier to their amelioration. Couples conflicts regarding parenting differences, money, sharing household or employment obligations, spending recreational time together, and other mundane matters may lead to chronic anger, resentment, and control struggles, and further erode communications and emotional intimacy. Other problems such as chronic jealousy, lack of trust, and resentment due to previous infidelities can become barriers to sexual enjoyment. A detailed functional assessment of the nature of the couples' sexual problems and formal diagnosis is also required.

Although Masters and Johnson (1970) are credited with emphasizing anxiety reduction and gradually increasing sensual pleasure through their pioneering "sensate focus" technique, current interventions have become more comprehensive. Overall, clinical reports and uncontrolled studies (e.g., Sarwer & Durlak, 1997) have shown that a multidimensional assessment and combination of cognitive-behavioral and medical intervention are the most promising strategies to reduce sexual dysfunction and increase sexual expressiveness between partners (LoPiccolo, 1994; Dzieglielewski et al., 1998; Rosen & Leiblum, 1995). These strategies focus on identifying and treating cognitive or interpersonal emotional barriers to intimacy; decreasing anxiety that may be inhibiting sexual arousal; gradually increasing sensual interactions through a combination of sexual stimulation aids (practicing sexual fantasy, use of adult videos, other sexual stimulation devices such as vibrators); increased sensual interaction between the couples leading to mutual masturbation; and other highly stimulating noncoital activities, and, ultimately, sexual intercourse. Social workers can enhance their work with couples by mastering assessment skills to determine couples' sexual well-being within the context of their relationship, and by incorporating some of these methods into their practice repertoire. Other interventions may require collaboration with specialists in this area, including medical personnel.

Interventions for Domestic Violence

Rubin (1991) and Abel (2000) have both noted the lack of evaluation research for interventions with battered women and other victims of domestic violence. Methodological limitations of the existing research include deficiencies in defining interventions and outcomes, few controlled trials, small samples, and little follow-up data. Nevertheless, some writers have made helpful recommendations based on their clinical experience. Jordan and Walker (1994) recommend thorough individual assessments for abuse history; multiple services, including consultation, education and prevention, crisis care, psychiatric services and inpatient facilities, counseling, and clinical and residential services; support services for the victims and close linkage with the police and criminal justice system to provide services to the perpetrators; availability of residential services for victims, including shelters, foster care as needed, and other transitional living arrangements; and endorsement of the assumption that domestic violence is a crime, and the safety of the victims is the number one priority. In addition to the immediate need to protect women and children from domestic violence, follow-up services are needed to maintain psychosocial improvements over time. Although there is a lack of research in this area, one promising uncontrolled evaluation of an intervention with twenty-eight battered women demonstrated significant improvements in both appraised social support and self-esteem (Tutty, 1996). Given the enormity of the problem, much more research is needed.

The literature comparing conjoint versus separate treatment for domestic violence is also sparse. Brannen and Rubin (1996) found no outcome literature to support the superiority of one modality over another, in general. Although using conjoint interventions for domestic violence is generally discouraged, there is some evidence to suggest that when the violence is less severe (i.e., pushing, slapping, often by both partners), with no evidence of serious injuries or of enduring psychopathy on the part of the (usually) male partner, couples therapy may be as effective as individual therapy and does not seem to result in any more risk to the spouse (Stith, Rosen, & McCollum, 2003). In their controlled study comparing two cognitive-behavioral approaches (conjoint group therapy versus gender-specific group therapy) as part of court-mandated services, Brannen and Rubin found that both groups made comparable gains, although there may have been some advantage for the conjoint group if the husband had an alcohol problem. However, caution should be exercised in treating couples where one member has been seriously violent. There are only six controlled studies to date, and many suffer from methodological weaknesses including high dropout rate, recidivism, and poorly defined outcome criteria. More research is needed to explore this approach as an option for less violent couples. Other approaches such as the Ackerman family model or solution-focused approaches have not been examined empirically.

Descriptions of Effective Interventions

Below, the basic steps for implementing EFT and BCT are presented. Practitioners should become familiar with both interventions, and examine possibilities for eclectic implementation.

The two major tasks in EFT are to access the couple's emotional experience and to change their interactional positions. S. M. Johnson and Greenberg (1988, p. 66) divide the descriptive intervention procedures into nine steps, usually lasting up to fifteen visits or so.

1. "Focus on the partners' experience of the relationship, particularly on their emotional responses to each other and how these responses mediate the closeness or separateness of the bond between them and the process of self-definition" (p. 83).

2. Identify the recurrent negative interactional cycle. The authors suggest that the "therapist must *see* the cycle" (p. 85).

3. Access unacknowledged feelings underlying interactional positions. The therapist must help the clients reenact the core emotional conflicts in the here and now.

4. Redefine the problem(s) in terms of underlying feelings. The explanation or interpretation of the couple's enacted experience should integrate their affective, cognitive, and behavioral experiences.

5. Promote identification with disowned needs and aspects of self by helping clients reconnect with thoughts, needs, and feelings that the partners have not been relating to their dysfunctional reactions and subsequent conflicted cycles. For example, a husband raised by hypercritical parents tends to be "thin-skinned" if his wife innocently queries him about when a home project might be finished. The practitioner can help him to identify the hurt feelings behind his angry and defensive responses.

6. Encourage acceptance by each partner of the other's experience. This involves helping a partner, listen, acknowledge, empathize, and accept the other's feelings and experience without needing to discount or criticize them.

7. Facilitate the expression of needs and wants to restructure the interaction. The partners move from defensive postures to openly expressing their desires in ways that may engender more caring responses.

8. Establish the emergence of new solutions. The couple solidifies gains by practicing more emotionally open communication of thoughts, feelings, and needs, and replaces old negative and dysfunctional interactions.

9. Consolidate new positions. Continue with new practices engendered above, but emphasize the before-and-after differences of a couple's interactive cycles. This review of progress should include an examination of future scenarios that may threaten their successes. Continue practicing clearer emotional expression to prevent returning to the old, negative interactive cycles.

Although there have been modifications to the basic BCT approach over the years (e.g., inclusion of explicit methods targeting changes in cognitions about the relationship), the basic behavioral methods of BCT are described in detail in Jacobson and Margolin 1979. In addition to a thorough assessment and relationship building with the client, practitioners should incorporate the following analysis, exchanges, and skills into their intervention.

Cognitive Analysis.   Practitioners should closely examine cognitive distortions and faulty attributions made by each partner about the other and about the relationship. Over the course of treatment, the practitioner should use the interactions in the sessions as well as homework to challenge these distortions, attempt to "disconfirm" them, and allow for alternative and more constructive cognitions to replace them.

Behavioral Exchange.   A key behavioral component to BCT is rooted in behavioral exchange, that is, an increase in engaging in behaviors that are positively reinforcing for the other partner. This behavioral exchange can not only reduce tensions and conflict, but also increase a sense of goodwill and caring, and lead to greater intimacy in the relationship. The rationale is simply to reduce costs in the relationship and to increase rewards (benefits). The practitioner must focus on identifying those positive behaviors that please the other partner. These hypotheses about what is pleasing or not must be tested out by the couple.

"Love days" are an effective way to highlight or concentrate on behaviors that are mutually pleasing. Couples must practice being clear and explicitly letting the other know what is pleasing and what is not. Behavioral exchange contracts (also called contingency contracting) can accompany this method and either be an explicit exchange of favors (known as the quid pro quo) or built upon a "good faith contract," where there is no specific contingency or timetable, but a general agreement by each partner that they will follow through on their end of the bargain. Ideally, contingency contracting should be a positive exchange as opposed to a form of coercion or threat ("If you don't come home on time, I'm leaving!")

Communication Skills. Communication skills (empathy, listening, reflecting and validating, accepting what the partner feels, responding clearly, expressing thoughts and feelings assertively) are key for each partner to examine the other's thoughts and feelings, and to create accurate expectations regarding what each partner likes and dislikes. Poor communication can easily lead to further misunderstanding and distress. The practitioner focuses on sensitively providing good feedback regarding the communication strengths and deficits of the couple, and gives instructions on how to improve communication. The couple must then rehearse these skills during sessions and practice more effective communication skills at home.

A hierarchy of topics should be addressed, gradually moving from moderately stressful areas of conflict to those that are more challenging as the couple increases their skills and capacity to tolerate talking about "touchy" subjects. Although maintaining effective communication skills appears to be an elementary aspect of intervention, they are challenging to maintain under stress, and are one of the more often cited problems that couples report about their relationships.

Problem-Solving Skills. Jacobson and Margolin (1979, p. 213) define problem solving as "the process by which change agreements are reached." Effective problem-solving skills are also necessary to weather normal stresses that can strain a long-term relationship from time to time. Although others have defined the steps of problem solving in behavior approaches somewhat differently (see D'Zurilla & Goldfried, 1971), the steps are similar to those recommended in BCT.

1. Define the problem(s) specifically.
2. Express one's feelings assertively.
3. Take responsibility for one's contribution to the problem and its solution.
4. Take turns briefly defining the problem.

5. Emphasize solutions (avoid attributing blame).

6. Work toward compromise and maintain a sense that we're in this thing together.

7. Record the agreements.

Combining the Best Couples Therapies: Theoretical Integration or Pragmatic Eclecticism?

Having noted the lack of clear superiority for any of the evidence-based interventions for couples work, several practitioner-researchers have recommended integrated or eclectic approaches drawn from psychodynamic, emotionally focused, and behavioral approaches (Halford, 1998; Lawrence, Eldridge, & Christiansen, 1998; Epstein, Baucom, & Diauto, 1997). However, the distinction made in chapter 3 between integration (common change processes) and eclecticism (combined techniques) should be kept in mind.

In explaining their rationale for EFT, S. M. Johnson and Greenberg (1988) cite attachment theory and object-relations theory (Bowlby, 1969; Guntrip, 1969), thus placing the theoretical foundation for EFT squarely in the psychoanalytic tradition. Snyder and Wills (1989) subscribe to a similar view regarding IOCT. Simply put, proponents of psychoanalytic couples theory aver that adult couples' problems are the consequence of disordered relational templates or prototypes laid down in early childhood that resulted from the failure of mothers (primarily) to adequately nurture their children. These disturbed early psychological templates are recapitulated in later relationships. This assumption is the cornerstone of psychoanalytic theory. Nevertheless, S. M. Johnson and Greenberg, (1988, p. 77) later assert that "the etiology of each couple's dance is a matter for speculation."

Other proponents of EFT (e.g., Lawrence et al., 1998) have elaborated on this theoretical premise. The emphasis on both the individual partners' relationship history and their dyadic development as a couple can provide a basis for identifying disordered attachment patterns based on the *apparent similarity between the way adults behave in interpersonal relationships and how infants behave.* References by Lawrence et al. to attachment theory, then, appear to be more analogous than explanatory, because causation cannot be inferred from "similarity," or correlation.

S. M. Johnson and Greenberg (1988, p. 29) also claim to have identified the theoretical change processes that are engaged in the implementation of EFT:

> Emotionally focused couples therapy is an affective systemic approach in which the emphasis is on changing interactional cycles and changing each person's intrapsychic experience, which maintains, and is maintained by, the cycle. In this treatment, the emphasis is first on identifying the negative interactional cycle early in treatment and then on accessing each partner's unexpressed underlying emotions, which serve to organize his or her views of self and partner. The problem cycle, the individuals, interactional positions, and

their behaviors are then redefined in terms of the newly experienced under-lying emotions. Thus, for example, the blaming of one partner may come to be seen as an expression of an underlying fear of abandonment, vulnerability or loneliness, while the withdrawal or rejection of the other partner may come to be seen as an attempt at self-protection or fear of engulfment. This approach is based on an integration of experiential and systemic approaches.

Although EFT techniques may, in fact, activate processes by which the couple better recognize their respective interpersonal "templates," there is no evidence that these templates were necessarily (or even primarily) created by disruptions in early childhood. In short, practitioners of different theoretical allegiances can agree that interpersonal change processes are related to "relational templates" without making the inference that these templates (interpersonal schemata?) were created primarily by mother-toddler experiences.

Given the absence of developmental research supporting attachment the-ory as a necessary or sufficient explanation for couples conflict, a more reason-able theoretical model would include multiple independent, additive, and inter-active influences on the emergence of interpersonal schemata over time: temperament, lifelong relationship experiences (including childhood family experiences, nonromantic friendships, adolescent and adult intimate relation-ships), and cultural disposition toward relationship roles (such as equality versus subservience), among other factors. In addition, practitioner-researchers should be open to the possibility that a number of change processes (alone or in com-bination) may be at work during the intervention itself: the emotionally correc-tive experience of the therapeutic relationship; better insight and increased empathy regarding each partner's respective concerns, fears, complaints, and relationship patterns; increased hope and better morale in dealing with marital distress; improved skill at problem solving; and increased self-efficacy as com-munications and problem-solving efforts improve. These explanations are not mutually exclusive, nor are they necessarily incommensurate with "early attach-ment" explanations. Given that relatively little research specifically targets change processes in couples therapy, however, it is currently not known *how or why couples interventions are effective*, even when they do work successfully.

It may be more fruitful for researchers and practitioners to focus on identi-fying and combining the most effective techniques of both EFT and BCT. These techniques include helping partners understand and clarify each other's cogni-tive appraisal and expectations; identifying and understanding emotionally charged interactional patterns; changing behaviors through improved communi-cation and problem solving to optimize interpersonal rewards; and ameliorating the impact of individual disorders such as substance abuse or depression on the relationship. Given the available evidence for effective couples work, flexible eclecticism seems to be a reasonable option. Further research on couples work should emphasize the identification of optimal combinations of intervention skills and matching them to client needs and preferred change modalities (e.g., emotionally focused analysis, behavioral contracting, or some combination).

Integrating Couples Therapy with Interventions for Child Behavior Problems

Couples dysfunction and problems in the couple's children often coincide. Although not all children's problems are the result of parental conflict, children's emotional and behavioral difficulties can be the direct result of parental conflict or be exacerbated by a conflicted couple. Child and adolescent behavior problems and disorders can also place considerable strain on a couple as intimate partners and as parents. Couples who are having trouble communicating and resolving other problems are likely to have difficulty cooperating as parents. Sanders, Markie-Dadds, and Nicholson (1997) point out the lack of controlled studies regarding childhood behavioral outcomes resulting from marital interventions. Nevertheless, some sensible guidelines are in order to address the challenging assessment issues when dealing with a family that is experiencing marital difficulties, parenting problems, and behavioral difficulties in the children.

Although sequencing the intervention is not easy to plan, addressing the conflicts in the couple is essential in order to help them "work from the same page" as parents. Some of the marital concerns may have to be temporarily put on the back burner. Sometimes getting together for the sake of the children can be a positive experience for the couple. Achieving some success in improving communication and problem solving regarding parenting may set the stage for improvements in their partner relationship as well. However, as Sanders, Markie-Dadds, and Nicholson (1997, p. 531) point out, "The key is to demonstrate rather than assume a functional relationship between child and marital problems. This requires close attention to the day-to-day co-variation between marital stress and child problems, as well as parents' own view of the relationship between parenting problems and their marriage." In the next few chapters, the emotional and behavioral difficulties of children and adolescents will be addressed. It is assumed that couple well-being and functioning as intimate partners and as parents (assuming a two-parent household) is a decided advantage (if not critical) for effective interventions with their children.

IMPLEMENTING AND EVALUATING THE EVIDENCE-BASED INTERVENTION PLAN

CASE STUDY: CONNOR AND LUIS

Connor and Luis arrived for their first visit with telltale signs of a serious problem: Connor sported a fat lip, and Luis wore a neck brace one usually sees on a person who's been in an automobile collision. First, they needed to explain. "This type of thing has never happened before. We frightened ourselves because of it. We don't want it to ever happen again." According to Luis, they had been arguing about "Connor's stonewalling over commitment. It's time we move in together." Luis, apparently, "got in Connor's face," and Connor went to push him back. Blows were exchanged, and Luis's hit his target. Connor lost his temper after he saw his own blood on his shirt, got one of his well-toned arms around Luis's neck, and threw him over a chair. Sitting in the hospital emergency waiting room gave them time to calm down and talk. They decided to get some help. Brad, the social worker, agreed that it was a good move for them to seek some help.

Connor, age thirty-six, came from a white working-class family. He has two younger sisters and two brothers. His father worked in a variety of blue-collar jobs, often two at a time, to support the family. His mom worked at home, but as the kids got older, she also supplemented the family income by taking in sewing work from the neighbors or helping out in a local catering service on weekends. Connor and his family all knew he was a little different. When he came home from school crying because the other kids called him "faggot" or "homo," his father and brothers would compensate by "showing me how to fight, to toughen me up." He has never discussed being gay with his family except for coming out to one of his sisters when she gently confronted him. His dad dismissed his lack of marrying as his being "just the bachelor type," and his mom was still waiting for him to "meet the right girl." Connor loves his parents and his family, although it had been difficult socially over the years to deal with queries from them about when he was "going to settle down." He never begrudged his family's lack of sensitivity to "gay issues." "I know they love me. That's just the way it is in their social circles." Connor himself still seemed to harbor some shame about being gay.

Luis, age thirty, grew up in a very poor section of Puerto Rico. He was the son of a Puerto Rican father and Mexican mother. They emigrated to the United States after they married. Luis was eight years old at the time. He grew up in poverty in a northeast American city, and left home at sixteen after being threatened by members of a rival gang. After two years of wandering, lying about his age, and working menial jobs, he joined the army, obtained his GED, and served overseas in the first Gulf War, during which he was awarded a Purple Heart (the army didn't "ask" and Luis didn't "tell" about his homosexuality). Luis met Connor in a gay bar outside of town. They hit it off immediately, and have seen each other steadily over the past two years. Luis worked his way up to become regional manager of a chain of men's clothing stores. Luis is openly gay, active in gay politics, and after his stint in the army became much less tolerant of people (like Connor) who are not "in-your-face gay." Luis also reported no notable grievances with his parents, "came out" a long time ago with his mom (whom he e-mails weekly), has been on a conversational basis with his dad, but has kept his distance from his brothers, who, he says, "have a major case of machismo."

Multidimensional/Functional Assessment: Defining Problems and Goals

Before the army "straightened me out," Luis had been a bit reckless over the years with drug use (injecting) and had been more active sexually, but in recent years he has maintained abstinence from drugs (although he occasionally overindulges in very dry martinis). He says he has been faithful to Connor for at least one year. Both partners have had HIV testing within the past year, and both are negative. Luis reports no specific mental health problems, enjoys his work, and is on good terms with his coworkers, family, and friends. He reports no specific health problems, although he has unsuccessfully been trying to quit smoking, another bone of contention between him and Connor.

Aside from an early bout with heavy drinking and some depression in his early twenties before he "came out to myself, at least," Connor presented no mental health problems other than his distress over his conflicts with Luis. He always took good care of himself physically, and continues in a well-paying career as a bank loan manager. He expressed the wish that he could be more open with his family about being gay, but was afraid that it would create distance.

The couple expressed to Brad many positives about their relationship, but they seemed to feel that it was seriously threatened if Connor remained unwilling to publicly acknowledge it. As the issue of commitment and living together continued to come up, the matter of "coming out" became a potentially more explosive catalyst for conflict. Any number of situations triggered this recurring patterning and sequencing of escalating tension and subsequent conflict. For example, Luis was invited to a management dinner where he was to receive an award for exceeding company production targets. He was quite proud of the honor, and felt it was going to provide some stability in his career. Connor was also pleased for him. But when Luis asked him to come to the event, Connor began to make excuses. Given that they both worked in the same community, it became apparent that Connor was concerned about running into people with whom he conducted business. Luis, in detecting this hesitation, became angry, began to object and quarrel vehemently, and provoked Connor, who admitted that he was concerned about being seen with Luis in public. "I also felt shame, guilt, and anger at being cornered." After these types of arguments, Connor tended to withdraw from Luis for a few days, and would wait for the anger to dissipate, until the next inevitable crisis. Although these confrontations were more easily avoided in the past when "we gave each other more space," they had become more frequent after the subject of living together was on the table. Over the previous two months, the couple had intense arguments at least once per week, with the residual anger lasting days at a time. The proportionate increase of angry and hurt feelings had begun to erode an otherwise loving and considerate relationship. The recent physical fight brought these matters to a head.

Luis saw Connor as not "serious about the relationship," and Connor saw Luis as "wanting too much too soon from me." They both said they loved one another but saw the relationship at a crossroads: either they would find some compromise, or the relationship was over. Given the recent fight, they were not strongly optimistic that a resolution could be found. They felt that this difference about "coming out" may have "poisoned the well," and had left only angry words and hurtful feelings. Although one of the goals of the intervention was to improve their ability to discuss this explosive issue without doing harm to one another, it was not clear at that juncture whether the goal was for Connor to become more openly gay.

Selecting and Designing the Intervention: Defining Strategies and Objectives

Brad discussed with the couple his thoughts about using an eclectic approach to their dilemma (table 11.1). He briefly described the emotion-focused analysis of EFT and the problem-solving/communications aspects of BCT. The couple agreed that they thought they could benefit from both. Luis preferred the emphasis on understanding feelings, Connor was a bit more analytical and liked the problem-solving emphasis of BCT. Brad helped Luis express his frustration more calmly and explain to Connor about how hurt he felt when Connor wouldn't show his commitment publicly. Conversely, the practitioner helped Connor identify his own fears that were provoked when Luis pressed him too hard to come out and say "the hell with what everybody else thinks." Connor needed to express to Luis that he felt his career and relationship with his family and other friends were at stake. The practitioner helped them identify and express these feelings, but also listen to the other partner without editing or contradicting him. He told them that they did not need to "buy into" what the other partner was saying, but simply accept it at face value though the problem remained unresolved for the time being.

BCT also provided a valuable complement to the initial progress with EFT. First, examining interpersonal misattributions (cognitive distortions about the other partner's motives or feelings) seemed to help clarify what the emotional conflicts were about. For example, in examining Luis's anger and hurt about Connor's reluctance to join him at his award ceremony, a cognitive analysis of "what's behind the feelings" revealed that Luis also thought Connor may have been seeing someone else. "If I'm at the award ceremony, where is he going to be? Does he have something more important to do or someone he'd rather be with?" Until that point, it had never occurred to Connor that his reluctance to "come out" was being interpreted as showing a lack of interest or faithfulness to Luis. Conversely, Luis's intense expressions of anger evoked a number of difficult feelings in Connor, including anger, fear, and shame. When the practitioner examined the cognitions behind these feelings, Connor said it was quite similar to a lifetime of subtle rejection and difference he had felt from other males (his dad, brothers, and schoolmates). As in the past, these feelings caused him to withdraw and "clam up." Improved communications and improved behavioral exchange may have helped to disconfirm these distorted attributions.

Second, the use of communication skills seemed to complement the goals of EFT, that is, to improve a consistent, honest, and open expression of emotions. Maintaining eye contact, active listening, not interrupting, and giving accurate feedback appeared to reduce the heat of an emotionally charged argument. Brad's coaching during sessions served as rehearsal for practice at home (three nights per week after dinner, for no more than half an hour, and before their favorite television shows).

Third, behavioral exchange activities were used to help them gradually solidify their commitment and express caring to one another as they temporarily accepted that coming out might not happen right away. In this way, the decision about if, when, and how to go public did not represent the only indicator of their feelings for one another, but rather, provided some breathing room as they learned how to discuss it in a more constructive light. They also agreed to a "good faith" commitment: Connor agreed to have Luis over for a dinner of his choice once a week, and Luis (at Connor's request) agreed to attend a "stop-smoking clinic," because, as Luis put it, "I plan on being with Connor for a while." In addition, on "love days" (Saturdays), they planned to do something together, and agreed not to discuss any timetable for Connor during that time.

As the couple became more comfortable accepting each other's present position for the time being, and as they were able to calmly and (more empathically) discuss each other's thoughts and feelings about their dilemma, it became clear that their desire to commit to one another grew. "If we can work through this, we can probably work through anything," said Connor. "This is the big test," Luis agreed. In a more analytical way, they began to address this challenge as a problem to be solved, rather than an unmovable barrier in their relationship. Brad encouraged them to address two questions in the session and during their planned discussions at home: using an accounting metaphor (since they are both in the business world), what were the costs and benefits of Connor's coming out versus the cost and benefits of staying in the closet? The couple were asked to "submit a report" in two weeks' time. As they made improvements in communicating and problem solving, the social worker felt that there was less of a need for weekly visits. Clearly this problem needed to be worked on by them together. Brad provided a list of gay support groups in outlying areas for Connor to consider, as others might be able to provide some advice and support on how to navigate the coming-out process. Connor agreed to consider it.

They returned two weeks later with a rather thoughtful analysis. Coming out would probably cause Connor some temporary discomfort, but in the long run, more problems if he didn't. "It's like a colleague of mine who goes to AA says: people change when they get 'sick and tired of being sick and tired.' Well, I'm sick and tired of hiding who I am. I don't know when I'm going to do this, or how I'm going to go about it, but I know I'm going to have to deal with it sooner or later. It might as well be sooner. Besides, I'm not the only gay guy working for my bank, and they seem to handle it OK. And when I come out, I want Luis to be there for me."

Selecting Scales and Creating Indexes to Monitor and Evaluate Client Progress

Perhaps, with minor modifications, any of the standardized scales for couples (e.g., MAT, MDS) could have been useful for examining overall relationship satisfaction or couple distress. But given the specific nature of the problem, other individual indexes were included to target problems and monitor progress (table 11.1): a self-anchored scale (1, "no discomfort at all," to 10, "extremely uncomfortable") to gauge the level of comfort each partner had in discussing coming

TABLE 11.1   The client service plan for Connor and Luis

Problems	Goals	Sample Objectives	Interventions	Assessment Tools
Intense conflict over one partner's reluctance to become openly gay	Improve their ability to communicate on emotional matters	Identify core emotional conflicts at the center of the couple's differences	An eclectic combination of emotionally focused therapy to identify emotionally charged patterns; and behavioral couples therapy with addition of a cognitive component: emphasis on communication skills and problem solving	MDS; monthly as a global measure of couple satisfaction/distress
Repeated pattern of explosive arguments about "coming out" with subsequent sullen retreats for days at a time	Improve intimacy Reduce level of anger Work toward a resolution of the problem on their own	Define the repeated interactional cycle the couple engages in repeatedly		Two self-anchored indexes (scored 1–10) to track weekly progress: level of comfort in discussing their mutual feelings about being more public with their relationship; level of commitment
		Examine cognitive distortions that are associated with intense feelings related to core conflict between them	Practitioner-provided information on gay men's support group to get "other points of view on the perils of coming out"	Self-developed chart to assess the pros and cons of coming out for Connor
		Improve communication skills to enhance discussion of emotionally charged issues (coach during sessions, and practice at home 3 times weekly)		
		Plan and agree to carry out "good faith" contract: Connor to cook 3 times weekly; Luis to attend "stop-smoking" clinic		
		Problem-solving plan: engage in a cost-benefit analysis of "coming out" and submit a report		

out, and a scale (1, "no commitment at all," to 10, "extremely committed") to assess their level of commitment to their relationship.

SUMMARY

Working with couples often reveals a range of both individual and interacting problems, including mental health disorders, substance abuse, domestic violence, child abuse and neglect, and the typical problems of the partners themselves: distrust, frequent arguments, parenting differences, money problems, difficulties with extended families, and sexual problems and dysfunctions, among others. Working with couples is also often the linchpin for working with children and families. A number of validated instruments can aid in the assessment of couples problems, and the body of research on effective couples practice has continued to grow. BCT and EFT provide sound approaches to helping couples enhance intimacy, improve communications, and become more adept at solving problems. Although little is known about how these interventions work, learning these methods is essential for social workers who work with adults, children, and their families.

CHAPTER 12

ANXIETY AND DEPRESSION IN CHILDREN AND ADOLESCENTS

Depression and anxiety disorders in children are often referred to as "internalizing disorders." Although this term is descriptively not quite accurate (some symptoms of depression and anxiety are externalized, that is, observable), children manifest many of the symptoms of depression and anxiety covertly. Thus, finding out what is troubling a child (especially very young children) can be a challenge for the social worker. In addition to being depressed, the same child may also be experiencing a combination of generalized anxiety, social phobia, school phobia, obsessional concerns and/or compulsions, and symptoms related to stressful or traumatic events. Variations in the course of both depression and anxiety disorders are common. A number of brief, valid and reliable scales for measuring internalizing disorders are available to enhance MDF assessment.

There is a range of effective cognitive-behavioral interventions for depression and anxiety disorders in children and adolescents. In addition to developing an empathic rapport with the child or adolescent, these methods include self-monitoring, anxiety management, and other coping skills often combined with contingency management techniques to be implemented by parents, teachers, and other significant adults in the child's life. It has been increasingly recognized that implementing these approaches within behavioral family therapy may be ideal for many children with internalizing disorders. Helping a child learn to cope better with depression and anxiety is challenging if the adults in their life are abusive, neglectful, apathetic, incompetent, or otherwise detrimental to the child's coping efforts.

Medications appear to have limited benefits for children and adolescents experiencing depression and anxiety-related problems, except for those suffering from OCD. Evidence-based interventions with children suffering from anxiety and depression have become a multifaceted strategy of relationship building with the child, the family, school personnel, and other influential people in the child's life. The approaches are effective for developing and enhancing the child's coping skills and improving psychosocial well-being. Because of the high rate of co-occurring symptoms in anxiety and depressive disorders and the similarity in key intervention skills, they are both addressed in this chapter.

ASSESSMENT OF ANXIETY DISORDERS

Background Data

It is common for children to be sad or afraid. Fortunately, children's episodes of sadness and fear are usually ephemeral, and most children learn to cope with life's stresses, losses, and disappointments without developing clinical disorders. Fears and anxieties are also developmentally linked. Fears in early childhood tend to be more discrete (animals, strangers, a dark basement) whereas fears among older children and adolescents are more likely to be a response to social inhibitions, school performance, and health concerns. Fear reactions may be linked to a combination of factors, including temperament, past experiences, and their social and environmental context. Fears (or the appraisal of fear) may also be linked to culture-bound beliefs and gender roles. Anxiety in children may be manifested by extreme behavior such as temper tantrums, clinging, and problems with peers. Given the ubiquitous nature of childhood fears, however, they should be seen as a "disorder" only if they cause significant dysfunction in the child's life (Last, 1989; Ronan & Deane, 1998; *DSM-IV-TR*; Fonseca & Perrin, 2001). These disorders include simple phobias, separation anxiety, OCD, PTSD, and generalized anxiety disorder. Childhood anxiety disorders constitute a significant risk factor for mental health problems in adulthood (Ost & Treffers, 2001).

Anxiety and depression are likely to co-occur with other problems in children and adolescents. This co-occurrence suggests that discriminating among internalizing disorders in children may not be a valid approach (Schniering, Hudson, & Rapee, 2000; Spence, 1997). From one-quarter to one-half of depressed youth also manifest an anxiety disorder, and about 10–15% of youth with anxiety disorders suffer from a depressive disorder as well. There are a number of suggested reasons for this co-occurrence: they share common risk factors, they are causally related, or they have independent but correlated risk factors. Other spurious reasons may include treatment-seeking factors (people who seek services for mental health problems are more likely to have other problems as well; Verhulst, 2001).

A thorough review of epidemiological research revealed prevalence rates for all the childhood anxiety disorders to be from 1% to 3% (Verhulst, 2001), but estimates of prevalence and incidence (including cross-cultural differences) vary across studies, probably because of methodological differences. Schniering et al. (2000) reported the following prevalence data for individual anxiety disorders: separation anxiety (children 3.5–4.1%; adolescents 0.6–2.4%), generalized anxiety (children 2.9–4.6%; adolescents 2.4–4.2%), social phobia (children <1%; adolescents up to 6.3%), simple phobia (children 2.4%; adolescents 5.1%), OCD (children 0.2–1.2%; adolescents 3%), and panic disorder ("rare" in children and young adolescents; older adolescents 0.3%). Rates of anxiety disorders for children exposed to severe stressors such as fires or sexual abuse can be considerably higher. Perhaps half of adolescents, especially females, have experienced panic attacks at one time (although few ever meet the criteria for panic disorder), and they appear to be related to life stressors such as family problems or school pressures (Ollendick, Mattis, & King, 1993). In an Australian study of 648 adolescents, female adolescents appeared to have more fears than boys, and younger adolescents reported more fears than older ones (Ollendick & King, 1994a). Most of these fears concerned physical danger and negative social evaluation.

Social phobia was not considered clinically substantive until recently. Although many young people are shy, most mature out of serious social inhibitions. More recently, social phobia has come to be seen as potentially debilitating, and may be a precursor for the later development of social inhibitions and related problems. Children who suffer from social phobia show considerable distress in a range of social situations, and this distress is likely to occur frequently as life demands more social interaction. Social phobia co-occurs with other childhood and adolescent phobias (e.g., avoidance disorder, separation-anxiety disorder) and with depression (Beidel & Morris, 1995).

Separation-anxiety disorder manifests itself as extreme anxiety when the child is separated from the primary caretaker. The symptoms include the full range of anxiety symptoms. School refusal appears to be a common manifestation of separation-anxiety disorder. The onset may be sudden or gradual, and it appears to be linked to the onset of adult agoraphobia and panic attack (B. Black, 1995). In separation-anxiety disorder, the child's behavior is marked by verbal and behavioral expressions of anxiety and fear, such as crying, clinging, screaming, tantrums, and phobic reactions to specific situations, and these problems are often accompanied by somatic complaints, such as stomach aches.

OCD in children and adolescents is similar to the diagnostic description for adults: unwanted obsessions, intrusive images, thoughts, impulses that cause distress, and compulsions such as repetitive thoughts or behaviors performed repeatedly or ritualistically in an effort to reduce the distress caused by the obsessions. Children may not recognize the obsessional thoughts to be irrational, excessive, or unreasonable. The preoccupation with ritualizing in a fruitless attempt to escape the anxiety associated with obsessions can be incapacitating for a child. Depression and social phobia often accompany childhood OCD. Children with OCD are likely to be anxious about germs, contamination, fears of harm to self or others, excessive religiosity, and guilt. The most common compulsions (in descending order) include washing and cleaning, counting, repeating, touching, and ordering/straightening up. These symptoms can be very disruptive and interfere with functioning at home, in school, and with friends. Mean age of onset for OCD is ten, more boys than girls manifest OCD symptoms, and the parents of a child with OCD are more likely to have OCD than other adults in the general population. There is considerable co-occurrence of OCD with other childhood disorders, including other anxiety disorders, depression, and specific developmental disorders. Many of these children also suffer from Tourette's syndrome and other tic-related disorders. OCD in childhood has a poor prognosis if left untreated, and at least half of these children will continue to struggle with it into adolescence and adulthood. Before the introduction of SSRI medications, the long-term outlook for a child with OCD was quite negative (March, Leonard, & Swedo, 1995; Shafran, 1998; Piacentini & Bergman, 2000).

Children may also experience the full range of symptoms associated with PTSD (Amaya-Jackson & March, 1995; Yule, Perrin, & Smith, 2001). Symptoms are similar to those experienced by adults (reexperiencing, avoidance, arousal), but are manifested somewhat differently. Children may reexperience the trauma through repetitive acting out, ritualistic play, or nightmares. Avoidance and numbing may manifest as regressive behaviors such as thumb sucking, detachment, and shutting down of feelings and expressiveness. Arousal is likely to be observed as nightmares, sleep problems, irritability, angry outbursts, depression, and poor concentration. Children suffering from PTSD are also likely to experience other anxiety disorders, depression, disordered behaviors including sexual and aggressive play, interpersonal difficulties, and conduct disorders.

PTSD in children can be precipitated by a wide range of events, including kidnapping and assaults, physical and sexual abuse, natural disasters, life-threatening illness, and medical procedures. There appears to be a dose-response relationship between the severity of the traumatic event and its effect on the child. Life-threatening events appear to be the most traumatic. As with adults, however, there is considerable variability in the way children respond to traumatic events. These mediating factors include differences in temperament, appraisal of the threat, and attribution of blame. Although there are few reliable data from large epidemiological studies on the prevalence and incidence of PTSD in children, Yule et al. (2001) estimate that about one-third or more of children who experience life-threatening accidents and more severe forms of trauma are likely to develop PTSD. Because not all children who are exposed to a traumatic event develop PTSD symptoms, clinicians should avoid overdiagnosing the problem by attributing all of a child's anxieties and related symptoms to trauma (Amaya-Jackson & March, 1995; Yule et al). Although diagnosing children with PTSD remains controversial, it has come to be seen as useful for theory development, assessment, and intervention planning (P. Smith, Perrin, & Yule, 1998).

Symptoms of anxiety and depression also vary by environmental stressors, including poverty and community violence. For example, given the disproportionate socioeconomic stressors experienced by many youth in racial minorities, it is reasonable to investigate whether children of color experience more severe and qualitatively different types of anxiety and related symptoms. In a thoughtful review of the literature, Safren et al. (2000) found mixed results but emphasized the need for more racially, ethnically, and culturally informed research. Treadwell, Flannery-Schroeder, and Kendall (1995), however, showed that African-American and white youth shared very similar fears (e.g., death or dead people, getting lost, getting poor grades, getting burned in a fire, failing a test, being hit by a car, falling from high places, not being able to breathe). Research on racial and cultural differences in depression and anxiety in youth is likely to reveal considerable overlap along with some differences.

Theories

Anxiety has been defined as a broad collection of distressing cognitive, behavioral, and physiological responses, and *fear* has been construed as a situation-specific event. However, research suggests that there is little theoretical or practical value in distinguishing the terms *fear* and *anxiety* (Barrios & Hartmann, 1997). Thus, they are generally used interchangeably in the theoretical literature.

Psychoanalytic theorists have noted that anxiety disorders often emerge during childhood and adolescence, and have emphasized inadequate nurturance in childhood as the primary cause (e.g., Erikson, 1950; Loevinger, 1976). Last (1989) suggested that the etiology of childhood separation anxiety, for example, is related to an overdependent relationship with the child's mother, although the theoretical mechanisms for this overdependency are open to explanation (e.g., common temperament, learning experiences, "hostile-dependent" relationship). Other psychoanalytic theorists have contended that anxiety disorders in children are symbolic expressions of early fears, but little evidence is offered to explain how anxiety disorders develop over time.

More recently, attachment theorists have argued that the roots of future anxiety disorders are related to anxious attachment style in early childhood (Bowlby, 1980; Ainsworth, Blehar, Waters, & Wall, 1978), an extension of earlier psychoanalytic theories. Cognitive maps of interpersonal relations between infants and their mothers (i.e., "internal working models") are presumed to be manifested in different attachment styles, such as secure versus avoidant, ambivalent, or disorganized. Proponents of attachment theory assert that anxiety originates in an infant's uncertainty about caregiver availability, and varied responses to that uncertainty account for different types of childhood anxieties. The early task of children is to gradually develop self-regulatory cognitive, behavioral, and physiological processes to cope with anxiety and stressful stimuli: "it is clear that caregiver-child social interactions are pivotal events that both exacerbate underlying constitutional problems and also function independently to produce difficulties in self-regulation" (Costanzo, Miller-Johnson, & Wencel, 1995, p. 87). Although childhood anxiety problems often continue into adulthood, however, the causal mechanism for this linkage is not well understood (Westenberg, Siebelink, & Treffers, 2001). Attachment style can be considered one risk factor (Manassis, 2001), but longitudinal data have never clearly demonstrated a substantive causal link between early childhood attachment and adult anxiety disorders. To establish such a link, one would have to account for a range of other independent and mediating factors (Costanzo, et al.). Generally, developmental research reveals a decrease in the influences of childhood factors as children grow older and as other factors begin to affect their development.

Biological temperament (e.g., proneness to anxiety, arousal) appears to make a significant contribution to the development of anxiety disorders (Oosterlaan, 2001; Kagan, 1989). Anxious temperament, manifested in shyness or social inhibition, appears to be largely inherited, and this inhibition appears to be stable over time and across situations. Children at higher risk of anxiety disorders show greater temperamentally related inhibition than children not at risk for anxiety disorders. In addition, it appears that parents of anxious children are more likely to have anxiety disorders themselves. The longer children remain temperamentally inhibited, the more likely they are to develop anxiety disorders in later childhood. However, not all anxious children develop anxiety disorders as they age. Temperament is mediated by a number of psychosocial influences that can exacerbate or diminish the predisposition to anxiety. Although there is now a general assumption regarding the neurobiological links in anxiety between childhood and adulthood, much less is known about the specific pathways for the development of individual anxiety disorders (Biederman, Rosenbaum, Chaloff, & Kagan, 1995). In addition to psychosocial influences, these physiological processes apparently involve the neurotransmitter systems and the hypothalamic-pituitary-adrenal system (R. Sallee & Greenawald, 1995). Research regarding the linkages between neuropsychological patterns in children and adolescents and specific anxiety disorders is in its early stages (Hooper & March, 1995).

As discussed in chapter 7, a multivariate model of anxiety disorders is slowly emerging (Craske, 1997; Rapoport, Swedo, & Leonard, 1992). Clearly a combination of interacting genetic, temperamental, parental/familial, psychological, and situational factors contribute to the development and maintenance of anxiety disorders in children. Genetic studies have shown a stronger tendency for developing anxiety disorders in monozygotic twins than in dizygotic twins. Behavioral inhibition appears to be a product of temperament and is characterized by "withdrawal, seeking comfort from a familiar person, and suppression of ongoing behavior, when confronted with unfamiliar people or novelty, as opposed to vocalizing, smiling, and interacting with the unfamiliar object or setting" (Craske, 1997, p.A14). Children with anxious temperaments are more likely to develop one or more anxiety disorders. Inhibited children also appear to be more prone to fears related to social situations and social evaluation, and these children's parents are more likely to have anxiety disorders as well. Nevertheless, the emergence of an anxiety disorder appears to depend on environmental factors, including childhood stressors and parental reinforcement of fears. A mother's ability to promote healthy attachment with her children is directly affected by the level of social supports (including a helpful partner) and other social and environmental stressors (Manassis, 2001). Extreme environmental stressors related to poverty, poor access to health care, fear of crime, and domestic and community violence are likely to have a significant impact on the parent's ability to nurture children in a constant and secure environment. Extreme stressors (early separation anxiety, other catastrophic trauma) can cause changes in neurocircuitry that may predispose a child to develop a specific anxiety disorder. Whether physiological or environmental factors predominate may determine the type of anxiety disorder that develops (e.g., separation-anxiety disorder versus PTSD; F. R. Sallee & March, 2001). More research is needed on the impact of social and environmental stressors on the development of specific anxiety disorders.

Within the context of this biopsychosocial framework, a good deal of theoretical work has been done on cognitive processes and anxiety disorders. Current theoretical formulations are the same as those for adults (see chapters 7–9), and these theories tend to favor social-cognitive and information-processing models. Anxiety disorders in children seem to develop from the interaction of cognitive, physiological, and behavioral components that reciprocally interact with stressful stimuli in the social environment (Ronan & Deane, 1998). Cognitive models focus on both negative schemata and maladaptive (dysfunctional) thinking, and information-processing models focus on how affective information is cognitively processed (Prins, 2001). Within this perspective, the original traumatic event (as in the case of PTSD, for example) is seen as a conditioned stimulus setting a process in motion whereby cognitive, physiological, and behavioral components of the response to the traumatic event become somewhat repetitive and reinforcing. The child seems incapable of resolving the meaning of the event, because of continued avoidance, emotional numbing, repetitive play, and other manifestations of the disorder. Cognitive, affective, physiological, and environmental cues accompanying the traumatic event then become conditioned stimuli often called "traumatic reminders." Through stimulus generalization, these reminders become capable of eliciting a conditioned response in the form of PTSD symptoms. By trial and error, children attempt to reduce PTSD symptoms through avoidance and other anxiety-dampening rituals (Amaya-Jackson & March, 1995, p. 288). These behaviors fail to extinguish the anxiety, however, and tend to reinforce and sustain it. Generally, anxious children tend to judge threats as more serious, underestimate their own coping abilities, report more catastrophizing thoughts than nonanxious children, and have more negative cognitions than nonanxious children (Prins, 2001). How these factors interact over time will vary among children, given their respective strengths and vulnerabilities.

The theoretical explanations for cognitive processes associated with OCD (discussed at more length in chapter 7) are similar for adults and children, and are closely tied to the rationale for effective therapy: graded exposure with response prevention until the obsessions and compulsions associated with anxiety are extinguished (Shafran, 1998). The behavioral model emphasizes anxiety reduction by the process of habituation, that is, exposing the child/adolescent to the feared situation and preventing the compulsive response. With repeated administration, children's fear that the anxiety will overwhelm them decreases. The core obsession appears to be related to children's exaggerated belief that they may be responsible for harm befalling someone, and that if they engage in certain repeated rituals, the likelihood of harm will be reduced (Salkovskis, 1985). Although their obsessional concerns may be broader than just harm occurring to others, the emphasis on cognitive constructions of OCD focuses on exaggerated and distorted belief in the oversignificance of one's thoughts, that is, *the belief that these thoughts have some influence on external outcomes.* Such preoccupations cause considerable psychological distress in young people with OCD. Effective treatment, however, tends to focus on the behavioral components (exposure and response prevention), although some literature addresses the use of overt cognitive challenges to the intrusive and irrational thoughts.

Ollendick and Hirshfeld-Becker (2002) reviewed the theoretical literature regarding social-anxiety disorder within the framework of developmental psychopathology. They note that all children do not "grow out of" early social inhibitions, and that children and adolescents who suffer from social-anxiety disorder show unreasonable responses to a number of often unavoidable social situations in which they feel they will be harshly evaluated. These sometimes incapacitating reactions include wariness, crying, and panic attacks. The average age of onset appears to be midadolescence. Although uncommon in younger children, social-anxiety disorder appears to be one of the more common disorders in late adolescence and early adulthood, with lifetime prevalence estimated between 5% and 15%. As with other disorders, developmental pathways can be diverse but appear to involve an interacting combination of temperament, parental and peer influences, and other social-learning experiences.

Regarding anxiety disorders in general, Kendall (1993) distinguishes between lack of cognitive skill and maladaptive cognitive processes and thought content. Cognitive distortions are presumed to start developing in childhood. Although innate temperament also plays a role, distorted cognition can develop as a result of adults communicating exaggerated threats of perceived danger to a child. Overprotection may also influence children to believe that they are not capable of coping with these perceived dangers, thus leading to deficits in self-confidence or self-efficacy. Anxious cognitions and negative affect appear to be common among children who experience anxiety or depression, and it is believed that anxiety and depression in children are closely related psychological processes.

Key Elements of Multidimensional/ Functional Assessment

The qualitative aspects of conducting an MDF assessment with children experiencing anxiety disorders and depression are quite similar. Thus, major aspects of assessing internalizing disorders will be addressed in this section. Special considerations for conducting qualitative assessment of depression along with a brief review of relevant instruments for measuring depression will be addressed in the second part of this chapter.

To conduct assessment with children, a basic developmental knowledge of their cognitive and emotional-processing capacities is required. Assessment of childhood internalizing disorders must take into account the child's "acquisition of specific cognitive and social cognitive skills . . . language skills, understanding of emotions, concept of self and self-awareness, and perception of others" (Schniering et al., 2000, p. 470). To the greatest extent possible, assessment of the child should use multiple informants: parents, family, the school, and other significant people in the child's life. In addition, it should be understood that not all symptoms of anxiety or depression (which are common in children) need to be resolved. A key benchmark should include some determination that depression or anxiety is having a significant impact on the child's psychological and social well-being (Barrios & Hartmann, 1997).

Diagnostic criteria for anxiety and depressive disorders in children are similar to criteria reviewed in previous chapters for adults (*DSM-IV-TR*) and need not be repeated here. However, there may be some differences in symptom presentation. Generalized anxiety disorder (including overanxious disorder of childhood) has symptoms like those in adults, including restlessness, trouble falling asleep, and chronic worrying, but may also include fears about unlikely or unrealistic occurrences. Although panic disorder with agoraphobia is not typically diagnosed in children, similar symptoms may express themselves as separation-anxiety disorder or school phobia. Symptoms of OCD in children mirror those in adults, but children may be less likely to think that their behavior is strange, whereas an adult may know "rationally" that the behavior makes no sense. In a similar manner, a child with a simple (specific) phobia may not find the phobia to be unreasonable. Children also experience many of the same symptoms as adults when suffering from PTSD or acute stress responses (e.g., hypervigilance, fear, avoidance, numbing), but manifest others differently (e.g., repetition of the experience through play). As with adults, differential diagnosis among depression and specific anxiety disorders can be difficult, yet fine-grained distinctions in diagnostic categories probably serve little heuristic purpose, given the often heterogeneous symptom profile of clients and the fact that effective intervention for these disorders uses similar methods.

Given the high co-occurrence rates between anxiety and depression, children and adolescents suffering from symptoms of either problem should be given a thorough MDF assessment. In addition to a detailed and thorough history (i.e., trauma, recent stresses, abuse and neglect, family history of depression or other mental illnesses), their distress should be examined across all areas of functioning. These areas include mental status, such as specific fears, cognitive distortions, mood disturbances, and somatic complaints; family and social functioning, for example, parental nurturance and discipline, abuse or neglect, relations with peers, and school performance; health; and general environmental stressors, such as poverty, violence, and adequacy of food, clothing, and shelter. MDF assessment will result in a unique portrait of each child's distress. For example, a shy child suffering from depression and obsessional worries may not outwardly manifest or verbalize serious concerns, but may be severely isolated from peers and suffering in quiet distress. Younger children experiencing separation anxiety are likely to show symptoms only under circumstances where they are confronted by the threat of being "left alone" or "taken" from their parent. A child who has been sexually abused may manifest any number of symptoms of PTSD, such as numbing or dissociation, but may not meet all criteria. An older child or young adolescent who has suffered similar abuse may be more outwardly aggressive toward peers. Children suffering from internalizing disorders are likely to manifest complex and somewhat unique combinations of cognitive, physiological, and behavioral signs and symptoms that do not fit neatly into diagnostic categories, and assessment should consider all potential symptoms of internalizing disorders as they are manifested across different social contexts.

A detailed functional analysis is essential to carefully map out how the child's anxiety and depression interact with everyday events in the context of family functioning, school, community, and social activities (Fonseca & Perrin, 2001; McGlynn & Rose, 1998). Multiple sources of information are essential, given many children's limitations regarding self-report, and attempts should be made to reconcile inconsistencies in collateral reports. Assessment of a child should become increasingly focused on the cause-effect details that appear to determine the child's daily distress across three key response modes: cognitions, physiological responses, and behavior. For a child suffering from an anxiety disorder, for example, these three response modes are likely to emphasize fear-related cognitive appraisal of events, physiological arousal indicated by overt signs of fear, and behavioral avoidance of people or situations that elicit the fear response (Ronan & Deane, 1998). This analysis will include a detailed cause-effect mapping of the relationship among antecedent events that the child appraises as frightening, physiological symptoms of anxiety, the resulting behaviors, and the ensuing social consequences that either mitigate or exacerbate the anxiety, as when parents reinforce the avoidance and worsen the anxiety over time. For example, a socially phobic child may dread going to a birthday party where she expects "nobody will like me." At the first sign of disinterest on the part of a fellow party-goer (antecedent), the child may become anxious, flushed, and panicked, and run into a bedroom to hide (behavior), a response that temporarily reduces some of the anxiety. An attending adult can either try to coax the child gradually back into the group by having her sit and fold party napkins with another child a distance from the screaming mob, or the child can be sent home with her parent, a move that would reinforce the child's expectations that "parties are not fun" and thus should be avoided. Sequential linking of cause and effect must be tied to specific events that have high salience for the child. In addition, the specifics must be examined within and across a variety of different contexts: home, school, the playground, after-school activities, and other relevant circumstances. As noted earlier, multiple sources of data from multiple points of view will help fill in a comprehensive picture of the severity and contextual specificity of the child's distress.

Additional assessment tools and procedures can enhance the MDF assessment. Silverman and Serafini (1998) recommend the inclusion of problem-behavior checklists (e.g., CBCL, depression and anxiety scales), observation in the natural environment, or analogue assessment (e.g., have the child role-play a problem on the school playground or at home with parents). Self-monitoring techniques may also be illuminating and could be a constructive way of engaging the parents and the child in treatment. Depending on the child's age, he or she may be willing and able to keep a diary, complete a chart, use self-anchored mood-rating scales, or engage in other self-monitoring activities collaboratively developed with the practitioner. Another useful approach to the functional assessment of anxiety disorders is the Behavioral Avoidance Test, whereby specific anxiety problems can be observed in vivo as they unfold (Fonseca & Perrin, 2001). The child who may be fearful of going outside (agoraphobia), approaching others in a social situation (socially phobic), or touching a "dirty" doorknob (obsessive-compulsive) can be placed in these situations and encouraged to "go as far as they can" before the anxiety becomes too uncomfortable for them. This test can be performed across different situations to determine whether the fear is contextually specific or more generalized. Close attention is paid to the antecedent events that appear to provoke the fearful or avoidant behavior and the ensuing consequences in specific circumstances.

MDF assessment is incomplete without conducting a thorough behavioral family systems assessment, either at home or in the consulting office. For children suffering from serious depression and anxiety disorders, a behavioral family systems assessment, at a minimum, should include the following considerations: quality of parental nurturance, disciplining and communication patterns and style with children, parental cooperation with one another regarding parenting matters, the quality of the couple's relationship, an examination of ongoing problems between parents and children or between siblings, other co-occurring difficulties experienced by the parents (e.g., mental illness, substance abuse, criminality), relations between the family and neighbors or the school, and general health of family members. The key assessment hypothesis regarding the identified child's well-being is straightforward: how do parental and family behaviors affect the day-to-day psychosocial functioning of the child, and, conversely, how does the child's behavior affect other family members? What factors within this family system, the school, and community directly and negatively affect the child, and what specific psychological and social supports are available to the child? A detailed functional assessment of these influences on the child often readily reveals those factors that have the greatest impact on the child's mood and behavior. Some of those problems may be readily amenable to change; others may be more challenging. If factors within the family and immediate social environment appear to cause or exacerbate the child's difficulties, however, it should not be assumed that they are the only causes. Temperamental influences as well as stressors external to the family should also be considered.

Instruments

Broad-band scales such as the CBCL (Achenbach, 1991) and the Shortform Assessment for Children (SAC; Glisson et al., 2002) measure both internalizing and externalizing disorders. These scales are discussed in chapter 2. A number of well-established narrow-band scales measure anxiety disorders and depression (Costello & Angold, 1988; Greenhill, Pine, March, Birmaher, & Riddle, 1998; W. M. Reynolds, 1994; P. Smith et al., 1998; Myers & Winters, 2002). Scales for measuring anxiety disorders will be discussed in this section, and scales for measuring symptoms of PTSD will be examined in chapter 14.

One of the most widely used scales for measuring anxiety in children is the Fear Survey Schedule for Children (FSSC; Scherer & Nakamura, 1968). The FSSC was originally developed for children ages 9–12, but later revised by Ollendick (1983) to make it applicable to a wider age range (7–18). The current version uses a three-point scale, and has been shown to have good internal consistency, good test-retest reliability, and adequate convergent and discriminant validity. Some studies showed good cross-cultural validity as well for the FSSC. The Spence Anxiety Scale for Children (SASC; Spence, 1997) has forty-five items and is scored "never to always" on a four-point (0–3) scale. Five subscales derived from factor analysis with a large community sample measure panic-agoraphobia, social phobia, separation anxiety, obsessive-compulsive problems, generalized anxiety, and physical fears. The SASC has good internal consistency, test-retest reliability, and solid evidence for construct validity. The Children's Yale-Brown Obsessive-Compulsive Scale (CYBOCS; W. Goodman et al., 1989) is the children's version of the YBOCS described in chapter 7, and is scored in a similar manner.

One of the more promising scales that combines good psychometric characteristics and practicality for use in clinic settings is the Screen for Child Anxiety-Related Emotional Disorders (SCARED) developed by Birmaher et al. (1997). The initial scale was developed with an item pool of eighty-five randomly ordered questions representing the different types of anxiety disorders in the *DSM-IV*. Three-hundred and forty-one children (ages 9–18, 59% female, 82% white, 18% African-American) and 300 parents completed the initial questionnaire. Factor analysis was employed to identify the major factors. This process resulted in almost identical five-factor solutions for the children's sample and the parent's sample. The five factors were somatic/panic, generalized anxiety, separation anxiety, social phobia, and school phobia. These five subscales were formed out of thirty-eight items scored 0 ("not true or hardly ever true"), 1 ("sometimes true"), and 2 ("true or often true"). Internal consistency for the final thirty-eight-item scale was .93, and subscale alphas ranged from .74 to .89. Test-retest reliability was .86 for the total scale, and subscale interrater reliabilities were .70–.90. The SCARED showed good discriminant validity among different anxiety disorders (using structured interview *DSM* criteria scales) and other diagnoses (e.g., depression). Very few differences were found in psychometric characteristics between gender, age, and race. In a replication study (Birmaher et al., 1999) with 190 outpatient children and adolescents and 166 parents (evenly split between boys and girls aged 9–18; a quarter of the sample African-American and Hispanic), a forty-one-item version of the SCARED demonstrated the same factor structure as the original with comparable evidence for reliability and validity. A brief (five-item) version of the scale was also developed by selecting the items that best predicted each anxiety disorder. The brief scale demonstrated psychometric characteristics comparable to the original scale, and performed well as a screening device. A score of 3 or more on the five-item scale indicates a serious problem with anxiety. The SCARED also showed good convergent and divergent validity with a sample of 295 children and adolescents in a mood-disorders clinic when the scale was correlated with the CBCL and the State-Trait Anxiety Inventory for Children (Monga et al., 2000). The forty-one-item SCARED is printed here (instrument 12.1) as an exemplar instrument given its

INSTRUMENT 12.1   Screen for Child Anxiety-Related Emotional Disorders (SCARED)

Below is a list of sentences that describe how people feel. Read each phrase and decide if it is "not true or hardly ever true," or "somewhat true or sometimes true," or "very true or often true" for you. Then for each sentence, fill in the answer (0-2) that corresponds to the response that seems to describe you for the last 3 months.

Client/parent scores the following items according to this scale:

  0 not true or hardly ever true
  1 somewhat true or sometimes true
  2 very true or often true

____ 1. When I feel frightened, it is hard to breathe
____ 2. I get headaches when I am at school
____ 3. I don't like to be with people I don't know well
____ 4. I get scared if I sleep away from home
____ 5. I worry about other people liking me
____ 6. When I get frightened, I feel like passing out
____ 7. I am nervous
____ 8. I follow my mother or father wherever they go
____ 9. People tell me I look nervous
____ 10. I feel nervous with people I don't know well
____ 11. I get stomachaches at school
____ 12. When I get frightened, I feel like I am going crazy
____ 13. I worry about sleeping alone
____ 14. I worry about being as good as other kids
____ 15. When I get frightened, I feel like things are not real
____ 16. I have nightmares about something bad happening to my parents
____ 17. I worry about going to school
____ 18. When I get frightened, my heart beats fast
____ 19. I get shaky
____ 20. I have nightmares about something bad happening to me
____ 21. I worry about things working out for me
____ 22. When I get frightened, I sweat a lot
____ 23. I am a worrier
____ **24. I get really frightened for no reason at all**
____ **25. I am afraid to be alone in the house**
____ 26. It is hard for me to talk with people I don't know well

_____ 27. When I get frightened, I feel like I am choking

_____ **28. People tell me I worry too much**

_____ 29. I don't like to be away from my family

_____ 30. I am afraid of having anxiety (or panic) attacks

_____ 31. I worry that something bad might happen to my parents

_____ 32. I feel shy with people I don't know well

_____ 33. I worry about what is going to happen in the future

_____ 34. When I get frightened, I feel like throwing up

_____ 35. I worry about how well I do things

_____ **36. I am scared to go to school**

_____ 37. I worry about things that have already happened

_____ 38. When I get frightened, I feel dizzy

_____ 39. I feel nervous when I am with other children or adults and I have to do something while they watch me (for example: read aloud, speak, play a game, play a sport)

_____ 40. I feel nervous about going to parties, dances, or any place where there will be people that I don't know well

_____ **41. I am shy**

Scoring guidelines: a score of ≥ 25 may indicate the presence of an anxiety disorder. Scores higher than 30 are more specific. A score of 7 for items 1, 6, 9, 12, 15, 18, 19, 22, 24, 27, 30, 34, 38 may indicate panic disorder or significant somatic symptoms. A score of 9 for items 5, 7, 14, 21, 23, 28, 33, 35, 37 may indicate generalized anxiety disorder. A score of 5 for items 4, 8, 13, 16, 20, 25, 29, 31 may indicate separation-anxiety disorder. A score of 8 for items 3, 10, 26, 32, 39, 40, 41 may indicate social-anxiety disorder. A score of 3 for items 2, 11, 17, 36 may indicate significant school avoidance. A score of 3 or more on the five-item scale (in bold print) indicates a serious problem with anxiety.

---

brevity, sound psychometric characteristics, and potential utility as a treatment outcome monitoring scale (Birmaher et al., 1997; Birmaher et al., 1999). The five-item version is highlighted in bold type. The child self-report version of the scale is presented here. (The parent version is identical, except that each item is prefaced with "My child"). Practitioners could use the scale in a face-to-face format with the child, reading along if necessary.

SELECTING EFFECTIVE INTERVENTIONS

The following review summarizes the outcome research on anxiety disorders in children and adolescents. It is understood that practitioners who intend to learn and apply evidence-based approaches for internalizing disorders in general will consult specific treatment manuals and practice texts, and adapt these methods as the client's individual assessment profile and circumstances necessitate.

Major reviews of the literature overwhelmingly support cognitive-behavioral interventions as the most effective methods for ameliorating anxiety disorders in children and adolescents. CBT for children addresses these problems through some combination of cognitive restructuring (reexamining and challenging anxiety-related thoughts realistically), relaxation and other coping methods, problem-solving strategies, guided exposure (imaginal or in vivo), and contingency management methods such as collaborating with the family to use positive reinforcement (Ollendick & King, 1994b, 1998; Kazdin, 1994b; Kendall, 1993; N. J. King, Hamilton, & Ollendick, 1988; W. M. Reynolds, 1992; S. N. Compton et al., 2002). Shaping children's behavior directly by guiding them into the anxiety-provoking situation until the fear extinguishes, and reinforcing these efforts, appears to be a well-established approach for achieving anxiety reduction even without the use of preliminary anxiety-reduction techniques such as relaxation training (Ollendick & King, 1998). Nevertheless, in actual practice, covert and direct methods are likely to be combined. It has also become increasingly evident that incorporating psychoeducation and cognitive-behavioral methods into family therapy may be a preferred approach under some circumstances, although more research in this direction is needed (Northey et al., 2003). Studies on the efficacy of childhood PTSD are also in the beginning stage of research development (S. N. Compton et al., 2002).

School Refusal

Last, Hansen, and Franco (1998) randomly assigned fifty-six children to twelve weeks (one-hour session each) of either cognitive-behavioral intervention (combined graduated exposure and coping-skills exercises, including self-talk carried out by parent and child) or an educational support group that combined information about school refusal, self-monitoring with diaries, and supportive listening. Unlike the CBT condition, no specific directives were provided regarding how to confront fear in the educational support group. Outcome measures included attendance records and standardized scales for measuring fear, depression, and other outcomes. There were no differences between the two groups in demographics or in dropout rates. At posttreatment and follow-up, there were no significant differences in either attendance or severity of symptoms between the two groups. The small sample size may have masked substantive clinical differences: posttreatment attendance was higher for the CBT group (65% versus 48%), a greater number of students in the CBT group maintained improvement from pretreatment to follow-up (65% versus 40%), and fewer students in the CBT group showed no improvement (14% versus 40%). Although these findings are suggestive, further controlled trials for school-refusal treatments are needed.

Barrett, Dadds, and Rapee (1996) conducted a similar test of CBT for children with a range of anxiety disorders (i.e., overanxious, separation, social phobia). The seventy-nine children ranged from seven to fourteen years of age, and were recruited from community centers, schools, and medical and mental health practitioners, or referred from parents in response to advertisements. The children were randomly assigned to three groups: individual CBT, CBT plus family involvement (in which each of twelve seventy-minute sessions were split between CBT and family sessions), and a wait-list control group (which received intervention after the waiting period). CBT was based on Kendall's work (1994, described in detail below), which combines a number of cognitive and behavioral coping-skills techniques. The CBT plus family intervention included the same CBT method, and parents were taught to actively reinforce "courageous" behaviors and ignore excessive complaining or anxious behaviors in their children. Parents were also taught how to deal with upsets, gain awareness of their own anxiety-coping abilities, and model better coping responses for their children through improved problem solving and communications. A battery of well-validated standardized measures were used, several of them identical to those employed in Kendall (1994).

Results clearly demonstrated successful outcomes for both active treatment conditions, and results were maintained at six and twelve months. Almost 70% of those who received CBT (with and without family involvement) no longer met the diagnostic criteria for the disorders, and only 26% of the wait-list clients no longer met the criteria. At one-year follow-up, results revealed that 95.6% of clients who received individual and family intervention no longer met diagnostic criteria for their disorder, and both self-report and clinician ratings showed significantly more improvement than did reports for the group that received only CBT. However, the addition of family therapy appeared to significantly benefit only younger children (ages 7–10) as compared to older children (11–14). It appears that in treating anxiety disorders, the addition of the family educational component may be particularly important for younger children. A six-year follow-up study with fifty-two of the original clients demonstrated that the vast majority of the children (85.7%) maintained their gains overall, but the results of CBT and CBT plus family were ultimately comparable (Barrett, Duffy, Dadds, & Rapee, 2001). Thus, these data suggest that the inclusion of family members may be helpful in the short run.

In a study with sixty children who met similar diagnostic criteria, Barrett (1998) compared group CBT with group family therapy that included parents and children. The sample comprised thirty-two boys and twenty-eight girls. About one-quarter of the sample was from non-English-speaking homes. Barrett employed the same intervention protocol (adapted to group format) and the same measures as used in Barrett, Dadds, and Rapee (1996). Children were randomly assigned to the three groups (group-CBT, group-family therapy, and wait-list, who were treated later). The interventions were conducted over twelve weekly two-hour sessions. As expected, the two active treatment groups saw significant improvement, with a marginally superior outcome for the family group. At twelve-month follow-up, 85% of the children who received the group family intervention no longer met their particular diagnosis for anxiety disorder. Overall, this and previously reviewed studies suggests that CBT is an effective intervention for children's anxiety disorders, it can be equally effective when administered in group format (Silverman & Berman, 2001), and the addition of parent education as part of the intervention may marginally improve outcomes. More research is needed to replicate these findings.

To examine whether CBT methods could be successfully implemented in a group format, Silverman, Kurtines, Ginsburg, Weems, Lumpkin, et al. (1999) compared a group format with a wait-list control group. Fifty-six children (thirty-four boys, twenty-two girls) with a mean age of ten, about half of whom were Hispanic, were randomly assigned to the treatment and control conditions (in a two-to-one ratio of treatment group to control). Children in the control condition were provided treatment within eight to ten weeks. The children had a variety of anxiety diagnoses, including overanxious disorder, social phobia, and generalized anxiety. A combination of broadband and narrowband measures was used. In the group CBT format, parents and children met in separate groups for forty minutes, and then children met with their parents together for fifteen minutes. The therapeutic content in the two separate groups was similar. The CBT group used contingency management approaches to help the parents reinforce the child's exposure to anxiety-provoking situations, and they practiced the use of coping responses. Results indicated that 64% of the treatment-group participants no longer met the diagnostic criteria, whereas only 13% in the control group did not. Based on CBCL scores, 82% of the children improved to within the cutoff range for internalizing disorders, whereas only 9% of the control group did so. Reduction in symptoms was maintained at twelve months. The authors concluded that CBT can be effectively implemented in group format with parents.

In a controlled trial to compare the efficacy of contingency management (CM) to self-control (SC) therapy and an educational support (ES) condition, Silverman, Kurtines, Ginsburg, Weems, Rabian, et al. (1999) recruited 104 children (ages 6–16; 54 boys) and their parents. About one-third of the sample was Hispanic American. Participants met *DSM* criteria for phobic disorder; most had simple phobias such as nighttime fears and small animals, and most had another anxiety disorder. The investigators used a battery of well-validated scales. Treatment manuals were employed to guide all three interventions, which lasted for ten sessions (forty minutes with child, twenty-five minutes with parents, and jointly for fifteen minutes). The contingency management condition emphasized teaching parents to use reinforcement principles to facilitate graduated exposure experiences for their child, using a fear hierarchy. Self-management skills were based on Kendall's work (1994), and the educational component included supportive listening and didactic material on phobias. Eighty-one percent of the original participants completed the study. All three conditions performed comparably well at completion, and at 3-, 6-, and 12-month follow-ups. These findings were comparable across multiple measures that reflected the points of view of child, parent, and practitioners. The authors speculated that it is possible that the participants in the ES condition took what they learned from the lectures and attempted self-directed exposure on their own. Future research is needed to replicate these findings and identify effective treatment components.

Obsessive-Compulsive Disorder

Cognitive-behavioral interventions and SSRIs alone or in combination have been demonstrated to be the treatments of choice for OCD (Piacentini & Bergman,

2000; Manassis, 2000; March & Leonard, 1996). Whether these work better in combination is a question that needs further research. March (1995) published a thorough review of the literature and identified thirty-two articles describing psychosocial interventions for OCD, twenty-five of which were qualitative case reports and seven single-subject designs. He concluded that exposure with response prevention (EX/RP) is the most effective method to date, and inclusion of the family may help facilitate the treatment process and improve outcomes. Psychodynamic therapies have been demonstrated to be ineffective with OCD, and the empirical literature provides no support for unfounded claims regarding symptom substitution, dangers associated with interrupting compulsive rituals, uniformity of learned symptoms, and an incompatibility between therapy and pharmacotherapy (March, 1995). Although responses to EX/RP are robust, many clients continue to improve after treatment as well (e.g., D. J. Fischer, Himle, & Hanna, 1998). However, over longer periods of time (e.g., 9–14 years after treatment) symptoms of the disorder can return for a significant percentage of clients (e.g., Bolton, Luckie, & Steinberg, 1995). More controlled trials with long-term follow-up are needed.

The techniques for treating OCD in children are quite similar to those for treating adults (Shafran, 1998). The child is gradually exposed to the feared situation that elicits the anxiety (e.g., touching a kitchen garbage can) and then prevented from engaging in the compulsive ritual (repeated hand washing). The length of time for exposure to the feared situation accompanied by response prevention is extended gradually, and (as with adults) the child monitors anxiety level with a self-anchored scale (the SUDS). A hierarchy of fears (from doorknob to garbage can to toilet bowl) is developed with the child, and family members are included in order to facilitate the treatment at home and to learn how to avoid reinforcing the child's ritualistic behavior. Material reinforcements can be incorporated into the treatment as a reward for substantial compliance with response prevention. A multimodal approach incorporates EX/RP, other cognitive coping and relaxation techniques, family psychoeducation, and medication (Shafran, 1998; Bolton et al., 1995). Children's significant others who have the opportunity to observe them on a regular basis should also be included. EX/RP is an effective intervention for many children and adolescents in the short run. However, many do not maintain those gains over time. Providing booster sessions and teaching family members to reinforce the client's skills may reduce recidivism.

Post-traumatic Stress Disorder

The procedure for graduated imaginal exposure for treatment of PTSD is quite similar to the process used for adults (P. Smith et al., 1998; see chapter 8). A script of the traumatic event is developed based on the account provided by the child (a tape may be made for use during homework exposure sessions). The child is also taught how to use the 0–10 SUDS scale to indicate level of anxiety so it can be managed during the covert exposure sessions. Care is taken not to overwhelm the child with anxiety during exposure in these sessions. The script should be developed with sufficient sensory detail to allow for a realistic mental reenactment of the event. The child's level of arousal is stepped up carefully based on level of tolerance, but the goal is to gradually elicit a high level of anxiety. The child is taught relaxation/breathing exercises so he or she can hold the image (ideally) for more extended periods of time in order to maintain imaginal exposure until the subjective level of anxiety decreases significantly. Homework for the child is to continue the imaginal exposure with the assistance of family members if possible. In vivo exposure to circumstances that remind the child of the traumatic event may become part of the treatment if behavioral avoidance of certain circumstances has become a significant problem (e.g., school yard where abduction took place). P. Smith et al. (1998) point out that, although uncontrolled studies of CBT for children's PTSD are generally positive, there are few data from controlled studies to date. Nevertheless, given the effectiveness of CBT for other anxiety disorders, it is considered the treatment of choice for PTSD at this time (P. Smith et al.).

Exemplar Study: Controlled Trial for Children with Anxiety Disorders.   Kendall (1994) conducted the first randomized clinical trial of cognitive behavioral intervention with children suffering from anxiety disorders. The methodology and the intervention have provided a foundation for many subsequent controlled trials. Forty-seven children referred from multiple community sources were included in the study. Twenty-seven children (ages 9–13) received treatment for sixteen to twenty visits, and after eight weeks, the twenty children in the control group were assigned to therapists for the same intervention. Of the initial treatment group, 52% were boys, 78% white, and 22% African American. All clients were diagnosed with one or more anxiety disorders, including overanxious disorder, separation anxiety, and avoidant disorder. More than half were given an additional diagnosis of simple phobia, and about one-third also experienced depression. There were no differences between the treatment and control groups on major characteristics noted above. Seven doctoral candidates provided the cognitive-behavioral intervention, and were trained in the procedure with an eighty-five-page manual detailing the following methods:

> a) recognizing anxious feelings and somatic reactions to anxiety, b) clarifying cognitions in anxiety-provoking situations (i.e., unrealistic or negative attributions and expectations), c) developing a plan to help cope with the situation (i.e., modeling anxious self-talk into coping self-talk as well as determining what coping actions might be effective), and d) evaluating performance and administering self-reinforcement as appropriate. (p. 103)

Findings of the study revealed significant improvements in almost all major indicators for the treatment group. Sixty-four percent of the treatment group versus 5% of the wait-list control group no longer met the criteria for anxiety disorders, and gains were maintained at one-year follow-up. A long-term (two–five years) follow-up study of 82% of the eligible study participants revealed stable maintenance of gains over that time. Participants reported specific cognitive-behavioral skills as well as the relationship with the therapist as important aspects of the treatment experience (Kendall & Southam-Gerow, 1996). In a second randomized control trial of cognitive-behavioral methods, Kendall et al. (1997) compared sixty children (treatment group) with thirty-four wait-list controls. The children (ages 9–13) had a variety of anxiety disorders, including overanxious, avoidant, and separation-anxiety disorder. After the intervention, more than half no longer met their pretreatment diagnosis, whereas only 6% of controls no longer met their diagnostic criteria. Gains were maintained at one-year follow-up.

In general, the program used in Kendall's studies (1992, 1994) combines traditional cognitive behavioral skills and adapts them for children and younger adolescents with anxiety disorders. Some of these techniques could be readily adjusted for older adolescents as well, or an adult protocol could be employed. The core skills include relaxation combined with imagery designed for the children's individual needs, problem-solving skills for difficulties that appear to cause anxiety, role-playing, modeling, in vivo exposure, and contingency reinforcement (using positive reinforcement to gradually shape successful coping with anxiety). *Therapists were encouraged to be flexible in the application of these skills to accommodate the needs of the individual child*, and upon review, the investigators deemed treatment fidelity to be adequate. A battery of well-validated measures was employed. In addition, other behavioral observations were made using a seven-item, five-point scale to measure the quality of the child's perception of the therapeutic relationship.

Kendall, Korlander, Chansky, and Brady (1992; Kendall, 1994) outlined the sixteen-week program schedule: Weeks 1–8 focus on four skill areas: an awareness of the physical sensations associated with anxiety; recognizing and evaluating self-talk when the child is anxious; learning problem-solving skills, including the use of constructive self-talk and coping skills; and engaging in self-evaluation and reward for overall performance. Skills are taught so that the children can demonstrate them through a series of "Show That I Can" tasks.

Session 1: The practitioner helps put the child at ease, gauges the child's understanding of the problem and readiness to engage in treatment, and develops a constructive rapport so the child and practitioner can collaborate on the problem in a nonpressured environment.

Sessions 2 and 3: The practitioner helps the child to identify and learn about their own emotional reactions. This may include some didactic methods such as looking at pictures of others and identifying what the person might be feeling, as well as role-playing to show how someone might act when they are sad, anxious, angry, and so forth. The ability of the child to tolerate and understand what is being demonstrated sets the pace for the intervention.

Session 4: Once the child has learned to identify anxiety more accurately, this skill is used as a starting point for learning how to use tension as a cue to engage in relaxation skills, including relaxing specific muscle groups and breathing exercises.

Session 5: The practitioner helps the child identify and articulate the self-talk they use when they are anxious (i.e., the content of their cognitive processes), challenge these cognitions, and replace them with coping self-talk that helps the child feel less anxious. One way to help the child articulate these "dysfunctional" thoughts and construct coping alternatives is with cartoon characters and thought balloons that the child can fill with coping statements.

Session 6: The child begins to engage in problem-solving strategies. The approach is to help the child identify situations, feelings, and thoughts regarding anxiety-provoking situations, and then to explore coping and problem-solving responses (actions) to a series of increasingly anxiety-provoking situations.

Session 7: The goal is to help the child learn to evaluate their performance fairly (anxious children tend to have high standards and judge themselves harshly), and then give themselves a "pat on the back" for making a good effort and achieving partial successes.

Session 8: The child reviews progress to date and solidifies what they have learned by summarizing the main points of the program using the acronym FEAR: Feeling frightened? Expecting bad things to happen (i.e., recognizing anxious self-talk)? Identifying positive actions and attitudes, and results and rewards. The acronym captures recognition of anxiety symptoms and the problem-solving and coping skills used to alleviate them, then uses self-evaluation and a pat on the back for a constructive response to the fearful situation. The steps learned in the first eight sessions are summarized on a wallet-size card, and the coping plan is shared with parents.

Session 9-16: The child learns to build on self-assessment and coping skills by implementing them with real anxiety-provoking problems covertly and in vivo in a graduated manner. The child is taught to use the SUDS, and after practicing covertly, they confront the fearful situation in vivo. The use of the SUDS helps the child gauge their fear and adjust the pace of exposure, so that it is challenging but not overwhelming. As they improve and achieve a tolerable level of anxiety at each stage by using their cognitive-behavioral coping skills to deal with their fear, they can reward themselves as planned. Imaginal and in vivo situations must be realistic and specific to the child's fear, and the child must experience significant degrees of anxiety in order to learn to successfully cope with the fears. Progress may be two steps forward, one step back, but practitioners should communicate optimism about the final outcome, and progress should always be rewarded. Termination should be a time of evaluation, reward for successes, looking ahead to further challenges, and (if needed) occasional booster sessions. As the family situation warrants, the parent(s) can continue to reinforce the child's progress.

ASSESSMENT OF DEPRESSION

Background Data

Symptoms of depression cut across an array of conditions suffered by children, and the indicators of depression are similar to those experienced by adults. They include sadness, dysphoric mood, pessimism, irritability, social withdrawal, loneliness, negative self-image, harsh self-criticism, sleep disturbances, and concerns about death. There are also differences between childhood and adult depressive symptoms. Symptoms such as somatic complaints, irritability, and social withdrawal may be more common in children, whereas psychomotor retardation, delusions, and hypersomnia are more likely to occur in adults. Depression may be associated with poor school performance and interpersonal problems. Other signs may be pessimism and social difficulties (Petti, 1989; Fonseca & Perrin, 2001). MDD appears to occur twice as frequently in adolescent females, but dysthymia appears to occur equally in children of both sexes. Adolescents with major depression are more likely to abuse substances, and those who do are more likely to exhibit conduct disorder and other psychosocial distress (C. A. King et al., 1996; Buckstein, Brent, & Kaminer, 1989; Buckstein, 1995). More than one-third of nonreferred children have been reported as experiencing significantly depressed moods, and between 10% and 20% of children in the community may meet diagnostic criteria for depression. The rate of depression among girls is proportionately greater than that of boys (Compas, 1997).

Theories

As with theories of anxiety, theories of depression have become developmentally multidimensional. Early psychoanalytic theories tended to overemphasize the role of early childhood trauma and frustration related to maternal neglect (e.g., introjected rage). Later formulations stressed interrupted attachment, separation, and loss (e.g., Bowlby, 1980). Cognitive theories including Beck's cognitive triad (1976; negative view of self, the environment, and the future) and learned helplessness (M. E. Seligman, 1975) focused primarily on the development of depression-causing attributions regarding one's ability to cope effectively with environmental challenges. Biological predispositions for disordered neurotransmitter dysfunction or hormonal changes during adolescence have been hypothesized to interact with environmental stressors over time (Garmezy, 1991). Although early loss may contribute to initial vulnerabilities to depression, temperament and other social and environmental stressors are probably at work in the etiology of childhood and adolescent depression (Harrington, 1995; Goodyer, 1995).

Cognitive theories of depression emphasize depression-causing cognitive structures and processes rather than developmental processes. However, whether children become depressed adolescents or adults depends on whether they develop a negative attributional style (Harrington, 1995; Harrington, Wood, & Verduyn, 1998). Developmental changes from early childhood into adolescence reveal a gradually increasing awareness of psychological states including an awareness of depression and other emotions. It appears that children have difficulty reflecting critically on their own cognitive schemata and "dysfunctional thinking" by comparing what they believe to be theoretically valid with verifiable evidence. Developmentally, they may not be ready or even amenable to critical cognitive self-appraisal until their early teens (Harrington et al.). Whether a negative attributional style is biologically predetermined or whether such cognitive structures are the result of a depression-prone temperament interacting with a harsh or critical environment is not known for sure. Evidence suggests that environmental stressors and maltreatment are likely to increase the risk for depression in children and adolescents, and are likely to have long-term effects that carry over into adulthood. However, the effects may also be mediated by a host of other social risk and protective factors. As with anxiety problems, this causal relationship between abuse and depression must be seen within its psychosocial context over time (Downey, Feldman, Khuri, & Friedman, 1994). Although cognitive theories provide a critical focal point for understanding how depression-causing processes mediate life events and depressive symptoms, their role is probably better understood when familial and community/environmental factors (acute and chronic stressors) are considered as well (Harrington, 1995).

Although there are both similarities and differences with regard to theories of anxiety and depression (Harrington, Wood, & Verduyn, 1998; Compas, 1997; Axelson & Birmaher, 2001), they appear to share a common multivariate framework for explaining risks and resiliencies related to depression by linking genetic predisposition, the quality of early-childhood family experiences, emergence of resilient or negative cognitive structures, and the development of skills for coping with environmental stressors. Longitudinal research provides the strongest argument for linking these biopsychosocial influences in a transactional-developmental framework. For example, Duggal, Carlson, Sroufe, and Egeland (2001) conducted a longitudinal study of 168 socioeconomically at-risk children who grew into adolescence. The researchers examined the associations among early family context, maternal depression, and development of depression in the child. They used videotaped observational data to measure maternal interactional behaviors during childhood and adolescence. Early maternal stress and child abuse were shown to be significant correlates of childhood depression accounting for 19% of the variance. Maternal depression predicted adolescent depression in females, but not in males. However, early abuse and both early and later maternal stress were not significantly predictive of depression in adolescence. Results showed only a modest continuity in depression from childhood through adolescence, suggesting that the causes of depression for children and adolescents may involve different factors and pathways.

Noting the consistent findings that females are diagnosed with higher rates of depression than males, Silberg et al. (1999) conducted a longitudinal study of twin males and females (at pre- and postpuberty), and demonstrated that negative life events contributed to depression in boys and had an even stronger effect on girls. For boys, any increase in depression appeared to be related to negative life events in the past year, whereas for girls depression increased despite the lack of any particular negative life event. Genetic influences appeared to account for about 30% of the variance for girls, suggesting that genetic factors play a predominant role in female depression. A one-year longitudinal survey of a mixed-race sample of 240 children and their mothers (Garber, Little, Hilsman, & Weaver, 1998) showed that a mother's depression alone did not predict suicidal symptoms in her child, but that the child's negative perceptions of family environment did, and these perceptions mediated the causal effects of the mother's depression. Finally, adolescent onset of a major depressive episode appears to have predictive value into early adulthood. Risk factors appear to be higher for females and for those with previous depressive episodes, depression in other family members, and co-occurring mental health symptoms (Lewisohn, Rohde, Seeley, Klein, & Gotlib, 2000).

Sorting out the relative effects of biological predisposition to depression and environmental effects continues to be a challenge for longitudinal researchers. Nevertheless, a model is emerging and includes the following factors: (1) biological vulnerabilities rooted in the limbic system and endocrine (hormonal) system, and biological rhythms that affect sleep patterns; (2) lack of early maternal care; maternal depression; abuse and neglect; and disruptive family relationships marked by lower levels of support and cohesion, conflict, hostility, rejection and criticism, parental conflict, and parental depression; (3) problems in cognitive schemata, reasoning errors, and attributional errors similar to those discussed with regard to adult depression; (4) development of poor coping strategies and interpersonal deficits; and (5) moderate to severe negative life events, including both traumatic events and common, everyday stressors (Cicchetti, Rogosch, & Toth, 1994; Duggal et al., 2001; Compas, 1997; Goodyer, 1995; Petti, 1989; Stark, Vaughn, Doxey, & Luss, 1999). One-factor theories for depression such as bad genes, bad mothering, or a traumatic event should now be considered a thing of the past.

Key Elements of Multidimensional/ Functional Assessment

MDF assessment of depression follows a deductive process similar to assessment of anxiety disorder, but is perhaps a bit more challenging. Unlike anxiety disorders, where key symptoms are more readily observable, thoughts and feelings of depression may be more covert, and behavioral symptoms of withdrawal may not be perceived as a problem in an otherwise "good" child. In addition, it may be difficult for children to conceptualize specific aspects of depression, gauge their own level of depression, or articulate the nature of their unhappiness. Drawing pictures, playing with toys, and other methods can be useful for engaging children in assessment and helping them express their feelings and daily concerns, although interpretations should be confirmed by more objective means.

Multiple observations of the child conducted across different situations with data obtained from multiple informants can provide an accurate portrait of a child's struggles with depression. As in the case of anxiety disorders, the functional assessment should cover the three major modes of expression: the child's cognitive appraisal of events in their life, including expressions of hopelessness, pessimism, and catastrophic expectations; physiological symptoms, such as somatic complaints and sleep disturbance; and behaviors often associated with depression, such as social withdrawal, suicidal threats, and aggression. Descriptively, the adult diagnosis of depression applies fairly well to children, and depressive symptoms are similar for both children and adolescents. Suicide, however, is more likely to occur in adolescents than younger children (Harrington, 1995; W. M. Reynolds, 1994).

About 2,000 adolescents commit suicide every year in the United States. Given the rates of co-occurring depression in childhood disorders, potential for suicide should be carefully assessed in both children and adolescents. Guidelines for screening and assessment of potentially suicidal youth are readily available (American Academy of Child and Adolescent Psychiatry [AACAP], 2001a; Greenhill & Waslick, 1997). Key risk factors for child and adolescent suicide include preexisting psychopathology (depression, bipolar disorder, aggressiveness, other mood disorders, substance abuse, personality disorder), stressful events, problems with the law, family difficulties, and previous suicide attempts. Other predictive factors include a history of running away, family history of suicide, history of child abuse, and being gay or lesbian. There is a particular need to be aware of the disproportionate risk of suicide in gay and lesbian youth, and a need for better organized social supports to prevent it (C. D. Proctor & Groze, 1994). With regard to cultural and racial differences, African-American suicide rates have been rising rapidly in recent years, and Native American youth historically have demonstrated higher suicide rates. Hispanic-American youth rates of suicide exceed that for non-Hispanics. Suicide is more common among young males than among females, and the ratio increases into young adulthood.

Assessing the potential for suicide in young people is quite similar to that for adults. In addition to the above risk factors, suicide risk falls on a severity continuum covering suicidal ideation, suicidal threats, and suicide attempts. Particular attention should be paid to the history of previous attempts and the degree of potential lethality of the means contemplated, frequency and intensity of the ideation, and whether the client has a plan in place and has contemplated the specific means of suicide. Intervention requires a continuum of options as well, beginning with acute emergency intervention, possible hospitalization followed by partial hospitalization (as needed), and follow-up outpatient intervention. As will be examined below, depressed children and adolescents respond quickly to CBT, and family psychoeducational methods may be a helpful adjunct to continued treatment. Referral and intervention decision points are all guided by consideration of the severity of the depression, co-occurring psychopathology, and available social supports.

Instruments

The Children's Depression Inventory (CDI) is one of the most widely used self-report measures for children (Kovacs, 1985). The CDI (derived from the BDI) includes twenty-seven items covering a broad range of depressive symptoms and related problems (Carlson & Cantwell, 1980; Kovacs). Each item comprises three statements describing symptoms at three levels of intensity. In a three-part study with a group of 216 children balanced by gender and race, four domains related to depression were identified through factor analysis: affective behavior, image ideation, interpersonal relations, and guilt-irritability (Helsel & Matson, 1984). Results showed no differences by gender and race, although age was directly predictive of greater depression. However, a more recent analysis of the scale employed a large community sample (more suitable for factor analysis than clinic samples), and demonstrated a somewhat different factor structure than had previous investigations (W. E. Craighead, Smucker, Craighead, & Ilardi, 1998). Results of the analysis suggested a five-factor scale that measured constructs related to depression (i.e., dysphoria and self-deprecation), but also measured externalizing symptoms, including school and social problems. Overall, the CDI is considered a useful and reliable instrument, but appears to measure constructs that extend beyond depression. Thus, discriminant validity of the scale has been questioned. Nevertheless, it continues to be widely used, has been translated into various languages, and has been used to examine depressive symptoms in minority youth (Myers & Winters, 2002).

The Depression Self-Rating Scale (DSRS; Birleson, 1981; Birleson, Hudson, Buchanan, & Wolff, 1987) is a self-report measure of moderate to severe depression in children and adolescents. It was initially developed with several samples of children, including those diagnosed as clinically depressed, residential patients, and a school-based population. The initial pool of thirty-seven items was reduced through statistical analysis to eighteen. Children rate whether they have experienced the symptoms "never," "sometimes," or "most of the time" within a week. The initial study demonstrated good discriminant validity between depressed and nondepressed children (ages 7–13), good test-retest reliability (.80), and good split-half reliability (.86). The advantages of the DSRS are that it is brief and may be useful as a treatment evaluation tool. Additional studies have demonstrated good utility and good sensitivity in that it correctly identifies children diagnosed as depressed (Birlson et al.). The factor structure of the DSRS was replicated and showed very good internal consistency with adolescents when compared with previous research (Ivarsson, Lidberg, & Gillberg, 1994; Ivarsson & Gillberg, 1997). A cutoff score of 15 is recommended to screen for clinical depression.

The Children's Depression Rating Scale (CDRS; Poznanzski, Cook, & Carroll, 1979) was derived from the HAM-D (see chapter 9). It was developed on the assumption that children's self-reports may not be as valid as the observations of experienced clinicians who use multiple sources of data. Because the assessment is conducted in an interview format, the practitioner can accommodate the child's cognitive level and language style. The initial study of the CDRS (Poznanski et al.) was conducted with thirty hospitalized depressed children, and demonstrated a high correlation between the scale and clinical diagnosis. The original version of the CDRS had fifteen items with a possible total score of 61. The items measured the following constructs: depressed mood, weeping, self-esteem, excessive guilt, morbid preoccupations, suicidal ideation, schoolwork, social withdrawal, irritability, anhedonia, speech tempo, appetite, sleep, hypoactivity, physical complaints, and fatigue. A revised version of the scale (Poznanski et al., 1984) includes seventeen items, correlates significantly with global ratings of depression, and reveals good interrater and test-/retest reliability. A five-item version that reflects *DSM* criteria measures dysphoric mood, anhedonia, social withdrawal, low self-esteem, and fatigue (Overholser, Brinkman, Lehnert, & Ricciardi, 1995). The CDRS (short form) was demonstrated to have high internal consistency ratings in two samples (.80 and .88), high interrater reliability (.93), high correlations between short and long forms of the CDRS for both boys (.89) and girls (.92), and significant correlation with other valid depression scales. The revised CDRS (short form) is reprinted here (instrument 12.2).

INSTRUMENT 12.2   Children's Depression Rating Scale–Revised Short Form
(CDRS-r)

For a general time frame, try to assess the child's symptoms as they occurred over the previous 2 weeks. If the child has been recently hospitalized and this has disrupted their life (e.g., not sleeping well because of the new surroundings), then try to evaluate their symptoms as they appeared during the 2 weeks prior to their hospitalization. Also, if a problem has occurred for a long time (e.g., chronic school problems), *only score symptoms that appear to be related to emotional distress*, not some other problem (e.g., learning disability, drug abuse).

1. Anhedonia (capacity to have fun): What do you like to do for fun? After school? On weekends? Do you have any hobbies? When was the last time you did the hobby? (Discuss the activities and note interest, involvement, enthusiasm.) How often do you have fun? (Note frequency of activities that are available.) When was the last time you really enjoyed yourself? Tell me about it. How often do you get bored? What do you do when you get bored? What do you like to watch on TV? Tell me about your favorite TV show. In the last month, has it been hard to get interested in most things? Have you still enjoyed the things you usually enjoy? Last week, did you find anything interesting? Enjoyable? Funny?

Scoring:
1___   Interest and activities are appropriate for age, personality and social environment. Shows no appreciable change with present illness. Any feelings of boredom are transient.
2___   Doubtful
3___   Describes some activities available several times a week but not on a daily basis. Shows interest but not enthusiasm.

4___ Mild to moderate

5___ Is easily bored. Complains of "nothing to do." Participates in structured activities with a "going through the motions" attitude. May express interest primarily in activities that are (realistically) unavailable on a daily or weekly basis.

6___ Moderate to severe

7___ Has no initiative to become involved in any activities. Primarily passive. Watches others play or watches TV, but shows little interest. Requires coaxing to get involved in activity. Shows no enthusiasm or real interest in activities.

So, it sounds like you have been feeling . . .

2. Social Withdrawal: Do you have many friends? Are they at school or home? What things do you do with your friends? How often do you see them? Do you have a really close friend? What is the name of your best friend? How long have you known this person? How often have you seen this person in the past month? (never, rarely, sometimes, frequently, always) In the past month, how often have you shared YOUR problems with him/her? (never, rarely, sometimes, frequently, always) In the past month, how often have they shared THEIR problems with you? (never, rarely, sometimes, frequently, always) Do your friends ever call for you when you don't feel like doing anything? How often do you just want to be left alone and be by yourself? What do you do when a friend calls you, but you don't feel like doing anything?

Scoring:

1___ Enjoys friendships with peers at school and home.

2___ Doubtful

3___ May not actively seek out friendships but waits for others to initiate a relationship or may occasionally reject opportunities to play without a describable alternative.

4___ Mild to moderate

5___ Frequently avoids or refuses opportunities for desirable interaction with others and/or sets up situations where rejection is inevitable.

6___ Moderate to severe

7___ Does not currently relate to other children. States s/he has "no friends" or actively rejects new or former friends.

So, it sounds like you have been feeling . . .

3. Excessive Fatigue: During the last month, what has your energy been like? How tired have you been feeling lately? Do you get tired more easily now than you used to? Have you been tired all the time? How often do you feel this way? Do you have little energy to do things or feel tired a lot? Do you feel tired even when you have had enough sleep? How often do you take naps during the day? How do you feel after a nap?

Scoring:

1___ No unusual complaints of "feeling tired" during the day.

2___ Doubtful

3___   Occasional complaints of fatigue that seen somewhat excessive and not related to boredom.

4___   Mild to moderate complaint

5___   Daily complaints of feeling tired.

6___   Moderate to severe

7___   Complains of feeling tired most of the day. May voluntarily take long naps without feeling refreshed. Fatigue interferes with play activities.

So, it sounds like you have been feeling . . .

4. Self-esteem: During the last month, how have you felt about yourself as a person? What are some things about yourself that you like? What kinds of things are you good at? What are some things about yourself that you do not like? Would you like to change anything about yourself? How do you feel about the way you look? How smart do you think you are compared to other kids your age? Have you been feeling down on yourself lately? Do you ever feel worthless as a person?

Scoring:

1___   Describes self in primarily positive terms.

2___   Doubtful

3___   Describes self with one important area where the child feels deficient.

4___   Mild to moderate

5___   Describes self in preponderance of negative terms or gives bland answers to questions.

6___   Moderate to severe

7___   Refers to self in derogatory terms. Reports that other children refer to him/her frequently by using derogatory nicknames and child puts self down.

So, it sounds like you have been feeling . . .

5. Depressed Feelings: How has your mood been lately? How often have you felt sad? In the past month, how much of the time have you felt sad? How long have you felt this way? What seems to make you feel like that? When you feel unhappy, how long does it last? One hour? A few hours? A day? What kind of things make you feel unhappy? How often do you feel like this? Every week? Every two weeks? When you've been feeling depressed, how bad has it been? Do other people know when you are sad?

Scoring:

1___   Occasional feelings of unhappiness which quickly disappear.

2___   Doubtful

3___   Describes sustained periods of unhappiness which appear excessive for the events described.

4___   Mild to moderate

5___   Feels unhappy most of the time without major precipitating cause.

6___   Moderate to severe

7___   Feels unhappy all of the time. Accompanied by psychic pain (e.g., "I can't stand it").

So, it sounds like you have been feeling . . .

SELECTING EFFECTIVE INTERVENTIONS

The following review summarizes the outcome research on treating depression in children and adolescents. Following that, the essential common elements of evidence-based practice for internalizing disorders are summarized.

CBT for children has shown solid benefits for moderately depressed children and adolescents, but results for seriously depressed young people are less impressive (Harrington, 1995; Stark et al., 1999; Curry, 2001; S. N. Compton et al., 2002). Using the methodological guidelines set forth by the Task Force on Promotion and Dissemination of Psychological Procedures (1995), Kaslow and Thompson (1998, p. 153) summarize the findings on psychosocial interventions for childhood and adolescent depression.

> [R]esults from this review reveal that several psychosocial interventions programs, the majority of which are based on the cognitive-behavioral model, are effective in reducing depressive symptoms and alleviating depressive disorders in non-clinical samples of adolescents. Positive treatment effects are noted regardless of treatment modality (group, individual or family therapy) or nature or extent of parental involvement. Treatment effects generally are maintained at follow-up. However, because most of the studies were conducted in schools with non-referred youth with depressive symptoms and used relatively inexperienced clinicians, the generalizability of the findings across populations, settings, and clinician-experience level remains unclear. Further, because few between-group design studies have compared different interventions, it is premature to conclude that any specific intervention approach is most efficacious in reducing depression in youth.

Reviewers also stress the need to address co-occurring problems such as anxiety disorders and to consider using family formats more often (Birmaher, Ryan, Williamson, Brent, & Kaufman, 1996). Given the possibility that more than half of children suffering from anxiety or depression may experience co-occurring symptoms of these disorders, practitioners must combine cognitive-behavioral methods (Kendall et al., 1992). Eclecticism may also extend to the inclusion of family-therapy methods in the treatment of depression in young people (Harrington, Whittaker, & Shoebridge, 1998). In a ten-year review, Birmaher et al. concluded that cognitive-behavioral and behaviorally oriented family systems approaches were shown to be efficacious for childhood depression. Harrington (1995) notes that family therapy could be useful in a number of applications: the practitioner could act as consultant to an otherwise healthy and intact family, and provide advice and guidance regarding how to help a son or daughter cope with depression; family members could participate as adjunct therapists by helping the child-client follow through on therapeutic "homework" or facilitate treatment in other cooperative ways; other problems in the family affecting the child's well-being, such as mental illness, substance abuse, domestic violence, marital problems, and other family dysfunction, could be addressed. As Kovacs and Bastiaens (1995, p. 298) point out, "treatment of the parents' own disorders should be seriously considered in tandem with the psychotherapy of the young-ster. It is difficult to see how one could expect a positive and lasting treatment response from a child whose parent is disturbed and is thereby probably unable to meet the youngster's needs." Lastly, although family factors have been associ-ated with contributing to depression and its relapse, more research on the use of family therapy for depression in young people is needed (Curry, 2001).

Interpersonal psychotherapy (IPT) may be another viable option for inter-ventions with depressed youths. Harrington (1995) notes that IPT may be use-ful, given its present and future focus and its emphasis on improving social rela-tionships and on dealing with interpersonal disputes and role transitions—all areas that are developmentally pertinent to children and adolescents. However, since the early 1990s, little outcome research had been conducted on IPT for children (Curry, 2001).

A series of key studies since the mid-1980s has shown modest support for the efficacy of CBT for depression and a growing interest in integrating CBT with family therapy. W. M. Reynolds and Coats (1986) randomly assigned thirty moderately depressed adolescents to three conditions: (1) CBT that included self-control skills (self-monitoring, self-evaluation, self-reinforcement); (2) relax-ation training; or (3) a wait-list control group. Both treatments demonstrated sig-nificant reductions in depression compared to the control group at five-week follow-up. Stark, Reynolds, and Kaslow (1987) compared two behaviorally ori-ented treatments for children ages 9–12 with a wait-list control group. The first behavioral treatment group consisted of self-monitoring and evaluation, and cop-ing skills practiced through homework assignments. The second group empha-sized problem-solving skills (feelings education, social skills, and planned activi-ties reinforced through homework assignments). Treatments were provided in small groups over twelve hourly sessions for five weeks. Both treatment groups resulted in positive outcomes (decreased depression) with results maintained at five-week follow-up. The control group showed little change. In a similar study, Kahn, Kehle, Jenson, and Clark (1990) showed that CBT and relaxation training had better outcomes than self-modeling over time. Fine, Forth, Gilbert, and Haley (1991) compared a social-skills training group with a therapeutic support group. Both groups were conducted over twelve weekly meetings, and showed com-parable improvements at nine-month follow-up. A. Wood, Harrington, and Moore (1996) compared an individual CBT model (cognitive restructuring, social prob-lem solving, coping skills for depression) with relaxation training with inpatient depressed children. In the short run, the CBT group showed better results, with improvements in symptoms and self-image. By six-month follow-up, however, some of the CBT group had relapsed, and the relaxation group continued to im-prove.

Some investigators have evaluated CBT approaches in a psychoeducational format. For example, Lewisohn, Clarke, Hops, and Andrews (1990) evaluated a school-based program for fifty-nine depressed adolescents (ages 14–18) in a cognitive-behavioral psychoeducational group (i.e., coping with depression) conducted over seven weeks of fourteen two-hour evening sessions. In one group, parents participated by receiving separate instruction in skills for coping with depression and family problems. Parents of the second group of adolescents did not participate. Wait-list controls received the intervention at a later date. Both treatment groups showed comparable and significant clinical gains, and outcomes showed continued improvements at two-year follow-up. In a more recent study, preliminary evidence of effectiveness was demonstrated for a five-week program that combined family psychoeducation and teaching depressed children CBT skills (Asarnow, Scott, & Mintz, 2002).

Exemplar Study: Cognitive-Behavioral Therapy and Family Therapy for Depression.   As with treatment of anxiety disorders in children and adolescents, recent controlled trials of CBT for depression have focused more on the differential effectiveness of family therapy alone or in combination with CBT. One randomized controlled trial (Brent et al., 1997) compared CBT, systemic behavioral family therapy (SBFT), and nondirective supportive therapy (NST). The sample included 107 clinically depressed adolescents treated over twelve to sixteen weeks. Participants were between 13 and 18 years old, met *DSM* criteria for major depressive disorder, and scored 13 or more on the BDI. Other serious comorbid psychiatric disorders were ruled out. Of the eligible 122 adolescents, 107 agreed to be randomly assigned to treatment conditions, and 78 completed the study. All participants were provided with free treatment. Therapists had six months of intensive training in the intervention method they provided, had master's degrees, and had a median of ten years' practice experience. CBT was characterized by collaborative empiricism, teaching the client about the CBT model, monitoring and challenging dysfunctional thinking, and enhancing problem solving and social skills. SBFT included functional family therapy (see chapter 13) combined with communication and problem-solving methods with an emphasis on homework practice. NST emphasized the core ingredients generic to most therapies: relationship building, empathic responding, and expression of feelings. Therapists in this condition refrained from providing directive advice of any kind. Close supervision and fidelity checks (use of videos to rate adherence to the respective models) demonstrated good adherence to each treatment approach. Well-validated instruments were employed at multiple points in treatment. These included standardized measures based on the *DSM*, the BDI, a global assessment of functioning for children, and other indicators. Results demonstrated markedly superior remission (60%) for the CBT condition, that is, absence of symptoms meeting the criteria for MDD, compared with the SBFT condition (38%) and the NST group (39%). There were no differences among the three groups on measures of suicidal risk or overall functional impairment. Parents' opinion of the credibility of CBT increased relative to that of SBFT.

The researchers noted a few limitations to the study. Because suicide attempters were referred out for emergency treatment, generalizations to suicidal adolescents are limited. In addition, given the need for experimental rigor in client selection, generalizations to young people with co-occurring disorders is limited as well. The intense amount of supervision and quality-control checks in this study are also difficult to transfer to typical clinical service environments. In comparing the results of CBT to SBFT and NST, they noted that "having a good therapeutic relationship ... may be necessary, but is not sufficient to result in optimal clinical improvement of adolescent depression ... results also indicate that insistence on the treatment of the family as a unit ... will cause a certain proportion of families to refuse treatment" (Brent et al., 1997, p. 883). They also noted that the rapid remission of depressive symptoms is critical in youthful depression, because depression too often precipitates suicide attempts. The greater credibility shown by parents for the CBT approach is important, because client satisfaction is linked to treatment adherence. Brent et al. recommend that future studies compare psychotherapeutic drugs with and without CBT, and test these methods in typical practice settings.

Follow-up studies with this same sample, however, suggested that after two years, results from CBT and SBFT were comparable. Most of the young people recovered with no discernable advantage from either of these two methods (Birmaher et al., 2000). Over the long haul, it may be that a good number of depressed adolescents may need more treatment, including, in some cases, antidepressant medication and continued family therapy. Their need is due to a number of predisposing factors, including severity of depression at intake, co-occurring disorders such as anxiety, maternal depression, and family difficulties (Brent, Kolko, Birmaher, Baugher, & Bridge, 1999; Renaud et al., 1998; Brent et al., 1998). Nevertheless, the superior short-term results of CBT should not be undervalued, given the importance of suicide risk early on in treatment. Future research should examine the differential contributions of CBT and family interventions for adolescents with and without the use of medication.

Finally, Kolko, Brent, Baugher, Bridge, and Birmaher (2000) conducted further analysis with these 107 depressed adolescents and found little evidence to link the specific therapeutic technique to the theoretically commensurate change processes (e.g., cognitive techniques should affect dysfunctional thinking, family techniques should change family functioning). They echo a point made throughout this text: *the evidence supporting specific cause-effect linkages between intervention methods and their commensurate theoretical change processes is far from compelling.* What we can tell, however, is that some psychosocial interventions are more effective than others, at least in the short run.

Descriptions of Comprehensive Cognitive-Behavioral Therapy for Treatment of Depression

CBT for children is based on the same theoretical and practice principles as is CBT for adults, but oriented to the child's age and circumstances (Harrington, 1995; Harrington, Whittaker, & Shoebridge, 1998; Kovacs & Bastiaens, 1995). In addition to challenging and changing maladaptive cognitions directly, CBT for depression in children and adolescents usually involves components such as goal directedness; self-monitoring and evaluating; learning specific skills such as social skills, self-reinforcement, and relaxation; and practicing the skills through role-play, rehearsal, and homework exercises to solidify and generalize their use. Self-monitoring may be the most important skill for a young person to learn as part of CBT. The emphasis is first on teaching children to accurately identify what they are feeling, and then on training them to focus on more positive thoughts and actions to break the cycle of negative thinking and reduce their depression. Identifying dysfunctional thoughts such as consistently devaluing oneself can be directly addressed through standard cognitive restructuring methods (e.g., Beck, 1976; see chapter 9). First, the child identifies the dysfunctional automatic thought and challenges it by answering the question, Where is the evidence to support this belief? Second, the child examines alternative explanations for upsetting thoughts or events. Third, the child is helped to challenge negative expectations about the future. These assignments should be followed by "experiments" creatively developed by the practitioner and the child to test and ultimately disconfirm these dysfunctional beliefs. Behavioral self-regulation skills (see Kanfer, 1970; Rehm, 1977) can help children reinforce themselves positively for successfully carrying out certain behaviors or activities that are purposeful and help them feel better about themselves. Helping children learn to structure their activities can also help them move away from the depressive rumination often associated with inactivity.

Building on these core cognitive-behavioral techniques, Stark, Rouse, and Kurowski (1994) outlined a comprehensive program for working with depressed children and (as needed) their family. Based on well-established self-control and cognitive-behavioral interventions, treatment aims to identify those core themes (i.e., cognitive schemata) related to dysfunctional thought processes. Key techniques include cognitive restructuring, cognitive modeling, self-instructional training, positive activity scheduling (e.g., fun activities, goal-oriented activities such as chores), relaxation training (muscle relaxation accompanied by imagery as needed), coping with behavioral problems including social-skills deficits (e.g., lack of assertiveness), problem solving, behavioral assignments, self-reinforcement, and behavioral disconfirmation tasks to challenge core negative schemata and dysfunctional thinking. Family interventions are employed as needed.

In the early phase of treatment, the practitioner takes much of the initiative in gauging the child's readiness to change and helping the child identify negative moods and the dysfunctional thoughts associated with depressive thinking, challenge these thoughts, seek alternative plausible explanations, and replace these dysfunctional thoughts with more positive ways of looking at a situation. As the intervention progresses, the child is encouraged to take more of the initiative at identifying dysfunctional thought processes, challenging them, and moving toward identifying core depressive themes presumably associated with core negative schemata. As these are identified and challenged, the most powerful part of the intervention is emphasized: *behavioral assignments to challenge and disconfirm these beliefs*. It is important that the practitioner work closely with parents and teachers particularly to support the goals of the intervention. If it becomes apparent that problems in the family are having a negative impact on the child, then these problems are addressed directly. For example, if the parent(s) are having trouble with parenting skills, they can be improved by demonstrating more supportive parenting and effective nonpunitive disciplinary practices. If the couple is having problems, a couples intervention should be implemented, focusing on problem solving and communication enhancement. In brief, an effective approach to depression in children combines effective CBT methods with behaviorally oriented family therapy.

Harrington, Wood, and Verduyn (1998) have also formulated a multimodal approach that includes a flexible application of cognitive-behavioral intervention methods tailored to the unique needs of the adolescent. Their program is designed for unipolar depressed adolescents between eleven and eighteen years of age. Ten to fourteen sessions take place over ten or twelve weeks (with four additional booster sessions). The adolescent is understood to have problems in three major domains: negative thinking (negative attributional style, low self-esteem), problems in social relationships (social inhibitions, withdrawal, conflict), and behavioral symptoms of depression (poor sleep, low activity). Following a broad multidimensional assessment including the detection of co-occurring problems, a functional analysis is undertaken to help the adolescent learn to assess troubling thoughts, feelings, and behaviors and link them to depressive mood. The adolescent is then encouraged to become more active, engage in more positive behavior, and reward himself or herself for efforts in this area. Social problem solving is a priority, and the practitioner helps the adolescent apply standard problem-solving techniques to social difficulties (i.e., brainstorming, coming up with possible solutions, putting them into action, evaluating them). As with the previous model, these methods are ideally suited to be tailored to the unique needs of each young person.

Medications for Internalizing Disorders

With the exception of using SSRIs to treat OCD (e.g., Castellanos, 1998), there is little research to support the use of antidepressants or antianxiety drugs for treating internalizing disorders in children and adolescents (Birmaher et al., 1996; S. N. Compton et al., 2002; Pine & Grun, 1998). Nevertheless, these drugs, particularly antidepressants, are commonly prescribed for young people. The prescribing of TCAs or SSRIs in children carries similar side effects as in adults: dry mouth, constipation, drowsiness, hypertension, and mania. Overdoses, possibly resulting in coma or death, are of particular concern with antidepressants. At best, antidepressants and anxiolytics may be useful as adjunctive treatments when combined with cognitive-behavioral interventions (Stock, Werry, & McClellan, 2001; Axelson & Birmaher, 2001).

Most recommendations for the use of benzodiazepines for anxiety disorders in children are based on case reports and guidelines that reflect adult prescribing practices even though there are significant differences in the way children and adolescents metabolize these drugs. Although prescribing for short-term reasons such as sleep problems is not uncommon, long-term prescribing is of greater concern, given the risks of tolerance. For problems with sleep, night terrors, or aggressive behaviors, psychosocial approaches are preferred. Side effects of these drugs for children may include sleepiness, poor concentration, decreased coordination, decreased school performance, and behavioral disinhibition. Discontinuation of benzodiazepines should be done gradually under medical supervision to avoid withdrawal-induced seizures. Buspirone, a drug that is chemically distinct from the benzodiazepine family, has not been subject to controlled trials with children, and is not recommended for anyone under the age of eighteen. Side effects based on case reports and uncontrolled studies include headaches, nausea, dizziness, drowsiness, and fatigue. Sedative hypnotics such as barbiturates are generally no longer recommended for children.

Reasons for variability in the findings of pharmacotherapy studies of children include biological differences in children relative to age and heredity, co-occurring disorders, and a host of methodological differences in relevant studies. Metabolic and other physiological differences make it difficult for physicians to predict blood levels or treatment responses to specific doses of medications. It is currently unclear what evidence-based medical standards guide the prescribing of these drugs for children (Harrington, 1995; Remschmidt & Schulz, 1995; Stark et al., 1999; H. I. Kaplan & Saddock, 1998; S. N. Compton et al., 2002).

Summary of Key Intervention Elements for Internalizing Disorders

Although every child's individual plan will be unique, effective psychosocial treatment for anxiety and depression should include some combination of the following elements:

Educate the children about their own emotional processes, by helping them identify, differentiate, and understand their feelings.

Teach self-monitoring of feelings and link children's feelings (including physiological/somatic sensations) to their anxious and depressive thoughts or situational factors.

Help children identify, examine, and challenge distorted cognitions associated with their anxieties and depression; help them learn to make the connections among situations, fears, depressive thoughts, and their behaviors.

If children suffer from low activity due to depression (perhaps combined with anxiety and fearful avoidance behavior), develop a step-by-step plan to increase their activity level.

Build hierarchies of the child's fears, worries, and perceived sources of anxiety.

Teach relaxation skills and key coping skills to be employed with covert and in vivo exposure and practice.

Use covert rehearsal skills to help children imagine how they can approach an anxiety-producing situation.

Help them develop an approach hierarchy; that is, break down their plan to confront their fear into small steps with a plan to confront each step one at a time.

Teach children the SUDS so they can gauge their level of anxiety as they approach fearful thoughts or situations covertly or in vivo.

Model the new behaviors children agree to try out.

Engage in role-playing that help children rehearse the new behaviors and prepare to address problems in vivo.

Guide children in gradually confronting the feared situation in vivo (if that is feasible), and work gradually up the fear hierarchy when they have successfully conquered each step. Successful efforts are very likely to enhance their sense of mastery (self-efficacy) in the problematic situation, and increase their confidence that they can do it again successfully.

Gradually increase the level of challenge (based on the fear hierarchy developed earlier). Children should practice their new coping skills (relaxation, breathing, self-talk) on their own or with significant others (as the situation dictates) in homework assignments.

Help children enhance their problem-solving skills in troubling or challenging situations related to their anxiety or depression. This includes brainstorming, considering possible solutions, testing out the strategy, and evaluating it.

Work with the family, teachers, coaches, and other collaterals to reinforce children's efforts to confront their fears and reduce feelings of helplessness or inadequacy.

Use family sessions when possible to identify interactional patterns and other problems in the family that may be contributing to children's distress or inadvertently sabotaging their progress.

Teach all collaterals how to use contingency management (giving or withdrawing tangible rewards) to reinforce the child's gains. Make sure all adults involved in the treatment plan understand the contingencies for rewards or sanctions. Depending on children's progress and age, they should be encouraged to gradually take over the control of some of these contingencies through development of their own self-evaluation and self-regulation skills.

Help collaterals avoid behaviors that may reinforce the child's anxiety and depression.

Use case management skills to co-ordinate the intervention with key collaterals to ensure continuity in delivering the intervention plan.

IMPLEMENTING AND EVALUATING THE EVIDENCE-BASED INTERVENTION PLAN

CASE STUDY: NOAH

Noah, a nine-year old African-American boy, was brought to the local mental health center because his aunt found him in his room sobbing. He was attempting to make a noose out of a bed sheet and, as he later admitted, was planning to hang himself in his closet. After disclosing his intentions to his aunt, she queried him about why he would want to do that. At about 4:30 Noah's mother came home from her shift as a nurse's aid in the local hospital, and they all sat down together. The aunt's son, Jared (eleven), also came home from school, and got busy doing his homework at the kitchen table.

Three months ago, Noah's cousin Damon (a nineteen-year-old son of another aunt) was killed as an innocent bystander in a drive-by shooting as a result of a feud between two rival gangs. Noah had been very close to him. He hung around Damon a lot and looked up to him. Noah's father had been out of the picture since Noah was about three. Noah had vague recollections of his father, sharpened over the years only through having seen pictures of him and overheard stories about him from his neighbors and his mom. Noah's mother and her sister agreed to share child-rearing and living expenses by moving in together, at least for a while. A while turned into a

few years. Noah and Jared got along well, and the two women, working different shifts, were able to cover child care, make ends meet, and develop a tight family unit.

Noah had always been somewhat anxious and quiet. He was not a problem, but caused his mother some concern because of his occasional odd behavior. He was shy, and did not like to be with other kids. He spoke about one friend in school with whom he had a relationship for three consecutive years in the same school. He played with his cousin Jared, but shied away from social events and school activities and never mentioned that he had been invited to other kids' birthday parties. He spoke about vague fears now and again, usually based on a TV show or something he read in a book (he was a good reader and had a complex and rich imagination). He complained of stomachaches off and on. His mother could never link his complaints to food, and they usually seemed to have something to do with going to an unfamiliar place or to the doctor or dentist for routine care. He was extremely methodical and orderly with his personal belongings. His mother always felt it was a bit extreme, but she was one of the few parents who never complained about their children being messy, not "minding," or not picking up after themselves. At times she checked on him if he were alone in his room (which he shared with Jared, who was often on the floor of the living room watching TV or playing video games). When she would knock and enter his room, she would find him deeply engrossed in his play, talking aloud, providing the voice for the characters in his imaginary playmate world of superheroes and villains. When his mother called him for dinner, he would often be hard to extract from his play. Once his mother, exasperated after having called him three times, stormed into his room and insisted that he come to the table immediately. When she went to prompt him by taking his hand, he started to scream that he could not leave until his work was done. "What work?" His toys had to be placed perfectly before he could let himself leave the room.

Although Noah was a good student, his mother noticed that he would get frustrated and bogged down in minutiae (e.g., getting a column of numbers perfectly aligned, perfect penmanship), and sometimes he would cry in frustration if he could not get it just so after spending hours trying. Another time she found him

sobbing on his knees next to his bed because "I can't get my prayers right. I can't get them to be perfect for Jesus." His mother and aunt, who both regularly attended services with their boys, were concerned that maybe they had overdone it, although they did not have prayer services at home, and Jared, bored by church, never indicated that he cared about prayers one way or the other.

But threatening to kill himself was another matter altogether. Although it had been three months since Damon had been buried, Noah seemed to be very upset about it all over again. Jared, a sharp listener, overheard them talking and offered an explanation: "They were talking about Damon on TV, and Noah was with me." As they talked to Noah they also found out that Damon had promised to take Noah to a baseball game when the season opened in the spring. When his mom spoke with Noah's teacher, she said that Noah had told her several times that he was going to a game with his cousin, Damon. Noah, who had never been to a game, was looking forward to it all winter. It was now baseball season, the kids in school were talking about their favorite players, but Noah would not be going with his best friend.

Multidimensional/Functional Assessment: Defining Problems and Goals

After several visits with Noah's mother and aunt, and a couple hours with Noah, the social worker, June, began to put together the pieces as best she could. It came out that Noah's father had been rather violent at home. He had been abusive to Noah's mother, and although Noah said he did not recall any of these events, his mother strongly suspected that it might account for some of his fears. As a little boy, he would come out of his room late in the night, apparently sleepwalking, after the couple had argued loudly (often with furniture being pushed, or thrown, and considerable screaming and yelling, sometimes hitting). He also tended to have nightmares during that time, and was often very afraid of being left with a baby-sitter or family member from age two and a half until age three. He would cry and scream if his mother left the house and, at times seemed inconsolable. After his father moved out, he settled down gradually, although some of his fears continued. Noah's mom reported alcohol problems on both sides of the family, as well as what appeared to be depression on her mother's side. She blamed herself sometimes because Noah did not have a father, and she was grateful when he was about seven years old that Damon took him under his wing. After Noah's father left, she was a "nervous wreck," and things were "unstable around here with baby-sitters and never knowing if I was going to be able to pay the rent." Things got better when she teamed up with her sister.

Based on more recent analysis, it appeared that Noah's depression, feelings of hopelessness, and thoughts of suicide may have resulted from a delayed reaction to the loss of Damon. He appeared to be somewhat emotionless, and numb during the wake and funeral. But his thoughts and feelings about the loss now seemed to be leaking out. In addition to his long-standing shyness, general fears, somatic complaints, and current stress response and grief, June was also concerned about Noah's extreme concern about orderliness and his distress about not being about to "make it perfect" with his tidying up, his homework, and his nighttime prayers. In sum, Noah appeared to have a predisposition toward anxiety disorders and depressive symptoms, all of which were now exacerbated by the recent trauma associated with the loss of his best friend, Damon.

Although there appeared to be a direct link between the increase in depression and suicidal thoughts and Damon's death, other problems appeared to be temperamental and the result of exposure to intense fighting and intermittent violence in the home when Noah was younger. In addition, his mother noticed an increase in his anxiety when he was expected to participate more socially in school or to make a presentation (show and tell), or after his mother worked double shifts (at which time both sisters hired a cousin as house-sitter for the evening). Changes in routine, unplanned events, and conflicts with another child in school, among other stressors, seemed to make Noah more anxious, as suggested by an increase in compulsive orderliness, somatic complaints (e.g., attempts to feign illness to stay home from school), and general restlessness.

The results of these discussions among June, Noah, and his mom seemed to indicate that helping Noah deal with his intense sadness and thoughts about killing himself were the top priority. Second on the list seemed to be his general fears about school and socializing with other children. Third was his mother's concern about Noah's need to be "perfect." All agreed on three main goals for the intervention: help Noah resolve his grief over Damon as best he could, improve his socialization skills (reduce his social anxiety to a manageable level), and help him "lighten up" on his obsessional tendencies to be "perfect."

Selecting and Designing the Intervention: Defining Strategies and Objectives

A series of step-by-step objectives were considered for each goal (table 12.1). To help Noah resolve some of his grief over Damon, the social worker planned a series of exercises that she and Noah started together to help him talk about Damon, his time with him, the good memories, and his fears and unspoken sorrow regarding how Damon died and how much he missed him. This process included putting together a scrapbook of Noah's time with Damon, with drawings and a few photographs that Noah's mother had saved, and talking about the things that they had planned to do together. His mom gradually participated in reminiscing with Noah at home. Objectives for reducing his shyness included gradually introducing him to some of the after-school programs that were available. Noah would be encouraged to stay at the program accompanied by an adult for a "couple of minutes" to look around, and this amount of time was gradually increased a few minutes until he became more comfortable and found some acquaintances with whom he shared common interests. The third series of objectives focused on gradually reducing his need for "perfection," modifying his extreme standards at homework, cleaning up, and prayer by setting more reasonable standards.

Interventions to address these objectives included a cognitive approach to grief work, graduated exposure to reduce shyness, and a combination of contingency management and EX/RP to reduce compulsive behavior. To facilitate these interventions, June worked closely with Noah to teach him anxiety-management coping skills, including identification of feelings, tracking his feelings over time and linking them to his behaviors in situation, and identifying some of his more troubling thoughts, such as nobody will like me if I don't tidy up just right, bad things will happen to mom and me, and it will be my fault. June worked carefully with Noah, using drawings and action figures to tease out a hierarchy of fears and help set a course for "conquering" these fears one by one. Showing him how to meditate, breathe, relax, and imagine himself more in control (just like one of his martial arts heroes) was a key skill necessary to give him the "superhero courage" to take on these other challenges. After he was taught the SUDS (to measure courage), Noah was taught imaginal exposure to prepare him to deal with his social anxiety, and to see himself (covert rehearsal) saying hi to other kids and practicing saying something positive to another child to initiate interaction ("That's a cool shirt."). The practitioner role-played some encounters with him, and rehearsed what to say if kids were mean or didn't want to play with him.

June, Noah, and his mother worked closely together on a careful hierarchy of steps for approaching other kids and for reducing his compulsive "perfect" behavior. Noah's aunt was included, so when mom was not around she could reinforce his "time limits" for cleaning up, writing out his homework, or saying his prayers at night. They all understood what the rewards were on a daily basis (e.g., praise, a little more TV time, etc.) if Noah stuck to the time limits and left things "just a little bit messy." A consultation was planned between the pastor at the local church, Noah, and his mother to talk about "prayer" (not to put Noah on the spot, but just to get an authoritative view of why "praying shouldn't be perfect, because only God is perfect"). The pastor and his wife (who was also a social worker) understood immediately what was needed, and made the encounter into a fun picnic on the church grounds with their own grandchildren. The meeting helped dispel some of Noah's more oppressive ideas about what he thought God wanted of him: "God wants you to have fun, Noah!" seemed to be a helpful injunction from the pastor.

June also had a phone conversation with Noah's teacher (with whom June collaborated regularly). The teacher, very familiar with classroom contingency management methods, immediately got on board with the reinforcement schedule to allow Noah only limited time to "tidy up" his work, and focused on praising the content of his work and discouraging him from being "too fussy." The after-school program monitor also agreed to estimate and record the number of minutes Noah played with other kids. This case management and networking paid off immediately, as there was little confusion among various players in Noah's life about what was expected of him. Over the next two to three months, Noah's mother and teacher reported considerable improvement. A sense of heaviness began to lift. He learned to live with "good enough" tidying-up, spent more time playing with other kids, and seemed less preoccupied with his grief.

Selecting Scales and Creating Indexes to Monitor and Evaluate Client Progress

The practitioner chose the revised CDRS (short form) because it seemed to address the right balance of anxious (social withdrawal) and depressive symptoms (anhedonia, depressed mood, self-esteem). It also has a conversational format that seemed to lend itself to assessment with Noah, who was fairly articulate once he felt comfortable with an adult. Specific indexes employed included (at different points during the intervention, depending on the achievement of different objectives): his intensity of sadness (0, "none," to 10, "extremely sad") regarding his grief over Damon, any indications of suicidal thoughts (0, "none," to 10, "all the time"), level of hopelessness (0, "none," to 10, "extremely hopeless"), the number of minutes he spent playing with another child in the after-school program, and the amount of time he spent trying to make his room or his homework "perfect" (table 12.1).

TABLE 12.1   The client service plan for Noah

Problems	Goals	Sample Objectives	Interventions	Assessment Tools
Depression, grief, stress-related symptoms resulting from the death of his friend	Provide some normative degree of resolution for grief; resolve any acute symptoms related to the death, the child's cognitive appraisal of the death, and further sense of danger	Carefully review his understanding of the circumstances of his friend's death and exaggerated fears of his own danger; review his time with friend and develop a scrapbook about their times together, what he means to him now	Cognitive therapy focused on resolving fears related to his friend's death and facilitating his grief Coping skills to enhance relaxation through imagery and muscle relaxation exercises; modeling and role-playing conversational/play skills; graduated exposure; contingency management with rewards for more play time in after-school program EX/RP exercised early on until he could "leave it alone." Implement daily rewards for reducing "organizing" time	CDRS-R (short form) to cover most target symptoms SUDS for level of anxiety if things not perfect Index of suicidal ideation; index of hopelessness Indexes used: number of minutes playing with other kids in after-school program; number of times he initiated conversation or play Number of minutes employed in "organizing" (at home and school)
Shyness, social anxiety with other kids at school	Increase his comfort level and improve socialization skills so he can play after school for at least 1 hour	Measure graduated objectives from a few minutes up to 60 minutes during after-school program; after-school instructors agree to record the number of minutes		
Moderate OCD symptoms; perfectionism, excessive "organizing" to get things "just right"; feelings of responsibility for external events	Reduce expectations to be perfect; tolerate "messiness" with reduced anxiety and compulsive behaviors	Use graduated objectives to reduce level of perfectionism with regard to tidying up his room, homework, prayer by reducing amount of "organizing" to 1–2 minutes daily at the end of each task		

SUMMARY

Many young people suffer substantial psychosocial disruption when symptoms of anxiety and depression are serious and chronic. These problems also co-occur frequently. A number of valid and practical scales are available to enhance assessment and evaluation for children suffering internalizing disorders, and interventions for these conditions are reasonably well developed and effective. Interventions for severe depression, however, lag behind. The key effective elements in treating these two disorders overlap considerably, and practitioners should develop eclectic treatment plans that address the unique needs of individual clients. Families and other participants in the child's life should be included in the treatment whenever feasible to provide consistency and follow-through. Practitioners who employ MDF assessment and evidence-based interventions for internalizing disorders can feel confident that many of their young clients will achieve substantial and lasting relief from anxiety and depression.

CHAPTER 13

CONDUCT DISORDER AND ATTENTION DEFICIT HYPERACTIVITY DISORDER IN CHILDREN AND ADOLESCENTS

Conduct disorder (CD) and attention deficit hyperactivity disorder (ADHD) are among the most common diagnoses applied to children and adolescents. As with internalizing disorders, the symptoms and problems associated with these externalizing disorders often co-occur, and the skills for effective interventions for these disorders overlap considerably. Thus, this chapter addresses them both.

Assessment for externalizing disorders emphasizes a detailed functional assessment employing data from multiple points of view. In addition to addressing behavioral problems across multiple settings, a comprehensive assessment of a child with ADHD requires testing for learning disabilities and academic deficits. Intervention with both disorders emphasizes a combination of cognitive-behavioral skills, behavioral family therapy, and contingency management techniques. In contrast to internalizing disorders, medications for young people with ADHD have been shown to be highly effective.

ASSESSMENT OF CONDUCT DISORDER

Background data

The *DSM-IV-TR* provides four main categories of behaviors indicative of CD: aggressive conduct that causes or threatens physical harm to other people or animals, nonaggressive behaviors that cause property damage or loss, deceitfulness or theft, and serious violations of rules. These behaviors often result in difficulties in social, academic, and occupational functioning. Young people who manifest these behaviors also show a characteristic callousness, lack of empathy regarding others' feelings, and little or no remorse concerning the effects of their behavior. These characteristics in children predict adult psychopathy (see chapter 10). Low frustration tolerance, temper outbursts, and risk-taking behaviors are common features and may be associated with lower academic achievement, precocious sexual activity, early use of drugs and alcohol, and higher suicide risk.

Oppositional defiant disorder (ODD, described in more detail below), is a likely precursor for CD and is characterized by chronic disobedient, uncooperative, and disruptive behavior.

Juvenile delinquency should be distinguished from CD. *Juvenile delinquency* is a general term referring to delinquent acts engaged in by young people. These are fairly common and usually do not lead to arrests. A subgroup of children and adolescents who engage in criminal activities including assault, robbery, animal cruelty, and rape are more likely to fit the criteria for CD. CD and juvenile delinquency are mostly associated with males, although female juvenile delinquency and CD should be considered equally serious. After a few offenses, it is likely that a juvenile is on the way to an enduring problem as an adult. Most offenses are committed by recidivists who started young and gradually engaged in more severe antisocial acts. Long-term outcomes for chronic offenders are generally considered bleak (Moore & Arthur, 1989).

Prevalence rates for CD are estimated at 2–9% and for ODD 6–10%, with boys outnumbering girls by a ratio of at least four to one. CD appears to account for about half of all referrals to clinics for childhood problems. Older boys are more likely to be diagnosed with CD than with ODD, and CD shows good stability over time from childhood, through adolescence, and into adulthood as APD (McMahon & Estes, 1997; Baum, 1989). The co-occurrence rates for ODD and CD are between 84% and 96%, and half or more of children with CD are likely to meet the criteria for ADHD as well. Children with CD appear to have academic deficiencies, problems with interpersonal relationships, and cognitive and problem-solving deficiencies (e.g., overinterpreting hostility in others). Animal cruelty is a particularly telling sign of CD (C. Miller, 2001). Children with CD, including some with ADHD, have increased risk of becoming antisocial adolescents and adults with co-occurring mental health and substance-abuse problems (Kazdin, 1997; Weinberg, Rohdert, Colliver, & Glantz, 1998; Disney, Elkins, McGue, & Iacono, 1999; Molina, Smith, & Pelham, 1999; Baily, 1998; P. D. Riggs, Baker, Mikulich, Young, & Crowley, 1995).

CD also appears to be a predictor of gang entry. This association is supported by a number of studies, including a six-year longitudinal survey (Lahey, Gordon, Loeber, Stouthamer-Loeber, & Farrington, 1999) that demonstrated that almost one-quarter of African-American boys, out of a sample of 347 children in first, fourth, and seventh grades, had entered a gang by age nineteen. Factors related to gang initiation included increased levels of CD symptoms prior to gang entry, having delinquent friends in early adolescence, lower family income, and lack of parental supervision. Juvenile offenders were also at higher risk than others in their age group for contracting HIV due to both drug abuse and risky sexual behaviors (Malow, McMahon, Cremer, Lewis, & Alferi, 1997).

Cultural factors may buffer or worsen the long-term outcomes for behaviorally disordered children and adolescents. Coatsworth et al. (2002) conducted a three-year longitudinal study with 150 low-income adolescent girls (ages 12–14) and their families from different Hispanic ethnic subgroups, and found family support to be a key factor in mitigating the occurrence of behavioral problems. However, peer conflicts and conflicts between family members and peer group predicted more externalizing problems. More research is needed to examine cultural risk and protective factors associated with CD and other behavioral disorders in youth.

Theories

Although it has been established for some time that conduct-disordered children are at increased risk to become antisocial adults (L. N. Robins, 1966), most children with ODD or CD *do not* become antisocial adults. Risk factors associated with CD include genetic predisposition, history of family psychopathology (psychopathy, substance abuse, criminality, mood disorder, schizophrenia, ADHD), disruptive parenting, conflicted family relationships, childhood abuse and neglect, early difficulties with behavioral self-control, problems with social competence resulting in peer rejection, academic difficulties, poverty, and exposure to community violence (*DSM-IV-TR*; Kazdin, 1997; Horne, Glaser, & Calhoun, 1999; Cadoret & Cain, 1980; Grilo, Sanislow, Fehon, Martino, & McGlashan, 1999). Signs of CD in younger children have more negative long-term outcomes than delinquency that begins in early adolescence (Herbert, 1998). "Late starters" tend to decrease these behaviors as they grow into adulthood (McMahon & Estes, 1997).

There appear to be major cognitive distortions and difficulties in social problem solving in conduct-disordered young people. These children lean toward action-oriented and physically aggressive solutions to problems, rather than talking things out (Herbert, 1998; Kendall, 1993). M. Fraser (1996) summarized the main points in emerging cognitive theories of aggression and antisocial behavior in children. These psychosocial processes take into consideration the child's innate arousal level (temperament) and social-learning experience, such as observing violent parents or other models, and witnessing substance abuse and associated negative consequences. These experiences can affect the development of cognitive appraisal of others' behavior (e.g., inaccurate appraisal of social cues such as seeing or exaggerating hostile intent when it is not present or significant), and failing to consider long-term consequences of aggressive action. In addition, youngsters may fail to learn the interpersonal coping skills necessary to engage in problem solving as a preferred method of resolving interpersonal conflict. In a violent home, for example, they may have learned that using force is an appropriate way of achieving one's short-term gains. Environmental factors that influence the development of aggressive behavioral style and CD also include exposure to community violence, poverty, and drug abuse.

Key Elements of Multidimensional/ Functional Assessment

CD is described in the *DSM-IV-TR* as a repetitive and persistent pattern of behavior that violates the basic rights of others or major age-appropriate societal norms or rules. The diagnosis requires three (or more) of the following criteria in the past twelve months (with at least one criterion present in the past six months): the adolescent is often aggressive toward people and animals; often bullies, threatens, or intimidates others; often initiates physical fights; has used a weapon that can cause serious physical harm to others; has been physically cruel to people; has been physically cruel to animals; has stolen while confronting a victim (e.g., mugging, purse snatching, extortion, armed robbery); has forced someone into sexual activity; has deliberately destroyed property; has engaged in deceitfulness or thefts; often lies to obtain goods or favors or to avoid obligations; and has stolen items of nontrivial value without confronting a victim. A young person who meets these criteria may also have engaged in serious violations of rules, often stays out at night despite parental prohibitions, has run away from home overnight at least twice (or once without returning for a lengthy period), and is often truant from school. These disturbances in behavior must have caused clinically significant impairments in social, academic, or occupational functioning. Some of these behaviors are likely to have begun before age thirteen. It is very likely that an older adolescent who has demonstrated a number of these behaviors with some consistency is likely to meet the criteria for APD at age eighteen. This diagnosis "should be applied only when the behavior in question is symptomatic of an underlying dysfunction within the individual and not simply a reaction to the immediate social context" (*DSM-IV-TR*, p. 96). How to make this determination is not clear.

ODD is a recurrent pattern of negativistic, defiant, disobedient, and hostile behavior toward authority figures that persists for at least six months. It is characterized by the frequent occurrence of at least four of the following behaviors: losing temper; arguing with adults; refusing to comply with authorities; deliberately annoying others; blaming others (not taking responsibility); being easily annoyed by others; demonstrating anger, resentfulness, and vindictiveness. The young person's behavior is particularly marked by stubbornness, unwillingness to compromise, ignoring directives of adult authorities, and failing to take responsibility for one's actions. To meet diagnostic criteria, these behaviors must result in problems related to social, academic, or occupational functioning. Adolescents who manifest these behaviors are also likely to suffer from low self-esteem, may have a history of high motor activity and poor frustration tolerance, are more likely to abuse alcohol and other drugs, and have a higher likelihood of meeting the criteria for CD. As with CD, ODD appears to be accompanied by a history of having at least one parent with similar behavioral disorders often accompanied by a substance-abuse problem, disruptive parenting, and a history of harsh, abusive, or neglectful parenting.

Individualized MDF assessment is necessary, given the heterogeneity of symptoms among behaviorally disordered children (Ashford, Sales, & Reid, 2001; Kazdin, 1997). Dimensional measures targeting the child's unique problems are also useful for measuring treatment outcomes. As with internalizing disorders, externalizing disorders in children have come to be better understood not as dichotomous conditions (i.e., diagnoses), but as multidimensional problems in which the child's thoughts, feelings, and behaviors are influenced by multiple developmental and environmental causes. Their psychosocial functioning is affected on every level to varying degrees of severity, and these problems are understood to interact in complex ways within family, school, and community environments (McMahon & Estes, 1997).

A functional analysis delineates the patterns and sequencing of the antecedents and consequences associated with conduct-disordered behaviors (Herbert, 1998). This functional analysis is conducted within the context of the child's expected achievement levels for cognitive, behavioral, physical, and social development (Rutter, 1997). Noting whether the child is an "early" or "late starter" regarding the behavioral symptoms may also be critical prognostically, as is the severity and types of conduct problems (e.g., school-yard fighting versus stealing or harming animals; McMahon & Estes, 1997). The functional analysis helps target goals and objectives for the individually tailored treatment plan. Therapeutic goals are likely to include changing cognitive distortions and attributional processes regarding a generally hostile or aggressive approach to family and peers, and improving social and general problem-solving skills to reduce conflict and increase prosocial behaviors.

A thorough examination of family functioning is also essential, given that some of the antecedents as well as the consequences of conduct problems are likely to be manifested in the home. Parenting skills (i.e., nurturance and disciplining methods) need to be given careful scrutiny, as well as the child's response to parents' behaviors in this regard. In addition, the couple relationship should be examined if relevant (see chapter 11), along with the presence of substance abuse, domestic violence, and other conflicts, such as custody battles. Foster and Robin (1997) summarize key areas of concern regarding parent-adolescent conflict: repeated, predominantly verbal disputes; disagreements that fail to resolve problems; unpleasant, angry interactions; and pervasive negative feelings about family relationships. Families prone to experiencing adolescent-parent conflict tend to have poor communications and problem-solving skills, cognitive distortions about family relations, poor cooperation between parents, and other dysfunctional coalitions among family members (e.g., triangulation, severe disengagement). During the family assessment, an effort should be made to forge a strong working alliance, so that the challenging work of changing the behaviors of both parents and children can be undertaken successfully. In addition to parental competence and overall family functioning, the assessment should take into account the larger social system: the child's functioning in school and the community, and any involvement in the criminal justice system (Baily, 1998).

Every effort should be made to employ multiple sources of data, such as parents, siblings, teachers, coaches, physicians, and law enforcement, and multiple methods. The latter include interviewing alone and with the family, direct observation in different settings, self-monitoring, and adjunct use of behavioral rating scales and other relevant instruments (Franz & Gross, 1998). The child may be an important informant, but the validity and usefulness of the data will depend on a number of factors, including age, cognitive capacities, and capacity for telling the truth. McMahon and Estes (1997) suggest that if children are younger than ten, their self-report may not be factually reliable, but much can be learned through brief periods of play or informal exchanges about their cognitive and emotional state. Particularly with older children, more can be learned from their point of view regarding home, school, friends, clubs, and so forth, and how they feel about themselves and their relationships with others.

Instruments

The Revised Behavior Problem Checklist (RBPC; Quay, 1983) is one of the most well-researched and widely used scales for measuring problem behaviors in children and adolescents. The eighty-nine items cover a range of behavioral dimensions: CD, personality disorder, inadequacy/immaturity, psychotic behavior, and socialized/delinquent personality. Test-retest reliability has been generally shown to be adequate, and like the CBCL, the RBPC discriminates between treatment and nontreatment groups. It can be filled out by parents, teachers, or other adult caregivers. Norms are available for teacher ratings from kindergarten through the twelfth grade, and ratings by mothers for children ages 5–16. However, one study of the RBPC demonstrated low interrater reliability among various informants (i.e., mental health professionals, special education teachers, classroom teachers) for all subscales (Cutchen & Simpson, 1993). Lack of congruence among different informants, however, is not an uncommon problem in the use of rating scales, including the CBCL and the SAC (noted in chapter 2).

The Eyberg Child Behavior Inventory (ECBI; Eyberg & Ross, 1978; Eyberg & Robinson, 1983) was developed to assess CD in children ages 2–12. Thirty-six items are rated on a seven-point scale. It gives an intensity score for frequency of occurrence, and a dichotomous score (yes/no) to indicate whether the respondent sees the behavior as a problem. The problem score thus ranges from 0 to 36, and the intensity score ranges from 36 to 252. Normative data are available. The parent and teacher versions (slightly different) of this proprietary instrument rate children's disruptive behaviors, and the scale takes less than ten minutes to complete. A number of studies have shown good psychometric properties, including excellent internal consistency, good to excellent test-retest and interrater reliability, good discriminant validity by distinguishing referred from nonreferred children, and good factorial stability by race and gender (G. L. Burns & Patterson, 1990; G. L. Burns, Patterson, Nussbaum, & Parker, 1991). A more recent analysis of the factor structure of the ECBI (G. L. Burns & Patterson, 2000) revealed three subscales that reliably measured symptoms of ODD, CD, and ADHD. The ECBI is a reliable, valid, and useful measure for these behaviors and for measuring treatment progress and outcomes, but differential diagnoses for these disorders should be made with formal diagnostic criteria. The ECBI may not be suitable for older adolescents with CD, because item content is oriented toward younger children (Collett, Ohan, & Myers, 2003).

The New York Teacher Rating Scale (NYTRS; L. S. Miller, Klein et al., 1995) is a very promising addition to the collection of scales available for measuring behavior disorders in youth. It is specifically designed to measure ODD and CD. The original scale consisted of ninety items gleaned from a number of existing scales (e.g., RBPC, Conners rating scales), and was administered by teachers to over 1,300 first through tenth graders and a small sample of children diagnosed with CD. The scale comprises four main factors: defiance, physical aggression, delinquent aggression, and peer relations. To add to the utility of the scale, two composite scores are computed (see directions below): the Antisocial Behavior Scale (ABS) and the Disruptive Behavior Scale (DBS). Means and standard deviations published in Miller et al. serve as normative data, and since there were no differences by class year, scores do not have to be adjusted. Internal-consistency ratings for all subscales were shown to be good to excellent with moderate to good test-retest ratings. As with other scales cited, interrater agreements tend to be moderate at best. The NYTRS has demonstrated good convergent validity with the RBPC, and accurately identifies young people with CD. It has also shown good sensitivity to behavioral interventions (L. Miller Brotman, personal communication, March, 2005) and would serve well as an evaluation tool. The teacher version is reprinted here (instrument 13.1). A parent version of the scale is also available (L. S. Miller & Kamboukos, 2000) as well as a preschool version from the first author (Miller).

INSTRUMENT 13.1   New York Teacher Rating Scale (NYTRS)

Please rate the child on the items below, using the average child in a regular classroom as your basis for comparison. Rate the child's behavior over the <u>previous four weeks</u>. Please answer all questions. For each item, indicate the degree of the problem. Not at all = 0; Just a little = 1; Pretty much = 2; Very much = 3.

	Not at all	Just a little	Pretty much	Very much
1. Defiant	0	1	2	3
2. Angry	0	1	2	3
3. Argues, quarrels with teachers	0	1	2	3
4. Acts "smart" (impudent or sassy)	0	1	2	3
5. Spiteful, vindictive	0	1	2	3
6. Loses temper	0	1	2	3
7. Disobedient, difficult to control	0	1	2	3
8. Tries to dominate others; bullies, threatens	0	1	2	3
9. Easily annoyed by others	0	1	2	3
10. Blames others; denies own mistakes	0	1	2	3
11. Deliberately annoys others	0	1	2	3
12. Lies	0	1	2	3
13. Breaks school rules	0	1	2	3
14. Destroys or defaces property	0	1	2	3
15. Acts violently to other children or adults (hits, pushes, etc.)	0	1	2	3

16. Starts physical fights	0	1	2	3
17. Gets involved in physical fights with peers	0	1	2	3
18. Physically cruel	0	1	2	3
19. Assaults others	0	1	2	3
20. Carries a knife or other weapon	0	1	2	3
21. Has used a knife or other weapon, in a fight	0	1	2	3
22. Has mugged someone	0	1	2	3
23. Sexual misbehavior (not masturbation)	0	1	2	3
24. Steals on the sly	0	1	2	3
25. Shakes down others for money or other belongings	0	1	2	3
26. Late to school or class	0	1	2	3
27. Truants	0	1	2	3
28. Others like to play with him/her	0	1	2	3
29. Peers seek his/her company	0	1	2	3
30. Is liked by peers	0	1	2	3
31. Helpful to others	0	1	2	3
32. Has at least one good friend	0	1	2	3
33. Is considerate with friends/companions	0	1	2	3
34. Shows remorse when does something wrong	0	1	2	3
35. How much of a conduct problem is the child at this time?	0	1	2	3
36. How much of an academic problem does the child have at this time?	0	1	2	3

Scoring instructions

Defiance scale = (items 1+2+3+4+5+6+7+8+9+10+11+12+13+14)/14
Physical aggression scale = (items 15+16+17+18+19)/5
Delinquent aggression scale = (items 20+21+22+23)/4
Peer relations scale = (items 28+29+30+31+32+33+34)/7 (Note: higher score indicates better functioning.)

Composite scales

Antisocial behavior scale = (items 15+16+17+18+19+20+21+22+23+24+25+26+27)/13
Disruptive behavior scale = (items 1+2+3+4+5+6+7+8+9+10+11+12+13+14+15+16+17+18+19+20+21+22+23+24+25+26+27)/27

Mean scores for conduct-disordered sample from L. S. Miller et al., 1995: Defiance, 1.75; physical aggression scale, 1.17; delinquent aggression, .11; peer relations, 1.0; for composite scales: ABS, .67; DBS, 1.53.

SELECTING EFFECTIVE INTERVENTIONS

A number of behavioral methods for treating ODD/CD, usually implemented in some combination, have acquired an impressive body of supporting evidence. These strategies include cognitive-behavioral coping-skills approaches (including cognitive restructuring, social skills, and behavioral self-control) to address the difficulties that conduct-disordered youth have in adequately perceiving others' behaviors and coping with their own anger and aggression; parenting skills; behavioral family therapy; and contingency management interventions employed by parents at home and by teachers, juvenile probation officers, and other collaterals in the community. Case management is essential to facilitating these multifaceted interventions.

Cognitive-behavioral treatment goals emphasize helping youths develop an improved ability to signal their arousal state, accurately label their feelings, use self-inhibitory messages, slow their responses, and better recognize hostile and nonhostile social cues. These approaches can be employed individually with the child, but have been incorporated more frequently into family approaches. The social worker plays an active role in modeling proper self-assessment and social responses and improving the child's ability to empathize with others (Webster-Stratton & Herbert, 1994; Kendall, 1993). Cognitive-behavioral programs have been successful in helping aggressive and antisocial children by using problem solving and parent behavioral management training that emphasizes the effective use of contingency management skills (i.e., learning how to provide nurturance and use rewards and sanctions more effectively; Kazdin, Bass, Seigel, & Thomas, 1989; Webster-Stratton, Kolpacoff, & Hollinsworth, 1988; Webster-Stratton, Hollinsworth, & Kolpacoff, 1989; Webster-Stratton & Herbert; Fraser, Day, Galinsky, Hodges, & Smokowski, 2004). Reviews of psychosocial interventions have outlined a well-established range of cognitive-behavioral methods for alleviating psychological and situational distress with children, adolescents, and their families (Kazdin, 1994b; Alexander & Parsons, 1982; Alexander et al., 1994; Webster-Stratton & Herbert; Ollendick & King, 1994a; Mann & Borduin, 1991; Kendall, 1993). Some research has demonstrated that successful interventions with children who have conduct problems also improve the mental health of mothers (Hutchings, Appelton, Smith, Lane, & Nash, 2002).

Cognitive-behavioral coping skills have been successfully implemented in the context of behavioral family therapy (Kazdin, 1994b, 1997; Webster-Stratton & Herbert, 1994; Alexander & Parsons, 1982; Alexander, Waldron, Newberry, & Liddle, 1988; McMahon & Forehand, 1984; Foster, 1994; Baily, 1998; Northey et al., 2003). These methods include helping parents to identify, relabel, and monitor child/adolescent problems and negotiate behavioral contracts with the child or adolescent. Psychoeducation is provided to help parents learn normative expectations for their child's behavior and develop more effective parenting skills. Therapeutic methods employed to this end include role-playing and modeling effective nurturing and disciplining behavior as well as effective parent-child communication, problem solving, and generalization of these skills across different situations.

Reviews of the literature have consistently demonstrated that structural and behaviorally oriented family therapies are the most effective for improving children's conduct problems and generalizing those benefits to the family system (Gurman, Kniskern, & Pinsof, 1986; Hazelrigg, Cooper, & Borduin, 1987; Alexander & Parsons, 1982; Alexander et al., 1994; Geismar & Wood, 1986; Lebow & Gurman, 1995; Kazdin, 1997). Estrada & Pinsoff (1995) found uniformly robust results supporting parent management training for improving long-term gains in children's behavior, parents' skills, and parents' positive perceptions of their children. However, clients who experienced greater social and economic disruption in their lives were not helped as much by these interventions, a problem that may underscore the limitations of even the most effective psychosocial interventions (Chamberlain & Rosicky, 1995; Kazdin, 1997).

Combining CBT with long-term family and systemic supports in the community (e.g., schools, juvenile justice systems) has been strongly endorsed over the years (Bramblett, Wodarski, & Thyer, 1991; Horne et al., 1999; Christophersen & Finney, 1999; Harnish, Tolan, & Guerra, 1996). Multisystemic therapy (MST), perhaps the most effective and well-defined comprehensive approach for conduct-disordered youth, combines individual CBT methods, behavioral family therapy, and community supports with contingency management strategies. MST has been shown to be effective at improving family functioning, and reducing psychiatric symptoms and recidivism in chronic juvenile offenders (Henggeler et al., 1986; Borduin, Henggeler, Blaske, & Stein, 1990; Borduin et al., 1995; Henggeler, Melton, & Smith, 1992; Henggeler, Melton, Smith, Schoenwald, & Hanley, 1993; Bourke & Donohue, 1996; Henggeler et al., 1998; Henggeler & Sheidow, 2003).

Brestan and Eyberg (1998) reviewed the intervention literature for eighty-two studies covering 5,272 children and adolescents with conduct problems. They used Chambless and Hollon's methodological criteria (1998) to rate studies as "established" effective treatments or "probably efficacious" (see chapter 3). Over half of the studies reviewed included at least one comparison group, random assignments to groups, and reliable measures; had at least twelve or more participants in each group; and reported the number of dropouts. Fewer than half of the studies reported using a treatment manual, conducted six-month follow-ups, or reported descriptive statistics on participants' gender, race/ethnicity, and other factors. Interventions deemed "established" had to meet the following criteria: positive results had to be demonstrated in at least two controlled studies in which treatment manuals were employed, and the replication study had to be conducted by researchers other than those who conducted the original controlled trial. "Probably efficacious" interventions were demonstrated effective by at least two controlled studies, but replication may have been conducted by the original research team. These reviewers concluded that only behaviorally oriented parent-training programs could be considered "established" treatments. "Probably efficacious" interventions included an array of cognitive-behavioral skill-oriented approaches (e.g., anger control, problem-solving therapy) and multisystemic interventions. The reviewer suggested that future research should include more girls with conduct disorders, and racial/ethnic-minority families and their children.

Farmer et al. (2002) came to very similar conclusions in a fifteen-year review of interventions for children ages 6–12: the data show consistent positive outcomes for cognitive-behavioral and family-oriented treatments. They added that combining child-focused and family approaches may have discernable advantages. With regard to a larger community psychosocial focus, multisystemic approaches clearly garnered the preponderance of evidence for effectiveness with emotionally and behaviorally disordered adolescents, although more research is needed with younger children and adolescents. Gacono, Nieberding, Owen, Rubel, and Bodholdt (2001) echoed these conclusions in a ten-year review of the literature: behaviorally oriented individual and family approaches (particularly MST) appeared to be most effective for conduct-disordered youth. Serin and Preston (2001) recommended that these interventions be modified, tested, and implemented with adult offenders.

Based on a comprehensive review of nine meta-analyses and twenty-three literature reviews spanning half a century, Palmer (1996) concluded that confrontation (e.g., "scared straight"), traditional social casework, counseling, and psychodynamically oriented therapies showed very little evidence of effectiveness in terms of recidivism. Programs that showed mixed results included diversionary programs, which combine case management, job program, and counseling; physical challenge programs such as Outward Bound; restitution; vocational and educational training; and enhanced probation and parole monitoring. Overall, these "mixed" results showed only modest reductions in recidivism. Programs judged to be successful were predominantly behaviorally oriented approaches that included family interventions, contingency management, and other life-skills approaches. Multidimensional and ecologically valid strategies such as MST (Henggeler et al., 1998) provide a comprehensive framework to guide effective eclectic interventions, and these approaches have also been applied to prevention programs for high-risk youths (Blechman & Vryan, 2000; Liddle & Hogue, 2000). Despite the advances made in treatments for juvenile offenders, however, one area has not been adequately addressed in outcome research: juvenile sex offenders. About one-fifth of sex offenses are committed by juveniles, and they are often diagnosed with co-occurring CD and ADHD (Bourke & Donohue, 1996). Nevertheless, evaluation research on the effectiveness of treatment programs for juvenile sex offenders has been largely descriptive, and thus a poor basis for making treatment recommendations (Becker & Johnson, 2001).

Exemplar Study: Multisystemic Therapy with Juvenile Offenders.
In their review of the literature, Borduin et al. (1995) pointed out that controlled studies of serious juvenile offenders have been relatively neglected. Although behavioral-skills approaches have been shown to be promising, long-term results have not been impressive. Long-term maintenance of gains is likely to require more extensive intervention with social systems that go beyond individual offenders and their immediate family. Such strategies, such as MST, include the school, community, criminal justice, and other systems that affect the lives of these young people. The Borduin et al. investigation was designed to have advantages over previous studies of MST by including a larger sample size, longer fol-

low-up measures, improved measurement tools, and comparable treatment groups with about equal amounts of intervention in both. The authors randomly assigned 176 clients (from a consecutive referral group of 200) to either MST or an eclectic individual therapy (a loosely defined psychodynamic, client-centered, and supportive approach). The juvenile offenders had at least one parent in the study (mostly mothers), were 70% white and 30% black, had been arrested about four times on average for serious crimes, and were mostly from the lower socioeconomic class. All clients were voluntary, but remained under the jurisdiction of the court during treatment. One hundred and forty clients completed treatment (with no significant differences between the two groups on completion rates), and the MST group had an average of about twenty-four visits whereas the individual eclectic intervention lasted almost twenty-nine visits, a statistically significant advantage. MST was provided by graduate-level practitioners who were trained and supervised in the approach by Borduin, and the individual eclectic control group was treated by practicing clinicians in local mental health agencies. In the MST condition, all clients received interventions that involved more than one social system, whereas 90% of those in the control group received only the individual therapy. Most assessments were conducted in the home for both treatment conditions, and both pre and post measures included an array of well-validated psychosocial measures including the SCL-90, the RBPC, the Family Adaptability and Cohesion Evaluation Scales (FACES-II), and an array of observational measures including videotapes of family interactions and checklists completed by the juvenile's teachers. State police records provided four-year follow-up data on arrests.

Results demonstrated that, compared to the control group, MST significantly and substantively reduced key family correlates of antisocial behavior in the youths, improved psychosocial adjustment in family members, improved family relations, improved psychological well-being of parents, improved behavior in youths, and resulted in a substantial reduction in rearrests after treatment. The success of MST did not vary by participant demographics (age, gender, race, income). The authors attributed the success of the model to its comprehensive nature and its ecological validity. Those who received individual therapy were arrested more than twice as often and for more serious crimes than were those who received MST.

Reducing aggressive behavior is also a primary target of concern among those who work in residential settings such as group homes or psychiatric hospital programs. Behavioral approaches using contingency management have been shown to be helpful in those circumstances as well. Wong (1999), for example, conducted an uncontrolled evaluation of a behavioral program in an inpatient multiservice treatment program with adolescents who had histories of severe emotional disturbance and violent behavior, three of whom had been adjudicated on homicide charges. These youths (ten females, nineteen males) were fifteen years old on average, were mostly of below-average intelligence, and had a mixed assortment of diagnoses, including CD, ADHD, major depression, and bipolar disorder. They also had numerous prior interventions. The behavioral intervention included structured teaching of prosocial interpersonal behaviors, which involved engaging the youth, identifying the problem behavior, providing a rationale, and demonstrating proper behavior to the youth who would then practice the behavior, providing corrective feedback and rewards as needed. It also included a reinforcement system by which clients could earn points to obtain small privileges; a privilege-level system for improved performance and responsibility (e.g., gaining off-site passes for better behavior and school performance); the use of minimally to moderately restrictive interventions for aggressive behavior (from verbal prompts to restraints for out-of-control aggression); implementation of an increasingly enriched daily schedule (e.g., movies, sporting events); and use of weekly community meetings. The findings demonstrated gradual and significant reductions in the most severe problem behaviors. Of course, due to the uncontrolled nature of the design, the relative effectiveness of the behavioral program cannot be judged, nor can specific effective elements of the program be identified. Nevertheless, the study serves as a good model for implementing behavioral-skills interventions in a residential setting with some of the most severely disturbed aggressive youth.

Conduct-Disordered Adolescents with Substance-Abuse Problems

In addition to substantial levels of co-occurring depression and anxiety disorders, about two-thirds of young people with substance-use disorders also demonstrate at least one externalizing disorder (Kandel et al., 1999). Structural and behavioral family therapy has been successfully employed with families of drug-addicted people (Stanton et al., 1982; Stanton & Shadish, 1997) and has been the subject of much outcome research (Weinberg et al., 1998). One meta-analysis of family interventions for a drug-abusing member focused on randomized controlled studies (Stanton & Shadish). A total of fifteen studies covering about 3,500 clients and significant others met suitable criteria. Results of the analysis showed that marital and family interventions produced outcomes superior to individual, peer group, or family psychoeducation. They also appeared cost-effective when combined with methadone maintenance. These strategies appeared to work equally well for both adolescent and adult abusers, and demonstrated relatively higher levels of client retention. A recent meta-analysis of adolescent substance-abuse treatments revealed that, on the whole, behaviorally oriented family therapies and cognitive-behavioral skills were most effective (M. G. Vaughn & Howard, 2004). Other narrative reviews of controlled trials of family substance-abuse treatments have provided concurring opinions (Liddle & Dakof, 1995; Waldron, 1997).

The results of structural and behavioral family therapies with substance-abusing youth and their families have not been uniformly positive, however. Szapocznik, Kurtines, Foote, Perez-Vidal, and Hervis (1983) compared conjoint family therapy with family therapy conducted with individuals. Clients were Hispanic families and individuals, and treatment included follow-ups of six to twelve months on some families. There was considerable attrition in the study, and results showed some advantage for the individual intervention. In a later replication study, Szapocznik et al. (1986) demonstrated similar results with another sample of Hispanic families. Santisteban et al. (1996) later demonstrated that more emphasis on early engagement efforts could substantially improve retention in treatment. In an uncontrolled trial of brief structural/strategic family therapy with 122 mostly Hispanic youngsters (ages 12–14) and their families, Santisteban et al. (1997) demonstrated that an ethnically sensitive intervention delivered in twelve to sixteen ninety-minute sessions over four to six months was moderately effective at reducing conduct-disordered behavior, improving family functioning, and reducing substance abuse. Practitioners made special efforts to address the cultural expectations of these primarily Hispanic families by being task-oriented and by showing an understanding of intergenerational tensions, family hierarchy, and acculturation stressors. Although more research is needed on culturally congruent interventions with conduct-disordered youth, evidence generally shows that outcomes of mainstream services for both minority and white young people may be comparable with regard to changes in delinquency, school performance, self-esteem, behavior, interpersonal problems, anxiety, depression, and family functioning, among other outcomes (S. J. Wilson, Lipsey, & Soydan, 2003).

Waldron, Brody, and Slesnick (2001) called for combining individual CBT methods and behavioral family therapy for substance-abusing adolescents. The objectives of this approach include reducing or eliminating substance use and other problem behaviors, and improving family relationships. They suggest three phases to the relatively brief (fourteen-session) intervention: Sessions 1–5 include engagement, motivational enhancement, and a thorough systems and individual functional assessment, targeting key problems for a skill-building intervention. The whole family is seen during the first few visits, with two visits reserved for the adolescent alone. Behavior-change interventions are the focus of sessions 6–10, with the hour divided (15 and 45 minutes) for the individual and family, respectively. These sessions include a combination of behavioral family interventions similar to those noted earlier (see, e.g., Alexander, Holtzworth-Monroe, & Jameson, 1994) and individual coping-skills approaches discussed in chapter 6 (see, e.g., Monti, Barnett, O'Leary, & Colby, 2001; Kadden, 1994). In the third phase (sessions 11–14), the intervention focuses on generalization of gains and relapse prevention.

Key Elements of Effective Practices with Conduct-Disordered Youth

Many practitioner-researchers have contributed to evidence-based practices with conduct-disordered children and their families. These approaches, for the most part, share common theoretical and practice elements, and have been incorporated and integrated into multilevel intervention strategies that are now likely to include methods for addressing the child's individual behavior, the parent's skills, family functioning and well-being, and the broader system within which the child's or adolescent's behavior has become a source of distress, such as the school and community.

Kendall (1993), Kazdin (1994b), and others contributed much of the research on individual CBT approaches for conduct-disordered children, and Hanf (1970), Forehand and McMahon (1981), Webster-Stratton and Herbert (1994), Patterson (1982), and others provided much of the foundation for parent management training and similar parenting-skills approaches that incorporate CBT skills. These methods are based on social cognitive and operant behavioral principles that stress the functional linkage between antecedent events and the child's behaviors, and subsequent reinforcement to increase prosocial behaviors and reduce negative or noncompliant behaviors. Parents learn about basic nurturing and effective limit setting through psychoeducation, modeling, and rehearsal with the practitioner (who provides verbal and/or video feedback). Clients then practice these skills at home, monitor the results, and evaluate their performance in subsequent sessions. Others such as Webster-Stratton and colleagues (e.g., see Webster-Stratton & Hancock, 1998) expanded these programs to incorporate additional communication and problem-solving techniques, marital therapy, stress management, and closer coordination with school personnel to maximize child and family well-being. In similar fashion, Henggeler et al. (1998) widened the scope of behavioral family-systems approaches to include community reinforcement and contingency management with key collaterals in the schools and the criminal justice system. Given that the adolescent's problems are often related to a host of factors, including family problems, associating with antisocial peers, school difficulties, substance abuse, criminal acts, and a lack of community support, it is the basic premise of MST that these problems be addressed through a multilevel intervention implemented in the youth's natural ecology.

Practitioners should become familiar with available clinical texts and treatment manuals for these evidence-based interventions. These approaches share common elements and are frequently combined. Although Kazdin (1997) rightfully cautions against simply combining treatments with the expectation that they will yield superior effects, practitioners should learn these methods "by the book," but should also be prepared to flexibly tailor the intervention plan to the needs and circumstances of each child or adolescent and their family. More research on matching eclectic models to problem type, severity, and other client characteristics is needed.

The core elements of evidence-based practice with conduct-disordered youth include CBT, parenting skills, behavioral family therapy, and systems/community-based contingency management.

Cognitive-Behavioral Therapy.   The child needs to more accurately read and interpret the behavior and feelings of others in social situations. The social worker

- uses Socratic questioning, clarification, gentle confrontation, and testing dysfunctional cognitions;

- teaches self-instructional training, including self-talk to identify and track problem circumstances and covertly reinforce behavioral self-control;

- employs cognitive restructuring to help correct the child's distorted expectations and misappraisal of social situations, and replace them with prosocial cognitions;

- through psychoeducation, modeling, role-play, and homework practice, helps the young person stop and think about immediate emotional reactions to social or other situational provocations in a more deliberate manner;

- emphasizes how to make self-statements about the problem, consider alternative responses, and engage in problem solving that will lead to solutions;

- teaches the young person to self-monitor their reactions and skills in these social situations;

- models cognitive processes by making prosocial verbal self-statements aloud in the presence of the child, helps the child rehearse these skills by prompting them with cues to practice the self-statements, and uses modeling and role-play to rehearse the prosocial behaviors while delivering feedback and praise for successful use of the skills;

- helps the child express feelings more effectively;

- teaches the child to control anger and related responses by early identification of anger-provoking cues and by using constructive responses to avert aggressive encounters;

- reinforces the use of standard problem-solving skills in response to provocation;

- teaches the young person covert desensitization to relax and visualize themselves identifying, processing, and responding to a potential problem situation in a prosocial manner;

- models and role-plays effective and assertive interpersonal skills;

- guides in vivo desensitization procedures and assigns homework to practice new skills in increasingly challenging social circumstances;

- shows the child how to reward themselves (self-reinforcement) for positive social responses and reductions in negative behaviors; and

- teaches parents how to reinforce these skills at home.

Effective Parenting Skills.   With parents, the social worker may need to demonstrate nurturance (e.g., emotional and physical caring and playing) and positive disciplining skills (giving directives calmly through simple communications). They may need to learn how to balance positive reinforcement for prosocial and constructive behaviors with proportionate sanctions or punishment as needed such as losing points as part of a contingency management contract, or temporary loss of privileges. Specific procedures employed for teaching parents more effective child management techniques include

> explaining the rationale for the approach: the parent will be using positive means to increase prosocial behaviors, reduce negative behaviors, and improve the child-parent relationship;
>
> demonstrating the skills via role-playing;
>
> asking parents to practice the skill while the therapist role-plays the child;
>
> explaining the desired behavior to the child until the child demonstrates understanding;
>
> having the child role-play the desired behavior;
>
> asking parents to demonstrate the approach with their child while being observed and coached by the practitioner;
>
> allowing parents to practice without direct coaching;
>
> assigning homework for parents to practice the new skills; and
>
> reviewing performance in the following session.

The social worker also teaches parents how to pinpoint the problem behaviors and record compliance versus noncompliance at home. Another skill parents learn is how to shape the child's behavior by stringing together rewards and sanctions to increase the child's constructive and otherwise prosocial behaviors. Parents are likely to need reminding that, at all times, their behavior must represent a model to their troubled child or adolescent; likewise, they should try to supervise their children at all times, even when they are away from home. This involves parents' knowing where their children are, what they are doing, who they are with, and when they will be returning. Children must be held accountable for these mini-contracts.

Social workers may need to demonstrate more subtle parenting skills, also. They can demonstrate to parents how to be somewhat flexible, particularly with older children, and practice problem solving and negotiating strategies. They should understand that being an effective parent does not always mean "winning" every battle decisively. Social workers should direct parent management techniques toward improving the child's school behavior and performance if needed, and arrange for regular communication between parent and teacher. As parents design goals for their children, they should keep the objectives achievable and specific. Parents, teachers, and other adults involved in the treatment should be trained to apply praise and tangible rewards for prosocial behaviors.

Behavioral Family Therapy Skills. Behavioral family therapy identifies problem behaviors between family members, negotiates solutions, and improves positive interactions (particularly by reducing coercive interactions). Social workers demonstrate communication and problem-solving skills among all family members, and continually monitor and evaluate improvements. They may need to provide couples interventions to improve communication and problem solving, including issues other than parenting differences. With the aim of improving communication, the practitioner facilitates the style, direction, and intensity of communications so they become increasingly constructive (e.g., one person speaks at a time, no interrupting, be specific about what you are saying, make no global accusations, no name calling). The practitioner negotiates straightforward contingency contracts to facilitate the couple relationship or parent management.

Systems/Community-Based Contingency Management. The practitioner may need to use assertive case management with social systems such as schools, law enforcement, and criminal justice, in addition to arranging for other instrumental and social supports. The practitioner actively includes teachers and other school personnel in the treatment plan to generalize and maintain prosocial behavioral improvements. It is important to get all parties on the same page with regard to the contingency management plan: it helps to have a consistent list of the problems and responses (contingencies) for positive and negative behaviors.

Various participants in the intervention must stick to the contingency management plan so responses can be swift, fair, and consistent. Rewards and sanctions based on the young client's behavior must be coordinated consistently to prevent the youth from becoming confused or allowing client to play one person against the other. As coordinators, social workers communicate often with collaterals to monitor intervention outcomes and to make suitable adjustments in the treatment plan. They coordinate the activities of teachers, physicians, law enforcement (e.g., juvenile probation), and the family, and keep all the parties focused on the intervention goals for the child or adolescent. All parties should use the same performance ratings for the child's behavioral goals in order to consistently judge cross-situational progress.

Finally, the practitioner makes arrangements for long-term follow-up, booster sessions, and other services to the extent that service policies and legal contingencies allow.

ASSESSMENT OF ATTENTION DEFICIT HYPERACTIVITY DISORDER

Background Data

ADHD is characterized by a constellation of cognitive and behavioral problems that cause dysfunction in social and academic roles. ADHD is marked by symptoms of inattention, hyperactivity-impulsivity, or a combination of both. The child or adolescent (ADHD can also be diagnosed in adults) demonstrates a number of problems such as lack of attention to tasks or inability to sustain attention for any length of time, lack of responsiveness to direct requests, trouble following through on chores or schoolwork, difficulty organizing tasks, avoiding activities that require sustained mental effort, disorganization and losing things necessary for completing tasks, being easily distracted by extraneous stimuli, and frequent forgetfulness in daily activities. Hyperactivity-impulsivity problems are indicated by the child's excessive fidgeting with hands or feet, trouble staying seated, difficulty quietly engaging in leisure activities, and difficulty waiting for a turn, among other signs.

Situational factors also have a significant impact on the frequency and severity of symptoms associated with ADHD (Barkley, 1987). Some factors that may affect the child's performance are time of day, fatigue, amount of restraint required, level of extraneous stimulation in the environment, reinforcement schedule associated with the task, and presence or absence of adult supervision. Children with ADHD appear most challenged when persistence is required to perform the task, or when they must restrain their behavior. In addition to academic achievement, other problems associated with ADHD include intellectual difficulties, slow language development, anxiety, depression, problems with peers, and a number of physical problems (Barkley, 1997a).

Age brings a different emphasis to ADHD symptoms. Children with ADHD are inclined to respond to the first thought that enters their mind, they do not consider sufficiently the effects of their behavior, and many find it difficult to delay gratification. The severity and frequency of these behaviors can vary over time in the same child. In addition to the impact on learning, speech, and language development, ADHD is also associated with sleep, emotional, interpersonal, and other behavioral problems (van der Krol, Oosterbaan, Weller, & Koning, 1998). Robin (1998a) notes that ADHD in adolescents may bring to light more serious problems related to conduct-disordered behaviors, including academic failure, serious behavioral problems in the family and the community (e.g., poor communications, frequent outbursts and arguments, physical violence, noncompliance with parent's expectations), and emotional disturbances such as depression, sadness, and low self-esteem possibly associated with constant frustration, repeated failures, and not living up to others' expectations. Impulsiveness in adolescents may also be associated with risk-taking behaviors that make them more prone to accidents and injuries. Robin (1998a) notes other developmental and medical problems associated with ADHD, including other developmental delays and mild neurological deficits.

Estimates of ADHD in the population vary from 3% to 10% of children (Pelham, Wheeler, & Chronis, 1998) and up to 6% of adults (Spencer, Biederman, Wilens, & Faraone, 2002). One of the problems with current diagnostic criteria is the lack of available norms for different age groups; this lack creates confusion in estimating prevalence and determining diagnosis. Estimates of the ratio of male to females diagnosed with ADHD range from 4:1 to 9:1 (J. D. White, 1999). ADHD co-occurs with CDs (van der Krol et al., 1998), bipolar disease, substance abuse, and other learning disabilities (Spencer et al.). ADHD symptoms also overlap with symptoms that characterize PTSD and thus suggest the need for a comprehensive assessment to rule out traumatic events that may be exacerbating problems characteristic of ADHD (Weinstein, Staffelbach, & Biaggio, 2000).

A childhood diagnosis of ADHD has a negative prognosis for future behavior problems (Pelham et al., 1998). M. Fischer, Barkley, Smallish, and Fletcher (2002) interviewed a group of young adults who had been diagnosed with ADHD as children. Over 90% of the original sample were located and interviewed (147 previously diagnosed with ADHD and 73 controls who were not). Although the follow-up data were based exclusively on self-reports, evidence suggested strongly that those who had been diagnosed with ADHD as children were much more likely to be diagnosed later with CD, a condition that also appeared to mediate a greater tendency to develop personality disorders (APD and BPD) as adults. The ADHD group appeared to have five times the risk of developing antisocial personality as the control group.

There is a lack of research on the relationship among ADHD, race, ethnicity, and socioeconomic factors (Gingerich, Turnock, Litfin, & Rosen, 1998). Research is hampered by a lack of culturally sensitive norms that has contributed to inaccurate estimations of rates of the disorder. However, some evidence suggests that ADHD is more likely to be diagnosed among African-American youngsters, perhaps as a result of socioeconomic and other environmental stressors that may affect the cause and course of the disorder as well as access to effective treatment.

Theories

ADHD appears to be partly caused by heredity, although an unstructured or chaotic environment can exacerbate the symptoms of the disorder (van der Krol et al., 1998). About 75% of the predisposition for the disorder may be explained by genetics, a rate higher than that of other disorders. Brain-imaging studies have demonstrated that areas of the brain that influence attention span are smaller and less active in people with ADHD than in those without the disorder (Spencer et al. 2002). Other factors potentially contributing to the causes of ADHD include parental psychopathology, low birth weight (possibly related to drinking or smoking during pregnancy), and brain injuries in utero. Although few research studies have focused on the links between personality traits and ADHD, some research suggests that children with ADHD appear more underaroused and more likely to seek external stimulation even to the point of engaging in risky behaviors compared to children without ADHD (J. D. White, 1999). People with ADHD also appear to have lower inhibitory control and are more likely to suffer from anxiety disorders. Other research has suggested links between ADHD and creativity, but data show lower levels of conscientiousness with a greater tendency toward behavioral disorders, including substance abuse. The link between temperament and ADHD (i.e., higher activity level, more distractibility and impulsivity) is well established. Longitudinal research on familial influences (including parental psychopathology) suggests that people diagnosed with both ADHD and CD may be a distinct subtype from those with ADHD alone, although sorting out the relative influences of genetics and environmental influences is still a challenge (Faraone, Biederman, Jetton, & Tsuang, 1997). Positive long-term outcomes, however, appear to be linked to higher levels of family cohesion, warmth, and support; higher socioeconomic status; and growing up in intact families with fewer children. The relationship among these biopsychosocial factors actually explains a substantial amount of the variance when accounting for ADHD (J. D. White, 1999).

There have been advances in process theories of ADHD as well. Although previous theoretical work has addressed problems in behavioral inhibition and information processing in people with ADHD, Barkley (1997a, 1997b) has offered a more unified and comprehensive approach to provide a sound theoretical foundation for further research. Poor behavioral inhibition related to neuropsychological dysfunction in the prefrontal lobes of the brain is specified as the central deficiency in ADHD. In Barkley's model, behavioral inhibition (which is needed to regulate performance) is the central construct related to four other executive functions, including working memory, self-regulation of affect, motivation and arousal, and internalization of speech and reconstitution (e.g., analysis and synthesis of behavior). Assumptions of the model include (1) the capacity for behavioral inhibition develops before the other executive functions; (2) these four executive functions develop at different times, have different trajectories, and are interactive; (3) if the capacity for inhibition improves, then these executive functions can improve (in other words, they are secondary to the primary role of inhibition); (4) dysfunction in behavioral inhibition is primarily genetic in origin, but its expression can be affected by the social environment; and (5) dysfunction in these four executive functions interacts reciprocally with deficits in the primary dysfunction in inhibition. These four executive functions regulate the relationship between cognitive information processing and behavioral performance (including sense of time and the influence of the future over immediate consequences). The result is a greater capacity for the individual to predict and control one's environment (and one's behavior within it), and to optimize performance and outcomes. The optimal interaction of these executive functions permits more effective adaptive functioning in general. For the person with ADHD, there is serious disruption in these regulatory processes, as evidenced by core clinical symptoms described above.

Barkley (1997a, 1997b) notes that the current descriptive clinical view does not consider an array of other cognitive deficits associated with the disorder. The purpose of the four main executive functions is to obtain better prediction and control over the individual's behavior, more influence over the individual's environment, and, ultimately, better influence on and prediction of future consequences. The difficulty in maintaining persistence in attention appears to represent impairment in task-directed behavior that is related to poor behavioral inhibition. This process results in the individual's difficulties in self-regulation. Distractibility in the child with ADHD appears to be related to difficulties in screening out interference, that is, internal and external events that disrupt executive functions necessary for regulating self-control and persistence. The difficulty in completing tasks appears to be related to a lack of reinforcement and a tendency to go from one uncompleted task to the next. Thus, inattention is considered a secondary symptom of ADHD, the result of poor behavioral inhibition and difficulty in screening out interference. Future research on this model could be improved with larger samples; an examination of gender differences, family history, and developmental factors; more consistency in defining ADHD; and more emphasis on the effects that these factors have on the performance deficits associated with ADHD.

Key Elements of Multidimensional/ Functional Assessment

Diagnostic criteria (*DSM-IV-TR*) for ADHD provide a choice of either multiple symptoms of inattention or multiple symptoms of hyperactivity-impulsivity. In either case, the child must exhibit six or more of the following for at least six months: For inattention, these may include failure to pay close attention to schoolwork or making careless mistakes, difficulty sustaining attention in tasks or play, not listening when spoken to directly, poor follow-through or failure to finish chores or schoolwork, difficulty in organizing tasks, avoidance of activities that involve sustained mental effort, frequent loss of things necessary for completing tasks, distraction by extraneous stimuli, and frequent forgetfulness in daily activities. For hyperactivity-impulsivity, the child often fidgets with hands or feet, has trouble staying seated when it's expected, runs around or "climbs excessively" in situations where such behavior is not expected, has difficulty engaging in leisure activities quietly, is often on the go or appears to be driven as if by a motor, talks excessively, blurts out answers before questions are completed, has difficulty waiting for a turn, and interrupts or intrudes on others. Other necessary criteria include the existence of some symptoms prior to age seven; presence of the impairment in more than one setting; symptoms causing dysfunction in social, academic, or occupational roles; and behaviors not caused by other disorders, such as pervasive developmental disorder, anxiety disorder, or PTSD.

There are problems in applying *DSM* criteria across the board with children and adolescents (Robin, 1998a). Symptoms may manifest themselves in different proportions with children versus older adolescents, and the criteria may result in fewer girls with mild to moderate ADHD being accurately diagnosed. Some critics have expressed concern that the use of *DSM-IV* criteria has led to an artificial inflation of the prevalence of the disorder, caused collectively by the educational system, mental health providers, and pharmaceutical companies. Further research is needed to elucidate the etiology of ADHD as well as to improve the reliability and validity of the diagnostic criteria.

Because of variability in the presentation of behaviors related to ADHD, MDF assessment is strongly recommended (Braswell & Bloomquist, 1991; American Academy of Child and Adolescent Psychiatry [AACAP], 1997b; Robin, 1998a, 1998b; Barkley, 1997a; Barkley & Edwards, 1998; Root & Resnick, 2003). Practitioners should include a careful diagnosis and assessment of academic performance and learning disabilities (with specialized testing and consultation). The assessment should also include the use of broadband and narrowband behavioral scales, input from multiple informants, an interview with the child, direct observation of the child, and a thorough medical examination to rule out any related physical problems (Barkley, 1997a). However, caution is in order with regard to the validity of much of the child's self-report. The child's behavior with the practitioner may not be a reliable indicator of behavior in other circumstances, and diagnosis should never be made based solely on the interview with the child. As part of the MDF assessment, careful attention should also be given to identifying co-occurring problems and disorders, such as effects of abuse or neglect, substance abuse, and anxiety disorders.

A careful functional assessment will help demonstrate any situational differences in the frequency and intensity of the child's or adolescent's behavioral problems over time. Identifying factors that precipitate an increase in problem behaviors and the situational factors that reinforce them can provide clues for effective intervention planning (Robin, 1998a, 1998b; Pfiffner & Barkley, 1998). A child who is well-organized and demonstrates sustained attention and good comportment in school, but is nervous, cannot follow through on homework assignments, or is behaviorally disruptive at home is less likely to have ADHD and more likely to be experiencing family problems, possibly psychological or physical abuse. Conversely, a child's behavior in school may suggest ADHD, but parents may see little evidence of distractibility or disruptive behavior in the home. Obtaining information from multiple informants in different situations can highlight these inconsistencies and avoid premature diagnosis and unnecessary or incorrect treatment.

The MDF assessment should also include a thorough analysis of family functioning. Parents may tend to blame themselves for the child's difficulties, may develop unrealistic expectations of the child, or have difficulty dealing with their anger and frustration with the child. Other parental difficulties that are likely to affect the child's behavior include unwittingly reinforcing the child's dysfunctional behavior or failing to reward the child for productive behavior. These patterns may be related to broader problems of parenting skill, including lack of effective disciplining techniques. Parental deficiencies in problem solving and communication may also interfere negatively with the intervention.

As with CD, developmental considerations should inform the assessment of ADHD (Barkley, 1997a, 1997b; Robin, 1998a). Restlessness and inattention tend to occur in young children. By latency and early adolescence, however, other behavioral problems may begin to emerge, including difficulties with peers and conduct problems at home and in the community (e.g., excessive argumentativeness, aggressiveness). Older adolescents have increased risk for becoming involved in delinquent behavior and dropping out of school. If an adolescent continues to manifest signs of ADHD and co-occurring behavior disorders (e.g., CD), family conflicts are likely to increase. Young adults who express signs and symptoms related to ADHD may be at greater risk for other mental health difficulties, substance abuse, interpersonal problems, and occupational frustrations. These problems are likely to negatively affect youthful developmental processes, including identity development, relationship building, and accomplishing academic and occupational tasks.

Barkley and Edwards (1998) emphasize the importance of interviewing the parents and suggest that they can provide the most ecologically valid account of their child's behavior. The main purposes of the parent interview are to (1) establish a good working rapport with the parents and child; (2) provide them with an opportunity to vent frustration regarding their attempts to cope with their child's difficulties; (3) obtain information about the family, in particular the parents' and child's behavior over time, as well as their health and academic history; (4) assess the psychological well-being of the parents, including the presence of other disorders, the quality of the couple's relationship, and the child's social functioning; and (5) observe family interactions.

Since the majority of children with ADHD have trouble with academic performance and classroom behavior, a detailed assessment of school performance is required. It should target specific areas of concern regarding the student's behavior and academic performance; include a formal diagnostic evaluation, testing for ADHD and any related learning disabilities; initiate the development of an individual education plan; and arrange for special accommodations for the student to optimize learning and facilitate resolution of behavioral difficulties in school. The intervention plan should be specific regarding the goals for enhanced academic achievement. Regular reports should pass from the school to the parents concerning progress toward those goals. The details of the plan for the student may include procedures for taking notes in class, homework completion, test preparation, improved study habits, better time management, and environmental changes at home (e.g., time and place to study, better organization in study/homework space). Case management should facilitate regular communication among all parties to ensure consistency, thoroughness, and follow-through with the overall plan.

Given that many children with ADHD are likely to experience specific learning difficulties and other academic deficiencies, specialized educational testing methods may be required to complete the assessment. Robin (1998a) points out that, in a practical sense, learning disabilities in the context of ADHD assessment refer to a significant discrepancy between scores on an IQ test and scores on academic achievement tests. The estimates of co-occurring learning disabilities and ADHD vary widely because of differences in definitions. Nevertheless, valid intelligence and achievement tests are available and are routinely used by specialists in educational testing. Social workers are likely to work with a school psychologist to coordinate the assessment and integrate these data into a comprehensive report. The Wechsler Intelligence Scale for Children may be used with standardized achievement tests that measure performance in verbal and written expression, mathematical reasoning, spelling, and other core academic performance domains. The continuous performance test (CPT) should be used in conjunction with other assessment data. It may also be used to monitor medication response. According to Root and Resnick (2003), the CPT provides important information that includes children's ability to sustain attention and inhibit impulsivity; their flexibility in thinking and reasoning; their ability to shift their attention; and their ability to perform tasks continuously. The CPT "is designed to be extremely boring. It requires the child to perform a repetitive activity (waiting for specific letter or geometric shape to appear on a computer screen) in a sequence of presentations that lasts for 10 to 20 minutes. The CPT measures a specific aspect of sustained attention (the ability to attend and respond to a stimulus in a boring, repetitive activity" (Swanson, 1992, p. 76; for a review see O'Laughlin & Murphy, 2000). A poor performance on a CPT may suggest, but does not confirm, a diagnosis of ADHD. Additional testing may be required to rule out other learning disabilities.

Based on data gleaned from diagnosis, educational and intelligence testing, classroom observation, and CPTs, students may be eligible for specialized services that would provide remedial assistance and other accommodations such as modifications to their schedule, alternative homework assignments and methods of classroom testing, special tutoring, and other adjustments. These accommodations can assist them in improving their learning experience and academic performance.

Instruments

Given the heterogeneity of symptoms and co-occurring problems associated with ADHD, the use of both broadband (e.g., CBCL, SAC) and narrowband scales is recommended. The CBCL subscale for measuring ADHD symptoms (W. J. Chen, Faraone, Biederman, & Tsuang, 1994) and the Child Attention Profile (Barkley 1995), which includes items from the CBCL (teacher report version) combined with items from the revised Conners rating scales (Conners, 1997), are considered among the most valid measures. Both parent and teacher versions of the Conners scale are also available in short and long forms. Internal consistency measures are good to excellent for the Conners subscales, and the scale distinguishes children with and without the disorder. A large normative database has been developed for the Conners subscales covering different age ranges, and it appears to be sensitive to change in symptom levels (Collett et al., 2003).

The Swanson, Nolan, and Pelham IV questionnaire (SNAP-IV) is based on *DSM-IV* criteria for ADHD diagnosis, is similar to other ADHD scales, and has been widely used in ADHD treatment research (Swanson, 1992; Collett et al., 2003). The short version of the scale focuses on symptoms of ADHD and ODD. Longer versions of the scale cover a broader range of symptoms and behaviors. Although few psychometric studies have been conducted on the SNAP-IV, it has been used extensively in clinical research including the multisite, multimodal treatment study (MTA; reviewed below), has been shown to have good to excellent internal consistency, and is sensitive to client changes in treatment (see Collett, Ohan, & Meyers, 2003, for a review).

The SNAP-IV, however, tends to overestimate the number of children in the general population with ADHD (Swanson et al., 2002). To correct this problem, a revised scale was developed that rates each item on a seven-point scale (from –3 to +3) indicating "far below average" to "far above average." The revised SNAP-IV, called the Strengths and Weakness of ADHD Symptoms and Normal Behavior Scale (SWAN; Swanson et al.), demonstrates improved distributional and structural characteristics, and is considered a reliable, valid, brief, and easy-to-use instrument that complements assessment and evaluation with children suspected of having ADHD. The brief SWAN rating scale is reprinted here.

INSTRUMENT 13.2   Strengths and Weakness of ADHD Symptoms and Normal Behavior Scale (SWAN)

Children differ in their abilities to focus attention, control activity, and inhibit impulses. For each item listed below, how does this child compare to other children of the same age? Please select the best rating based on your observations over the past month. Compared to other children, how does this child do the following:

	Far below	Below	Slightly below	Average	Slightly above	Above	Far above
1. Give close attention to detail and avoid careless mistakes							
2. Sustain attention on tasks or play activities							
3. Listen when spoken to directly							
4. Follow through on instructions and finish schoolwork/chores							
5. Organize tasks and activities							
6. Engage in tasks that require sustained mental effort							
7. Keep track of things necessary for activities							
8. Ignore extraneous stimuli							
9. Remember daily activities							
10. Sit still (control movement of hands/feet or control squirming)							
11. Stay seated (when required by class rules/social conventions)							

12. Modulate motor activity
    (inhibit inappropriate running/climbing) _____ _____ _____ _____ _____ _____ _____

13. Play quietly (keep noise level reasonable) _____ _____ _____ _____ _____ _____ _____

14. Settle down and rest
    (control constant activity) _____ _____ _____ _____ _____ _____ _____

15. Modulate verbal activity
    (control excess talking) _____ _____ _____ _____ _____ _____ _____

16. Reflect on questions
    (control blurting out answers) _____ _____ _____ _____ _____ _____ _____

17. Await turn (stand in line and take turns) _____ _____ _____ _____ _____ _____ _____

18. Enter into conversations and games
    (control interrupting/intruding) _____ _____ _____ _____ _____ _____ _____

The seven-point response is scored +3 to –3 accordingly: far below average = +3, below average = +2, slightly below average = +1, average = 0, slightly above average = –1, above average = –2, far above average = –3. Subscale scores on the SWAN are calculated by summing the scores on the items in the specific subset (ADHD-Inattention and ADHD-Hyperactivity/Impulsivity), and by dividing by the number of items in each subscale to express the summary score as the average rating for all items in the subscale. Use the scorecard below to calculate each subscale. The average scores have been designed to reflect population norms. Scores "above or far above" average may indicate a problem in that area. Diagnosis is not confirmed by these scores, which give a relative measure of performance in each area (i.e., Inattention and Hyperactivity/Impulsivity). Changes in scores that increase over time would indicate a greater problem; scores that decrease would indicate improvement.

	ADHD-Inattention	**ADHD-Hyperactivity/Impulsivity**
	1_____	10_____
	2_____	11_____
	3_____	12_____
	4_____	13_____
	5_____	14_____
	6_____	15_____
	7_____	16_____
	8_____	17_____
	9_____	18_____
Total score =	_____	_____
Average =	_____	_____

SELECTING EFFECTIVE INTERVENTIONS

The outcome literature largely suggests that ADHD is optimally treated with psychostimulant medication combined with individual, family, and classroom-based behavioral interventions. Specifically, effective psychosocial interventions include cognitive-behavioral skills for the child to engender better self-regulatory skills, such as anxiety management, getting better organized, staying on task, and controlling disruptive or aggressive behaviors; behavioral family therapy; and classroom contingency management procedures (Kazdin, 1994b; Kendall, 1993; Braswell & Bloomquist, 1991; Rapport, 1992; Pelham et al., 1998; Root & Resnick, 2003; Barkley, 2002; Hinshaw, Klein, & Abikoff, 1998; Anastopoulos,

1998; Anastopoulos, Smith, & Wien, 1998). Although there is strong consensus for the use of behavioral family therapy and classroom-based contingency management, evidence is mixed with regard to the necessity of adding individual cognitive-behavioral coping-skills therapy (Root & Resnick, 2003).

Farmer et al. (2002) identified over 130 studies of treatment outcomes for ADHD for youth of ages 6–12. Based on twenty-eight studies that met strict methodological criteria, they concluded that the most effective psychosocial interventions were CBT (including social-skills training), parent management training, and contingency management programs. Although effect sizes were fairly large, indicating clinically significant results, data demonstrating generalization and maintenance of gains were less impressive. Farmer et al. recommended more research on minority children (who are very underrepresented in the research overall), more replication of studies, more follow-up data beyond six months, and more ecological validity in the studies.

Recent controlled studies demonstrated the efficacy of combined behavioral programs as well as their limitations when applied to more challenging populations. Barkley, Edwards, Laneri, Fletcher, and Meevia (2001) compared eighteen sessions of problem-solving and communication intervention, behavior management training (nine sessions), and a combined intervention group (total of eighteen sessions) with adolescents diagnosed with ADHD and ODD. At midpoint of treatment (nine weeks) and endpoint (eighteen weeks), there appeared to be some improvement overall, but results were modest. Outcome measures were mixed and depended on who provided the behavioral ratings (mother, father, or adolescent). In addition, considerable attrition occurred by the end of treatment, particularly for the problem-solving and communication group (38%). In a randomized study of preschoolers identified as having high levels of aggression, hyperactivity, and other behavioral problems (Barkley et al., 2000), 158 students were randomly assigned to four conditions: parent training, classroom behavioral management, combined parent training and classroom management, and no treatment. Ratings included the CBCL and several standardized and well-validated behavioral and academic performance measures. Results showed that classroom behavioral management resulted in observable behavioral improvements in parent and teacher ratings. The parent-training module revealed no significant effects; however, results appeared to be largely due to high rates of attrition during the study. When parent-training conditions were combined, 25% of all parents assigned to that program had attended 1–4 sessions, (29%) 5–8 sessions, and (13%) 9–14 sessions. Those who did not attend the parenting sessions, however, did not differ significantly on several variables from those who did attend at least one session. Although the contingency management procedures were shown to be effective at reducing hyperactive, impulsive, inattentive, and aggressive behaviors, the lack of response to the parent training was discouraging. These problems underscore the challenges of implementing such programs in typical school settings where the parents have not voluntarily sought treatment, but where it has been offered to them because their children were screened as "high risk." A two-year follow-up study revealed no lasting positive effects for the classroom behavioral management program (Shelton et al., 2000). Clearly, there is a need to improve long-term follow-up in the homes and classrooms of children and adolescents with CD and ADHD. In addition to effective skill-based interventions, families with greater psychosocial and financial challenges in their lives will need greater instrumental and social supports as well as better linkages between the parent(s), schools, juvenile law enforcement, health care, and other community resources (Webster-Stratton, 1997).

Families and Schools Together (FAST) is one example of a program that combines therapeutic techniques and community support for early intervention programs in low-income settings (McDonald, Billingham, Condrad, Morgan, & Payton, 1997, p. 153). The FAST program has been widely implemented in at least twenty-six states. Components of FAST include identifying at-risk children, sending paraprofessionals (FAST graduates) to the respective parents' homes to exhort them to join FAST, and engaging in multifamily gatherings for eight sessions at the child's school. The gatherings follow a structured agenda of family activities, parental mutual support, parent-child play therapy, singing, sharing a meal, and other expressive activities. Incentives to attend the program include a free meal and transportation if needed. A formal graduation ritual is provided to enhance the status of being FAST graduates. As graduates, participants may continue as members of FASTWORKS, a series of monthly meetings intended to enhance social and family supports and maintain the social network. Over time FASTWORKS evolves into a self-generating, self-governing social-support network intended to enhance linkages among family, schools, and the community. Uncontrolled outcome evaluation and testimonials provide only suggestive evidence for the effectiveness of these programs in improving child behavior, family functioning, and social supports.

Exemplar Study: The Multisite Multimodal Treatment Study of Children with ADHD.   At the time of the study, the MTA project was the largest study of its kind on any childhood disorder. Its main purpose was to compare the relative efficacy of medication, home- and school-based behavioral programs, and a summer program with children diagnosed with ADHD (Arnold et al., 1997; Richters et al., 1995). In response to the existing literature showing somewhat variable responses to stimulant medications and psychosocial interventions either alone or in combination, given different client characteristics, a five-year multisite multimodal investigation was conducted to address the following unanswered questions regarding the treatment of ADHD:

> Under what circumstances (co-morbid conditions, age, gender, family background) do which treatment combinations (medication, behavior therapy, parent training, school-based intervention) have what impacts (improvement, stasis, deterioration) on what domains of child functioning (cognitive, academic,

behavioral, physical, peer relations, family relations), for how long (short- versus long-term), to what extent (effect sizes, normal versus pathological range), and why (processes underlying change)? (Richters et al., p. 996).

Understanding the role of socioeconomic status and co-occurring disorders was also an important goal of the study.

The MTA study was a randomized controlled trial of the treatment of over 500 children (ages 7–9) with ADHD. It was conducted at six sites in the United States and Canada. Four treatment groups were developed for the study: (1) a community care (CC) control group of "treatment as usual" in local community mental health agencies (where about two-thirds of those referred received medication); (2) a medication-only group (MED) that received one month of medication; (3) a behavioral intervention group (BEH) that received a three-part behavioral intervention; and (4) a combined behavioral intervention program (same as group 3) and medication group (COMB) (Root & Resnick, 2003).

The multivariate design called for a comprehensive multidimensional assessment battery at baseline, at 3, 9, and 14 months, and at 24-month follow-up (Arnold et al., 1997), which allowed for an examination of the following variables and their relationship to treatment: severity of the disorder, role of co-occurring disorders, gender, socioeconomic status, ethnicity, parental psychopathology, domains of functioning on outcome, acceptability of treatment, and compliance with the intervention. Interventions were selected for the study based on the following criteria: they must be state-of-the-art, as demonstrated by evidence supporting at least short-term efficacy, manualized and conducive to implementation in real practice settings, and "sufficiently intense, integrated, and flexible to credibly stand alone" (Arnold et al., p. 867). Great efforts were made to design programs that had high ecological validity and could be applied flexibly to accommodate the vagaries of practice in real-world settings with real clients.

The design of the BEH reflected the findings from existing outcome literature (K. C. Wells et al., 2000) and consisted of behavioral parent training, an eight-week all-day summer session for the children, and a school-based contingency management intervention. The parent-training classes were a combination of group and individual sessions over the course of twenty-seven weeks and included the skills reviewed above (based on the works of leading experts in the field, such as Patterson, Forehand and McMahon, Webster-Stratton and Herbert, and Barkley). The training consisted of introduction and overview, setting up school-home report cards, principles of learning and reinforcement, playing and learning how to reward children in a timely manner, giving effective commands, time-out procedures, token economy, stress/anger management (for the parents), helping the child deal with peer relations, and several weeks of review and generalization of these skills.

The school intervention included consultation with teachers and an eight-week summer training program. The therapist-consultants who provided the parent training also served as teacher consultants, and paraprofessionals trained to support the classroom-based program also served as counselors in the summer program. Therapist consultants met with the teachers about twenty-six times overall. During that time, they set up the daily report card that the parents learned how to use in the parent-training program, and the therapist-consultants provided the link between the parent and the teacher. The teachers were also taught basic behavior management skills to be implemented in the classroom (similar to the skills taught to parents for home-based intervention): how to implement and enforce classroom rules, giving attention to positive behaviors, ignoring annoying negative behaviors, giving clear commands and soft reprimands, giving individualized instructional materials as needed, altering class structure, reinforcement procedures including the establishment of token economies, and use of time-out procedures.

The paraprofessionals also received extensive training in behavior management techniques to help in the classroom and to serve as counselors in the summer program. Only two children were assigned to each paraprofessional counselor. Specific target behaviors were itemized for each child, based on consultation with the therapist-consultant. The paraprofessional's goal for each child was to shape and fade his behavior so that the teacher and parent could increasingly concentrate on tasks evaluated with the daily report card (while simultaneously decreasing the paraprofessional's attention). The summer treatment program consisted of an intensive group-oriented combination of both academic and recreational activities that filled the day from 8 to 5. Token economy and behavioral management methods were employed in a highly supportive atmosphere to improve behavioral and interpersonal performance. Well-established social-skills training methods (i.e., instruction, role-playing, modeling) were emphasized to improve peer relations. The program included a buddy system in which each child was paired with another and had access to a buddy coach to work on relationship difficulties. The children were also taught group problem-solving skills when difficulties arose, and were provided with "sensitive" sports coaching. The daily report card was used during the summer program as well. A heavy emphasis throughout this multicomponent behavioral module was on developing good alliances with the parents and teachers especially, and establishing a balance between adhering to the treatment model and being flexible enough to adapt the interventions to the needs of individual children and their parents.

Root and Resnick (2003) summarized the results of this ambitious study. The COMB group performed significantly better than behavioral treatment alone or treatment as usual in the community. At first look, the MED group and the COMB group appeared to be about equally successful. However, when Conners, Epstein, and March (2001) combined teacher and parent measures, the COMB intervention revealed the best outcomes overall. Combining behavioral programs and psychostimulant medication may be advantageous when dealing with co-occurring problems associated with ADHD (e.g., conduct problems, depression, family problems, interpersonal difficulties), problems that may not be optimally addressed by stimulant medication alone.

Descriptions of Effective Interventions

Although CBT skills alone do not appear robust enough to improve the behavior problems and academic performance of children with ADHD, these skills may add to the overall effectiveness of a comprehensive approach that includes home- and school-based behavioral (contingency management) programs combined with medication. Many of the CBT skills reviewed in chapter 12 for anxiety and in this chapter for addressing ODD and CD may be useful for children and adolescents with ADHD. Cognitive behavioral coping skills include self-talk, self-monitoring and self-evaluation, cognitive modeling, problem solving, and other self-regulatory strategies. Braswell and Bloomquist (1991) and Van der Krol et al. (1998) suggest combining the following skills: anxiety reduction to reduce stress and improve concentration; basic problem solving to approach daily problems in a more organized, focused, and systematic manner; and environmental management (at home and in the classroom) to reduce distractions and facilitate self-control, attention, and problem solving. Parents should be taught to coach their children in self-regulation skills at home, and help them create an environment conducive to quiet concentration.

Parent training in contingency management methods have been shown to be very successful in reducing behavior problems and improving academic performance, primarily in younger children with ADHD. Parents are taught in the clinic setting (through reading, direct instruction, modeling, role-playing, videotapes) the basic effective parenting techniques examined in detail earlier in this chapter. Practitioners should coordinate home-based behavioral parenting skills with a complementary contingency management plan in the classroom through consultations with the child's parent and teacher. A consistent evaluation-feedback system should be set up among social worker, parent, and teacher to reinforce classroom performance through the use of daily report cards. More intensive contingency management approaches may be carried out in a specialized treatment facility or by specialists in a classroom setting. The key elements of effective psychosocial interventions for ADHD are summarized below (Barkley, 2002; Anastopoulos et al., 1998; Anastopoulos, 1998).

Psychoeducation is provided to teach parents about the causes, developmental course, and prognosis for ADHD. Books and videos may be recommended or provided as well.

The causes of oppositional/defiant behavior are explained. Parents are taught to understand the systemic and interactional nature of behavioral problems in the home. These factors include child and parent characteristics, situational factors including consequences for defiant behavior, and the role of stressful family events. The practitioner helps the parent understand especially how negative coercive interactions reinforce oppositional/defiant behavior.

Parents are taught more effective ways of attending to a child's behavior to reduce off-task or negative behaviors and increase on-task and positive behaviors. The technique consists of verbal narration and occasional positive statements to the child. Attention is applied strategically only when on-task, prosocial, and otherwise positive behaviors are displayed. Parents are taught to ignore unwanted behaviors.

Parents are taught how to attend to child compliance and independent play by breaking down complex tasks, managing environmental distractions, and giving simple, direct commands while providing immediate reinforcement for prompt compliance. Positive reinforcement is provided frequently to shape the child's ability to engage in longer periods of nondisruptive activity.

A token home economy is established by which a menu of rewards is negotiated, and tokens are given only when the child promptly obeys the parent's directive. Chips or tokens are forfeited if the child does not comply with the first command. Additional chips may be awarded for the child's initiative or particularly positive attitude.

Parents are taught how to implement time-out procedures for noncompliance. Two serious violations are defined, based on discussions regarding the child's particular disruptive behaviors. Parents are taught to issue a command, wait five seconds, issue a warning, and wait another five seconds. If the child has not complied, the child is taken to time-out. During the time-out, the child must meet three conditions: (1) remain in time-out for roughly two minutes per year of age (e.g., twenty minutes for a ten-year-old); (2) be quiet during the time-out; and, (3) agree to comply with the original command. More time-out may be instituted should the child continue to be oppositional or disruptive. When time-out procedures and previous lessons are reviewed, time-out may be extended to more behaviors if needed.

Parents learn to manage noncompliant behaviors in public places. They learn to review basic rules of conduct for the child prior to entering a public place, give the child an activity to keep them occupied, reinforce good behavior, and institute punishment should the child engage in disruptive behavior. The time-out or loss of privileges is instituted immediately upon returning home.

Parents collaborate with the school to improve the child's school behavior. Rewards and punishments are instituted based on daily reports from school. The report card is designed to address specific behaviors of concern, and rewards and punishments are dispensed by the same principles noted above. In the classroom, contingency management is implemented (by the teacher or an assistant) following these general guidelines: (1) the learning tasks are broken down into smaller components; (2) stimulation in the learning environment is increased (e.g., use of more colorful or otherwise more visually stimulating materials); (3) on-task behavior is rewarded; and (4) off-task or disruptive behaviors are sanctioned through time-out or loss of privileges.

Parents review what they have learned, entertain scenarios about future problems, and discuss how they might handle them. A one-month follow-up or booster session may be planned to review any additional problems that arise after the program.

Pfiffner and Barkley (1998) recommend some refinements in implementing contingency management programs, methods that can be applied in the classroom and at home. Instructions must be given in a concise, clear, and somewhat exaggerated manner, followed by the child's repeating the instructions to demonstrate that they were heard and understood. Consequences (positive and negative) must immediately follow the specific target behavior in order to be effective; they must also be more frequent and of greater magnitude than would otherwise be expected for "normal" children. Positives are preferred over negative reinforcers. Reinforcers should be changed every two or three weeks so that they do not lose their influence on the child's behavior. A specific reward can be returned to after it has been set aside for a while. Anticipating changes in environment or other contingencies, and helping children to review rules of their own conduct is important for them to cope adequately with transitions. Parents help the child anticipate and plan ahead. They use a strategy that combines positive consequences (praise, tangible rewards, token economies) and negative consequences (reprimands, revoked privileges, time-out). For maximum effectiveness, consequences must be immediate, brief, consistent, salient, and, in the case of positive consequences, delivered frequently. On-task behaviors should be immediately rewarded with warmly delivered praise or other tangible reinforcement, while negative behaviors should be responded to with withdrawal of attention. Token economies are effective; negative consequences include reprimands or revoked privileges. Punishment must be immediate, unemotional, and consistent; overall, positive reinforcement is much preferred and should be used more frequently than negative reinforcers or punishment. Time-outs can also be used in a variety of ways: the child may be isolated or moved to the periphery of the "action," and thus is unable to obtain rewards; their work materials may be put away, or a clock that earns rewards during productive activity may be stopped during off-task or otherwise disruptive behavior.

These same principles are used at home as well, and ideally, are coordinated between teachers and parents via the daily report card, which eventually becomes weekly. A list of target behaviors are on the report card, rated on a scale (e.g., poor, fair, good, excellent) that can be scored with points and summed to a total score. Expectations of the child's behavior and academic performance (e.g., completed homework) must be made clear. The rewards and sanctions at home for improvements and agreed-upon ratings must be made equally clear. Rewards could include pizza, movie, TV or video-game time, or a special trip for long-term major goal achievement (e.g., four weeks of 90% adequate ratings).

Robin (1998a, 1998b) has noted that there is little research regarding the pragmatics of how to sequence interventions with an adolescent and family dealing with ADHD, but experience and judgment can serve as guides. Priority should be given to acute behavioral problems (e.g., CD, substance abuse), moving toward a family psychoeducation model, arranging for medication evaluation, and directly improving the child's behaviors through family behavior therapy (including parent management training) and contingency management intervention in the classroom. Parents' efforts at home must be carefully coordinated with the classroom intervention (via the daily report card) to focus on the child's social behaviors and academic performance. The intervention tends to be intensive in the beginning, lasting from ten to twenty visits, and ideally shifts to a long-term follow-up model with intermittent checkups. In addition to coordinating both home-based and classroom efforts, close coordination should include the efforts of other participants in the intervention: the prescribing physician, teachers, guidance counselors, special education personnel, school administration, and testing specialists.

Robin (1998a, 1998b) also recommends some general implementation guidelines for behavioral interventions particularly with older children and adolescents. Practitioners, parents, and teachers should strive to be somewhat flexible and willing to negotiate on some matters with the adolescent. Adults should also give immediate and frequent positive feedback and encouragement when it is earned, as well as negative feedback (e.g., mild rebukes) when warranted. Adults should be consistent and follow through with feedback and contingencies (e.g., when you finish your homework, you can visit your friend or spend time on the phone), keep to a plan of action, avoid giving lectures and unnecessary arguments, avoid personalizing the conflict or tension, and be ready to forgive. The adults should focus on achieving successes, move forward, and avoid getting bogged down by holding grudges. They should take the long view of the child's progress, and see the goals of day-to-day interventions as enhancing the adolescent's accountability, responsibility, and independence. The parent, particularly, should strive to gradually relinquish directives and punishments as the adolescent "earns" independence and learns by coping with the consequences of their own behavior. Adults should model accountability and follow-through. With children and adolescents, adults should clearly discriminate between those matters that are negotiable and those that are not, and be flexible when possible. Always give a good reason for directives or requests of the child, and explain one's rationale for sanctions, restrictions, or punishments. Model good communication skills, and monitor the young person's behaviors. Ask, Where are you going? Who are you going to be with? What are you planning to do? When will you be back? and be ready to confront serious discrepancies between the adolescent's words and deeds (should you ever find out about it).

Social workers, whether working in community agencies, private practice, or the schools, should be prepared to work in an interdisciplinary environment to help provide a thorough MDF assessment and collaborate with a range of other professionals to facilitate implementation of these evidence-based practices for children, adolescents, and their families. This collaboration is critical if evidence-based psychosocial interventions for ODD, CD, and ADHD are to be implemented successfully and maintained over time (Tourse & Sullick, 1999).

Much work is left to be done to enhance interprofessional collaboration in social work in the schools (Mooney, Kline, & Davoren, 1999) and elsewhere.

Medication for Attention Deficit Hyperactivity Disorder

The use of stimulants for children diagnosed with ADHD is perhaps the most well-established use of medication for children both clinically and empirically. These medications include dextroamphetamine, methylphenidate, and pemoline (H. I. Kaplan & Saddock, 1998). The clinical usefulness of stimulant medication with "ADHD children" has been known since the 1930s (AACAP, 2001b), and a virtual consensus has been reached regarding the efficacy of these drugs for reducing the primary symptoms of ADHD, that is, improving on-task behavior, academic performance, and disruptive behaviors (AACAP 1997b; Hinshaw et al., 1998; Farmer et al., 2002; Barkley, 1997a).

> In the classroom, stimulants decrease interrupting, fidgetiness, and finger-tapping and increase on-task behavior. At home, stimulants improve parent-child interactions, on-task behaviors, and compliance. In social settings, stimulants improve peer nomination rankings of social standing and increase attention during sports activities. Stimulants decrease response variability and impulsive responding on laboratory cognitive task, increase the accuracy of performance, and improve short-term memory, reaction time, math computation, problem-solving in games and sustained attention. (AACAP, 2001b, p. 1353)

Greenhill (1998) cites over 160 studies demonstrating the efficacy and effectiveness of amphetamine drugs for the treatment of ADHD. Data reveal that between 50% and 70% of children show marked improvement in cognitive functioning, on-task concentration, disruptive behavioral indicators, and to some degree, social functioning.

Despite the success of stimulant medications for ADHD, there are some serious limitations in the use of these drugs. Many children do not approach "normal" levels of functioning, although most are rated improved. Long-term benefits are often not evident. Drugs do not appear to improve peer relations in the long run, nor are they likely to resolve the family problems that often accompany the lives of children diagnosed with ADHD. Drugs do not help a sizeable proportion of youngsters (10–20%) even in the short run, and almost one-third show adverse responses. Many parents find drug treatment unacceptable for a variety of reasons, and will not comply with medical recommendations (K. C. Wells et al., 2000; Pelham et al., 1998). Although debate continues as to whether medication alone is sufficient to reduce the main symptoms of ADHD, there is notable evidence that psychosocial interventions reduce the need for medication (AACAP, 1997b; Farmer et al., 2002).

Other factors to consider when prescribing medication for children with ADHD include age, duration and severity of the problems, history and success of prior treatment efforts, normal levels of anxiety in the child, parental motivation, absence of stimulant abuse in the home, and likelihood of compliance with the regimen (Barkley, 1997a). Since little evidence clearly guides prediction of the correct dose, physicians generally begin with a low dose and increase it gradually until an optimum balance is struck between therapeutic effectiveness and side effects (Greenhill, 1998; AACAP, 1997b). Immediate-release stimulant medication acts for three to five hours, so multiple daily dosing is required. Practical concerns include administering the drugs at different times during the child's school day. In addition, the rapid rise in the prescribing of these drugs in the United States presents a risk of overprescribing primarily to control behavior, without a thorough diagnostic assessment. Contraindications include evidence of previous sensitivity to stimulants, heart disease, glaucoma, drug abuse, hypertension and hyperthyroidism, motor tics, and family history of Tourette's syndrome or other tic disorders. Although these drugs are very safe, potential side effects include irritability, moodiness, headaches, abdominal pain, and loss of appetite. Side effects can often be avoided or reduced by gradual adjustments in the dose. Withdrawals may result in rebound effects such as excitability, talkativeness, irritability, and insomnia (AACAP, 1997b, 2001b). Despite these concerns, stimulant medications have provided relief for many young people with ADHD and their families. Nevertheless, many who could benefit from them do not receive proper care. A large seven-year multistage survey of over 100,000 client records demonstrated that almost half of the clients eligible for psychostimulant medication were not prescribed these drugs. In addition, at least one-quarter of the clients who were prescribed these medications did not receive follow-up care (Hoagwood, Kelleher, Feil, & Comer, 2000).

IMPLEMENTING AND EVALUATING THE EVIDENCE-BASED INTERVENTION PLAN

CASE STUDY: RICKY

Ricky was a nine-year old boy of Native American and Hispanic descent. His parents were never married, but he had met his father informally once or twice when he was younger. His father, of mixed Native American ancestry, was something of a drifter, having left the reservation in the Southwest years ago, and periodically moved around to follow his work. His mother, Margarita, raised Ricky by herself, but received help from family members, particularly her mother. Although Margarita had a serious problem with alcohol and other drugs when she was younger (including when she was pregnant with Ricky), she had been "clean and sober" for the past six years, and was an active member of her Pentecostal church, which she credits with her new life. Nevertheless, raising Ricky without his father had been challenging. Although he had always been "un jalapeño pequeño," it wasn't until the past year or so that Margarita realized she could not handle him by herself, and it was getting tougher to find people she could ask to watch him now and then. Complaints from the teachers at his school were on the increase. Her friends, who had always said he was a handful when they baby-sat for him, heard about his conduct in school, and counseled Margarita to get help for him. She had been reluctant and unwilling to acknowledge his escalating behavior and problems with schoolwork because she felt somewhat guilty regarding his problems. In previous counseling, a therapist had told her that Ricky's problems were the result of "poor attachment," because Margarita had been "unavailable" to him due to her early drug problems. Her friends were more pragmatic: Ricky was getting older, having more problems adjusting to his new school, and becoming more difficult to handle. In addition to having difficulty sitting still and focusing on his schoolwork in class and at home, Ricky had recently gotten into fights with the other kids at school, usually during lunch or on the playground after school ("they deserved it for calling me a 'coyote' "). He had also become somewhat belligerent with his mom when she asked him to do chores at home or to turn off the TV to finish his homework.

As for his schoolwork, he had been tested by the school psychologist, who said Ricky had trouble with math and reading, but that if he were a bit more in control, some of these things could be improved through tutoring. Margarita had managed over the past few years to get an associate's degree in administration from a community college, and landed a good job in a university as assistant to a dean and, later, assistant to the university president. She was fortunate to have good benefits to cover services for Ricky, who now attended a school that could provide them. During the conversation with the psychologist, she discussed her early drug problems and expressed guilt over that period in her life, wondering if she had not been a good mother to Ricky. The psychologist pointed out that she should be proud of how she thrived under duress without a partner, and how difficult it must have been to turn her life around. By observing Ricky with her in the office, the psychologist also noted that he could tell how close they were. She must have done more than a few things right.

Ricky, based on his recent physical, was very healthy, but did appear (based on the testing and the psychologist's diagnosis) to have all the signs of ADHD, and was certainly becoming a behavior problem. There was every reason to be optimistic that if he started a program of medication, behavioral therapy at home and in the classroom, and some tutoring for his academic challenges, he could get better. If they stuck with it, the intervention might also prevent future problems. Because he was becoming somewhat belligerent and getting into fights with other kids in his class (sometimes being the bully), the psychologist was concerned that he might become increasingly conduct-disordered. Dan, the social worker on the team, would teach behavioral management skills to Margarita and coordinate the treatment with the school psychologist (who would supervise a tutor on staff), the consulting psychiatrist (who would provide the medication), and the teacher (who would implement a contingency management plan in the classroom).

Multidimensional/Functional Assessment: Defining Problems and Goals

Dan thought that Ricky met many of the criteria for ADHD and ODD. These problems had persisted for some time and appeared to be getting worse. Ricky demonstrated a consistent pattern of being argumentative and conflictual with other children, and stubborn and oppositional when dealing with his mother and other adult authority figures, particularly his teachers. He appeared easily frustrated when things didn't go his way. Many of these problems overlapped with his learning and behavioral problems in school. He was often very fidgety and "always in motion" (according to his teacher), had a hard time focusing on one task at a time and finishing his work, often blurted out responses to questions out of turn, and had trouble waiting his turn in general. He was disorganized in his work, often complaining that someone took his materials or saying that he had lost his materials, and he did not respond readily to commands from the teacher when she attempted to set limits on his behavior or tried to help him focus on his work. He clearly had become disruptive to those around him, and was taxing the patience of both his mother and the teacher. The fact that Ricky had moved to a new neighborhood and school may have disrupted his sense of security and consistency. Although he had been a handful in his previous school, complaints from the teachers and the assessment of the current school psychologist seemed to be more serious than before. Margarita did not know whether this change was because the school personnel felt differently about her son (who was one of few children of color or mixed race) in the school, or whether there had been a real change in his behavior.

In addition to the recent uprooting and changes in Ricky's life, Dan and Margarita speculated whether this inability to focus on tasks and control his behavior was "in the blood," given the problems of Ricky's father, or whether Margarita's substance abuse problems during pregnancy may have caused some subtle neurological problems. Since Ricky had no overt signs of fetal alcohol syndrome, this was mere speculation, and the social worker did not overemphasize it. While the history of impulse problems and substance abuse in Ricky's family history was of concern as a possible explanation for his troubles, the assessment turned to more current and functional aspects of his difficulties.

As Dan discussed Ricky's behavior over the course of a typical day with his mom and teacher, they noticed some patterns. Ricky's mom reported that he was more cooperative in the morning, getting ready for school, and she had less trouble getting him to get dressed, eat breakfast, and so forth. The teacher also noticed that he was quieter in the morning, and that as lunch approached he became more restless, showed less ability to focus on his work, and began to interact negatively and more frequently with his classmates. The afternoons appeared to be the most difficult, as he would often sigh loudly, and writhe and fidget in his seat as though he were going to come out of his skin. It seemed that he could not wait for the end of class. During this time he was the most difficult to control and the most likely to be sent out of the classroom.

His mother noted that when Ricky got home, he often seemed angry and depressed and could not bring himself to start his homework. He often procrastinated well past dinner time. He would bargain with his mom to watch TV or play video games "just for a little while, then I'll start my homework." His mom, who often took work home from her new job, was stressed herself, and often did not have the energy or patience to maintain limits and structure with Ricky. She often "caved in," giving in to him so she could finish her own work, make dinner, clean up, and get him ready for bed. One complaint of Ricky's teacher was that his work was often carelessly completed, incomplete, or simply not done. These problems and complaints appeared to be occurring with increasing frequency and severity. He seemed to be more easily provoked in school. One playground monitor started to refer to him as the "playground bully." When he came home from school, his mother was increasingly alarmed at the degree of his anger and his defiant posture when she asked him to pick up his room or start his homework. She was also concerned because Ricky was growing quickly, and seemed to be developing his father's physical build, and she was very worried about being able to handle him in a couple of years as he entered adolescence. The school psychologist and social worker also confirmed that this was a good time to get these problems under control.

After meeting with mother and son and consulting with the school psychologist and teacher, Dan set up a meeting to discuss a service plan to address Ricky's difficulties. They all agreed that first his belligerent behavior had to be reduced. The second priority was to help Ricky improve his work and study skills, both at home and in the classroom. They all agreed that through weekly school reports and occasional meetings coordinated by the social worker, they could help Ricky get more control over his behavior and improve his grades. Dan also suggested a consultation with the psychiatrist to consider medication. As for Ricky's view of the problem, he just "wanted the other kids to like me better" and felt that if they did, his problems would all go away. Improving Ricky's social skills was added to the list of improvements that would become a part of his service plan.

Selecting and Designing the Intervention: Defining Strategies and Objectives

Dan explained to Margarita that Ricky's difficulties with focusing his attention, staying on task, controlling his behavior, relating better to the other kids, and improving his mood and sense of well-being overall were somewhat related. In addition, the interventions that had been shown to be most effective for these problems were also quite similar and could be easily integrated. He explained that, in addition to possible medication for Ricky, behavior therapy and contingency management, when applied by Margarita and the teacher in a coordinated and consistent way, were very likely to help Ricky improve control over his behavior and his school performance. The social worker also suggested that Ricky's mom learn some stress-management skills (brief meditation and breathing exercises) for her own benefit and so she could teach them to Ricky to help him settle down and concentrate before he started his homework. Dan spent an entire session providing psychoeducation to Ricky's mother on what ADHD was and what the entire behavioral program would entail. Since Dan and the teacher had collaborated on classroom contingency management skills before, the teacher was well prepared to carry out her part of the plan, and would report to him and Margarita on a regular basis.

Dan reviewed a plan with Margarita that would include psychoeducation for her about clinical behavior therapy, parent management training (clarity and consistency in communicating expectations), contingency management (consistent use of rewards and sanctions with short- and long-term rewards), coordination with Ricky's teacher (who would use similar behavioral and contingency management skills), and medication procedures (table 13.1).

The plan included relaxation and playtime after school. Margarita would pick Ricky up around 4:30 from the after-school program (which was near the campus where she worked). She would then devote her sole attention to Ricky for about twenty minutes, asking him about his day, providing some nurturance (perhaps a snack), and (if he wanted to) engaging in a game of some kind. This time would help her to check on his mood, and his needs and prepare him for a more structured schedule in the evening. A reward would be planned for the end of the evening if all tasks were accomplished satisfactorily. This time also was used to review the reports from school (she retrieved a simple scorecard every day from the school secretary), and his progress toward long-term rewards.

Margarita would "meditate" with Ricky for a few minutes before he began his homework. During this time, she could teach him some basic relaxation and meditation skills to "settle down and be cool" before starting his work. Five minutes per day at that time were allotted to this activity before be began his homework and chores. Margarita would also have Ricky talk aloud about his plans to organize and complete his homework ("First, I'll do my spelling homework, 'cause that's easy; then I have to draw a map of Italy and show where the big cities are; then I'll do my math homework, that's the hardest part.").

Dan reviewed parent management training to help Margarita focus on structuring Ricky's late afternoon and evening. He reviewed how to issue simple commands with assertive follow-through. She would also learn to ignore some of the less important but annoying behaviors (whining, complaining, loud sighing), to reduce overall negativity that had begun to define their time together at home. Margarita and Ricky agreed to the following: "I will ask you once to do a specific chore, I will ask you to repeat it to me to make sure you understand, and I will wait three minutes to see if you begin the chore. Depending on what it is, we will also agree on how long it will take, and I will hold you to that."

Implementing a contingency management plan would help Ricky better self-regulate through a home economy by which he could earn points for accomplishing schoolwork and home chores. The rules were spelled out clearly and posted on the refrigerator. A similar plan with the same scoring guidelines would be applied by the teacher, and the overall score combined so Margarita could issue the larger rewards or sanctions on the weekends. If Ricky did not comply with the rules regarding how he accomplished chores and homework at school, he would lose a point for the day. If he had trouble completing some of the homework (e.g., a particular math problem), he had to show partial work on it. On the advice of the school psychologist, Ricky was encouraged to do as much of the work as he could, and return later to the more challenging problems to avoid getting overly frustrated. A special education intern would provide extra tutoring during the after-school program.

If Ricky resorted to negative attention-getting, bothering other students, getting into physical fights, not responding to his mother's or teacher's commands readily at home or in school, he would lose points. Physical fighting would cost him 5 points. Ricky's teacher agreed to use the same point system for his classroom tasks. He could achieve a maximum of 10 points per day in school and 10 points per day at home if he accomplished all his tasks. For a five-day school week, he could achieve a total of 100 points. The team and Ricky all agreed that, at this point, they would start by expecting Ricky to get 15 points per day to obtain his daily rewards at home, such as TV time, video or computer time, and modest monetary rewards, and 75 points would be expected for a larger weekend reward (having a neighborhood friend stay over, renting a movie with pizza). Margarita and the teacher discussed how these points would be applied or withdrawn, given their slightly different circumstances, to maintain some consistency. Later, the point level was raised to 85%, then 90% of goals.

Dan devised a stress management plan for Margarita, so she could feel less overwhelmed and more in control. As Ricky became more cooperative, she was able to relax more, get her own chores done, and occasionally get baby-sitters so she could have an evening out (the same reward system applied when the baby-sitter was in charge).

Finally, Ricky would be sent to a consultation to see if medication for ADHD symptoms would be of assistance.

Selecting Scales and Creating Indexes to Monitor and Evaluate Client Progress

To establish a useful baseline for Ricky, a trained teacher's aid used the NYTRS and the SWAN to measure behavior problems and ADHD symptoms (table 13.1). Dan showed Margarita how to use the SWAN at home so they could have one

TABLE 13.1   The client service plan for Ricky

Problems	Goals	Sample Objectives	Interventions	Assessment Tools
Belligerent, oppositional, defiant behavior with adults (mother, teacher); not responding to reasonable commands to attend to tasks	Minimize oppositional behavior; increase cooperativeness to level suitable to age	Initiate response to requests within 5 seconds; be consistently engaged in request until task is accomplished (75% of the time based on weekly scorecard)	Psychoeducation with mother regarding parent management and contingency management skills	NYTRS and SWAN for assessing classroom behavior and ADHD symptoms at home and school
Frequent fidgetiness, difficulty concentrating and attending to tasks; disorganized at work; often "on the go" when in the classroom	Reduce fidgetiness, restlessness and improve concentration and organizational skills to accomplish tasks	Consistently complete work 75% of the time when tallied weekly	Implementation of parent management skills at home along with contingency management plan; similar contingency management plan implemented in the classroom by teacher experienced in the technique	Indexes for daily performance developed by mother and teacher (combined 20 points per day, total weekly 100-point scale): items include accomplished in-class schoolwork, lack of negative social behaviors, including fighting; homework and chores
Poor school performance; possible learning deficits in math, reading skills	Improve math and reading skills; obtain passing grades in all classes	Attend tutoring sessions consistently to identify specific learning problems and learning/study strategies	Mother will implement relaxation/ meditation skills to prepare son for homework and chores after school daily	Standardized tests for intelligence, math, and reading aptitude provided and analyzed by school psychologist
Social problems with other children; bothering them, provoking negative interactions, fighting	Reduce/eliminate fighting; improve social ties with classmates	Obtain no negative scores on weekly tally for provoking negative interactions with other children	Psychiatric consultation for possible ADHD medication	
		No specific prosocial objectives suggested, pending initial results of contingency management intervention, which may eliminate negative interactions and improve overall relations with classmates	Psychological testing for assessment of learning disabilities/deficits; psych intern tutor half-hour 3 times weekly	
			Teacher will continue to observe; social-skills training considered if problem behaviors do not abate	
			Case management and coordination of total service plan to be conducted by social worker as team leader	

baseline measure for each situation. The school psychologist performed a couple of CPTs and standard academic tests to assess Ricky's learning problems and recommend remedial exercises to the special education intern. These indexes would be used to gauge his academic progress. As for idiographic measures of behavioral comportment, completing chores, homework, and so forth at home and in the classroom, Margarita and the teacher agreed to use the same indexes on their daily scorecard (rated -1, 0, +1) for chores completed in a timely manner, completed homework, completed in-class work, and maintaining good relations with others in class. Zeros would be applied for not completing tasks or work, and points could be taken away for actively negative or oppositional behavior at home or school: -1 for being "mouthy" and defiant, or -5 points for fighting or being belligerent. Margarita picked up the simple scorecard when she picked up Ricky after school. They would sit and discuss his experiences and scores every day. The social worker compiled all the data from standardized scales and specific indexes to monitor and evaluate behavioral and academic progress over the course of the intervention.

SUMMARY

Conduct problems and ADHD are among the more common and distressing problems for children, adolescents, and their families, and have a major impact on schools and the community. MDF assessment will reveal many factors that are amenable to effective intervention through a combination of individual skill building, family behavior therapy, and contingency management methods employed consistently at home, in the classroom, and in the community. Medication is also likely to be of considerable help to children with symptoms of ADHD. Effective case management is essential to ensure consistent collaboration with the overall service plan. Social workers are in a position to take on important leadership roles in implementing evidence-based practices for these troubled children and their families.

CHAPTER 14

CHILD ABUSE AND NEGLECT

This chapter examines the biopsychosocial factors associated with the abuse and neglect of children, describes some of the more immediate consequences of abuse and neglect, examines the clinical and forensic aspects of assessment, and reviews the literature on intervention and prevention strategies. Internalizing and externalizing disorders may be, in part, a consequence of abuse and neglect; chapters 12 and 13 describe interventions for these problems. Current interventions are probably best seen as a continuum of prevention, early intervention, and intervention to stop abuse and neglect and help the victims cope with the psychosocial consequences. The demarcations along this continuum of care often overlap in the literature.

ASSESSMENT

Background Data

Childhood abuse and neglect are co-occurring and overlapping constructs. A review of the literature reveals various definitions of child abuse and neglect (e.g., D. A. Wolfe & St. Pierre, 1989; S. J. Kaplan, Pelcovitz, & Labruna, 1999; Pecora, Whittaker, Maluccio, & Barth, 2000). *Physical abuse* includes both minor physical harm (scratches, bruises) and major physical harm, meaning broken bones, head injuries, wounds, burns. *Psychological and emotional abuse* includes verbal abuse and harsh physical punishments, such as tying up, emotional neglect, exposing a child to domestic violence, and deliberately impeding normal emotional and psychological development with inconsistent limits or unreasonable expectations. *Child physical neglect* includes a failure to provide basic care (e.g., food, clothing, shelter, hygiene, basic medical care if available). Definitions of *sexual abuse* vary considerably, but a general consensus includes a range of increasingly severe forms: voyeurism or exhibitionism; deliberately exposing a child to pornographic material; sexualized touching or kissing; masturbation with, by, or in front of a child; giving or receiving oral sex; vaginal or anal penetration with fingers or objects; vaginal or anal intercourse. These events may be brought about through enticement, various forms of persuasion, threats, or physical force. Child psychological, emotional, physical, and sexual abuse often occur within the context of various forms of family violence, and researchers are beginning to acknowledge that it may make more sense to look at them as interrelated phenomenon rather than as discrete entities (Slep & Heyman, 2001). Nevertheless, there are advantages to examining these forms of abuse separately for a variety of clinical and forensic reasons.

Based on a review of extant data (D.A.Wolfe & McEachran, 1997; S.J. Kaplan et al., 1999; Pecora et al., 2000; USDHHS, 1996a, 1996b; Putnam, 2003), approximately one million cases of child abuse and neglect are confirmed annually in this country. Estimates of child deaths resulting from abuse range from 1,500 to over 2,000 children per year, and these rates have increased since 1990. Roughly half these cases are identified as neglect, one-quarter as physical abuse, one-eighth to one-tenth as sexual abuse, and about one-twentieth emotional maltreatment. Definitions of abuse and neglect vary considerably in incidence and prevalence studies, and it is unlikely that these experiences are mutually exclusive, as these categories suggest. Different forms of abuse and neglect are likely to overlap in a substantial proportion of cases, and reoccurrence of abuse probably exceeds 50%. About one-half of these children will enter foster care at some point, and close to three-quarters of a million children will be served annually by the child welfare system.

American consciousness regarding sexual abuse of children has been raised significantly over the past twenty years (Wolfe & Birt, 1997). However, because of high-profile cases involving false accusations of abuse and the popularization of bogus treatment methods, public backlash has dampened community concern and engendered considerable skepticism regarding the real neglect and violence perpetrated by some adults upon millions of children in the United States. Approximately 100,000 to 200,000 reports of sexual abuse of children are documented annually, and prevalence estimates (based on adult retrospective reports) have ranged from 15% to 30% of children (less than age 18), 12–35% of females and 4–9% of males (Pecora et al., 2000; Putnam, 2003). Based on a random sample of 930 adult women in one western city, Russell (1983) estimated that 16% of women had experienced at least one episode of intrafamilial sexual abuse and 31% had experienced extrafamilial sexual abuse before the age of 18. Stepfathers were about eight times as likely to abuse their daughters as biological fathers (17% versus 2%), and stepfathers' abuse tended to be more severe (Russell, 1984). In the first national survey of sexual abuse, Finkelhor, Hotaling, Lewis, and Smith (1990) estimated that up to 27% of women and 16% of men experienced sexual abuse during childhood.

Increases in estimates of violence toward children may not be merely the result of increased reporting (Gelles & Straus, 1987). Rates of childhood sexual abuse are most likely underestimated because data more likely reflect confirmed cases (C. C. Swenson & Hanson, 1998). Surveys of adolescents and adults that look at retrospective accounts of abuse give much higher rates than other estimates. For example, in a survey of ten- to sixteen-year-olds, Finkelhor and Dziuba-Leatherman (1994) found that 3.2% of girls and 0.6% of boys are sexually abused every year, and about 15% of girls and about 6% of boys are reported to have been sexually abused in their lifetime. Based on a thorough review of forty-seven surveys of clinical and community samples, Fergusson and Mullen (1999) found average rates of childhood sexual abuse to be within 8–62% for females and 3–29% for males. Regarding children having experienced intercourse, rates were 1–28% for females and 1–14% for males. Divergent estimates of abuse are attributed to a lack of reliable definitions of the problem, lack of reliable measures, sampling differences, and other methodological problems. Based on the results of several studies reviewed by V. V. Wolfe and Birt (1997), family members accounted for less than half the incidents of sexual abuse of girls and less than a third of boys. More than one-half of sexual abuse appears to be a one-time event, and girls are more likely than boys to be abused (roughly 2 or 3 to 1). Girls are also more likely than boys to be abused by a family member over a protracted period of time. There appears to be no compelling data to suggest that socioeconomic status, race, or ethnicity predict which child is likely to be abused sexually, although data appear to suggest that sexual abuse among the middle class is less likely to be reported. About a third of cases of sexual abuse are disclosed during childhood, and those who do not disclose are motivated to keep silent through fear of retribution against themselves or family members. Others keep silent due to shame, guilt, or a lack of understanding that the act was wrong, a belief often engendered through indoctrination by the abuser.

Risk factors correlated with child abuse and neglect are well documented and include single-parent households, lack of parental knowledge and skill in child care, maternal depression and other psychopathology on the part of the adult caretaker, substance abuse, the presence of couples violence, lack of social support, low educational status, unemployment and poverty, homelessness, lack of access to basic health care, living in crime-ridden neighborhoods, parental stress and poor coping skills, and having an above-average number of children (Gaudin, 1993; D. A. Wolfe & McEachran, 1997; Smokowski & Wodarski, 1996; Gelles, 1997; Dore, 1999; Zlotnick, Robertson, & Wright, 1999; Appel & Holden, 1998). Generally, one can assume that the greater the number of risk factors in a family, the greater the risk of abuse or neglect. However, correlated risk factors are not proof of child abuse or neglect. In addition, there are no consistently identified differences in rates of abuse or neglect by race when socioeconomic factors are statistically controlled. Definitions of abuse and neglect are also subject to considerable variability by local statutes, community, and cultural norms. For example, views regarding the "acceptable" use of corporal punishment range considerably, depending on cultural and religious norms (Gelles, 1997).

In addition to general risk factors for child abuse and neglect, correlates of sexual abuse include being female, median age of 10–11, being prepubertal, living in an otherwise dysfunctional family environment (e.g., marital conflict, lack of supervision of children), and experiencing other forms of emotional and physical abuse (Fergusson & Mullen, 1999). To repeat, however, these correlated factors are not confirmatory of abuse, and determinations of sexual abuse must be made through careful clinical and forensic evidence gathering. Nevertheless, a confluence of multiple risk factors for child abuse and neglect in general should prompt practitioners to carefully pursue more in-depth assessments.

Evidence strongly suggests that the consequences of child abuse and neglect, in general, do increase risk for child maladjustment and future psychopathology as adults (Putnam, 2003). These problems include depression, anxiety, PTSD symptoms, CD, substance abuse and other high-risk behaviors, ADHD, social and interpersonal deficits (including difficulties developing trusting relationships with others), and other intellectual and academic deficits. Adults who were sexually abused as children may be at greater risk for substance-abuse problems, eating disorders, BPD, PTSD, and depression. Gender differences reveal a greater likelihood of emotional disturbances (internalizing disorders) in girls and more behavior problems (externalizing disorders) in boys (Kazdin, 1994b; Dore, 1999; S. J. Kaplan et al., 1999; D. A. Wolfe & St. Pierre, 1989; Widom, 1998). These various problems may also be related to witnessing violence in the home. Probably more than half of children in violent homes have witnessed their father's assaults on their mother, have been exposed to an array of psychologically and physically abusive behaviors, and are more likely to be abused themselves. In addition to the emotional problems listed above, they are also more likely to engage in aggressive or violent behaviors. The intensity of the child's response may be related to the intensity and frequency of the violence, the quality of their relationship to their caregivers, the content of the disagreements, whether the parents can demonstrate satisfactory problem solving and conflict resolution, and whether the child gets directly involved with the conflict (see review in S. A. Anderson & Cramer-Benjamin, 1999). The effects of witnessing couples violence can have long-term impacts on children, well into adulthood. Research on these and other traumatic events and their effects on children have demonstrated a direct relationship between the degree of victimization and severity of the child's emotional and behavioral symptoms (Milgram, 1989).

Children who have been sexually abused are at increased risk for many of the same emotional and behavioral symptoms suffered by other abused children, with the possible addition of sexualized behaviors (e.g., public masturbation, flirtatiousness), adolescent promiscuity, running away, engaging in prostitution, and perhaps symptoms of PTSD (V. V. Wolfe & Wolfe, 1988; V. V. Wolfe & Birt, 1997; Kendall-Tackett, Williams, & Finkelhor, 1993; C. C. Swenson & Hanson, 1998; V. V. Wolfe, Gentile, & Wolfe, 1989; Friedrich, 1993; O'Donohue, Fanetti, & Elliott, 1998; Putnam, 2003). Sometimes there are no indications of psychosocial consequences of sexual abuse at the time of assessment, and most abused and neglected children do not develop formal PTSD (Widom, 1999). As for the long-term effects of child sexual abuse, there is clear evidence that, based on severity, type, chronicity, and social response to the abuse, people who experienced sexual abuse as a child are at increased risk to develop emotional, behavioral, and interpersonal problems in the long run. *However, there is no direct link between child sexual abuse and the development of any specific disorder. As of yet, there is no homogeneous set of core symptoms that can be identified as "sexual abuse syndrome"* (Alter-Reid, Gibbs, Lachenmeyer, Sigal, &

Massoth, 1986; C. C. Swenson & Hanson; Fergusson & Mullen, 1999). It is also not empirically justified to draw the conclusion that sexually abused children are likely to suffer more psychosocial difficulties than children who suffered other forms of physical abuse (see review in C. C. Swenson & Hanson).

A host of moderating and mediating factors account for the lack of a simple linear relationship between the experience of child abuse (including sexual abuse) and the development of psychopathology in children (and later as adults; Ammerman, Cassisi, Hersen, & Van Hasselt, 1986; V. V. Wolfe & Wolfe, 1988, V. V. Wolfe & Birt, 1997; Kendall-Tackett, Williams, & Finkelhor, 1993; Milgram, 1989; Fergusson & Mullen, 1999; Briere, 1992; Conte & Schuerman, 1987; Widom, 1998; C. C. Swenson & Hanson, 1998; McGloin & Widom, 2001). The factors include

the existence of other chronic adversities that often exist in multiproblem homes, including poverty, unemployment, and parental substance abuse;

the type, frequency, severity, and duration of the abuse;

whether the abuse included sexual abuse (e.g., forcible oral, anal, or vaginal penetration);

the relationship of abuser to victim;

severity level of threats used at the time of abuse;

innate resilience or vulnerability due to temperament and child's coping abilities;

cognitive appraisal of the abuse, the abuser, and related factors; and

response of familial and social supports around the child.

In general, multiple types of maltreatment, duration of abuse, and the associated severity of events predict greater long-term psychosocial effects in adulthood (D. J. Higgins & McCabe, 2001). Manifest symptoms and behavioral consequences are also relative to developmental level. For example, younger children may experience night terrors and somatic and externalizing problems, and adolescents are more likely to exhibit depression, suicidal behaviors, and substance abuse (C. C. Swenson & Hanson, 1998). Although child abuse in its various forms appears to have some "dose-response" relationship to future psychopathology and violence, most abused children do not become abusive parents or violent members of society. A host of factors noted above may increase or decrease the likelihood of predicting who will succumb to the impact of childhood victimization and who will not. However, interpreting the findings of this research is hampered by a number of methodological shortcomings (Widom, 1989; Milgram, 1989; S. A. Anderson & Cramer-Benjamin, 1999; Fantuzzo & Mohr, 1999; R. M. Johnson et al., 2002; D. A. Wolfe & McEachran, 1997).

Theories

D. A. Wolfe and St. Pierre (1989) identified three major categories of relevant theories of child abuse and neglect: the psychiatric model, which posits that child abuse and neglect are predominantly the result of parental mental health problems; the sociocultural model, in which parents succumb to some of the negative influences of social and economic deprivation; and the social-interactional model, whereby the abusive parent's psychological state mediates environmental stressors that may lead to abuse. However, the distinctions among these theories have faded as research has become more multidimensional (D. A. Wolfe & McEchran, 1997). The factors that explain the causes of child abuse and neglect and the consequences of abuse in the short and long term include a range of biological, familial, social, environmental, and economic factors as they interact over time (Azar, Povilaitis, Lauretti, & Pouquette, 1998; Belsky, 1993). Theories that overemphasize one group of factors must be qualified. Despite the assertion, for example, that environmental factors are predominantly to blame for child abuse and neglect (e.g., Garbarino, 1977, 1997; Garbarino & Kostelny, 1992), there is no reason to assert that child abuse is predominantly the result of social, political, economic, and cultural conditions. This emphasis on the "ecosystem" is apparently intended to take responsibility for child abuse off the shoulders of the individual parent (and affiliated adults), and place it exclusively on society as a whole. However, evidence demonstrates that no specific psychosocial factors are necessary or sufficient to account for child maltreatment. The combination and interactions of factors are complex, and they include the psychological characteristics of the parent, based on their own temperament, learning history, childhood experience, modeling of their own parents, beliefs about child-rearing practices, and mental health problems; characteristics of the child such as behavioral disorders or temperamental problems related to prenatal conditions, and other health problems; parent-child interactions such as an irritable mother with a history of abuse in her own childhood attempting to discipline a naturally rambunctious child; sociocultural factors that condone violence; social stressors related to poverty, overcrowding, crime, and violence, and the impact of these factors on the parents and their ability to cope. Intergenerational effects of these personal, interpersonal, and contextual factors have also been recognized. Recent longitudinal data, for example, has demonstrated that the more risk factors present (e.g., poverty, young single mother, poor maternal mental and physical health, lack of paternal involvement, difficult childhood temperament) the more likely (by several orders of magnitude) that maltreatment is likely to occur (e.g., J. Brown, Cohen, Johnson, & Salzinger, 1998). Although there is little doubt that poverty and the effects of living in a crime-ridden neighborhood can thwart efforts to adequately raise children, engaging in child abuse and neglect is not the private domain of the poor.

Other theories have focused on the psychological processes that account for pathological outcomes in children who have been sexually abused. Psychodynamic theorists such as Hartman and Burgess (1990, borrowing from Horowitz 1997 and others) have offered their theories regarding how the abuse event is psychologically processed. They build on a foundation that considers pretrauma factors, characteristics of the abuse event, the quality of the disclosure experience, and postdisclosure outcomes. They explain: "The premise of informational processing gives some clues to the intensity of defensive adjustment made by children who are assaulted over a prolonged period of time. Their initial distress is subdued by a level of cognitive operations that allows the abuse activities to be stored partially in past memory. It is merely speculation as to what the child goes through to do this" (p. 116). Hartman and Burgess then use the psychodynamic concepts of "encapsulation of the event, dissociation, splitting, ego fragmentation, and drive disharmony . . . which shows how the traumatic event is processed and provides the conceptual link between the event experience and patterns of post-abuse adjustment" (p. 117). Encapsulation of the event involves the child's keeping the event (which may still be in progress) to themselves. Because this encapsulation requires considerable psychological energy, the effects disrupt normal psychosocial development, including sense of self, and other self-regulatory activities. They theorize that the child then relies on the defense mechanisms of dissociation, splitting, denial, and "ego fragmentation" to deal with the psychological stress associated with the abuse. They further aver that a number of possible outcomes to the event may ensue. (1) In the integrated pattern, a child sees the abuse realistically and is able to discuss it with some objectivity. (2) In the avoidant pattern, the child denies the event and refuses to discuss it. Avoidance may lead to stress and later psychological and social problems. (3) In the symptomatic pattern, the child develops long-term difficulty coping with the event, feels guilty and responsible, and may experience behavioral problems, including sexual acting out. Should identification with the abuser occur, the child eventually impersonates the aggressor and masters the anxiety by antisocially exploiting others.

The problems with this formulation are, first, the stages of the theory and possible outcomes are largely descriptive and simply reflect possibilities that are documented in the empirical literature. The explanations regarding "how" these processes occur, however, refer to theoretical constructs and processes that are largely inferred from case-study observation. Little evidence has been forthcoming to substantiate psychodynamic explanations for why some children develop problems and others do not. No prospective research has identified these unconscious processes as predictive of child or adult psychopathology in abused versus nonabused groups.

Finkelhor's traumagenic model (Finkelhor, 1988; Finkelhor & Browne, 1985) proposed that four psychosocial dynamics associated with sexual abuse distort cognitive and emotional processes in children. These dynamics are traumatic sexualization (causing distorted views of sexual feelings and behavior), betrayal (causing general distrust of various people associated with the abuse or the community response to it), powerlessness (a sense of learned helplessness, depression, and fear), and stigmatization (guilt and shame leading to other problems such as withdrawal from others and substance abuse). Although a thoughtful theoretical model and perhaps a useful way to organize potential long-term effects of child sexual abuse, there is little empirical evidence to support the model or to say these concepts reliably predict the behavioral outcomes associated with them. Again, the long-term consequences of child sexual abuse will be affected significantly by many factors, noted earlier.

Some theoreticians have emphasized the PTSD model to account for the long-term effects of child sexual abuse (e.g., Kendall-Tackett et al., 1993). Certainly, severe abuse, including sexual abuse, is a traumatizing event, and children have been shown to manifest the core symptoms of PTSD in response to it, including intrusive thoughts, numbing, hyperarousal, and avoidance. In their review, however, Kendall-Tackett et al. suggest that the PTSD model is not always a good fit for a number of reasons: sexual abuse produces no traumatic symptoms that are unique compared to other traumatic events; other non-PTSD problems (e.g., running away, promiscuity) may result; and many victims of child sexual abuse do not develop PTSD symptoms. Nevertheless, O'Donohue et al. (1998) consider that the PTSD theory of child sexual abuse is still evolving, and provides a useful model for understanding the consequences of abuse.

Key Elements of Multidimensional/ Functional Assessment

The initial identification of suspected child abuse or neglect may come from a number of sources, including a hospital emergency room staff, police officer, physician, school nurse, social worker, another professional, or a private citizen in the community. Many professionals, including social workers, are "mandated reporters": they are legally required to report suspected incidents of child abuse or neglect to the state child protective services or the police. Once the report is filed, a child protective services worker will initiate a more formal intake and investigation. Should an initial screening produce evidence of child abuse or neglect, a more thorough assessment should follow (Pecora et al., 2000).

Two major purposes of the child abuse and neglect assessment include the *clinical assessment* to prepare the child and other family members for psychosocial intervention if needed, and the *forensic investigation* to assist in the prosecution of the person who abused the child. These methods may be applied in parallel fashion or be conducted simultaneously by an interdisciplinary child-abuse investigatory team. Regardless of what specific role or combination of roles the social worker takes on, competent assessment of child maltreatment requires clinical and legal knowledge, use of evidence-based risk-assessment data, and implementation of valid instruments to augment the qualitative assessment (Milner, Murphy, Valle, & Tolliver, 1998).

Assessment of child abuse and neglect requires an MDF perspective to capture all relevant data related to the child, the parents, the child-parent relationship, and the relationship of the family to their social environment. With the primary concern being the child's safety and well-being, the interacting causes and consequences of abuse or neglect need to be linked over time. Input is required from multiple sources, including the child and family members, teachers, child protective workers, social workers, psychologists, physicians, teachers, law enforcement personnel, and neighbors. Data must also be obtained and collated with multiple methods, including face-to-face interviews, medical exams, observation of the adults and their children individually and together in the home and the consulting office, behavioral performance tests of parenting skills, observations of the couple's communication and problem-solving skills, and standardized scales. Gradually, a more detailed and fine-grained idiographic analysis focuses on the behavior of the parents and other important adults in the child's life, the child's behavior, and an analysis of parent-child interactions to determine the nature of their relationship and the parents' capacities for providing nurturance and positive disciplining over time (D. A. Wolfe & McEachran, 1997).

An assessment of overall family functioning includes identifying evidence of domestic violence, evaluating basic conditions of the home environment (e.g., safety, adequacy of the structure, overall cleanliness), and socioeconomic conditions (e.g., adequacy of food, clothing, shelter). An evaluation of overall family structure, communication styles and patterns, problem-solving skills, and coping capacities with crises and everyday stressors can be very telling. The use of a global family functioning scale such as the FACES (Olsen et al., 1989) can provide useful insights. The family's quality of relationships with extended family, level of social supports, friends, and other relations in the community can indicate their level of social integration, whether they allow themselves to be observed or have become increasingly isolated.

Assessment of individual adults in the household should include psychosocial history, including evidence of their own experiences as victims of abuse and neglect; history of domestic violence and substance abuse in their respective families of origin; and other traumatic events, sudden losses, and the like. Practitioners should examine the parents' relationships with family and peers during their adolescence, the quality of their relationships through adolescence and early adulthood, and their engagement in abusive behaviors, violence, criminality, or drug abuse (or successful adaptation in healthful relationships and educational and occupational achievements). Any history of family members' prior involvement in mental health, substance-abuse, criminal justice, or child protective services should also be identified and explained. A review of the parents' adult relationships and marital history should include evidence of couples conflict, domestic violence, substance abuse, parenting style, custody arrangements, infidelities, financial problems, and so forth (see chapter 11 on couples assessment).

A thorough psychosocial assessment of the parents' behavior should include their level of parenting skills (both nurturance and positive discipline procedures), and any evidence of outright abuse (psychological abuse or emotional negligence, physical and sexual abuse) of other children previously or currently in their care. A thorough examination of each parent's relationship with their children should include the degree of empathy and caring the adult shows for the child, hostility, and evidence of harsh verbal or physical discipline. The practitioner should assess each adult's expectations of the children and their perception of what behavioral norms apply to their children, given their respective ages. Practitioners can observe parenting skills (either in the consulting office or, preferably, in the home) by asking parents to engage in play activities, provide normative discipline for some infraction of house rules, or demonstrate how they make a request for a child to accomplish a household task. Despite the seemingly contrived nature of this request (and expecting that parents would strive to perform at their best), these demonstrations can be quite telling, particularly if the practitioner is adept at putting the adults somewhat at ease. Observation and demonstration of parent-child interactions can be accompanied by videotaped role-play to assess parenting style or the manner in which parents communicate with each other about their children or how they communicate with their children directly. Immediate triggers for child abuse are often attributed by the parents to the child's behavior (e.g., difficult or oppositional behavior, excessive crying, screaming).

When interviewing the adult suspected of child abuse, there is good reason to be concerned (as with many "mandated" or involuntary clients) about the validity of their self-report. In assessing the validity of the initial report of abuse, the practitioner should pay particular attention to the following data: a known history of abuse, any delay in obtaining assistance for the injured child, any incongruity between the client's assertions and the known evidence of abuse, and any variation in the client's narrative about what actually occurred with regard to the allegations of abuse (D. A. Wolfe & McEachern, 1997).

The assessment should cover the individual child's psychological and social functioning commensurate with their age and developmental level. Evidence of internalizing and externalizing disorders should be examined (see chapters 12 and 13), and adjunct instruments used as needed. The SAC (appendix B) can provide a relatively brief yet comprehensive overview of significant symptoms. Although children may suffer from anxiety, depression, and behavioral disorders for a variety of reasons, one can make tentative cause-effect inferences about children's functioning and the behavior of their parent by observing the quality of parent-child interactions, the parents' communication style and disciplining practices, whether children appear to be receiving sufficient emotional nurturance, the expectations the children feel the parents have of them, and the emotional expression of the children and their parents in each others' presence. Other important indicators of a child's well-being include school performance, relations with peers, and overall health and adequate physical care, including food, clothing, and basic medical care; regular adult supervision and/or school attendance; adequate personal hygiene; and evidence of physical or sexual abuse (D. A. Wolfe & McEachern, 1997; S. J. Kaplan et al., 1999; Pecora et al., 2000). Although psychological, behavioral, and situational problems among family members including the children can have multiple causes and can co-occur for a variety of reasons, practitioners must build a case for child abuse by carefully linking the parent's behavior to evidence of psychological and physical abuse and/or neglect of the child in a gradual, logical, and evidence-driven fashion.

Again, collating the results of multiple sources of data using multiple methods can go a long way to determining whether the child's problems are associated with parental neglect or physical abuse.

Although many medical examinations do not reveal confirmatory evidence of child abuse, they are an essential part of the assessment process. Reichert (1992) emphasizes the need to examine the child carefully for unexplained burns, bruises, scars, and torn, stained or bloody clothing. Lesions, warts, abrasions, lacerations, and the like in the genital/anal areas may be readily observed. One should note any difficulty walking or sitting, pain with diapering or when held, bowel dysfunction (constipation, encopresis), somatic complaints, and behavioral changes. Other medical indicators include marks of physical trauma near the child's mouth or genitals, evidence of abnormalities resulting from an anal examination, and positive test results for sexually transmitted diseases. The chances of obtaining compelling forensic evidence increase with a timely medical examination. Should a practitioner suspect abuse, she should make the referral as soon as possible. Most often the indications of abuse can be observed externally by the attentive medical professional, and many signs can be readily observed by nonmedical practitioners (marks on a child's face, arms, and legs).

Depending on the type and severity of abuse, a range of intervention options may be available. These may include simple monitoring of the case and family counseling at a local family service center, specialized services for the child and/or other family members (e.g., mental health, substance-abuse treatment), and intensive home-based multilevel treatment (e.g., intensive family preservation services). In cases where the immediate safety of the child is a concern, other services may be available: temporary out-of-home placement, foster and kinship care, residential care for the child, family reunification at some later date, or termination of parents' rights and permanent removal of the child to foster care, kinship care, or adoption. This continuum of services is likely to vary considerably from case to case as well as from state to state, given the variability in the application of assessment protocol and standards, regional benchmarks for what constitutes levels of abuse and neglect, and the availability of services all along the continuum of care (Pecora et al., 2000).

The Sexual-Abuse Assessment

Should sexual abuse be suspected during the initial child-abuse screening and assessment process, a specific sexual-abuse assessment and investigation should follow. It is best to approach the assessment of child sexual abuse as a special evaluation procedure nested within a comprehensive child-abuse and neglect assessment (O'Donohue et al., 1998; C. C. Swenson & Hanson, 1998; V. V. Wolfe & Birt, 1997). However, blending the roles of clinical practitioner, advocate, and forensic evaluator is generally not advised, given the need for the evaluator to consider several hypotheses and examine all relevant evidence as objectively as possible. There is also considerable overlap in the requisite knowledge and skill between a valid clinical and forensic assessment, although the data gleaned from the clinical assessment and forensic investigation are applied to somewhat different purposes. As with a child-abuse and neglect assessment in general, the state-of-the-art sexual-abuse evaluation requires a comprehensive (multidimensional) and interdisciplinary team approach that uses multiple sources of data. These include clinical interviewing, use of scales, direct observation, medical and other physical evidence, and the self-reported observations of multiple sources including the child, the parents, the child with each parent, and significant others knowledgeable about the child.

The clinical assessment focuses on identifying and gauging the impact of sexual abuse on the psychosocial well-being of the child, family functioning, and other indications of abuse or neglect in order to plan the intervention (C. C. Swenson & Hanson, 1998). A team approach is likely to increase cross-validation of observations and to help avoid biases interjected by one practitioner's taking on different roles with different interviewees. If an allegation of abuse is made, the abuser should be interviewed by a practitioner with expertise in interviewing child sexual abusers (McGleughlin, Meyer, & Baker, 1999). The forensic investigation may be conducted by a law enforcement professional, child protective worker, social worker, or other mental health professional or team of professionals. The forensic assessment focuses on determining the validity of the accusation. The investigators also strive to determine the frequency, severity, and duration of the abuse; whether force or other forms of coercion were used; the relationship of the alleged abuser to the child; the time, place, and other situational factors associated with the abuse; current safety of the child; ability of other caretakers to protect and support the child; and potential for any further abuse.

Anywhere from one-fifth to one-half of initial allegations are ultimately not confirmed, and (contrary to common opinion) only a small percentage of allegations are related to custody conflicts (and these are no more likely to be confirmed than allegations of sexual abuse in general). When allegations are confirmed, many cases are not prosecuted for a number of reasons, including poor cooperation from the alleged victim and the family, variations in state jurisprudence, and ambivalence regarding whether child abuse is a crime or a mental health problem. The investigation and trial experience for children can be very stressful, but most children report after the fact that it was worth doing, and there appears to be little long-term harm from the judicial experience itself (V. V. Wolfe & Birt, 1997).

A detailed history should be taken to cover the child's normative development and to identify problems, specifically any that appear to be directly related to sexual abuse (e.g., evidence of sexual trauma, exposure to pornography or adult sexual behavior, precocious sexual behavior), and details about the parents' mental health, substance abuse, level of intimacy, and sexual history (McGleughlin et al., 1999; C. C. Swenson & Hanson, 1998). The History of Victimization Form (V. V. Wolfe, Gentile, & Bourdeau, 1987) covers a list of specific sexual-abuse indicators, including solicitation to abuse, exhibitionism and forced viewing of sexually explicit material, sexual kissing, touching and fondling, digital penetration, giving/receiving oral stimulation to genitals, and intercourse. The relationship of the perpetrator to the child is identified, along with the duration and frequency of each type of abuse, and the degree and types of coercion employed (e.g., blackmail, rewards, threats of various kinds). Although there has been much controversy regarding the validity of children's memories of alleged sexual abuse, their memories of these events are generally considered to be accurate, although the degree of accuracy depends on a number of factors, including age, type and style of interview, and other situational factors. Prompts to anchor memory (e.g., Where were you? Who was there? What were you wearing?) can help a child recall events more accurately. Controversies regarding the problems with assessing the validity of memory and "recovered" memory are considered below.

There appears to be some consensus regarding forensic and clinical evaluations of allegations of sexual abuse. Presented below are recommendations for the practitioner conducting a sexual-abuse assessment (American Professional Society on the Abuse of Children, 1990; AACAP, 1990; American Academy of Pediatrics, 1991; American Psychological Association, 1994; Kuehnle, 1996; McGleughlin et al., 1999; Saywitz, Goodman, & Lyon, 2002; O'Donohue & Fanetti, 1996).

Build good rapport with the child and other principals.

Be clear about whether the interview is forensic or clinical in nature and what the importance of the content of the interview will be in the context of the legal process.

Communicate the limits of confidentiality.

Obtain multiple reports from significant others: parents, teachers, police, doctors, school nurses, coaches, and so on.

Include interviews with the child alone and not in the presence of the alleged perpetrator of the abuse (except with very young children).

Orient the interview to the correct developmental (cognitive, verbal) level of the child.

Proceed from general to more specific questions without leading or suggesting the answers.

Use open interviewing techniques that avoid leading, suggestive, or coercive persuasion methods.

Consider the timing and circumstances of the allegations, the disclosure, and the function and impact on the family or the divorce process, to bring up opportunities for the child's being led or used as leverage in a custody battle.

Consider whether children's sexual knowledge is congruent with their developmental level, or whether other circumstances may have exposed them to sexual material (e.g., videotapes, magazines, witnessing adults having sex or children being abused).

Judge whether the child's disclosure is congruent with the child's own language or with vocalizations mimicked from an adult.

Examine whether the child's report is consistent within and between interviews.

Determine the quality of the child's emotional response to the report.

Videotape the investigative interview to avoid the stress of repeated interviewing.

Recognize the ability and limitations of a child's testimony in court and the potential for negative effects of testifying on the child.

Make an effort to determine the child's ability to tell the truth and accurately recall events.

Elicit facts about the abuse: what happened, how, when, where, under what circumstances? Have the child report other relevant details, such as clothes, smells, identifying body parts or unique physical details such as moles or tattoos. Query the child for circumstantial facts such as what was on the television, whether it was night or day, who was home, and so on.

Ask the child to describe other details about the abuser's behaviors, such as bribes or threats of reprisal.

Determine the basic plausibility of the alleged abuse by comparing the report to other known circumstantial facts (e.g., the abuser may have been out of town that week).

Be alert for denials of abuse, signs of coercion, or pressure to claim or deny abuse originating from others.

Recognize the limitations and fallibility of memory, suggestibility of changing memories, and the fact that memories are subject to distortion, and assess the child's overall competency and credibility.

Understand that many problems children have are not unique indicators of sexual abuse, and that their distress or symptoms may indicate other problems.

Use valid scales as adjuncts to the multidimensional interview.

Obtain a thorough medical examination of the child.

Despite these well-documented guidelines, the empirical evidence supporting the validity of child sexual-abuse assessments is lacking (McGleughlin et al., 1999). There is no consistent symptom profile or valid "syndrome" for sexually abused children. Such symptoms are found in many nonsexually abused children as well. Conversely, the absence of these symptoms does not suggest that a child was not abused, because many sexually abused children manifest no symptoms. In addition, empirical examinations of interviewing skills related to child sexual abuse demonstrate a high degree of inaccuracy in determining whether sexual abuse has occurred, in part because child self-report can be vague. The testimony of sexual-abuse experts cannot be taken at face value or dismissed out of hand. Standardized assessment protocols are not available for any specific age group, and instruments cannot be confirmatory, any more than the self-report of individuals. Although careful reviewing of a child's narrative account may increase the validity of recall, suggestibility in children remains a serious concern. Research findings based on confirmed cases of abuse can be misleading, because they are based on nonrepresentative groups of abused children. Overall, although a well-trained sexual-abuse evaluator using evidence-based protocol can accurately identify many cases of child sexual abuse, there is still considerable room for false positives (false accusations of abuse) as well as false negatives (not confirming abuse when it happened). Although the validity of assessment for mental health problems in general falls well short of 100% accuracy, the clinical and dispositional implications of these problems are not nearly as profound as they are in making decisions that may permanently alter the lives of children and parents (O'Donohue et al., 1998). *Social workers who perform clinical or forensic child sex-abuse assessments and interventions would be well-advised to obtain specialized training from recognized professionals who engage in evidence-based assessment and intervention practices.*

Controversial Methods of Child Sexual Abuse Assessment

Reliability and Validity of Memory and Recovered Memories.   The reliability and validity of children's memories and the phenomena of repressed and recovered memories have been controversial topics in clinical practice for some time. In general, children's memories, particularly memories that have been consistently maintained over time, are considered fairly resistant to distortion. The likelihood of memory distortion is related to the following factors: preschool age, intimidation by authoritative people, delay between the event and the time of recall, the suggestions of others, retroactive interference (e.g., memories of a previous abusive situation affects recall), autosuggestion (e.g., previously held beliefs about sexual abuse), and confabulation of information in order to fill memory gaps (G. Goodman, Bottoms, Shaver, & Qin, 1995; V. V. Wolfe & Birt, 1997). The controversy in eliciting children's memories about abuse seems to lie on a continuum from the use of nonleading open-ended questions, to the use of prompts, to the asking of leading questions. At the extreme, children can be pressured to answer questions a certain way if they are cross-examined like an adult witness in a criminal trial. There is compelling evidence that memory can be unreliable and that children's reports of abuse (or absence of it) can be influenced or distorted through pressure, coercion, and other ways. Even highly detailed investigatory interviews are fraught with reliability and validity problems, because children's reports and memories can be manipulated. Most experts understand that validating an allegation of sexual abuse in either a clinical or forensic assessment is very challenging (e.g., O'Donohue & Fanetti, 1996; Loftus, 1993, 1994; AACAP, 1997a). These experts also recognize that, although many memories of abuse are accurate, people do often forget or distort memories, and the recollection of memories once forgotten is a possibility.

The problem with assessing repressed memory lies not in its possibility, but in determining whether recovered memories can be accurately determined through clinical assessment techniques, ranging from ordinary interviewing to "memory regression" work. These questions are important and must be determined by scientific inquiry, not through uncontrolled case studies or conference testimonials. Given the fact that even the most skilled investigators employing "objective" evidence (e.g., medical evidence, eye witnesses) have trouble making highly confident allegations of abuse, those who make their allegations based on highly questionable assumptions, unsubstantiated theories, and untested interviewing and diagnostic techniques are more likely to make false allegations and to inaccurately dismiss the possibility that abuse actually has occurred. Basing one's assessment on false assumptions (e.g., satanic ritualistic abuse is common), confusing correlation with causation (e.g., depression and low self-esteem are obvious indicators of sexual abuse), or using assessment techniques that lack scientific merit (e.g., "body work," memory regression, dream analysis, projective testing, interpretation of children's drawings) make allegations of sexual abuse in general and recovered memories in particular much more risky. A good rule of thumb in making allegations of sexual abuse should be to use evidence-based assessment guidelines that have been promoted by leading professional groups, use a range of conventional assessment tools and protocols based on data gathered from multiple points of view, and, above all, be conservative in making criminal allegations of child abuse. For a more thorough discussion of this critical topic see Loftus 1993, 1994.

Despite much of the distortion promulgated in the child welfare field, a scientific consensus regarding the repressed-memory phenomenon has emerged (Knapp & VandeCreek, 2000; M. L. Eisen & Goodman, 1998). In brief, child abuse in all its forms is harmful in the short run and often in the long run, satanic ritual abuse of children is rare, continuous memories of abuse are likely to be accurate, some memories can be lost and recovered, memories from infancy are highly unreliable, false memories can be created, traumatized children are no more suggestible than nontraumatized children, memory-recovery techniques are not reliable, child and adult emotional and behavioral disorders can be successfully treated without having first established whether sexual abuse actually occurred, and the complex processes involved in the interaction of traumatic events and memory are not sufficiently understood to justify much confidence in "recovered memory work."

Projective Techniques. Projective testing is at best a questionable approach to mental health assessment. Its use in child abuse assessments (particularly sexual abuse) is highly controversial. These techniques include drawing methods (e.g., House-Tree-Person, Draw-A-Man), free-hand drawing, interpretation of children's play, and Rorschach testing. The fundamental problem with such tests (given their psychoanalytic origins) is that they require the practitioner to make cause-effect interpretations from highly ambiguous data that can usually be interpreted in any number of ways. Although a denotative drawing by a young child (e.g., two people having sex) is reason for concern, interpretations of ambiguous material are more likely to be influenced by the expectations of the interpreter than what is in the child's mind or relevant to the child's experience. Reviews of methodologically sound research (e.g., Veltman & Browne, 2002) conclude that, although projective tests may be useful for stimulating discussion and evoking emotional expression, there is no evidence that the interpretation of children's impressionistic drawings, paintings, dreams, or play is a reliable or valid method for establishing allegations of sexual abuse, for diagnostic purposes or for prognosis of psychosocial interventions. The risks for false positives and false negatives are unacceptably high. Employing these tests as diagnostic tools in sexual-abuse assessments adds little to the overall validity of a comprehensive assessment and should be strongly discouraged.

Anatomically Correct Dolls.   Use of anatomically correct dolls has come to be considered a useful device when employed by well-trained interviewers as part of a comprehensive evidence-based assessment (C. C. Swenson & Hanson, 1998; Everson & Boat, 1994). According to V. V. Wolfe and Birt (1997, p. 595), "Recent research evidence has quelled many of the concerns about anatomically correct dolls. Dolls do not elicit unfounded reports of sexual behavior or elicit excessive sexual behavior in free-play conditions with non-abused children; they are also useful in discriminating abused from non-abused children in terms of both sexual abuse disclosures and sexual play with the dolls." Generally, proper use of dolls will elicit more valid disclosures of sexual abuse than will open-ended questions. When using the dolls to interview children, interviews should occur as soon as possible after the alleged event, use just one interviewer, avoid leading questions, use open-ended questioning, use developmentally sensitive questions with younger children (under six years of age), and be videotaped (M. Lamb, 1994).

V. V. Wolfe and Birt (1997) concluded from their review of the empirical literature that anatomically correct dolls should be used to identify body parts, clarify previous statements, and help nonverbal or low-verbal children express themselves and describe an event after there has been indication of abuse activity. "*However, though unusual behavior with dolls may be worthy of note in an evaluation report, such behavior without a direct report of sexual abuse should not be considered conclusive evidence of abuse*" (V. V. Wolfe & Birt, p. 597; emphasis added). The use of dolls to comfort a child, to help break the ice in an interview, to facilitate conversation, to stimulate emotional expression, and to help stimulate memory when narrating experiences is generally accepted as useful and reasonably valid, as long as the interviewer does not lead the child. When used for these purposes, suggestiveness and interviewer error are considered relatively unlikely (C. C. Swenson & Hanson, 1998; Everson & Boat, 1994).

Cultural Aspects in Assessment of Child Abuse and Neglect

Although genuine efforts have been made to examine racial and ethnic differences regarding child abuse and neglect (e.g., Meston, Heiman, Trapnell, & Carlin, 1999; Moisan, Sanders-Phillips, & Moisan, 1997), research is marked by a number of methodological shortcomings, including lack of representativeness in samples; problems in defining ethnic subgroups, abuse, and neglect; and lack of adequate statistical controls. Thus, caution should be taken in drawing conclusions about ethnic differences, given the stigmatizing nature of child-abuse allegations.

Despite the lack of consistent evidence in linking cultural factors to child abuse and neglect, there are important general recommendations that apply to social work practice with diverse populations. It is important to consider the cultural milieu of the community before engaging in child-abuse and neglect interventions. The lack of compatibility between practitioners' beliefs, attitudes, and behaviors and those of their clients on matters of child-rearing practices, family norms, and rituals can impede efforts to help. Practitioners should strive to understand the cultural processes of the communities they intend to assist (O'Donnell, Wilson, & Tharp, 2002).

For example, noting the lack of research on family preservation services with Native Americans, Coleman, Unrau, and Manyfingers (2001) provided some thoughtful suggestions. Assessment and successful engagement of Native American families requires some basic understanding of the particular tribe, the importance of family (particularly with regard to intergenerational relationships that include ancestors), the communal view of extended family and their responsibility for raising the children, and the role of spirituality and importance of symbol, ceremony, and rituals (which can be readily incorporated into family interventions). Broader social and historical matters need to be understood and recognized as well. These include a keen sensitivity to the history of oppression and dislocation experienced by many tribes, the continuing poverty and protracted periods of unemployment for many Native Americans, and the devastation wrought by addiction to alcohol and other drugs. An awareness of clients' tribal history, sense of frustration, distrust, humiliation, and disempowerment is vital before one should expect any level of acceptance. Specific knowledge and skills apply even on the microlevel of engagement, requiring basic familiarity with communication norms such as significance of eye contact, acceptability of asking personal questions, and readiness to endure long periods of silence during conversations.

As indicated in chapter 2, given the variability among people of color, no standard "diversity" methods will apply to all relevant cases. Yet one can open doors with patience, appreciation of history and culture, and learning a bit of language *before* attempting to engage. The practitioner should be willing to ask questions and listen to answers before presuming to help.

Current Status of Risk Assessment of Child Abuse and Neglect

Currently, risk assessment of child abuse and neglect is in an embryonic stage. Most evidence suggests that even experienced practitioners do not accurately predict the likelihood of abuse, given current practices in child welfare. In one prospective study of 446 at-risk families positively identified for child abuse and followed for five years (DePanfilis & Zuravin, 1999), results demonstrated that family stress, partner abuse, social-support deficits, and child vulnerability factors were significantly predictive of later abuse. Further analysis of decisions to close these cases showed that workers were not using evidence-based criteria to support their decisions about the likelihood of future abuse. In addition, workers tended to concern themselves less with child neglect than with child abuse, despite the potentially greater consequences associated with neglect (DePanfilis & Zuravin, 2001).

In a three-wave survey of 432 children alleged to have been abused or neglected, Camasso and Jagannathan (2000) tested the reliability and predictive validity of a structured assessment tool (the Washington State Risk Assessment Matrix) for predicting reoccurrence of abuse. They found poor reliability ratings and little reason to believe that reoccurrence could be predicted with any confidence. However, they suggested that risk assessment scales be improved by shortening them to focus on items that have been shown to be predictive of abuse (e.g., chronicity of abuse, substance-abuse problems), and by applying more rigorous psychometric standards to the selection of instruments, to ensure reliability and validity. A convergent validity study of 261 cases in the northwestern United States (English & Graham, 2000) showed insignificant and otherwise weak correlations between child protective workers' judgments and research interviewers' ratings taken with an extensive battery of valid instruments for measuring multiple domains of child and parent well-being and functioning. Finally, a recent examination of decision-making patterns in child protective services highlighted further concerns about accurately identifying child abuse and neglect. P. H. Rossi, Schuerman, and Budd (1999) compared the decisions of 27 child welfare experts with those of 103 child protective service line workers, and based their coded decisions on seventy actual case summaries. Findings revealed little relationship between level of professional experience and pattern of decision making. The authors underscored the obvious risks inherent in making false positive and false negative decisions, and noted the need for evidence-based standards to be developed for child protective service assessment, evaluation, and decision making.

Despite all that has been written regarding the importance of improving assessment in child protective services, there has been little or no research on the matter. The first substantive descriptive survey of child protective evaluations in Illinois was conducted by Budd et al. (Budd, Felix, Poindexter, Naik-Polan, & Sloss, 2002; Budd, Poindexter, Felix, & Naik-Polan, 2001). A random sample of about 200 cases of African-American, Hispanic, and Caucasian children was selected from child protective case rolls, and evaluations were conducted largely by doctoral-level psychologists. Based on case data using rigorous coding methods, Budd et al. demonstrated that (1) multidimensional assessments that included a range of methods and sources of data collected over multiple sessions were not the norm; (2) there was a disproportionate focus on the child's attributes or developmental functioning, with little ecological validity in the assessments (getting collateral reports and/or observing the child in a range of settings such as school, with peers); (3) despite their lack of validity, projective assessment methods were used in almost 90% of cases; (4) many reports did not make any assessment regarding the credibility of the data collected; and (5) whether the evaluation was clinical or forensic was often not made clear. To improve the ability of child protective workers to make informed decisions and reduce risk of harm to children, more aggressive efforts must be made to incorporate the training and use of evidence-based assessment tools into child welfare services.

Instruments

A number of standardized measures may enhance the assessment of risk for child abuse and neglect (P. Lyons, Doueck, & Wodarski, 1996; T. McDonald & Marks, 1991; Camasso & Jagannathan, 2000), but they must be used as part of a comprehensive MDF assessment. In addition, broadband and narrowband scales are useful for measuring baseline severity of children's problems (whether related to abuse or not), and for monitoring and evaluating changes in the child's problems. PTSD scales, in particular, have become widely used for children who have suffered traumatic stressors such as child abuse. Other adjunctive tools should be considered for assessing mental health, substance abuse, and other problems in children and adult family members, along with tools that measure family functioning (Combs-Orme & Thomas, 1997). Many relevant scales have been noted or more fully described in other chapters.

The Child Abuse Potential Inventory (CAPI; Milner, Gold, & Wimberley, 1986; Milner, 1994; Milner et al., 1998) is a widely used child-abuse screening device that is self-administered by the parent. It has 160 items, and it contains a 77-item physical-abuse scale (but is not intended to detect sexual abuse), and six other subscales: distress, rigidity, unhappiness, problems with child and self, problems with family, and problems with others. It also contains scales to detect lying or other inconsistencies. Overall reliabilities (internal consistency, split-half, test-retest) for subscales have been in the good-to-excellent range, and the CAPI accurately classifies physical abusers and nonabusers better than 80% of the time with various abusive populations. The scale also correlates with perception of behavior problems in the child, negative parent-child interactions, weak social supports, family conflict, and a lack of cohesion in the family. The CAPI also correlates with abuse-related life stress, and physiological and psychosocial indicators of abuse. Although more research is needed to determine its predictive validity for abuse, the scale does appear to be sensitive to change in clients when administered over time. Thus, the CAPI seems to be a useful adjunct to an MDF assessment for screening, monitoring, and evaluation.

Although not all abused and neglected children would meet criteria for PTSD, even subclinical signs and symptoms (e.g., avoidance, arousal, numbing, dissociation) may be an indication that a child is under significant duress as a result of psychological or physical abuse and neglect. The revised Children's Impact of Traumatic Events Scale (CITES-R; V. V. Wolfe & Gentile, 1991; Nader, 1997) is a structured interview instrument designed to measure children's cognitions regarding the effects of abuse. It is intended to be used with children from ages eight to sixteen, and comprises seventy-eight items (eleven subscales). With older children, it may be administered as a paper-and-pencil self-report scale. It takes from twenty to forty minutes to administer. Many of the items were borrowed from related scales, and several subscales were derived from factor analysis. The scale measures a number of important constructs, including PTSD symptoms, perceptions of social support following abuse, abuse attributions (e.g., guilty feelings), and eroticism. Scale items are scored (0–2), "not true," "somewhat true," "very true." Internal consistency reliabilities generally are in the acceptable range, although inadequate alpha coefficients have been noted for a couple of the subscales (e.g., "dangerous world"; Crouch, Smith, Ezzell, & Saunders, 1999). Other data have shown moderate support for both the internal consistency and concurrent validity of the CITES-R subscales with sexually abused children (Chaffin & Shultz, 2001).

The Trauma Symptom Checklist for Children (TSCC; Briere, 1996; Nader, 1997) is a fifty-four-item scale intended to measure the effects of trauma and child abuse in 8–16-year-olds. Subscales include measures of anger, anxiety, depression, dissociation, PTSD symptoms, and sexual concerns. Items are rated on a four-point frequency scale (0–3) ranging from "never" to "almost all the time." Subscales are in the acceptable range for internal consistency reliability, have shown good concurrent validity with other validated scales, and have demonstrated good discriminant validity with sexually abused (versus nonabused) females. Population norms are available. With a group of 119 hospitalized adolescents, the TSCC subscales were shown to be reliable and correlated well with other independent measures of psychiatric distress. The PTSD subscale accurately distinguished sexually abused adolescents from those who were not sexually abused (Sadowski & Friedrich, 2000).

The Post-Traumatic Stress Disorder Reaction Index (PTSD-RI) is one of the most widely used and validated instruments for measuring PTSD symptoms in children and adolescents. Developed in the mid-1980s (Frederick, 1985), the PTSD-RI was initially administered in response to a fatal sniper attack on a children's playground (Pynoos et al., 1987; Nader, Pynoos, Fairbanks, & Frederick, 1990). The PTSD-RI has been translated into several languages and has been used in many nations to assess trauma symptoms in children who have been subjected to natural disasters, sniper attacks, political violence and terrorism, exposure to atrocities, witnessed sexual assaults of their mother, witnessed suicide of an adolescent peer, life-threatening medical illnesses, and severe burn injuries (Steinberg, Brymer, Decker, & Pynoos, 2004).

Evolving with changes in *DSM* criteria for PTSD, the current PTSD-RI (revision 1) is designed as a paper-and-pencil instrument to be used for screening young people for PTSD symptoms. It is also useful for monitoring and evaluating the effects of intervention. The items are thoughtfully designed to be easy to read with little or no prompting from the interviewer. It is divided into three parts. Part 1 contains dichotomous (yes/no) items that screen for lifetime traumatic events. Part 2 provides an assessment of *DSM-IV* criteria: intense fear response to a traumatic event (items 15–21) symptoms of reexperiencing (items 22–26), and dissociation (item 27). These thirteen items relate directly to the traumatic event referenced in part 1 that the respondent marked as having bothered him or her "the most." The list of traumatic events includes items related to child physical and sexual abuse. Part 3 addresses symptoms of PTSD that correspond to *DSM-IV* criteria of intrusive thoughts, avoidance, and arousal. These twenty questions are designated to correspond with specific PTSD criteria. These items are scored on a continuous frequency scale (0–4), from "none" to "most," indicating the relative frequency with which the symptoms occurred during the past month. A frequency scale sheet is included to help the child anchor frequency estimates. A scoring sheet is also included (appendix G) to tabulate the total score and subscale scores corresponding to *DSM-IV* criteria.

The children's version (instrument 14.1) is intended to be used for those 7–12 years of age. A parent version closely mirrors the children's version. There is also an adolescent version (minor alterations in language) for those older than twelve. Practitioners can administer the scale in a face-to-face format and detach the frequency rating sheet so the child can easily follow along. The "past month" criteria can be modified as needed to suit the time frame relevant to the traumatic event (e.g., "since the traumatic event" or "in the past week since 'X' occurred"). Under most circumstances, the scale can be administered and scored in less than an hour. The scale should be administered by someone who has some training and familiarity with PTSD and *DSM-IV* criteria, and is at least a graduate-student intern under the supervision of a licensed master's-level clinician.

The scoring guidelines for parts 1 and 2 are straightforward. In part 3, only the seventeen items corresponding to the *DSM-IV* criteria are scored. Three of the items have alternate forms, and the one scored higher by the child is counted in the final scoring. The scoring guide helps the practitioner calculate the total PTSD severity score and scores for each *DSM-IV* criteria (B, C, and D). A cutoff score of thirty-eight or more has been shown to have optimal sensitivity and specificity for detecting PTSD (Steinberg et al., 2004). The PTSD-RI has been shown to have very good to excellent internal consistency (e.g., Layne et al., 2001), good to excellent test-retest reliability (Pynoos et al., 1987), and good convergent criteria with *DSM* diagnosis (e.g., Pynoos et al., 1993). The PTSD-RI is an excellent screen and treatment evaluation tool. The different formatted versions of the PTSD-RI, associated training materials, and scoring aids are available from the authors.

INSTRUMENT 14.1   Post-Traumatic Stress Disorder Reaction Index (PTSD-RI)

Below is a list of VERY SCARY, DANGEROUS OR VIOLENT things that sometimes happen to people. These are times where someone was HURT VERY BADLY OR KILLED, or could have been. Some people have had these experiences, some people have not had these experiences. Please be honest in answering if the violent thing happened to you, or if it did not happen to you.

FOR EACH QUESTION: Check "Yes" if this scary thing HAPPENED TO YOU. Check "No" if it DID NOT HAPPEN TO YOU.

1. Being in a big earthquake that badly damaged the building you were in.   Yes [   ]   No [   ]

2. Being in another kind of disaster, like a fire, tornado, flood or hurricane.   Yes [   ]   No [   ]

3. Being in a bad accident, like a very serious car accident.   Yes [   ]   No [   ]

4. Being in a place where a war was going on around you.   Yes [   ]   No [   ]

5. Being hit, punched, or kicked very hard at home. (DO NOT INCLUDE ordinary fights between brothers & sisters.)   Yes [   ]   No [   ]

6. Seeing a family member being hit, punched or kicked very hard at home. (DO NOT INCLUDE ordinary fights between brothers & sisters.)   Yes [   ]   No [   ]

7. Being beaten up, shot at or threatened to be hurt badly in your town.   Yes [   ]   No [   ]

8. Seeing someone in your town being beaten up, shot at or killed.   Yes [   ]   No [   ]

9. Seeing a dead body in your town (do not include funerals).   Yes [   ]   No [   ]

10. Having an adult or someone much older touch your private sexual body parts when you did not want them to.   Yes [   ]   No [   ]

11. Hearing about the violent death or serious injury of a loved one.   Yes [   ]   No [   ]

12. Having painful and scary medical treatment in a hospital when you were very sick or badly injured.   Yes [   ]   No [   ]

13. OTHER than the situations described above, has ANYTHING ELSE ever happened to you that was REALLY SCARY, DANGEROUS OR VIOLENT?   Yes [   ]   No [   ]

14. a. If you answered "YES" to only ONE thing in the above list of questions 1 to 13, place the number of that thing (1 to 13) in this blank. _____

    b. If you answered "YES" to MORE THAN ONE THING, place the number of the thing that BOTHERS YOU THE MOST NOW in this blank. _____

    c. About how long ago did this bad thing (your answer to a or b) happen to you? _____

    d. Please write what happened: _____

_____

_____

FOR THE NEXT QUESTIONS, please Check "Yes" or "No" to answer HOW YOU FELT during or right after the bad thing happened that you just wrote about in Question 14.

15. Were you scared that you would die?   Yes [   ]   No [   ]

16. Were you scared that you would be hurt badly?   Yes [   ]   No [   ]

17. Were you hurt badly?   Yes [   ]   No [   ]

18. Were you scared that someone else would die?   Yes [   ]   No [   ]

19. Were you scared that someone else would be hurt badly?   Yes [   ]   No [   ]

20. Was someone else hurt badly?   Yes [   ]   No [   ]

21. Did someone die?   Yes [   ]   No [   ]

22. Did you feel very scared, like this was one of your most scary experiences ever?   Yes [   ]   No [   ]

23. Did you feel that you could not stop what was happening or that you needed someone to help?   Yes [   ]   No [   ]

24. Did you feel that what you saw was disgusting or gross?   Yes [   ]   No [   ]

25. Did you run around or act like you were very upset?   Yes [   ]   No [   ]

26. Did you feel very confused?   Yes [   ]   No [   ]

27. Did you feel like what was happening did not seem real in some way, like it was going on in a movie instead of real life?   Yes [   ]   No [   ]

Here is a list of problems people sometimes have after very bad things happen. Please THINK about the bad thing that happened to you that you wrote about in Question 14 on page 2. Then, READ each problem on the list carefully. CIRCLE ONE of the numbers (0, 1, 2, 3 or 4) that tells how often the problem has happened to you in the past month. Use the Rating Sheet on page 5 to help you decide how often the problem has happened in the past month. PLEASE BE SURE TO ANSWER ALL QUESTIONS.

HOW MUCH OF THE TIME DURING THE PAST MONTH

		None	Little	Some	Much	Most
1D4	I watch out for danger or things that I am afraid of.	0	1	2	3	4
2B4	When something reminds me of what happened, I get very upset, afraid or sad.	0	1	2	3	4
3B1	I have upsetting thoughts, pictures, or sounds of what happened come into my mind when I do not want them to.	0	1	2	3	4
4D2	I feel grouchy, angry or mad.	0	1	2	3	4
5B2	I have dreams about what happened or other bad dreams.	0	1	2	3	4
6B3	I feel like I am back at the time when the bad thing happened, living through it again.	0	1	2	3	4

7C4	I feel like staying by myself and not being with my friends.	None 0	Little 1	Some 2	Much 3	Most 4

8C5	I feel alone inside and not close to other people.	None 0	Little 1	Some 2	Much 3	Most 4

9C1	I try not to talk about, think about, or have feelings about what happened.	None 0	Little 1	Some 2	Much 3	Most 4

10C6	I have trouble feeling happiness or love.	None 0	Little 1	Some 2	Much 3	Most 4

11C6	I have trouble feeling sadness or anger.	None 0	Little 1	Some 2	Much 3	Most 4

12D5	I feel jumpy or startle easily, like when I hear a loud noise or when something surprises me.	None 0	Little 1	Some 2	Much 3	Most 4

13D1	I have trouble going to sleep or I wake up often during the night.	None 0	Little 1	Some 2	Much 3	Most 4

14AF	I think that some part of what happened is my fault.	None 0	Little 1	Some 2	Much 3	Most 4

15C3	I have trouble remembering important parts of what happened.	None 0	Little 1	Some 2	Much 3	Most 4

16D3	I have trouble concentrating or paying attention.	None 0	Little 1	Some 2	Much 3	Most 4

17C2	I try to stay away from people, places, or things that make me remember what happened.	None 0	Little 1	Some 2	Much 3	Most 4

18B5	When something reminds me of what happened, I have strong feelings in my body, like my heart beats fast, my head aches, or my stomach aches.	None 0	Little 1	Some 2	Much 3	Most 4

19C7	I think that I will not live a long life.	None 0	Little 1	Some 2	Much 3	Most 4

20AF	I am afraid that the bad thing will happen again.	None 0	Little 1	Some 2	Much 3	Most 4

Frequency Rating Sheet

How often or how much of the time during the past month, that is since _____, does the problem happen?

None 0							Little 1							Some 2							Much 3							Most 4						
S	M	T	W	T	F	S	S	M	T	W	T	F	S	S	M	T	W	T	F	S	S	M	T	W	T	F	S	S	M	T	W	T	F	S
								X									X		X			X		X		X		X	X	X	X	X	X	X
																	X				X		X		X			X	X	X	X			
																						X		X		X		X	X	X	X			
													X				X				X		X		X		X	X			X	X	
																X		X		X	X	X				X	X	X	X	X	X	X

Never	2 times a month	1–2 times a week	2–3 times a week	Almost every day

SELECTING EFFECTIVE INTERVENTIONS

This section provides a critical overview of prevention, early intervention, and reactive interventions. The methods used include residential programs, individual treatment of the child affected by abuse and neglect, interventions with parents to improve their child-care skills, and ecosystem programs that employ multiple modalities in both the home and the community. If parental rights are terminated, children may be referred to foster care or kinship care or be made eligible for adoption.

Interventions targeting child abuse and neglect must be understood within the context of child welfare policy. Pecora et al. (2000) summarize important principles and notable legislation. The main principles include ensuring child safety; promoting the psychosocial and economic well-being of child and family; empowering the family in directing their future well-being; paying due attention to the unique cultural context and needs of families; providing access to services; making the child welfare system accountable; and facilitating efficient coordination of system resources.

The goals of the child welfare system are to balance child psychosocial and physical well-being with permanency planning for the family, a difficult and often contentious balance. Modern child welfare policy in the United States began to emerge in the 1960s in response to growing national awareness of abused and neglected children, captured by the phrase "battered-child syndrome" (Kempe, Silverman, Steele, Droegemueller, & Silver, 1962). This growing awareness inspired legislation to cope with the prevention of child abuse. The Child Abuse Prevention and Treatment Act (1974) mandates reporting of child abuse and neglect, and provides funds for prevention and treatment demonstration projects. Title XIX of the Social Security Act enhances health-care services for low-income individuals and bolsters early-childhood health-care services. The Adoption Assistance and Child Welfare Act of 1980 promotes permanency planning for children. The Family Support Act of 1990 gave further financial assistance for low-income families. The Adoption and Safe Families Act (1997) promotes the safety of children by procedures aimed at reducing child abuse and neglect.

In addition to a burgeoning body of research on the causes, prevention, and treatment of child abuse and neglect, all fifty states now have mandatory child-abuse reporting laws (Mattaini, McGowan, & Williams, 1996).

Residential Programs

Reviewers have noted that twenty-four hour residential treatment services serve a purpose in the child welfare system by providing a haven of last resort for many children, and giving them distance from abusive, neglectful parents and intense emotional conflict. This time-out gives them a chance to obtain emotional and psychological support, and provides an opportunity to affiliate in a peer environment. Ideally, such stays are time-limited, and parents are concurrently involved in treatment. Despite the rapid increase in small residential facilities for placement of abused and neglected children, relatively little research of adequate methodological quality has been conducted on such services. Therapeutic programs in the residential treatment facilities do not appear to result in sustainable benefits when children are released to the community (Smokowski & Wodarski, 1996; Pecora et al., 2000).

Child-Focused Interventions

Relatively little emphasis in the literature has focused on treating abused and neglected children directly to improve coping skills. Two prominent efforts are reviewed here.

Fantuzzo et al., (1988) demonstrated that positive and prosocial peer-mediated play can result in more responsiveness in maltreated and withdrawn children. Thirty-nine children (about half non-Hispanic whites and half African Americans) who were brought to the attention of child welfare professionals were randomly assigned to three groups. In group 1, "normal" children were taught to initiate prosocial behaviors toward the withdrawn child. In group 2, adult teacher aids prompted social interaction between the maltreated child and the peer. Group 3 served as a control condition. All treatment conditions included eight brief play sessions spread out over three to four weeks. Several observational measures rated four types of social interaction: behavioral initiations and responses and oral initiations and responses. By viewing videotaped samples, measurements were made by raters who were blind to the purposes and hypotheses of the study. Six-month follow-up data from classroom settings was available for about half the sample. Results showed statistically significant improvements for children in the peer-initiation treatment condition in both verbal and behavior initiations and significant improvements in oral verbal initiations in the classroom setting. There were no significant effects in either the adult-initiated or the control condition. Overall, the results support the use of peer-initiation strategies to help withdrawn, neglected children.

Culp, Heide, and Richardson (1987) conducted a controlled experiment in which thirty-five maltreated children were enrolled in a multiservice day treatment program. These children were matched on age, gender, race, and problem category (i.e., abuse, neglect) with thirty-five maltreated children who did not receive these services. Of the seventy children, 43% were female, 63% African American, and 37% (non-Hispanic) white, and the mean age was thirty-six months. The program emphasized a strong teacher-child relationship and activities that focused on self-esteem building, enhancement of caring peer relationships, coping with feelings, and multiple learning activities typical of preschool programs. The program was conducted for six hours a day, five days a week. Other services included individual child treatment, parent group counseling and educational services, individual therapy if needed, and a twenty-four-hour telephone crisis service. Using cognitive, behavioral, interpersonal, and language-development indicators, results demonstrated that the treatment group improved significantly more than the control group. Percentile improvement scores were on average about ten to fifteen points higher posttreatment for the treatment group. In a related study with a similar population and program, Culp et al. demonstrated that improvements were not related to the race of the child, but that girls benefited more than boys for reasons that were not explained. Although many of the skill-based programs to enhance the coping skills of children were reviewed in chapters 12 and 13, the programs above are highlighted here because they were tested specifically with children who were known to have been abused or neglected. It is reasonable to suggest that interventions designed for internalizing and externalizing disorders in children would be beneficial for abused and neglected children as well. Nevertheless, there is a lack of practice research that incorporates these skill-based approaches for these children.

Behavioral Parenting Skills

An extensive literature tests interventions designed to improve behavioral parenting skills for parents who have been identified as being abusive or neglectful (Gershater-Molko, Lutzker, & Sherman, 2002; D. A. Wolfe & Wekerle, 1993; Kazdin, 1994b). Some of these intervention methods have also been incorporated into broad-based ecobehavioral or other multimodal programs. These interventions have characteristics like those of the parent-child training programs reviewed in chapter 13 for conduct-disordered children and adolescents. Behavioral techniques such as psychoeducation, modeling, role-playing, practice, feedback, and reinforcement principles are intended to reduce risk of abuse by helping the parent to be more nurturing and to use more positive disciplining methods with their children. Later developments in behavioral parent training include anger management, stress management, coping skills, anger control, and cognitive interventions to address the erroneous and unrealistic expectations some parents set for their children's behavior. Practitioners employing cognitive behavioral interventions can help parents avoid taking the child's provocative behavior as a personal affront, and develop a more empathic understanding of the child's emotional, physical, interpersonal, and situational needs (Corcoran, 2000). Controlled studies have shown that increasing parental self-control and other skills results in a significant improvement in emotional rapport between child and parent and a decrease in the child's negative and aggressive behaviors.

D. A. Wolfe and Sandler (1981) conducted a single-subject design with three parents referred through child protective services to evaluate the use of behavioral parent management techniques. Contingency management was also used, to reward parents for consistent use of their newly learned parenting techniques. The three case analyses revealed excellent results, which were maintained up to twelve months posttreatment. Watson-Perczel, Lutzker, Greene, & McGimpsey (1988) demonstrated with three single-subject evaluations of neglectful families that standard behavioral interventions (teaching, support, reinforcement, contingency management) could be used to successfully help severely neglectful families (e.g., evidence of excrement, dead animals, swarms of cockroaches, decaying food) improve the safety, cleanliness, and health of the child's environment.

Schinke et al. (1986) conducted a matched-pairs experiment in which the treatment group received ten weekly two-hour sessions teaching stress-management skills geared toward improving parents' self-control, interpersonal communication, positive disciplining skills, and skills for enhancing social supports. Although the authors reported significant improvements at posttest and six-month follow-ups, there were few details regarding measures employed. Nevertheless, the study offered one of the few skill-based brief interventions that could be readily employed in typical agency settings, and the results did include some follow-up data.

Several controlled trials provided substantial evidence for the potential of behavioral interventions to reduce abuse and neglect. Brunk, Henggeler, and Whelan (1987) compared group parent training to a multisystemic intervention for abusive and neglectful parents in an eight-week randomized controlled trial with an equal mix of white and African-American parents. Results based on standardized scales and videotaped observational measures showed significant improvements in both groups. There were some differences, however. Positive outcomes for multisystemic intervention included observational ratings showing significantly greater reduction in child abuse and neglect. Group parent training enhanced social support for these parents and reduced isolation. Group parent training showed greater reduction in social isolation and improvement in parents' social well-being, whereas multisystemic group showed more improvements in parent-child relations. No follow-up measures were taken, and the overlap in the results for both groups suggest considerable similarity between the two approaches, particularly in addressing parent-child management practices.

Whiteman, Fanshel, and Grundy (1987) investigated the effectiveness of a three-part cognitive-behavioral intervention with abusive parents who had trouble controlling their anger, often an antecedent to abuse. The investigators devised a skill-based intervention that exclusively targeted the parents' thoughts, feelings, and behaviors related to anger control. Three specific cognitive-behavioral skills were investigated: cognitive restructuring (CR) to change the parent's negative attributions regarding the child's behavior, stress management (SR) to reduce arousal associated with anger, and problem-solving skills (PS) to find more constructive ways of dealing with the stresses of child rearing. Fifty-five subjects were randomly assigned (about evenly) to five groups: CR; SR; PS; combined CR, SR, and PS; and agency treatment as usual. Participants were, on average, thirty-three years of age and, poor. They were about one-quarter non-Hispanic white, one-quarter Hispanic, and half African-American, and 91% were female. Realistic scenarios that would typically provoke an angry reaction by the parent were portrayed and role-played. A scale that measured various dimensions of anger was developed as part of the study to evaluate the effects of the intervention. In addition, items adapted from previously published reliable scales were employed to measure affection, discipline, empathy, and irritating behaviors. Results suggested that the composite treatment package was the most effective intervention overall, although the relaxation training component probably did not account for much of its positive impact. The authors concluded that since the current study included only six sessions of treatment, CBT packages that are provided for longer duration would likely yield even greater outcomes.

D. A. Wolfe, Edwards, Manion, and Koverola (1988) conducted a randomized trial comparing a child-care educational program (agency treatment as usual) with an education plus parent training program based on Forehand and McMahon's model (1981). Thirty young, poor, single mothers with young children (ages 9–60 months) completed the program, which lasted a median of nine sessions. Trained graduate-level therapists with no prior parenting experience of their own provided the parent training interventions. Bachelor-level paraprofessionals conducted the educational component. Self-report measures included standardized instruments for quality of parenting and level of depression, observational measures of mother-child interaction, and standardized measures of child behavior at pretest, posttest, and follow-up. The parent training intervention took place in a clinic setting. Education groups included eight to ten mothers and were conducted at the agency. Parent training included in vivo practice and an opportunity for parents to observe their own performance with their child on videotape, accompanied by constructive feedback. They were also trained in anxiety management and coping skills to improve interactions with their child. At three-month follow-up, results indicated that parents who received the behavioral parent training improved significantly more than those who received just the educational component. However, observational measures in the home were modestly positive for both groups and not significantly different. One-year reports by child welfare workers on indicators of child care or abuse showed improvements for both groups as well. Overall, results strongly suggest that the addition of behavioral parent training to standard agency intervention improves outcomes for mothers of at-risk children. It is important to point out, however, that these mothers, while needy, were carefully screened to rule out domestic violence, unsuitable housing, serious psychopathology, and substance abuse. In short, generalizing to more severely troubled situations may not be warranted.

In a randomized controlled design, Meezan and O'Keefe (1998) compared an eclectic combination of behaviorally oriented psychoeducational multifamily group therapy (MFGT) with traditional family services for eighty-one abusive and neglectful white, Hispanic, and African-American families. Both groups also received case management to ensure adequate instrumental supports. Using a range of psychometrically sound scales to measure social supports, problem-solving skills, attitudes toward child rearing, knowledge of child development, family structure, and child-abuse risk, both groups showed improvement, but the MFGT group showed more areas of improvement in child-abuse potential and in attitudes toward child rearing. It was difficult to discern whether the differences were due to differences in programmatic content or the overall amount of service (the MFGT conditions received three to five times as much face-to-face and phone contact during the study). Because there were no follow-up measures, it is hard to determine how durable the changes were. Nevertheless, one could argue the MFGT condition engendered better engagement in treatment than traditional services.

Ecosystem Approaches: Family Preservation, Family Reunification, and Other Models

Comprehensive multiservice ecobehavioral methods are typically some combination of home-based child and parent-focused interventions, enhancement of social and instrumental supports, and other case management activities that may include interactions with schools, medical professionals, and law enforcement personnel. The basic rationale of ecological approaches emphasizes the need to address the problems of the family in their ecology in an integrated fashion on several interacting levels (i.e., individual, familial, community). In recent years, these methods have been provided within the context of the family preservation/reunification movement, where temporary placement of the child is sometimes part of the intervention.

Family Preservation.   The Homebuilders model (Kinney, Madsen, Fleming, & Haapala, 1977; Kinney, Haapala, & Booth, 1991) is perhaps the most recognized "brand name" of family preservation interventions. This model, started in 1974 in Tacoma, Washington, is an intensive, in-home, brief, multiservice effort aimed at stabilizing the family of the abused or neglected child by improving parenting skills, addressing mental health and substance abuse of individual family members, and providing case management to interface with larger social systems. As described in the initial program evaluation (Kinney et al., 1977), one driving rationale for the development of this family preservation model was to prevent removal of family members and avoid institutionalization of the child, given the associated emotional and financial costs. The Homebuilders concept was informed by research that showed home-based interventions with families in crisis could prevent placement and institutionalization of the child. In that uncontrolled evaluation, eighty families were recruited who met the following criteria: they were in crisis, it seemed highly likely that some member would be removed, one member had to express a strong desire to keep the family together, and staff would not be placed in a highly dangerous situation. After initial emotional and physical crises ebbed, workers focused on defining behavioral problems. These problems included (in descending order of frequency) running away, truancy, school disruption, child abuse, other physical violence in the home, high suicide potential, and substance abuse. The intervention comprised behavioral problem solving and skills training, advocacy and case management to improve community resources, and follow-up services for booster sessions if needed. Over 90% of the participants were followed up in a year. Virtually all cases avoided placement, the main goal of Homebuilders. Many methodological weaknesses however, precluded definitive conclusions about the effectiveness of this program. These weaknesses included a lack of control group, poorly defined interventions, and a lack of standardized outcome measures to evaluate the psychosocial functioning of children, adults, and overall family functioning.

Walton (1997) conducted a posttest-only experimental comparison between child protective services (CPS; i.e., treatment as usual) and CPS combined with eleven hours of family preservation services (FPS) with 132 randomly assigned cases. While the CPS investigators focused on allegations of abuse and neglect, the collaborating FPS workers emphasized strength-based approaches to help the family take responsibility for strengthening itself, provided support, encouraged problem solving and decision making, accompanied the parents to court, and established a network of services to increase child safety. Results showed that the FPS cases were open for fewer days. Walton concluded that home placement "hastened the closing of the case and the returning of total responsibility to the caregiver" (p. 456). Based on interviews six months after case determination, experimental services were deemed to have improved the attitudes of the caregivers toward the agency. The participants said they were more satisfied with services, used more services, found counseling and other services more helpful, appreciated the FPS services more than standard CPS services, and were more likely to use services.

In a replication of this study with a similar randomized posttest-only experimental design (Walton, 2001), follow-up interviews were conducted with caretakers, caseworkers, administrators, and supervisors. Additional data were gleaned from agency databases (e.g., abuse, neglect status, services used, custody history, caseworker demographics). Instruments included the Index of Parental Attitudes and another interview questionnaire with no known psychometric qualities. As in the original study, the FPS intervention comprised engagement, problem solving, and case management interventions provided in tandem with CPS services for an average of fourteen hours. Attrition reduced the 97 experimental cases to 65 and the control cases from 111 to 60 families. Results demonstrated that, although there was no significant difference between the two groups in the number of children remaining in their homes, children in the FPS group were more likely to return to their home and stay longer. There was no difference between the two groups in the number of cases of substantiated abuse or services employed. The parents in the FPS group had significantly more problems regarding the parent-child relationship, yet expressed more satisfaction with the FPS workers, were more likely to view the services as helpful, and rated the FPS caseworkers higher. A number of other service-related data were reported, but no tests of significance were provided. There was no difference between the groups on additional referrals during the six months following the intervention. Although these attempts to improve FPS services should be encouraged, there appears to have been relatively little methodological improvement in the research, frustrating any attempts to determine the actual superiority of FPS over standard child protective services.

Family Reunification.   Pecora et al. (2000) outline the principles and assumptions of family reunification. The biological family is the preferred context for child rearing. The family of origin is the best place to raise a child when the family is given adequate assistance. Separation from the biological family can have long-term negative consequences. Extended-family members should be considered part of the family unit. Reunification ranges from partial to full reconnection with the child's family. Children should be reunited in a timely manner, and early and consistent contact with their families of origin should be brought about as soon as is feasible. If it becomes clear that the risks of reunification to the child's well-being far outweigh the potential benefits, termination of parental rights remains an option, although some connection may still be maintained. Evaluating whether children should be reunified with their biological families requires a thorough assessment of the following considerations:

- the parents' and child's mutual expectations and willingness to be reunified with one another;
- a thorough reevaluation of the parents' skills and competencies, expectations, adequacy of the home, and ability to care for the child's psychological, emotional, and physical needs;
- resolution of the problems that brought about placement initially;
- a gradual reintroduction of the child into the home with progressively longer visitations;
- dealing with temporary setbacks; and
- continued liaison with social service professionals, legal monitoring, and involvement with the foster parents and other social supports.

Overall, outcomes of family reunification programs are indeterminate at this time (Pecora et al., 2000). However, in one combined quantitative/qualitative study on the effectiveness of family reunification, Terling (1999) examined data collected on over 1500 cases over four years. An in-depth case-record analysis on 59 randomly selected cases was also conducted to provide a more fine-grained view. Of reunified cases, 37% were shown to reenter child protection services within 3.5 years. No differences in reentry rates were shown between whites and African Americans. One disturbing finding revealed that assessments by child protection service workers did not predict whether a child was likely to be further abused or neglected. In addition, when serious risks were documented in the case record, they were sometimes ignored. The in-depth examination revealed a number of factors that were associated with reentry into the system: previous and repeated involvement with child protection services; substance abuse by the parent or partner and a lack of sufficient time to succeed in recovery; an inability to grasp basic parenting competencies; and inadequate social support. The study also pointed up one particularly illuminating fact: if the perpetrator of child abuse were removed from the home, the risk of that child's being abused again was virtually eliminated.

Other Models.   Project 12-Ways (Lutzker & Rice, 1984; Lutzker, Bigelow, Doctor, Gershater, et al., 1998) is an ecobehavioral approach whereby assessment and intervention are conducted in the client's living environment. The intervention may include a number of services such as parent-child training, stress management, homemaker skills and budgeting, marital counseling, and infant health care. Some evidence suggests that families benefit from participation in Project 12-Ways. Lutzker and Rice (1987) compared outcomes (further abuse and neglect) between Project 12-Ways and child protective services (treatment as usual) with ninety-seven randomly selected families. Results showed some slight advantage for Project 12-Ways clients, but other methodological problems preclude definitive answers.

Lutzker, Bigelow, Doctor, Gershater, and Greene (1998) reported two replications of Project 12-Ways: Project SafeCare and Project Ecosystems. Project Safe-Care included three of the twelve components of Project 12-Ways: home safety, such as identifying and correcting hazards; infant health care, such as recognizing problems and seeking prompt treatment; and bonding and stimulation, aimed at increasing positive parent-child interactions (Lutzker, Bigelow, Doctor, & Kessler, 1998). Five weeks of service were provided for each component consecutively, for a total of fifteen weeks. In the evaluation, two groups of predominantly Hispanic families were served: a nonabusive at-risk group and a confirmed abuse/neglect group referred by child welfare staff. Four single-subject case studies were conducted to test the efficacy of the program. Results indicated modest improvement in safety, health care, and parent-child behavior. Due to the methodological limitations, results must be viewed with caution. Project Ecosystems was implemented with developmentally disabled children in an urban setting. Single-subject studies showed it to be reasonably effective (Lutzker, Bigelow, Doctor, Gershater, & Greene, 1998). Both studies provided modest support for integrating behavioral interventions within a more ecologically valid systems approach (Lutzker, Van Hasselt, Bigelow, Greene, & Kessler, 1998; Gershater-Molko et al., 2002).

Overall, ecosystem approaches to child welfare show mixed results. Those approaches that incorporate behavioral skill-based interventions have shown considerable promise. Given the lack of clearly defined interventions, of standardized measures, and of randomized trials, however, firm conclusions cannot be drawn regarding the effectiveness of these models (K. Wells & Biegel, 1992; L. H. Friedman, 1991; McDonald and Associates, 1990; AuClaire & Schwartz, 1986).

Interventions with Sexually Abused Children

A small research literature on interventions with sexually abused children has begun to emerge. It is understood that, although the child's problems may be the direct result of sexual abuse, other contextual factors have probably contributed to their distress. Nevertheless, C. C. Swenson and Hanson (1998) make some basic recommendations regarding the unique practical aspects of treating a child who has been sexually abused: assuming that the child's safety has been secured, practitioners complete a thorough forensic and clinical assessment and aim to stabilize any crises. An empathic and sensitive relationship is developed with children to help them express their feelings regarding the abuse. Psychoeducation and cognitive interventions are provided to help the child resolve erroneous beliefs about the abuse, such as "He told me it was my fault." Anxiety- and stress-management techniques are used to help children cope with residual anxiety and depression. Structural and behavioral family interventions are implemented to cope with other co-occurring problems through communication and problem-solving techniques, and substance-abuse treatment of adolescents or adults who remain in the home. A broader multisystemic approach includes clinical case management to pursue evidence of other abuse, neglect, and problems the child may be having in school and the community.

Critics of the sexual-abuse field have accurately noted the lack of evidence to support the psychodynamic approaches to treating sexually abused children (Conte, 1984). However, based on reviews of the literature that include randomized controlled trials, interventions that have been shown to be effective with other internalizing and externalizing childhood disorders are also effective in reducing problems that are presumably the result of sexual abuse (O'Donohue et al., 1998; Fergusson & Mullen, 1999; Finkelhor & Berliner, 1995; Nader, 2001; Saywitz, Mannarino, Berliner, & Cohen, 2000). Single-subject designs with multiple baselines have revealed similar results (e.g., Farrell, Hains, & Davies, 1998). Finkelhor and Berliner noted a number of limitations in the sexual-abuse treatment literature. In addition to the paucity of randomized trials, they noted the heterogeneity of problems experienced by children who have been abused sexually, the asymptomatic response of some who have not yet or will not develop symptoms, and the multiproblem context within which sexual abuse often occurs.

Nonoffending parents may require intervention for any number of problems: reassessing their role in their family as parent, coping with the loss of their partner, and improvement in their relationship with the child victim. Treatments for the offending parent are typically court mandated. As for some offending parents who remain or return to the home, anecdotal literature on family therapy has described interventions whereby offenders recount their actions in manipulating the victim, apologize and take full responsibility for their behavior, redefine their role, and articulate different guidelines for their relationship with the victim and other family members. Given the high rates of co-occurring psychopathy in adult sex offenders, one must weigh carefully the likelihood of rehabilitation versus the risk of renewed abuse. Little research has been conducted on these types of postoffense family interventions (C. C. Swenson & Hanson, 1998).

Exemplar Study: A Controlled Trial of Cognitive-Behavioral Therapy and Family Therapy for Sexually Abused Children.　This controlled study illustrated an effective intervention for children who have been sexually abused. Thirty-six sexually abused children (ages 5–17), some of whom had PTSD symptoms, participated in a clinical study in which CBT with parent or caregiver involvement was compared to CBT without family involvement and a wait-list control group (N. J. King et al., 2000). The child received twenty fifty-minute sessions of CBT that focused largely on anxiety management, including hierarchical imaginal exposure and anxiety coping skills to address stressful memories and images related to the abuse. Assertiveness and psychoeducation components were also included to help the children learn personal safety skills and improve their sense of confidence. For the family treatment condition, problem solving and communication skills were emphasized for the family members, and the caregiver was taught contingency management skills to improve parenting. Parent/teacher training sessions were also coordinated by the practitioner. All treatments were geared toward the developmental stage of the child. Fidelity checks revealed high agreement between instruction manual and actual implementation. A range of standardized and validated indexes were employed to measure baseline assessment and outcome. These instruments measured the degree of PTSD symptoms, self-rated fear and anxiety, depression, and the child's perceived ability to cope with abuse-related symptoms.

Results demonstrated very good improvement for both treatment groups compared to the control group. Although both the individual CBT and the CBT plus family conditions showed comparable results in reduced PTSD symptoms, fear and anxiety, and global functioning at posttest and follow-up (twelve weeks), practitioners found the family format more satisfying overall. In short, as with previous studies, CBT (with or without direct family involvement) was shown to be substantively effective in reducing symptoms associated with sexual abuse of children.

Related Needs of Clients Receiving Child Welfare Services

Substance-Abuse Services.　Substance abuse and associated criminal problems among the parents of abused and neglected children co-occur with a wide range of other difficulties, including mental illness, health problems, and domestic violence. The consequences of children's exposure to the effects of substance abuse and addiction include increased risk of depression, anxiety problems, low self-esteem, learning difficulties, behavioral disorders, interpersonal problems, and substance abuse (Dore, Kauffman, Nelson-Zlupko, & Granfort, 1996). Child protection services can be improved by training workers in valid assessment and monitoring of substance abuse in their clients, improving integration with substance-abuse services, and developing better collaboration with law enforcement and the criminal justice system (Semidei, Radel, & Nolan, 2001).

To date, little research on coordinating substance-abuse services and child welfare has been conducted, although anecdotal evidence suggests it is feasible (McAlpine, Marshall, & Doran, 2001; Gruber, Fleetwood, & Herring, 2001). In one study, substance-abusing women with children who were involved with child protective services were surveyed during or soon after receiving substance-abuse services. In spite of a low response rate to the survey and concerns about self-reporting bias, some evidence suggested that matching services to the needs of the clients could result in better outcomes (B. D. Smith & Marsh, 2002). Some of the evidence-based approaches to treating couples or adolescents with a substance-abuse problem could be readily incorporated into an ecobehavioral approach to dealing with child abuse and neglect. These methods include motivational enhancement therapy, coping-skills approaches, behavioral couples and family interventions, and community reinforcement and contingency management approaches (see chapter 6).

Foster Care, Kinship Care, and Adoption.   Foster care, long-term group home, or other residential treatment programs may be an option should attempts fail to "preserve" or reunite a family. Termination of parental rights and adoption of the child by permanent foster parents is one possible outcome. Smokowski and Wodarski (1996) found that placements of long duration are associated with a combination of more severe child behavior problems, parental skill deficits, poverty, and lack of social supports. Although there are considerable methodological weaknesses in the data regarding psychosocial correlates of children in foster care, Horan et al. (1993) demonstrated in a review of the literature (from 1974 to 1989) that children who entered foster care have very high rates of serious mental health disorders and are in need of much more care than is currently available.

About half a million children are in foster care in the United States at any given time. They are taken from their families of origin for reasons ranging from inadequate parenting skills to serious physical or sexual abuse. The number of children in foster care continues to grow, and children of color, particularly African Americans, are disproportionately represented and are likely to remain in foster care longer than their white counterparts. Foster care is intended to be a temporary placement, and refers not only to family foster care but also to temporary placement of a child in a group home or other residential setting. During this time, the initial problems that prompted the child's removal from the home could be ameliorated through psychosocial intervention, social services, and possibly adjudication, if criminal acts such as sexual abuse have occurred.

Problems that have plagued the foster-care system include excessive lengths of stay, drifting from one foster home to another, disproportionate representation of children of color, and long-term disruption in relationships with members of the families of origin. Policies and procedures vary considerably from location to location. To improve consistency in foster care, more coordination is recommended among child protective services, the legal system, and other community service agencies.

There has been increasing discussion regarding the professionalizing of foster parenting. Such a strategy would involve improved recruitment, training, and evaluation of prospective foster parents; increased compensation for greater expertise; greater specialization in foster care of children who have special medical or psychological needs; and greater liaison between professional foster parents, agencies, and perhaps the biological parents (Pecora et al., 2000). It has become widely accepted that, despite the problems and shortcomings of the foster-care system in this country, foster parents provide a critical service for children in need. However, there is little solid systematic evaluation research in the foster-care field.

Kinship care (foster placement with relatives) has gained increasing interest as a viable alternative to placement of a child. The challenges of kinship services are similar to those of nonrelative foster care: initial assessment of caretakers, adequacy of the relative's home situation, and the need for greater professionalization of kinship caretakers. In addition, evaluation has revealed similar mixed outcomes (Pecora et al., 2000). Kinship care appears to account for a good portion of the increase in foster-care placements over the past twenty years, and a number of factors (e.g., child's age, gender, family income, geographical location) have been shown to be related to the likelihood of kinship placement (Grogan-Kaylor, 2000).

Should reunification efforts fail, adoption may be the ideal permanent-placement alternative, although not all child welfare professionals share that view. Although prospective adoptive parents outnumber available children, many children are not adopted because of the general preference for healthy, white babies in contrast to older children from racial minorities or those with special needs (Mather & Lager, 2000). Although prospective adoptive white parents may desire to adopt a child from another race or cultural background, such arrangements have met with considerable resistance. Many in the minority community feel it is not in the best interests of children to be raised in a cultural environment that is not indigenous to them. For example, the Indian Child Welfare Act (1978) was passed, in part, to stop the adoption of Native American children by non–Native American parents (Mather & Lager, 2000). Similar controversies have arisen in recent years regarding gay couples adopting children. Many in the heterosexual community object to such an arrangement, stating their opposition in ostensibly religious or psychological terms. There appears to be little evidence (perhaps due to a lack of research) that having been raised by otherwise nurturing adoptive parents of a different background is in any way detrimental to a child's psychosocial development. Those who wish to influence child welfare policy must weigh the risks and benefits of raising a child in a "different" family against significantly reducing the chances of a child's ever having a home and a family.

Preventing Child Abuse and Neglect

Wekerle and Wolfe (1993) examined over thirty controlled studies evaluating prevention efforts primarily to improve young mothers' parenting skills and secondarily to improve child developmental and behavioral competencies. The prevention efforts are premised on the notion that while there may be no obvious signs of neglect or abuse by (typically) poor, young single mothers, prevention may guard against problems that might arise later and interfere with the child's healthy psychosocial development. The studies were divided into three main categories: those that focused on parent competencies, using intensive group intervention or home visits to provide support and parenting skills; parent-child support for new parents, using home visits to provide information and support; and parent-child support for teen parents, using group intervention or home visits to help improve attitudes and parenting skills. Although the data were compromised by methodological limitations, it appears that behavioral skills approaches that continue for up to three years hold more promise as compared to general supportive, educational methods. Results seem to show greater improvement in mothers' attitudes and skills as compared to improvements in children's well-being and development.

A meta-analytic review (MacLeod & Nelson, 2000) tested a number of related hypotheses for fifty-six proactive and reactive programs designed to prevent or reduce child maltreatment. Proactive programs are designed to begin when the mother is pregnant, immediately after the birth of the child, or during early infancy. These interventions include home visiting and multicomponent social support and mutual aid. Community-based proactive programs include family support, child care, preschool education, and community development. Reactive programs are usually employed in early childhood in response to indicated child abuse or neglect. These programs include intensive family preservation (e.g., Homebuilders), multicomponent interventions (e.g., Project 12-Ways), social supports, and specific parent-training programs. The methodological criteria employed in the search included studies of children up to twelve years of age, prevention programs only (excluding sexual-abuse programs), the use of prospective controlled designs, the use of studies published in journals, books, and dissertations; outcome measures that included indicators of out-of-home placement, child maltreatment, parental attitudes, observations of parents' behaviors, and measures of the home environment.

The authors of the review had expected the following findings to emerge from the analysis: programs using an ecological framework would be more successful than more targeted programs; "empowerment and strength-based" interventions would be more effective than "expert-driven, deficit-based" interventions of longer duration and higher intensity; and interventions that employed both social and instrumental (concrete) supports would be more effective than those that employed a more targeted "professional helping approach." Findings of the meta-analysis revealed a total mean effect size for these programs of .41, meaning that outcomes for clients in the experimental groups exceeded outcomes for 66% of those in the control groups, and longer interventions generally resulted in better outcomes overall. Effect sizes for proactive interventions tended to be higher at follow-up than when measures were taken postintervention. However, the converse was true for reactive interventions. Interventions based on an "ecological" framework were not more successful than microlevel interventions. Although empowerment/strength-based approaches showed higher effect sizes than deficit-based approaches, many of these programs (e.g., family preservation services) used placement status as an outcome measure, and used few indicators of family, parent, or child well-being to measure outcomes. Lastly, social supports appeared to improve outcomes for proactive programs, but showed less impact for reactive programs, possibly because the social supports added an element of surveillance in cases where abuse had yet to occur. Overall, this meta-analytic review sheds a positive light on efforts to prevent and intervene with child abuse and neglect, but conclusions must be tempered with caution due to poorly defined program components and outcome measures.

One major review of outcome studies that focused exclusively on primary prevention programs for child neglect and physical abuse (nonsexual) revealed eleven studies that met rigorous methodological criteria (MacMillan, MacMillan, Offord, Griffith, & MacMillan, 1994a). Findings showed strong support for home-visitation programs primarily targeted at the prenatal and early postnatal needs of poor, unmarried young mothers. In a second study focused on sexual abuse, MacMillan et al., (1994b) showed that educationally oriented prevention programs can increase knowledge and safety skills regarding sexual abuse, but there is little evidence that these programs actually result in reduced rates of childhood sexual abuse.

School-Based Strategies.   Although not explicitly developed for the purpose of reducing child abuse and neglect, programs that foster better integration of school and community services may reduce some of the environmental risk factors that can lead to the neglect and abuse of children. These risk factors include inadequate adult supervision of children, poor-quality day care, and parental stress symptoms due to overwork, poverty, single-parent status, and other causes. The School of the 21st Century (Zigler, 1989) was developed as a comprehensive year-round program of child care, early parent education, and family support for parents and their children from prenatal care to age twelve.

The program is based on several principles: creation of a stable and reliable child-care system, equal access for all children to quality child care, and adequately addressing children's developmental (cognitive, emotional, social, and physical) needs. Finn-Stevenson, Desimone, and Chung (1998) reported that there are currently more than 500 Schools of the 21st Century, operating in at least sixteen states and serving more than quarter of a million families. The programs run year round and are implemented after school lets out for the day, and during school vacations and summers. The program includes outreach services into the community to provide in-home parent education and referral for other needed services. The results of a recent evaluation of two such schools covering the second to fourth years of the program (Finn-Stevenson et al.) demonstrated a number of positive outcomes, including a reduction in child-care costs to parents, reduction in lost work hours, a decrease in parental stress, and improvements in the parent-child relationship. These outcomes imply promising influences on children's academic and psychosocial development and well-being.

Home Visiting Programs.   Paraprofessional home-visiting programs can reduce the rates of child abuse (I. Roberts, Kramer, & Suissa, 1996). Social workers often play a key role in home-visiting programs, sometimes teaming up with nurses or other health professionals. A narrative review of early intervention "support services" for vulnerable families with young children in the United Kingdom and the United States (Armstrong & Hill, 2001) found that while "voluntary" attendees (mostly young mothers and children) found the experience satisfying, "referred" clients found them to be stigmatizing, often viewing them as a "dumping ground." Nevertheless, these programs show some improvements in psychosocial adjustment for mothers and children. Longer-term programs (two years or more) that provided education, occupational counseling, health education, and social support were found to be generally helpful. Among home-visiting programs, home-health visitors give priority to the health of the young child; they also provide emotional support and general advice on child rearing. Some of these programs have focused on at mothers suffering from postpartum depression or other psychiatric problems, as well as low-birth-weight babies or those showing indications of failure to thrive. Overall evidence from a number of quasi-experimental studies suggests strongly that children who are targeted in these programs make significant improvements in health and psychosocial adjustment in the long run. Development of networking strategies, enhancement of social supports, and inclusion of paraprofessionals have been accepted positively by many mothers in need. In addition, the findings of uncontrolled studies suggest an increase in feelings of support and self-confidence, and reduction in incidents of child abuse and neglect.

In one Australian study (J. A. Fraser, Armstrong, Morris, & Dadds, 2000), researchers conducted a controlled trial comparing in-home services with access to standard clinic health services in a group of young at-risk mothers. One hundred and eighty-one mothers met the following criteria for being "high risk": single parent, victimized by domestic violence, screened positive for child abuse or neglect, financial stress, and unstable housing. These cases were randomly assigned to an experimental early-intervention home-visiting program intended to improve family and parent adjustment and to reduce incidents of child abuse and neglect. The program was specifically designed to promote a good working alliance with the mothers, improve mother-infant attachment, enhance parenting skills, promote healthful behaviors in child, reduce parental stress, promote the use of social supports, and reduce child abuse and neglect. The experimental program included intensive in-home services provided by a nurse, social worker, and paraprofessional assistants. A designated pediatrician coordinated services and provided care in both a clinic setting and in-home crisis situations. The experimental group received twenty or more home visits on average, and more home visiting was given to mothers with acute needs (e.g., low-birth-weight babies). Information about the availability of health and social services for the mother and child served as the control group. Although the study demonstrated positive results in child, parent, and home adjustment measures after six months, there were no substantive differences in outcomes between the experimental and control interventions at twelve months. In the comparison group, only about one-fifth of the women consistently availed themselves of clinic services. No specific demographic factors predicted superior adjustment overall. In this case, it appears that access to standard child health care services is as effective as intensive in-home care. Both interventions, when analyzed separately, also demonstrated a comparable reduction in the potential for child abuse.

Leventhal (1996) suggests a strategy for home visiting to prevent child abuse and neglect.

Visits should begin early and occur frequently.

Practitioners should emphasize the development of a sound working relationship.

The home situation should be closely monitored, including the child's needs for safety, health, and nutrition.

Practitioners should provide concrete services and supports for the family, such as transportation, housing, and budgeting.

Modeling techniques should be used to teach effective parenting skills.

Men should be included in the overall strategy, if possible.

Interventions should be tailored to fit the needs of the particular family.

Given the reduction in available funds for such services, Leventhal suggests that the real question is "not whether we . . . can prevent these types of maltreatment from occurring (because the answer is yes), but whether we, as a society, can afford the resources to provide the necessary preventive services to families" (p. 647).

Description of Effective Interventions for Child Abuse and Neglect

Unlike most of the other chapters in this book in which there are clear models of "best practices," the literature in the child welfare field is rather fragmented and inconclusive. What follows is an overview of effective intervention "ingredients" for addressing child abuse and neglect. These elements could be applied in various combinations, depending on the severity and complexity of a case, after determining whether the case requires prevention, early intervention at the first signs of abuse, or reactive care for documented serious cases.

Conduct comprehensive forensic and clinical assessment for the child and the family, incorporating the inputs of multiple sources and employing multiple methods, both qualitative and quantitative.

Teach behavioral parenting skills (see chapter 13 for details).

Teach and monitor adequate standards for maintaining the orderliness, safety, and cleanliness of a home, and maintaining basic hygiene of the child.

Teach awareness of and responsibility for monitoring the safety of the child in the presence of other members of the family and in the community.

Teach stress-management skills to parents to better cope with anger and frustration, especially when dealing directly with children.

Teach problem solving and communications skills as part of behavioral couples therapy and structural/behavioral family therapy to improve marital relations and overall family functioning.

Provide case management services (including advocacy, schools, health-care professionals, other social services) to help the parent by enhancing social and instrumental supports. Facilitate the exchange among service providers of information regarding the welfare of the child and family, to promote generalization of improvements. Facilitate contingency management programs to ensure adherence to drug-treatment protocol and compliance with other court-ordered mandates as required to maintain or regain custody of a child in placement.

Use integrated or contracted mental health and substance-abuse services for parent(s) and for adolescents as needed.

Facilitate placements such as brief hospital or residential stays and temporary foster and kinship care.

How these services are applied will depend on state child welfare policies, funding, and the structure and organization of private, public, and contracted services. A key point is the need for close interservice collaboration among child welfare agencies, mental health services, substance-abuse services, law enforcement, and criminal justice.

IMPLEMENTING AND EVALUATING THE EVIDENCE-BASED INTERVENTION PLAN

CASE STUDY: MIKEY AND JANET

Janet, a twenty-eight-year-old waitress at a rural highway diner, was driving home about midnight after her shift when she was pulled over by a local police officer. She was arrested for driving under the influence of alcohol. Since the officer had a suspicion that Janet was also using other substances, he shined a flashlight on the passenger side floor and noticed an empty rolling-papers wrapper and small squares of tin foil. After further investigation, Janet admitted that she had a "very small" amount of cocaine in her possession, but that it belonged to her boyfriend. She was arrested and brought to the local police department for processing. The officer allowed her to contact her sister to come and pick her up. Upon arriving at home, her sister, Kara, discovered that Janet's son, Mikey (aged five), was home alone. She also noticed drug paraphernalia and beer bottles strewn about, the house dirty and in disarray, and Mikey sleeping on the couch with his wrist tied with a piece of rope to the couch leg. Very upset, she argued with Janet, and insisted that Mikey come home with her to stay at her house. Janet tearfully agreed. The next day, Kara contacted the child welfare department, and an investigation was immediately conducted.

The social worker from child welfare, Rachel, saw the same disarray in the house the next day. Kara kept Mikey out of school for the day, and met the social worker at Janet's home to discuss the situation. Janet apparently had left Mikey, as she often had, with her live-in boyfriend, who she thought was taking care of him. On further investigation, it came to light that he seemed to have a serious problem with alcohol and other drugs. The social worker took a close look at Mikey, rolled up his sleeves, and noticed welts and bruises up and down his arms. She found the same types of marks on his legs. When she asked Mikey if Bret hit him, holding back tears he sniffled, "He's mean. He hits me all the time." Janet objected, saying, "He does not, he only hits him when he's being bad .... when he doesn't do what we say." The child welfare worker informed her that a full investigation would have to be conducted. In the meantime, she recommended that Mikey stay with Kara until the investigation was completed.

Further assessment of the situation revealed that the boyfriend had been living with Janet for about eighteen months. Prior to that time, there had been no indications of abuse. After he moved in with Janet, their occasional drug use began to escalate, and things got out of hand. Janet worked evenings, and Bret, in the beginning, was pretty good about staying at home and looking after Mikey. As drug use increased, they became more negligent with everyday duties, including housecleaning, taking care of Mikey, and making regular meals. The school nurse and Mikey's teacher had sent home notes of concern about Mikey's appearance and his behavior. He was becoming increasingly withdrawn from the other children and, at times, became oppositional about "clean-up" duties for which each child was responsible.

Rachel's concern grew, and she sent Mikey for a medical evaluation to rule out any serious injuries, nutritional deficiencies, and other health problems. Although she had yet to detect any indicators that Mikey had been sexually abused, she asked the physician to include those considerations in her examination. Discussion with Janet revealed that, while Bret did have "sexually explicit materials around and did look at porn movies," none of them had anything to do with children, and she didn't think that he exposed Mikey to it. As Janet put it, "He may be a jerk, but he's not a pervert." Nevertheless, the social worker kept the possibility of sexual abuse in mind as she planned a more in-depth assessment.

Since the social worker became involved and Janet had to go to court for driving under the influence and drug possession, Bret left town and had not been seen for over a week. The police indicated that a warrant had been issued for his arrest on suspicion of child abuse and drug possession. The social worker accompanied Janet to court, and the judge put her on probation for one year with the stipulation that she cooperate with child welfare services and obtain treatment for her drug abuse. Since her arrest for driving under the influence was her first such offense, she was fined and told to attend mandatory substance-abuse classes as well. Rachel was told that reports on Janet's progress would be expected periodically over the course of the next ninety days to determine whether Janet would regain custody of Mikey. Kara agreed to take her nephew for that time, and Janet could have visits if accompanied by the social worker.

Multidimensional/Functional Assessment: Defining Problems and Goals

Rachel was employed in a small rural agency that delivered most child-welfare services to clients. Over the next couple of weeks, Rachel spent a few hours further assessing the situation by conducting interviews and making observations in Janet's home. She was also able to interview Mikey in private in Kara's home, observe his behavior in Janet's presence, and assess Janet's parenting skills. In addition, Rachel, who was well known in the community and had good collegial relations with other professionals, readily communicated with Mikey's teacher, physician, the court, and law enforcement to continue the assessment and evaluation of the case.

In addition to her substance-abuse problems, Janet had a range of other troubles: her conflicted and sometimes violent relationship with Bret, her family history of emotional neglect, having witnessed domestic violence between her parents, poor parenting skills, and financial problems. She was also considerably depressed. She did, however, appear to genuinely love her son, was remorseful about her neglect of him, and felt very guilty about the abuse he had received at the hands of Bret. She also felt somewhat complicit in that she had gone along with Bret's "old-school discipline," as he called it. She regretted ever having let him punch Mikey on the arms and legs. (Bret was careful not to hit Mikey in the face so as to not leave any obvious bruises or wounds.) Janet also seemed to have few social supports. She had drifted away from her sister over the years; her sister was "the perfect one" with a comfortable home, three children, and a stable marriage.

A combination of assessment strategies was employed: observation of Mikey at home alone and with his mom, "play assessment" (drawing and playing with action figures and other toys), and discussions with Janet and with Mikey's teacher. Rachel determined that Mikey was somewhat depressed, anxious, withdrawn, had some difficulties getting along with his peers in kindergarten, and demonstrated occasional outbursts in school, especially when asked to carry out a required task. He also wet his bed at night, which had been a source of provocation for Bret. Sometimes he went to school smelling of urine ("to teach him a lesson," reasoned Bret), and because of his occasional dirty appearance and difficulty relating to the other kids, they shunned him and made fun of him. Mikey was lonely much of the time, and didn't know where he fit in with the other kids. The medical tests came back negative, and further examination of additional traumas including sexual abuse turned up no substantive data. (Child trauma checklists were used as a guide to consider other forms of abuse.) He did see Janet and "stupid Bret" arguing vehemently sometimes, and "Bret hit mommy too . . . I wish I could beat Bret up."

Janet began receiving substance-abuse treatment at the local mental health center and attending her classes, which were held there as well. She had not shown signs of withdrawal, and her heavier drug use was a relatively recent development. She did not think she was going to have a hard time "giving it up . . . I'll do anything to get Mikey back," but did confess to missing Bret. She knew, however, that if he came back there would be trouble again. The social worker strongly encouraged Janet to continue with her treatment for substance abuse, and obey the court mandate "to the letter" if she wanted to get Mikey back. Rachel was clear about her role as both therapist and court liaison, stressing that if Janet wanted to get Mikey back, she was going to have to work hard not to relapse, eliminate any use of corporal punishment, and take better care of his emotional and physical needs. Janet said she understood what was expected, and thanked Rachel for "being straight with me."

A functional analysis of Janet's situation revealed that, even without the influence of Bret, her parenting skills could use considerable improvement. Part of the difficulty seemed to stem from the poor model provided by Janet's parents, "although I can't blame them completely since, I admit, little-miss-perfect [her sister, Kara] is a pretty good mom. I just become so frustrated at times. I never feel like I have enough time to do anything with him, and I lose my temper and start yelling. Then he cries and I feel bad about losing my cool." On one of the supervised visits, Kara dropped Mikey off with Janet and the social worker, and Janet was instructed to play a game that Mikey liked. She then helped Mikey clean his room. After that, they made lunch together. As Janet engaged in these activities with Mikey, Rachel made herself relatively unobtrusive (catching up on progress notes at the kitchen table), but she could observe the impatience in Janet's face during her playtime with Mikey, trying to orchestrate his every move rather than hanging back and just "being there" with him, as Rachel put it. Later, when Janet went to coach Mikey in cleaning up his room, she demonstrated a similar lack of patience. Although things remained relatively calm, Janet admitted when questioned that if the social worker hadn't been there, these situations would have turned into yelling matches. If Bret were around, then the hitting would start. A concise functional analysis revealed serious difficulty in Janet's ability to provide a calm, nurturing, and fun environment for Mikey even for a brief period of playtime. She showed an abrupt impatience when it came time for tasks or setting limits. These situations had become a daily event, would quickly escalate into a reciprocal negative exchange (with yelling and hitting becoming somewhat serious). Janet's reactions would upset Mikey and reinforce Janet's sense of incompetence as a parent.

After a couple of weeks and several hours of assessment, Rachel discussed their time together so far, and with Janet's input, summarized the problems and goals: Janet loved her son but had problems of her own, including substance abuse, depression and low self-confidence, a short temper, and proneness to involve herself in psychologically and (sometimes) abusive relationships. Her parenting skills needed considerable improvement, and she was under much stress financially, which contributed to her "feeling stuck." Janet felt that, first, she had to get off drugs and alcohol. To earn her son back, she would have to demonstrate that she could provide better nurturance and positive discipline for Mikey. She also agreed that in the long run, she probably needed to upgrade her criteria for selection of romantic partners.

Selecting and Designing the Intervention: Defining Strategies and Objectives

The overall service plan included a multifaceted approach in the tradition of an ecobehavioral framework, but with specific attention paid to integrating evidence-based interventions within this framework (table 14.1). Components of the plan included development of a solid relationship with Rachel, who was clear about her combined role of clinician, advocate, and liaison to the court; teaching behavioral parenting skills; contingency management contracting with the courts; case management with court, school, medical, and substance-abuse services; and improving social supports.

Parenting skills intervention included psychoeducation to provide Janet with developmental information regarding normative expectations for Mikey, and to instruct Janet in better child nurturance and limit setting. Rachel also provided her with brief cognitive therapy to help her understand and cope better with negative feelings associated with her own abuse as a child. Janet and Rachel spent considerable time engaging Mikey in play and in task-oriented activities to teach Janet how to put Mikey at ease, make him feel loved, and "invest in good feelings between them," so that getting him to obey the rules (e.g., clean-up, keeping his bedtime) would go more smoothly and be less of a source of anger and conflict. Specific objectives were to successfully spend ten, twenty and eventually thirty minutes of play-time a day with Mikey, and to deliver calm, clear directives for accomplishing his daily tasks. Rachal and Janet developed a chart to track his progress every day. If he did well, he received a five-minute bedtime story with a "special present" at the end of the week if he did a "very good" job (met expectations for four out of five days). Although the groundwork for improving parenting skills was done during visits with Mikey at her sister's home, Janet did not fully practice and carry out all the components of the plan successfully until Mikey returned to Janet's home. During this time she reconciled somewhat with Kara, and was able to implement some of the bedtime rituals at Kara's house.

Rachel also taught Janet some basic stress management (brief meditation and imagery) to use when she felt "like I'm going to lose it." She practiced three times a day, and used imagery of being with Mikey when he returned home, images associated with remaining calm during playtime, helping him cooperate with her around the house, or getting him ready for bed. After Mikey returned home, she was able to keep a chart of stressful situations when caring for Mikey, what her actions were, what the outcomes were (of both her behavior and Mikey's), and how she evaluated her performance afterward. Her goal was to keep her verbal outbursts to a minimum and to reduce any pushing, pulling, or hitting to "zero." After Mikey returned and Janet had more opportunity to practice her new skills, she worked on the finer points: giving praise when Mikey did well (stressing the power and superiority of positive reinforcement over punishment), ignoring little annoying things, and taking time out for activities she enjoyed (all this with her sobriety in mind). Rachel also stressed the importance of maintaining a reasonably neat home and paying attention to Mikey's hygiene, clean clothing, and appearance. Rachel helped Janet design a simple time-management chart to complete basic household chores in a timely manner. Communication between Janet and Mikey's teacher was designed to get feedback about Mikey's behavior in school and in the after-school program.

Rachel examined the potential for additional income supports and discovered that Mikey was eligible for health-care coverage at no cost with a state-sponsored health clinic. Nevertheless, she was going to continue to struggle to get by unless she increased her income. Rachel and Janet discussed making some adjustments and budgeting decisions. Now that Mikey was in school full time (including the after-school program), Janet decided to work full time and give up working evenings. She also found a more affordable apartment and decided to move ("and I am not telling Bret where I'm going"). Consultation with Mikey's teacher revealed that there were two bachelor-level volunteers (teachers in training) in the after-school program who were willing to work with Mikey on alternate days to help him with his social and behavioral problems (shyness, oppositional behavior). The social worker discussed a plan with them to help

Mikey initiate cooperative play with one or two other children with whom he wanted to make friends, and record (monitor and evaluate) their efforts. They would also record how Mikey obeyed the rules of the after-school program.

After the sixty-day period, Janet and the social worker returned to court to give a generally positive report to the judge regarding some of the adjustments she had made. There appeared to be no further instances of substance abuse, she was no longer consorting with drug users in her personal life, and she felt she was ready to take her son home. Although Janet felt some lessening of anger toward her sister, she needed to make some new friends. New prospects included some of the other single mothers she was meeting at the after-school program and women whom she met in the single-mothers support group she occasionally attended at the mental health center. The court mandated that her case remain open for the remainder of the year, and Rachel was required to file quarterly reports. Custody of Mikey would remain contingent on Janet's continued progress.

Selecting Scales and Creating Indexes to Monitor and Evaluate Client Progress

The PTSD-RI was employed to screen Mikey for traumatic events and symptoms and the SAC to measure internalizing and externalizing symptoms at the start of the intervention and at three-month intervals (table 14.1). In addition, a number of idiographic monitoring indexes and charts were employed to gauge Mikey's progress at home and in the after-school program, to help Janet improve her time-management skills, and to engage in self-monitoring to complete household chores in a timely fashion.

TABLE 14.1 The client service plan for Janet and Mikey

Problems	Goals	Sample Objectives	Interventions	Assessment Tools
Mikey Bruises up and down his arms	*Mikey* Eliminate all forms of neglect and abuse; restore custody when situation is resolved	Paraprofessionals: model and coach Mikey to offer some specific help to another child with whom he wanted to "be friends"	Child welfare placed child with sister for 60 days; court-ordered interventions for Janet Coach paraprofessional students to help Mikey improve his social skills through gradual exposure Use prompts and rewards to help reduce oppositional behavior directed toward teacher	*Mikey* PTSD-RI to screen for traumatic events and related symptoms SAC to assess for both internalizing and externalizing symptoms and problems Behavioral observation to test his social skills in school Design and implement a monitoring chart for his suc-
Signs of depression and anxiety at home and in school; oppositional (angry) at times in school	Alleviate depression and excess anxiety, improve his ability to socialize with other kids	Social worker: instruct sister how to use the "bell and pad" method (available commercially), and Kara would pay for it and implement it with Mikey; praise		
Bedwetting once or twice a week	Eliminate his enuresis			

Problems	Goals	Sample Objectives	Interventions	Assessment Tools
Janet Abuse of alcohol, marijuana and, on occasion, cocaine	*Janet* Abstain from marijuana and cocaine use (one stipulation for regaining custody); strongly encouraged to abstain or, at least, minimize alcohol use	him for dry days, and provide encouragement for "mishaps" (Initially, during visits when Janet, Mikey, and the social worker were present at home): Play board game for 10 minutes (even if "bored"), and gradually increase to 30 minutes; plan one directive to give to Mikey (e.g., clean up plate after lunch) during visits and follow up with either praise or one calm reminder; begin using chart to record his successes	Use "bell and pad" home kit; work with sister to use the device and reward Mikey for successful "dry" mornings Janet to attend mandatory mental health/substance-abuse treatment at CMHC Cognitive therapy to address depression and examine abuse experiences and beliefs, expectancies these experiences created regarding current relationships; educational women's support at same clinic Behavioral parenting-skills program carried out at home by social worker during visits and continued after custody restored; stress-management skills included Free budgeting counseling; full-time job Case management: referrals, networking, advocacy and coordinating services through contacts with court, schools, health care, and mental health center; court liaison to ensure compliance with contingency management plan and periodically report results of treatment to court	cesses in responding to mother's directives Paraprofessionals chart his social skills and positive responses to classroom directives *Janet* Self-monitor completion of domestic duties, including physical care of Mikey's hygiene and appearance
Signs of depression	Further assess depression and treat pharmacologically if needed			
History of being abused in her family, in other relationships, and occasionally pushed, hit by Bret	Help her better understand effects of abuse history, current repetition, and seek alternative type of relationship			
Serious deficits in parenting skills, both nurturing and positive disciplining skills	Improve her parenting skills and eliminate need to use coercive methods			
Financial problems commensurate with being "working poor"	Long-term, reduce expenditures and improve her working situation (i.e., work full-time)			

SUMMARY

The physical and sexual abuse of children along with the neglect of their physical, psychological, and emotional needs remains a prevalent problem. Multiple factors contribute to the likelihood of child abuse and neglect. Qualitative and quantitative methods are available that could improve both risk assessment and clinical assessment of abuse and neglect in child protective services and in clinical practice with children and adolescents who have been abused and neglected. Broad-based ecobehavioral interventions have been shown to be promising, but are more likely to be effective over time if they include behavioral parenting skills; integrated substance-abuse, mental health, and foster-care services; and consistent follow-up with contingency management programs linked with the criminal justice system. Even with improvements in child welfare assessment, intervention, and evaluation methods, however, improving child welfare policy will require much greater national commitment to protect children and adolescents from abuse and neglect.

CHAPTER 15

EATING DISORDERS IN ADOLESCENTS AND YOUNG ADULTS

Eating disorders, generally categorized as anorexia, bulimia, and binge-eating disorder, constitute a continuum marked by cognitive, behavioral, and physiological symptoms, including preoccupation with body image, problems with appetite, and dietary regulation. A range of other problems often co-occur with eating disorders. The seriousness of eating disorders can range from mild and transitory to severe and chronic. A significant proportion of people with primary anorexia are likely to die from the disorder, even with aggressive medical care. However, most people struggling with an eating disorder are very likely to recover substantially, regain the ability to regulate dietary practices, and improve overall self-image and interpersonal adjustment. A range of well-developed assessment protocols and evidence-based practices for eating disorders include cognitive-behavioral interventions and interpersonal psychotherapy. In recent years, it has been recognized that early intervention with adolescents and young adults may effectively interrupt the onset of an eating disorder.

ASSESSMENT

Background Data

The literature amply describes the characteristics of eating disorders (*DSM-IV-TR*; Fairburn & Wilson, 1993; Foreyt & Mikhail, 1997; Shekter-Wolfson et al., 1997; Fairburn, Cooper, Doll, Norman, & O'Connor, 2000). Three categories of eating disorders have emerged in the empirical literature: anorexia nervosa, bulimia nervosa, and binge-eating disorder.

Anorexia Nervosa.   People diagnosed with anorexia have a morbid preoccupation with staying extremely thin, refuse to gain weight (remaining below the eighty-fifth percentile for their weight class), and demonstrate a serious cognitive disturbance in the way they see their own body shape and size, with a particular fear of becoming "fat" (G.T. Wilson & Fairburn, 1998; *DSM-IV-TR*). If the onset of anorexia precedes puberty, a young woman may not achieve menarche.

489

Should the onset follow puberty, the female may develop amenorrhea. Often these clients do not see their preoccupation with ultrathinness as a problem. The *DSM* provides two subtypes of anorexia nervosa: "restricting type," which is characterized by an almost exclusive emphasis on dieting, fasting, or excessive exercise, and a binge-eating/purging type, where the client binges and then purges through self-induced vomiting, laxatives, diuretics, or enemas. Most people with anorexia who binge eat also purge, although there are some who purge without bingeing. People with anorexia are often clinically depressed, and many show signs of OCD. They often suffer from poor self-esteem, appear to be emotionally restricted, are often preoccupied with a need to control their environment, and can be somewhat inflexible in their thinking and adherence to perfectionist standards. Anorexia can result in a long list of medical problems, many of which can be detected in laboratory workups (e.g., electrolyte abnormalities). In addition, clinical problems may include constipation, emaciation, dry skin, hypotension, cardiovascular problems (e.g., arrhythmias), and osteoporosis. The onset of anorexia usually begins between fourteen and eighteen years of age, and may require hospitalization at some point. Even with aggressive medical intervention, the mortality rate for people with anorexia is over 10%. One ten-year prospective study of thirty-nine adolescents with anorexia showed a 69% remission rate over ten years (including all seven males in the sample), and many continued to have other psychiatric difficulties, including depression, anxiety, and substance-abuse disorders (Herpertz-Dahlmann et al., 2001). Although anorexia appears to be a clinical syndrome in predominantly industrialized countries where thinness is prized as a sign of beauty, people from other cultures who assimilate and acculturate to these ideals may also become anorectic.

Bulimia Nervosa.   Bulimia nervosa is characterized by binge eating and compensatory methods to avoid weight gain (e.g., self-induced vomiting, laxatives, enemas) (*DSM-IV-TR*; G. T. Wilson & Fairburn, 1998; Foreyt & Mikhail, 1997). A binge is eating a greater than normal amount of food within a discrete period of time (less than two hours), often with an emphasis on high-carbohydrate, high-caloric foods (e.g., one dozen donuts or a whole layer cake). Usually people with binge-eating disorder are ashamed of their behavior in this regard, and bingeing often takes place in secret. Often the binge-eating episode is precipitated by emotional upset, dysphoric mood, or interpersonal conflict. Binge eating is typically accompanied by a feeling of loss of personal control. Vomiting is employed by 80–90% of binge eaters as a way of avoiding weight gain. They are also preoccupied with body shape and weight. Their appearance plays a disproportionate role in self-evaluation.

There are subtypes of bulimia: in the purging type, in which the person regularly engages in vomiting or other compensatory behaviors, and in the nonpurging type, the person attempts to compensate for bingeing through excessive exercise or fasting, but does not regularly engage in vomiting, use laxatives, or apply other methods to eliminate what they consume. Those with bulimia tend to be within their normal weight range (more or less), and may experience other problems such as depression, poor self-image, social-anxiety disorder, and other anxiety problems. People with bulimia appear to be disproportionately more likely to have a substance-abuse problem, and stimulants are often employed in appetite suppression. Medical examination and laboratory findings are likely to detect other problems such as electrolyte abnormalities, loss of enamel on teeth (gastric fluids eat away tooth enamel as a consequence of vomiting), and menstrual irregularities. Bulimia tends to begin in late adolescence or early adulthood, and may have a variable course over time. If symptoms remit for one year, long-term outcomes are quite positive. Although some practitioners see similarities in excessive drinking and eating disorders as addictive processes, there are significant differences in etiology, psychophysiological, and behavioral mechanisms (G. T. Wilson, 1993b), not the least of which is the absence of any classic dependence syndrome (tolerance and withdrawal).

Binge Eating Disorder.   Binge-eating disorder is similar to bulimia. In binge-eating disorder, however, the person does not engage in compensatory behaviors on a regular basis (*DSM-IV-TR*; G. T. Wilson, 1993; G. T. Wilson & Fairburn, 1998). Binge-eating disorder is more likely to be associated with people who are overweight or obese. Many of the clinical samples for this disorder are drawn from weight-control clinics. As with bulimia, binge-eating episodes are often precipitated by depression, upsetting events, interpersonal conflict, or feelings of tension that are relieved by bingeing. Often a weight problem is associated with poor self-image, low self-esteem, depression, anxiety, and dissatisfaction with work or relationships. There is also a disproportionate risk for personality disorder or substance-abuse diagnoses. The problem appears to begin in late adolescence or early adulthood. Long-term prognosis for binge-eating disorder appears to be better than that for bulimia. In the first prospective study to compare long-term (five-year) outcomes of these two disorders, about half of those with bulimia retained an eating-disorder diagnosis, whereas only about one-fifth of the binge-eating group did so (Fairburn et al., 2000). Binge eating is an important health risk to focus on with young people, because it is the core component of both bulimia nervosa and binge-eating disorder, and may also be related to a subtype of anorexia nervosa.

Epidemiological Data for Eating Disorders

Community studies have revealed prevalence estimates for anorexia nervosa at about 1%, bulimia nervosa at 1–3%, and binge-eating disorders at 2–5% (Johnson, Tsoh, & Varnado, 1996). The vast majority of people suffering from eating disorders (90% or more in the United States) are female. However, the rates of subclinical symptoms that include extreme dietary restrictions, binge eating, and purging behaviors have been estimated at 15–40% (W. G. Johnson et al.), and unhealthy dietary practices have been estimated to be as high as almost 80% of young people (Fairburn & Beglin, 1990). Early symptoms of eating disorders appear to have significant prognostic value. In a longitudinal study of 800 children and their mothers in the community, data on risk factors and symptoms associated with eating disorders were collected over four time periods between the mid-1970s and early 1990s. Symptoms in early adolescence are strongly predictive of the development of bulimia nervosa in later adolescence and adulthood. Bulimia in late adolescence is even more predictive of adult bulimia. Early-childhood conflicts around eating and mealtime appeared to have prognostic value for the development of later eating disorders (Kotler, Cohen, Davies, Pine, & Walsh, 2001). Young women in college may have comparable rates of eating-disorder attitudes and other symptoms as they did in senior year of high school, as shown in one prospective study, but there may be an increase in dissatisfaction with body shape and size (Vohs, Heatherton, & Herrin, 2001).

These behaviors co-occur with a range of other psychosocial problems, including depression, anxiety disorders, substance abuse, OCD, personality disorders, PTSD, and interpersonal problems. In addition, the behavioral consequences of eating disorders disrupt work and school functioning (Kashubeck-West & Mintz, 2001; Pratt, Phillips, Greydanus, & Patel, 2003; O'Brien & Vincent, 2003). Although depression and anxiety appear prominent in both binge and nonbinge disorders, substance abuse and BPD seem to be more prominent in binge disorders. Despite the correlations between eating disorders and these other conditions, causal explanations remain a subject of speculation.

Theories

Evidence suggests that eating disorders are the result of a number of interacting biopsychosocial factors (Striegel-Moore, 1993; Foreyt & Mikhail, 1997; Striegel-Moore & Cachelin, 2001). Developmental trajectories of these disorders can be highly variable for individuals, and these factors may combine cumulatively to provide a dose-response relationship with eating disorders. Identified risk factors include genetics and other biological predispositions, gender, race, early maturation for women, high body-mass index, body size and shape, excessive dieting, and family problems, as well as childhood sexual abuse for bulimia (Pratt et al., 2003). Family and twin studies demonstrate that eating disorders run in families where a first-degree relative had an eating disorder (potentially supporting both social-learning and genetic theories). Other biological evidence suggests that eating disorders are also correlated with hormonal changes during puberty, depression (as a result of genetic transmission), and metabolic dysfunction in the individual. Case-controlled studies, which match people with and without an eating disorder on several variables such as age and gender, also suggest that personal risk factors (e.g., low self-esteem) are also somewhat predictive. Developmentally, binge-eating behaviors emerge during late adolescence, perhaps motivated by dissatisfaction with body image and shape. Some feminist theorists have asserted that these factors are linked to the negative stress women bear regarding gender-role expectations, idealized images of feminine beauty, and social acceptance. Extreme dieting, binge eating, and purging may be attempts to ensure acceptability and to affirm identity. These difficulties may emerge in adolescence due to the cascading and interacting effects of biological changes, social stressors, struggles with self-esteem and identity development, conflicts with parents, and perfectionist demands to cope with academic performance and the drive toward independence.

Psychodynamic theorists have hypothesized that eating disorders are an expression of unresolved unconscious childhood conflicts and, as such, are a defense against oral impregnation by the father, overidentifying with a negative maternal introject, or the result of unresolved dependency needs, among other explanations. There currently is no scientific evidence that supports these hypotheses. Sociocultural-based psychodynamic formulations have examined the different developmental roles expected of adolescent females versus males, to account for the onset of eating disorders as a compensatory effort to achieve an idealized norm of female beauty in a defense against rejection (Slater, Guthrie, & Boyd, 2001). However, this formulation is not uniquely psychodynamic in origin.

Cognitive theories have gained prominence in the theoretical and empirical literature regarding the cause and maintenance of eating disorders (e.g., Fairburn, 1997). Cognitive distortions regarding body shape and weight, chronic negative self-evaluation, and poor self-esteem seem to dominate the thought processes of people with eating disorders. These distortions are directly related to false beliefs about the value of highly restrictive diets, the "goodness" or "badness" of certain foods, and the assumed benefits of purging after eating as a form of weight control. Negative schemata and dysfunctional thinking may extend to other aspects of life, including beliefs about interpersonal relations. The false beliefs among those with eating disorders regarding dieting can be seen as a generalized manifestation of two dysfunctional forms of cognitive processing: dichotomous thinking and perfectionism. When clients with an eating disorder view their eating patterns in such rigid terms, these rules become fragile and easily broken, thus reinforcing the cycle of dietary restrictiveness and binge-purging. These lapses in keeping to the rules are often precipitated by periods of emotional stress associated with a conflict situation, such as a fight with boyfriend. Positive and negative reinforcing behaviors meant to accommodate these beliefs (binge eating to cope with stress or feelings of inadequacy, purging to cope with fears of weight gain) help maintain the dysfunctional cognitions.

Racial and cultural factors in research on eating disorders have gained more attention in recent years, given that eating disorders are more prevalent among white women (Pratt et al., 2003). Race is most often used for classification, rather than cultural and ethnic groupings that may have more salience. Cultural beliefs may be related to negative cognitive schemata about body image, and research on cultural influences may have implications for the etiology of the disorder. Observing that eating disorders are among the most common problems for college women, Arriaza and Mann (2001) compared samples of young white, Hispanic, and Asian university women and found that, while all groups have concerns about their body shape and overall appearance, white women engaged in more dietary restrictive behaviors commensurate with eating disorders. In the first community comparison between a recruited sample of African-American and white women (mean age thirty-one) with binge-eating disorder, Pike, Dohm, Striegel-Moore, Wilfley, and Fairburn (2001) used matched samples of black and white women with and without an eating disorder to demonstrate that white women were more likely to demonstrate more frequent binge eating, dietary restrictiveness, and concerns about weight, body shape, and eating. The authors surmised that, as a result of less concern in these areas, black women are at lower risk for developing bulimia nervosa. Black women, were more likely to be overweight, however, and less likely to seek treatment for obesity, thus putting them at greater risk for other health problems. In the first college-based study to examine diagnostic rates of eating disorders in a representative sample of African-American young women, Mulholland and Mintz (2001) found rates of anorexia (1%) and bulimia (1%) and symptoms of eating disorders (23%) to be comparable to estimates in the literature on white college women. Mixed findings on race may be explained, in part, by the use of different diagnostic criteria or inclusion of subclinical symptoms (Kashubeck-West & Mintz, 2001).

Key Elements of Multidimensional/ Functional Assessment

The diagnostic criteria (*DSM-IV-TR*) for anorexia nervosa and bulimia nervosa are described above. Binge-eating disorder is described provisionally in *DSM-IV-TR*. In addition to the criteria for eating large amounts of food within a discrete period of time and a sense of lack of control over eating during the episode, the diagnosis includes three or more of the following: eating much more rapidly than normal, eating until uncomfortably full, eating large amounts when not physically feeling hungry, eating alone because of embarrassment about one's eating behavior, and feeling disgusted at oneself, guilty, or depressed. The person meeting this provisional diagnosis has engaged in binge eating at least twice weekly for six months.

Foreyt and Mikhail (1997) suggest that people with binge-eating disorder may be somewhat secretive and embarrassed about discussing their problem, may be somewhat reluctant to cooperate with the assessment or preliminary recommendations, and can be somewhat oppositional and rebellious about treatment in general. Medical assessment is essential to avoid problems, including dental enamel erosion, electrolyte depletion (possibly related to cardiac arrhythmia or kidney disorder), gastrointestinal disturbances, and menstrual irregularities. Clients' weight history should be examined carefully, and some estimate made of what clients' notion of their "ideal" weight should be (relative to an estimate of the ideal weight for their age and body type). Clients' and their family's beliefs about nutrition and dieting should be explored. Additional questions regarding dieting include duration of dieting behaviors, when the dieting began, with whose encouragement, and for what reason. The extent and function of weighing and exercise behaviors are also of interest, for they can often become ritualistic and self-defeating (Foreyt & Mikhail). Assessment should, at a minimum, capture the following data: weight history (highest, lowest, ideal), bingeing (types of food, triggers, patterns), weight-control methods, overall eating patterns (caloric intake, weighing practices), menstrual history, co-occurring problems, previous treatments, childhood abuse or neglect, and a physical exam (U. Schmidt, 1998; Fairburn & Wilson, 1993).

Self-monitoring is an indispensable and reasonably accurate tool, and should be employed to enhance assessment, provide ongoing monitoring of treatment progress, and evaluate treatment outcomes. In order to obtain a reliable and valid self-report, however, the client should be actively encouraged to learn and use self-monitoring techniques, not passively expected to do it spontaneously (G. T. Wilson, 1993b). Self-monitoring is usually conducted with a chart that can be tailored to the needs and expectations of the client. As part of a comprehensive and ongoing assessment, self-monitoring of binge-eating episodes can create an accurate data trail that describes days of the week, the time of day, the situation (where, with whom), state of mind and emotional distress of the client (e.g., response to a negative event), substance use, the type and amount of food consumed, response to the binge (e.g., client purged or refrained), and so forth. Monitoring begins as part of the initial assessment, and continues throughout treatment. Self-monitoring may also add to the client's sense of participation and control as a collaborative participant in treatment. Benefits to the intervention for binge eating often occur quickly in treatment, and some of these benefits appear to be associated with clients' self-monitoring activities, which they can use to track and make cause-effect connections between antecedent situational, cognitive, or emotional events and bingeing. When applied skillfully within the context of a sound working alliance, self-monitoring can provide an invaluable adjunct to the assessment, monitoring, and evaluation of treatment with clients who are struggling with binge eating (G. T. Wilson & Vitousek, 1999). Foreyt and Mikhail (1997) offer a version of a commonly used daily chart to help the client participate in the assessment and self-monitoring process (figure 15.1).

Self-monitoring provides a framework for functional analysis of the binge-purging pattern. The functional analysis informs the intervention plan by defining a chain reaction of interacting cognitive, behavioral, physiological, and situational factors. Accordingly, the client's anxieties about body shape and weight may trigger dieting behavior, then bingeing, then purging to compensate for overeating (U. Schmidt, 1998; Fairburn & Wilson, 1993). Treatment targets both the cognitive and behavioral aspects of the disorder directly. First, practitioners in collaboration with the client must make a detailed analysis over the course of a week or two of events that appear to precipitate the binge-purging episode. These may include troubling thoughts, feelings, behaviors, or situations that cause distress or emotional upset that precipitate the binge. A client may simply be feeling generally stressed or may have had a fight with a friend, been rejected

FIGURE 15.1   Daily chart for self-monitoring eating patterns

Time of day	Place	With whom	Associated activities	Foods/liquors (include amounts)	Feelings before, during, and after eating	Purge yes/no: if yes, how? (vomiting, laxatives, diuretics, etc.)	Feelings before, during, and after purge

by a boyfriend, been turned down for a job, or failed an exam. Second, a detailed analysis should be conducted on the thoughts associated with the decision to binge-purge, the type of food, and the amount of food. Third, any consequences that ensue after the binge-purging episode should be recorded and reviewed as well. These might include feelings after binge-purging, substance abuse, suicidal thoughts, use of laxatives, or other reactions to the episode.

Instruments

The Eating Disorder Examination (EDE; Z. Cooper & Fairburn, 1987; D. E. Smith, Marcus, & Eldredge, 1994; G. T. Wilson, 1993a; Grilo, Masheb, & Wilson, 2001) is considered by most experts in the field to be the gold standard for assessment of binge eating and other eating disorders. The EDE is a semi-structured interview schedule that examines signs and symptoms of eating disorders retrospectively over the course of twenty-eight days, and includes time frames commensurate with *DSM* categories in order to provide diagnostic data for clinical and research purposes. For binge-eating disorder, the criteria have been adapted to *DSM-IV-TR* six-month criteria as well (Grilo et al.). The EDE divides overeating into several categories, including objective bulimic episodes (ingestion of large quantities of food with a subjective loss of control), subjective bulimic episodes (eating quantities of food that are generally not considered extreme, but the client reports feelings of losing control), and objective overeating episodes (overeating without a subjective sense of losing control). The EDE comprises four subscales: dietary restraint, eating concern, weight concern, and shape concern. Items are rated 0–6 with higher scores indicating greater severity or frequency.

The EDE-Q (Fairburn & Beglin, 1994) is the self-report version of the EDE. Both scales have excellent psychometric properties—good internal consistency of subscales, good interrater reliability, and discriminant validity for diagnosing those with eating disorders. In a study using both community and patient samples, the self-report EDE-Q compared well with the EDE structured interview (Grilo et al., 2001). Agreement was very good on the more unambiguous behaviors of self-induced vomiting and laxative use, and "close agreement" on dietary restraint. There was more disagreement on "concerns about weight," although not clinically substantive, however, and even more disagreement on concerns about shape. Overall, the EDE-Q provides a sound basis for conducting an initial screening commensurate with a provisional diagnosis.

In addition to the EDE, Kashubeck-West, Mintz, and Saunders (2001) reviewed a number of scales with solid psychometric properties, including the Eating Disorder Inventory (Garner, Olmsted, & Policy, 1983) and the Bulimia Test–Revised (BULIT-R; Thelen, Farmer, Wonderlich, & Smith, 1991; Welch, Thompson, & Hall, 1993), perhaps one of the better-known scales. The Yale-Brown-Cornell Eating Disorder Scale (YBCEDS; Mazure, Halmi, Sunday, Romano, & Einhorn, et al., 1994) was designed to identify and measure a client's unique eating-disorder symptoms, using eight core items. The scale also contains six items that measure motivation for change. The scale has shown good reliability and concurrent validity with other eating-disorder scales (Mazure et al.), and effectively distinguishes normal controls from restrained eating dieters (those with preoccupations about controlling food intake, but who generally do not meet *DSM* criteria for an eating disorder) and those who have recovered from eating disorders (Sunday & Halmi, 2000).

A recent addition to the collection of eating-disorder scales is the Eating Disorder Diagnostic Scale (EDDS), reprinted here (instrument 15.1). Scores on the EDDS can be used to diagnose anorexia, bulimia, and binge-eating disorder, and the scale provides a composite score that is useful for measuring overall symptoms and detecting changes in symptoms over time. If the scale is primarily used to measure overall symptom level and to monitor changes during intervention, however, the composite total score should be used. This global symptoms measure is calculated by simply summing all items (except height, weight, and birth control). Yes is equal to 1, and no is equal to 0.

The EDDS was initially developed in two consecutive studies (Stice, Telch, & Rizvi, 2000). In the first study, items derived from the EDE, the *DSM*, and the structured interview version of the *DSM* were compiled and examined by twenty-six experts on eating disorders. The scale was then piloted with a combined group of college and high school students and clients in an eating-disorders clinic. The second study examined reliability and validity with a combined community and clinic sample of 367 females. Internal consistency reliability for the composite scale was .91 for the full sample. Overall accuracy rates for test-retest reliabilities exceeded 90%, and test-retest reliability for the composite score was very good (.87). Criterion validity was supported with data showing the EDDS diagnoses to be congruent over 90% of the time with diagnoses based on interviews. Correlations among the EDDS composite scores and subscales of the EDE and the YBCEDS were moderate and significant.

Four studies reported simultaneously (Stice, Fisher, & Martinez, 2004) further supported the reliability and validity of the EDDS, including its predictive validity and sensitivity to change. Study 1 essentially replicated Stice et al. (2000) with over 700 adolescent females who were somewhat younger than those in the original study. Study 2 demonstrated that the EDDS was sensitive to change with undergraduate women enrolled in an eating-disorders prevention course. Study 3 demonstrated that the EDDS was sensitive to clinical change resulting from an intervention with 181 adolescent females with concerns about body image. Study 4 demonstrated that the EDDS predicted increased risk for the onset of binge eating and compensatory behaviors and the onset of depression. In sum, the EDDS shows excellent reliability, construct, and criterion validity; is sensitive to clinical change; and has a high degree of utility in that it can be completed within the parameters of a typical interview with people suffering from a range of eating-disorder symptoms.

INSTRUMENT 15.1   Eating Disorder Diagnostic Scale (EDDS)

Please carefully complete all questions.

Over the past 3 months . . .	Not at all	Slightly		Moderately		Extremely	
1. Have you felt fat?	0	1	2	3	4	5	6
2. Have you had a definite fear that you might gain weight or become fat?	0	1	2	3	4	5	6
3. Has your weight influenced how you think about (judge) yourself as a person?	0	1	2	3	4	5	6
4. Has your shape influenced how you think about (judge) yourself as a person?	0	1	2	3	4	5	6

5. During the past 6 months have there been times when you felt you have eaten what other people would regard as an unusually large amount of food (e.g., a quart of ice cream) given the circumstances?   Yes   No

6. During the times when you ate an unusually large amount of food, did you experience a loss of control (feel you couldn't stop eating or control what or how much you were eating)?   Yes   No

7. How many DAYS per week on average over the past 6 MONTHS have you eaten an unusually large amount of food and experienced a loss of control?   0 1 2 3 4 5 6 7

8. How many TIMES per week on average over the past 3 MONTHS have you eaten an unusually large amount of food and experienced a loss of control?   0 1 2 3 4 5 6 7 8 9 10 11 12 13 14

During these episodes of overeating and loss of control did you . . .

9. Eat much more rapidly than normal?   Yes   No

10. Eat until you felt uncomfortably full?   Yes   No

11. Eat large amounts of food when you didn't feel
    physically hungry?   Yes   No

12. Eat alone because you were embarrassed by how much
    you were eating?   Yes   No

13. Feel disgusted with yourself, depressed, or very guilty
    after overeating?   Yes   No

14. Feel very upset about your uncontrollable overeating
    or resulting weight gain?   Yes   No

15. How many times per week on average over
    the past 3 months have you made yourself
    vomit to prevent weight gain or counteract
    the effect of eating?   0 1 2 3 4 5 6 7 8 9 10 11 12 13 14

16. How many times per week on average over
    the past 3 months have you used laxatives
    or diuretics to prevent weight gain or
    counteract the effects of eating?   0 1 2 3 4 5 6 7 8 9 10 11 12 13 14

17. How many times per week on average over
    the past 3 months have you fasted (skipped
    at least 2 meals in a row) to prevent weight
    gain or counteract the effects of eating?   0 1 2 3 4 5 6 7 8 9 10 11 12 13 14

18. How many times per week on average over
    the past 3 months have you engaged in
    excessive exercise specifically to counteract
    the effects of overeating episodes?   0 1 2 3 4 5 6 7 8 9 10 11 12 13 14

19. How much do you weigh? If uncertain, please give your best estimate. ____lbs.

20. How tall are you?   ___ feet ___ inches

21. Over the past 3 months, how many menstrual periods
    have you missed?   1 2 3 4 na

22. Have you been taking birth control pills during the
    past 3 months?   Yes   No

SELECTING EFFECTIVE INTERVENTIONS

Controlled studies of CBT and IPT have demonstrated these methods to be effective approaches for bulimia nervosa and binge-eating disorders (R. I. Stein et al., 2001; U. Schmidt, 1998). Although there has been more research on CBT, direct comparisons of CBT and IPT have produced comparable outcomes. Feminist therapy, family therapy based on communication models, and psychodynamic therapies have not been shown to be effective overall. More research on the efficacy of treatments for eating disorders among racial minorities is needed (Stein et al.).

Findings from several reviews of the outcome research on eating disorders have demonstrated that CBT is effective for over three-quarters of clients, and over half report successfully abstaining from bingeing and purging. Long-term maintenance of gains is also well-established. CBT is considered the first-line treatment for bulimia nervosa and binge-eating disorder, and shows superior outcomes when compared with medication. In direct comparisons to CBT, IPT has been shown to be comparably effective. However, the specific change processes for both CBT and IPT are still undetermined (G. T. Wilson & Fairburn, 1993, 1998; D. E. Smith et al., 1994; Shekter-Wolfson et al., 1997). There is less evidence of effectiveness for either CBT or IPT with anorexia nervosa (Vitousek, 2002; G. T. Wilson & Fairburn, 1998). Relatively little controlled intervention research has been conducted with anorexia nervosa in general.

Although most of the research on the treatment of eating disorders has occurred with adults, these treatments are readily adaptable to adolescents (Bowers, Evans, & van Cleve, 1996). Cognitive-behavioral interventions for eating disorders focus on "identifying and changing specific beliefs, attributions, expectations, values, and cognitive distortions that contribute to the eating disorder. Cognitive and behavioral techniques are employed to teach adolescents to be more aware of their thoughts, feelings, and behaviors . . . they learn to identify and label their emotions, as well as recurrent patterns of thinking" (Bowers et al., p. 236). Examining and challenging distorted dysfunctional cognitions related to bulimia is a key component in CBT. Behavioral changes in eating habits are planned carefully and in specific, graded steps to help the adolescent achieve optimal success.

IPT has also been shown to be helpful with bulimia nervosa and binge-eating disorder. Originally developed for treating depression (Klerman, Weissman, Rounsaville, & Chevron, 1984; Weissman et al., 2000), IPT focuses on interpersonal conflicts, usually a role dispute or role transition, and associated emotional distress that may precipitate binge eating. According to Weissman et al. (p. 318), "Subjects benefit from exploring their interpersonal options, practicing them in therapeutic role playing, and then trying them out with significant others. As the interpersonal problem area is addressed, bulimic symptoms resolve."

A series of controlled studies directly compared IPT with CBT (e.g., Fairburn et al., 1991; Fairburn, Jones, Peveler, Hope, & O'Connor, 1993; Fairburn et al., 1995). These investigations assessed the relative efficacy of three interventions: behavior therapy (BT) that focused exclusively on dietary changes, CBT, and IPT. Although initial outcomes showed CBT to be the superior treatment, follow-ups demonstrated comparable results for IPT. Although clients who received BT originally did well, results deteriorated over several years. Although IPT has been shown to have results comparable to CBT for reduction of binge eating, there is considerably less research on the efficacy of IPT for bulimia nervosa and binge-eating disorder overall. IPT and CBT for eating disorders have also been

visits may be modified should a more severely disturbed client need more intensive treatment (e.g., twice weekly at first). Normally, weekly visits are sufficient.

The main elements of current effective CBT approaches (G. T. Wilson & Fairburn, 1993, 1998;) are, briefly, (1) develop a good therapeutic relationship; (2) educate the client about the CBT model of bulimia nervosa and the need to reduce dysfunctional cognitions about the self, and dietary restraint, and the need to change actual eating behaviors; (3) teach self-monitoring skills to the client regarding thoughts, feelings, behaviors, and situations associated with eating habits as well as the eating habits themselves; (4) develop an established routine of weekly weigh-ins; (5) educate the client about regulating body weight, and the potentially negative consequences of both dieting and purging; (6) develop and follow through on a plan of regular healthful eating habits; (7) teach self-regulation skills; (8) teach problem-solving skills; (9) modify rigid rules concerning "forbidden" foods; (10) challenge and change cognitive distortions regarding eating habits, body shape, and weight; (11) teach and carry out graduated exposure methods to increase acceptance of body weight and shape; and (12) instruct the client in relapse-prevention skills (i.e., identifying triggers and having planned responses to at-risk situations). What follows are more details on how to implement CBT for bulimia nervosa and binge-eating disorder.

In stage 1, the practitioner presents the CBT model and modifies dietary practices (visits 1–8, approximately). First is a thorough assessment (see the MDF assessment points above).

Educate the client about the problems associated with binge eating and dietary restraint, how these practices are linked to mood and self-image problems, and why both practices need to be changed in order to overcome the problem. In brief, the interactions of extreme dietary restrictions, bingeing (and perhaps purging), mood disturbance, and low self-esteem constitute a vicious cycle that may persist until extreme dietary practices are brought under control. Help the client understand that cognitive-behavioral treatment works by changing dysfunctional beliefs and attitudes about eating, body shape, and weight, and reinforcing those changes through improved and less restrictive dietary practices.

Teach self-monitoring skills to the client to track eating behaviors and associated thoughts, moods, behaviors, circumstances, and episodes of binge-purging. This classic functional analysis helps both the practitioner and the client get a clear picture about the sequential patterned linkages among binge eating (and purging), mood, self-image concerns, emotional distress, interpersonal problems or other stressors that may trigger binges, the role of substance abuse, and so forth. Develop a daily monitoring sheet with the client; it may help to enhance compliance. Weekly detailed discussions of the monitoring sheets are important.

Conduct weekly weigh-ins. Clients should be encouraged to weigh themselves weekly; the practitioner may weigh the client only at the first and last sessions of the intervention.

Clients and practitioner should work together to develop a new dietary plan that is healthier and less restrictive (e.g., three regular meals with in-between snacks). The client must eliminate all purging behaviors, and throw away laxatives. Continue to educate the client about the importance of normal eating and the avoidance of extreme dieting practices that tend to perpetuate the problem. Vomiting practices should be adamantly discouraged. This practice usually disappears without much struggle when normal eating patterns return.

Instruct clients in the use of coping skills. Distractions such as pleasant activities or seeking social supports can be planned as a way of reducing the risk of bingeing and purging. Clients can learn to anticipate at-risk times such as late in the afternoon after classes or work, and plan healthful alternative activities.

Significant others and social supports should be included in the intervention. At this point, interviewing friends and relatives can help the clients be less secretive about the problem and provide social support. It also can be used to see if clients understand the treatment procedures, by having them explain the intervention to their friends and family.

In stage 2, dietary modification continues. Intensive cognitive interventions are used to modify dysfunctional beliefs regarding dietary practices and self-evaluation (about eight more visits). More healthful eating is still addressed, as is the problem of avoiding "forbidden" foods. These foods are gradually reintroduced into the client's diet. The average amount of food increases, to avoid "fasting" and to improve energy level. Clients should be less scrupulous about every calorie eaten, and should eat in a wider array of circumstances. Overall, this stage concentrates on returning clients to normal eating habits and helps modify their overly restrictive dietary rules.

Continue practicing coping skills. Review basic problem-solving processes to help the client cope with situations that can lead to relapse. These skills include identifying thoughts, feelings, behaviors, and circumstances that put them at risk, and finding alternative healthy coping responses.

Teach and emphasize standard cognitive therapy techniques (e.g., Beck, 1976) to identify and disconfirm irrational thoughts through rational argument. For example, if the client thinks "People think I am ugly and dislike me because I am not thin," this belief is challenged by questions such as, "Where is the evidence to support this belief? What evidence discounts this belief?"

Another step is enacting behavior changes through practice and graduated exposure to disconfirm dysfunctional beliefs. Although cognitive challenges can be posed to confront dysfunctional beliefs about dieting and self-image, graduated exposure using behavioral "experiments" will be necessary to convincingly disconfirm these beliefs. Not gaining weight on a normal diet while engaging in normal exercise (e.g., jogging a reasonable distance two or three times per week) as well as being less inhibited in one's dress or appearance in public will help solidify gains in self-image and help maintain normal dieting and reduction or elimination of binge-purging.

Stage 3 works on maintenance of gains and relapse prevention (three visits at two-week intervals). In this final stage, clients are assisted in standard relapse-prevention practices. Clients should be taught to expect relapse and to avoid overreacting to it. Encourage clients to quickly resume their normal eating regimen where they left off. A written plan may be a useful way to prepare for at-risk situations. Brainstorm possible coping responses, such as reaching out to helpful social supports to avoid potential pitfalls.

For binge eaters where obesity is a key concern, CBT methods are basically applicable, but modifications are in order (see Fairburn, Marcus, & Wilson, 1993). Because those with binge-eating disorder present a different problem profile than those who have bulimia nervosa (i.e., less cognitive distortion about body shape and absence of purging), they have somewhat *different intervention goals*. The initial emphasis for obese clients is to stop binge eating, rather than to lose weight, and to develop realistic goals regarding weight loss. Nutritional counseling based on current scientific data is important, and it is critical to reinforce the avoidance of extreme diets of any kind. Healthful, regularly scheduled meals and regular exercise are strongly recommended. Clients should be helped to avoid popular "addiction" metaphors regarding food, and focus on regular healthful eating habits with a wide variety of foods. Concern about body image and self-appraisal of attractiveness should be addressed realistically with attention paid to exercise, feeling better about oneself, avoiding unrealistic comparisons to ultrathin and idealized images of female beauty, and emphasizing aspects of one's self-worth other than physical attractiveness. Broad and long-term improvements in healthful living should be established during the last visits of treatment.

Incorporating Elements of Interpersonal Therapy

Symptoms related to binge eating and purging (cognitive distortions about self and body image) may be exacerbated or directly precipitated by interpersonal stressors. Although much less research has been conducted with IPT than with CBT, it has been shown to be effective with binge-eating disorder without employing the techniques of CBT. Thus, it is possible that IPT may be effective by activating change processes related to cognitive distortions regarding interpersonal relations. It seems reasonable to integrate IPT into a CBT approach with a specific focus on resolving cognitive distortions and emotional distress regarding interpersonal conflicts.

The format for IPT has been described in several sources (Weissman et al., 2000; Fairburn, 1993; see chapter 9). The therapist is active in the early sessions, conducts a thorough assessment, and provides psychoeducation about eating disorders and the rationale for the intervention. During the first four sessions or so, the therapist takes a history of eating patterns, weight changes, bingeing, purging, and interpersonal functioning, and *notes any apparent connections between interpersonal distress and the eating-disorder behaviors.* Significant life events and any problems with depression or self-esteem are explored. The emphasis in treatment then shifts to an examination of efforts to constructively address the identified interpersonal conflicts, on the assumption that relationship distress serves as a precipitant to binge-eating episodes (sessions 5-16). The onus of responsibility is placed on the client to address these problems between sessions, and little attention is explicitly focused on the eating behaviors themselves. In the final two or three visits, the client and therapist review their progress, prepare to cope with possible relapses, and terminate.

Prevention and Early Intervention with Binge-Eating Behavior

With adolescents and young adults, there are good reasons to consider prevention and early intervention for eating disorders. There is a high rate of subclinical symptoms in young women, particularly, and some may be in the early stages of developing a serious eating disorder. In addition, co-occurring problems (e.g., substance abuse, depression, social anxiety) are amenable to screening and early intervention. Some of these clients may be helped significantly with early identification and intervention, whereas others may be referred for primary intervention.

Levine and Piran (2001) reviewed twenty-two outcome studies of programs for the prevention of eating disorders. All studies were at least quasi-experimental in design, used repeated measures, and included at least one-month follow-up measures. The prevention programs included some combination of education, skill building, and environmental changes. Overall, results were modest but demonstrated that prevention programs could increase knowledge and improve attitudes and behaviors related to eating disorders. The authors called for more research and prevention programs that include efforts to improve organizational and community attitudes regarding healthful eating and general physical well-being.

In a review of twenty investigations of programs designed to prevent eating disorders, Austin (2000) concluded that few firm recommendations could be made because of programmatic weaknesses and methodological flaws in the research. Feminist models, for example, used didactic and broad-based educational efforts to focus on environmental, cultural, and political factors that potentially increase a woman's risk for developing eating disorders. But primary prevention methods have not been shown to be particularly effective at changing individual problem behaviors (e.g., college alcohol abuse; see chapter 16). Other studies focused on making changes in the social environment, but methodological flaws again muddled the findings. Austin recommended further research to consider implementing prevention programs that might have a direct effect on the social environment, such as addressing social norms, changing curriculum content to target health-related issues, and providing healthier eating choices in schools and universities.

Winzelberg et al. (1998) conducted an initial controlled trial of a psychoeducation and behavior-change program called Student Bodies, an Internet-based prevention program designed to improve body image among university women. Initial results with fifty-seven undergraduates demonstrated improvements in body image and problem behaviors associated with binge eating. After making improvements in both the program and the study methodology, Winzelberg et al. (2000) conducted a second controlled trial of the same program with forty-eight undergraduates. The program lasted eight weeks, and students were reassessed at three-month follow-up. The program was educational, and included information on the cultural determinants of beauty and CBT self-help methods for improving body satisfaction. The program consisted of interactive software that featured text, audio, and video components. Participants also used on-line self-monitoring devices, used behavior-change exercises, and posted their reactions to the lessons each week. On-line discussion groups enhanced social supports during the project. As for results, there were no immediate significant differences in concerns about body shape as measured by standardized scales, but statistical differences did emerge at three-month follow-up, although they were clinically modest in magnitude. Nevertheless, the Internet-based program demonstrated promising results and the feasibility of engaging young people in an interactive program. In a related study, Celio et al. (2000) demonstrated that the Internet-based program described above was substantially more effective than a class-room-based didactic program that did not include the CBT skills of the Internet-based program.

Exemplar Study: A Controlled Trial of Student Bodies.   In a subsequent trial of the Student Bodies program (Zabinski et al., 2001), the investigators narrowed their selection criteria to those students deemed to be at risk for an eating disorder. The sixty-two participants were randomly assigned to the Student Bodies program or to a no-treatment control group (who were offered the same program after the study). Measures were taken at baseline, posttest (eight-weeks), and ten-week follow-up. Measures included the EDE-Q, a social-support scale to test whether the program would negatively impact subjects' exposure to "live" social supports, and other measures. Fifty-six (twenty-seven experimental, twenty-nine control) participants completed the whole program, including follow-up assessments. The program components are described in Winzelberg et al. (2000).

Both groups improved significantly on self-assessment of body image and eating-disorder pathology. There were no significant differences between the two groups. But the reports from the treatment group indicated that they benefited from the intervention, and felt a good deal of social support from the Internet-based bulletin board. The treatment group also showed slightly more improvement in body satisfaction, although the difference was not statistically significant. How does one account for successful outcomes in both the treatment and nontreatment groups? Zabinski et al. (2001) suggested that small sample size and much variability in reported problems may have reduced the statistical power needed to demonstrate significant results. In addition, these clients were screened for higher severity of symptoms than the general college population, and some of these symptoms may have regressed to the mean over time in both groups. Despite these modest results, this study of high-risk young college women supports the utility and potential efficacy of using an Internet-based skill-oriented program to reduce cognitive and behavioral symptoms of eating disorders.

IMPLEMENTING AND EVALUATING THE EVIDENCE-BASED INTERVENTION PLAN

CASE STUDY: TINA

Tina was a young white woman (nineteen) from a large working-class family (she was the youngest of seven children). She was referred to a social worker, Peggy, by her family physician because her mother caught her vomiting in the bathroom. After a brief discussion, her mother discovered that Tina had been binge eating and purging for almost two years. Alarmed, her mother sent her to the family physician, who felt she needed counseling or psychotherapy. Despite this problem, Tina presented herself as cheerful and positive, and reported that she did not see her binge-purging as a big problem, because she knew "lots of girls" who were doing it. She attended community college, and worked part-time in a dress store. She was involved in a romantic relationship with a young man whom she cared a lot about, and wanted very much to please him. She had also been using cocaine on the weekends, along with alcohol. She said her cocaine use was not a problem, and did not see what the big deal was. Tina also was saving up her money for

plastic surgery to improve her appearance, although her friends wondered aloud what she was concerned about.

Tina had recently returned home after living away for a couple of years. She said she had money problems, and just needed some time to get back on her feet financially. As the children had gradually left home, her mother went to work full-time as a cashier in the local grocery store, following her career as a full-time homemaker. Tina's dad had always worked hard, sometimes two jobs when all the children were at home, and he had not been around much. On the weekends he was often with his pals at the local tavern. Mom and dad generally got along, if for no other reason than to cooperate in raising their children, but they sometimes argued on the weekends. Two of Tina's brothers had substance-abuse problems, and one of her sisters had been diagnosed with schizophrenia. Two of her sisters had finished college, and the rest of her siblings seemed to be working steadily and starting families of their own.

Multidimensional/Functional Assessment: Defining Problems and Goals

Tina's bingeing and purging apparently had been relatively continuous for two years. She reported that she had started bingeing and purging after a sleepover with a girlfriend when she was sixteen or seventeen. She was impressed by her girlfriend's conviction that the only way to get a guy was to stay "as thin as possible." In addition to bingeing on "junk foods" and purging, she began to take laxatives and, about that time, met Steve, who became her steady boyfriend. Steve used drugs and introduced Tina to cocaine, which she referred to as the "ultimate diet drug." She also smoked pot and drank too much on the weekend, although this was more intermittent. Steve sold cocaine to support his own drug habit. During the week, Tina would not drink or smoke pot while she was working and going to classes at the local community college (she wanted to become an executive in the fashion industry), but occasionally she would use cocaine to keep herself going. During her visit with the doctor, she discussed her drug use and a constant burning in her esophagus. The doctor explained that if she did not stop her bingeing and purging, she would develop problems that would require serious medical attention. Tina had also not had a regular menstrual cycle for several months, a problem that caused her much concern. The physician gave her some medication for her esophageal irritation along with some supplements (she was also anemic), and referred her to a social worker who specialized in treatment of eating disorders.

As Tina discussed her problem history with Peggy, she began to cry. Peggy, taking a more detailed history, realized that Tina had apparently been unhappy with her relationship for a while, was worried about her binge-purging and cocaine use, but was afraid that she would not be able to stop. She appeared to be depressed and had not been sleeping well. The social worker told her she would have to stop using the cocaine before her symptoms could be sorted out and before she could develop a more healthful dietary plan. In summing up her situation, it appeared that Tina had a number of interacting co-occurring problems that needed to be dealt with: she had a long-standing lack of self-confidence, low self-esteem, and distorted body image. Her bingeing and purging was starting to take a toll on her physically and was causing havoc with her sense of well-being. She was somewhat depressed, she was in a relationship with someone who was exploiting her, and her substance abuse was exacerbating her psychological, emotional, and interpersonal problems. On the plus side, she had some good friends who were willing to give her support despite being increasingly puzzled by what they saw as self-destructive behavior. She was ambitious and disciplined enough to hold down a steady job and take classes, and was doing reasonably well. She was not suicidal and had never engaged in self-mutilating behaviors. She wanted to change what she was doing, but wasn't sure where to begin.

Peggy suggested that they discuss in more detail what Tina wanted to accomplish in the intervention. The social worker laid out what she saw as the major problems, and discussed how she thought Tina's eating disorder, drug problem, unhappy relationship, and self-image were somewhat related. Tina agreed with these connections, and got the clear impression from her discussions with the doctor and social worker that she had to first stop using drugs, because they were "messing me up." She had not yet developed a clear dependence syndrome, as her use was fairly intermittent, but her drug use was affecting her mood preventing her from dealing constructively with her other difficulties. Peggy and Tina decided that a good course of action would be for Tina to spend time at home in a period of supervised abstinence from drug use to clear her head, and then undertake a more detailed assessment of her binge-purging habit. Once Tina felt that she was in more control of the recreational drug use and her eating habits, she could take on the more long-standing concerns about her lack of self-confidence and the quality of relationships that she wanted to have in her life. In the meantime, Tina agreed that it might be a good idea to reduce her contact with Steve by explaining that she needed some time to herself.

In coordination with the physician, who would continue to monitor Tina's physical symptoms, Peggy, with Tina's approval, had her parents come to the next session. Since Tina was living at home and was not prepared to live independently just yet, they agreed that having her parents involved in her treatment, at least initially, might be helpful. With the support of her social worker, physician, and parents, Tina felt more confident that she could make some of these initial changes in her life.

The first step was to stay at home for a week to detoxify. Because she was between semesters, she did not have to miss classes. She told her employer that she had some "personal problems" to work out, and she requested a week off from work. Her mom took time off from her job at the supermarket. Tina scheduled two brief visits with her social worker during this first week, and had a follow-up visit with her physician. In the evening her dad spent some time with her. They went out to see a movie together, something she had never done alone with him. Her dad discussed his off-and-on drinking problems with her, and stunned her with a confession that years ago, when he was working as a boiler maintenance service man in a hospital, he had become dependent on "uppers" to keep him going between two full-time jobs. She was open with him for the first time about her relationship with Steve, and her dad suggested that she think about choosing a better boyfriend. Her mom and dad got along well that week, and seemed to be exclusively concerned about her well-being. As the week wore on, she became somewhat bored but noticed that she was sleeping better and her spirits were lifting. Her physician had also prescribed an antidepressant, but she did not expect to feel the effects for another week or so. She spent much of the time helping her mother around the house.

After her "detox week," Tina worked with Peggy to develop a more detailed assessment of her binge-purging cycle and to come up with a more healthful dietary schedule. An analysis of her "typical week" showed that she had developed a fairly predictable pattern of getting herself "stressed out" at work, and in school, and then trying to balance these demands with "making Steve happy." This last challenge was apparently very difficult, because Steve was never satisfied with her looks, their sex life, or anything else that Tina did. He was particularly uninterested in her schooling, often describing it as a "waste of time," and made fun of her job. Sometimes they drank or used cocaine together. If she was feeling down after a long day or had an argument with him on the phone, she was particularly likely to go home and binge on junk food and purge afterwards. She always felt worse after purging, but felt she did not have any choice. Otherwise she feared she would "get disgustingly fat" and be even less acceptable to Steve. Often, after dealing with him, her mood swings, and daily stressors, Tina felt out of control and that she was just surviving from one day to the next. Although each week was a little different, the pattern was a variation on the same themes: keep going, get stressed out, feel badly about herself, binge and purge, use alcohol or coke to cope, and so on. She was bingeing and purging about three to four times per week. At some point she knew that this routine had to come to an end, and felt she was ready to do something about it.

Selecting and Designing the Intervention: Defining Strategies and Objectives

After identifying the problems and general intervention goals, Peggy discussed intervention options with Tina, and suggested they choose a number of initial objectives (table 15.1). Tina already felt very much involved, and having survived the first week at home using the self-monitoring chart, felt that she was collaborating well with Peggy. She already felt she had some basic understanding of how her problems were related to one another, and this gave her some sense of control over some of the changes she was about to embark upon. Although Peggy had touched upon it initially, she provided Tina with a more detailed explanation of how her mood, self-image, drug use, and binge-purging cycle were related, and how her bingeing and purging actually "kept the pattern going." They reviewed the details of the types of food Tina binged with, how much and how often, and then discussed in detail what a healthful "normal" diet would look like. Tina was encouraged strongly to discontinue all bingeing and purging immediately and begin her "normal" diet. Given her distorted expectations about gaining weight and becoming "fat," her social worker discussed with her how her distorted view of herself might be related to how she felt about herself in general, her feelings of not being acceptable or "good enough" for others.

Tina continued to self-monitor over the next couple of weeks and track her mood, her negative cognitions about herself and her physical appearance, and her urges to binge and purge. Although she made progress, she did "slip" a couple of times, once after she was confronted by Steve after she came out of class.

She did not resume cocaine use, but came home upset because he was very angry with her and "made me feel like a traitor." After discussing her momentary relapse with Peggy, however, she felt less guilty about it. Her social worker congratulated her for getting back on the plan with her new eating regimen and not resuming cocaine use with Steve. Tina weighed herself weekly, and did not see any substantive change in her weight. This alleviated any fears she had that she was going to put on a lot of weight if she didn't purge. She began to exercise with a friend of hers, running once or twice during the week and alone on the weekend. She began to feel better about her body, beginning to see herself as "fit" rather than feeling the need to be "ultrathin." She spent more time with friends from whom she had drifted since she started dating Steve, and she was feeling better about herself. Steve had called her several times, and with the exception of the episode when he confronted her after school, Tina had not seen him. She was bargaining for more time when he angrily told her not to come around anymore. Although upset, she refrained from bingeing and purging, and stayed on her regimen despite doubts about her decision not to see him.

As she continued to follow her dietary regimen, more or less, Tina's fears of relapse began to abate, and she became less concerned about gaining weight. More of her focus during visits turned to her feelings about herself and the types of relationships she had had over the past few years. She had felt for a long time that something was missing, that she was not satisfied, and that she spent too much time worrying about whether the other person was happy even when she was not. Peggy went with this new direction, and felt that as long as Tina's self-monitoring and dietary regimen continued, and as long as she stayed away from cocaine and marijuana, it might be helpful that she examine her self-image and her relationship with Steve. This emphasis on interpersonal relationships revealed a distorted or disproportionate belief that it was basically all up to Tina to make a relationship work, with little expectation of return on her part. As they examined these long-standing beliefs, Peggy challenged them and encouraged Tina to begin actively putting these beliefs to the test in everyday circumstances.

As the weeks passed, Tina seemed to gain confidence that relapse was not going to be a major problem. The more she stayed with her current eating regimen and exercise, the better she was feeling about herself. She was keeping very busy as a way of coping, but felt that this was all right for now. She was not ready to take on a new relationship, and felt good about herself for not "caving in" when Steve called again. She surprised herself when she told him over the phone that she really didn't want to spend much more time with a "pot head." Although she felt a little guilty afterwards, the feeling didn't last long. After sixteen visits or so, Tina and Peggy agreed that it was time to back off from regular visits to once per month for a while. Tina was planning to stay at home for the rest of the school year, and then think about her next move. She wanted to keep in touch with the social worker in the meantime (just as a safety net) until she felt she was ready to go it alone.

Selecting Scales and Creating Indexes to Monitor and Evaluate Client Progress

In addition to using the EDDS to monitor specific symptoms (using individual items) as well as the overall composite score to track progress, the social worker decided to use the HAM-D (see chapter 9) to keep an eye on Tina's level of depression (table 15.1). The development and use of a daily self-monitoring chart was an integral part of Tina's role in the intervention. The chart helped keep her on track and, as a self-monitoring tool, helped hone her self-regulatory skills in the following ways: not overreacting to upset; stopping to consider what she was thinking and feeling; gauging the degree of risk for binge-purging; considering healthier alternatives to binge-purging; and thinking about the negative consequences she would experience if she did give in to the urge (as well as the feeling of satisfaction and progress she would feel if she successfully bypassed the urge). Other indexes could have been used to monitor co-occurring substance use.

SUMMARY

Depending on type and severity, anorexia nervosa, bulimia nervosa, and binge-eating disorder can be among the most challenging disorders to treat. In addition, they often co-occur with other serious problems, including depression, anxiety disorders, and substance abuse. Assessment protocol emphasizes detailed functional analysis of thoughts, feelings, and behaviors related to bingeing and purging. A number of valid eating-disorder scales can enhance assessment and provide a measure for monitoring progress. CBT and IPT are comparably effective for bulimia nervosa. Although binge-eating disorder may respond well to behavioral dietary management strategies, anorexia nervosa remains a difficult, often intractable, disorder.

TABLE 15.1   The client service plan for Tina

Problems	Goals	Sample Objectives	Interventions	Assessment Tools
Intermittent drug abuse: alcohol, marijuana, cocaine	Eliminate drug use; refrain from all illicit drug use; social drinking to be reconsidered at later date	Refrain from drug use immediately with supervision of family, physician, and social worker; begin self-monitoring urges to use and identifying feeling states	Combined CBT and elements of IPT to address interpersonal distortions and how they affect her self-image and mood Psychoeducation to help her better understand how problems are linked, and how eating normally and exercising will help her stop the urges to binge/purge	EDDS to assess and monitor individual and global symptoms of bulimia HAM-D to monitor depression Self-monitoring chart with self-anchored indexes to measure stress level, emotional antecedents to binge/purge, actual episodes of binge-purging; chart could be used to monitor any use of alcohol or other drugs
Binge-purging 3–4 times per week	Eliminate all binge-purging and associated use of laxatives	Self-monitoring thoughts, feelings, situations associated with urge to binge/purge		
Poor self-esteem and distorted body image (thinks she is fat)	Improve self-esteem and develop healthier and more realistic body image through healthful diet and exercise	Eat normal amounts and types of food daily; have weekly weigh-in at home; begin exercising 2–3 times per week	Brief behavioral family therapy to incorporate parents' social support to help her detox for further assessment of mental status and mood	
Unassertive in relationships; allows herself to be exploited; feels she is not "good enough"	Develop better understanding of her interpersonal distortions and reasons for being unassertive; improve quality of interpersonal relationships	Identify in daily chart thoughts, feelings about her relationship and how it seems related to urges to binge/purge or "get high"; select daily opportunity to "assert herself" and discuss with social worker	Help her develop detailed eating and exercise regimen; report weekly weigh-ins; develop self-monitoring chart with social worker and use daily Interpersonal psychotherapy to examine distorted beliefs and expectations and understand how her behavior in relationships affects her mood; role-play and practice in community to be more assertive and less compliant with others Case management with physician re health status, testing and medication	

CHAPTER 16

SUBSTANCE ABUSE AND RISKY SEX IN ADOLESCENTS AND YOUNG ADULTS

Late adolescence and young adulthood are particularly potent times for psychosocial development. Changes include greater emotional and sexual involvement with others, increases in academic or occupational responsibilities, taking control of one's own physical and economic survival, and, eventually, achieving emancipation from one's parents. The outcome trajectory for this dynamic period, which bridges adolescence and adulthood, eventually moves toward psychosocial growth, stagnation, or decline. Two of the most salient and risk-prone behaviors ushered in during this period are substance abuse and unplanned/unprotected sex. Although responsible drinking and sexual activity are generally accepted as enjoyable aspects of adult life, the abuse of alcohol and drugs and risky sexual behaviors can result in negative short- and long-term consequences. Patterns of drinking and sexual behavior developed during this time can portend problems well into adulthood.

This chapter summarizes what is currently known about assessment and early intervention with substance abuse and risky sexual activities engaged in by young people. Early intervention is also referred to as secondary prevention. In the public health lexicon, primary, secondary, and tertiary prevention efforts reflect a continuum of methods for preventing, interrupting, and treating psychosocial dysfunction and disease. Primary prevention efforts for substance abuse and risky sex include broad-based informational strategies meant to reduce substance use, such as media exhortations to "be smart, don't start," and messages that urge young people to abstain from sex or use condoms. Tertiary interventions for substance abuse include treatment for more serious substance-abuse problems. Secondary prevention (i.e., early intervention) includes psychosocial interventions for people who have shown "early indications" of a potentially more serious problem. This case identification may occur in a number of ways: a female college student is positively screened for depression and co-occurring substance abuse in a college health clinic; a male high school student is arrested for vandalism and underaged drinking; a young person is diagnosed as having contracted a readily curable sexually transmitted disease through unprotected sex. These cases would be good candidates for early intervention efforts, an arguably more efficient approach than primary prevention efforts, in that resources can be targeted at those who have begun to manifest clear signs of a problem. The motto for early-intervention experts could be "the squeaky wheel gets the grease."

Evidence-based early interventions with substance abuse and risky sex have come to be associated with harm-reduction principles (Marlatt, 1996; Marlatt & Witkiewitz, 2002). The goals of harm reduction are to reduce both the problem behaviors and the negative consequences associated with them. Harm-reduction principles are based on the following assumptions: problems are determined by multiple biopsychosocial and environmental processes; problems exist along a continuum from mild to severe; the development or trajectory of most behaviorial problems is not linear, but follows peaks and valleys of severity and attenuation; the problem may be accompanied by an array of co-occurring difficulties and consequences that may be amenable to harm-reduction efforts. Early intervention often follows a "stepped" trajectory. It starts with moderate and attainable goals (e.g., reduced drinking) and increases the intensity of treatment until more ambitious outcomes are achieved (complete abstinence), should attempts to moderate or attenuate the behavior fail. Although some prohibitionist prevention experts opine that it is better to "aim high" by stressing abstinence initially, evidence suggests that such an approach may discourage young people from engaging in and persisting with early-intervention programs, thus reducing the chances for avoiding risky behaviors in the long run (Sanchez-Craig, 1980).

ASSESSMENT

Background Data

People between the ages of eighteen and twenty-nine account for almost half (45%) of adult drinking in the United States (Greenfield & Rogers, 1999), and college drinkers consume as much if not more than their noncollege cohorts (Gfoerer, Greenblatt, & Wright, 1997; O'Malley & Johnston, 2002). Research has catalogued an array of problems related to excessive drinking by college students (e.g., Wechsler et al., 2002; Wechsler, Davenport, Dowdall, Moeykens, & Costillow, 1994; O'Hare, 1990b). These problems include negative psychological consequences (depression, suicide, anxiety), interpersonal problems (fights, unplanned and unprotected sex), community disturbances including criminal behavior, and other acute consequences (death by excessive alcohol consumption during fraternity hazings, alcohol-related accidents). A recent review of five national college drinking surveys (O'Malley & Johnston, 2002) summarized the major findings and trends over the past twenty years.

More than two thirds of college students drink alcohol.

Forty percent are considered binge drinkers, that is, they consumed five or more drinks at one sitting within the past two weeks.

Rates of alcohol use have not changed substantially since the 1950s.

Males are about one and one-half times as likely to be binge drinkers as females.

Differences in alcohol consumption by gender have narrowed over the past ten years.

In addition, women are known to be at greater risk for the consequences of excessive drinking. These include more co-occurring depression and anxiety, higher blood-alcohol levels, and greater vulnerability to being victimized through sexual assault (Wechsler, Dowdall, Davenport, & Rimm, 1995; O'Hare, 1997a, 2001a; Amaro, 1995). Despite evidence for widespread heavy drinking among young people, most will not develop long-term addictions (K. Chen & Kandel, 1995; Fillmore, 1974, 1988), although it is hard to predict which individuals will. Young people tend to underestimate the short-term acute risks involved with substance abuse (Wechsler & McFadden, 1979; Wechsler et al., 1994; O'Hare & Tran, 1997; Perkins, 2002). Awareness of youthful problem-drinking patterns and associated risk factors such as disinhibited drinking, stress-related drinking, and high expectations of positive reinforcement from drinking may also have prognostic value for future alcohol dependence (M. E. Bennett, McCrady, Johnson, & Pandina, 1999; Schuckit, 1998).

Perhaps because of their relative inexperience and recent emancipation from parental oversight, freshmen in college appear to have more problems related to drinking than upper classmen. Drinking in senior year of high school is significantly predictive of college drinking (Yu & Schacket, 2001). According to the Monitoring the Future report (USDHHS, 1999c), rates of binge drinking increased successively from 14% to 24% to 32% in eighth, tenth, and twelfth graders, respectively, and jumped to 39% when they enter college. It is not until they move beyond this important transition from high school to college that problem drinking begins to decline through senior year and beyond (O'Neill, Parra, & Sher, 2001). These changes include a reduction in overall consumption, greater discretion regarding risky drinking situations (e.g., driving under the influence), and development of other skills that may attenuate some of the negative consequences associated with excessive use. It seems that freshman year may present a critical opportunity to reduce future harm associated with excessive drinking.

Drugs other than alcohol continue to be a significant matter of concern. According to the Monitoring the Future report (USDHHS, 1999c), although there were some reductions in illicit drug use into the midnineties, it has increased in the 19–28-year-old group on the whole. Recently data have shown increased use of marijuana among college students as well as MDA/MDMA and similar drugs, and cocaine. Between 1991 and 1998, the rates of marijuana use among eighth graders nearly tripled (from 6% to 17%), nearly doubled among tenth graders (from 15% to 31%), and grew by 80% among twelfth graders (from 22% to 38%).

Among high school seniors, the use of any illicit drug rose from 15% to 21% between 1992 and 1998. Among young people, African-American students use drugs at significantly lower rates than whites and binge drink less (12%) than Hispanic students (28%) or whites (36%). Whites use other drugs at higher rates, including marijuana, inhalants, LSD, heroin, barbiturates, amphetamines, and tranquilizers. However, Hispanics in the senior year have the highest rates of use for some of the most dangerous drugs, including cocaine and crack. Students and practitioners should be cautious when interpreting trend data from one year to the next. Use of one class of drug or another comes in and out of fashion. One must examine substance-use trends over time, particularly data that describe heavy and problematic use.

Substance-abuse problems in young people are accompanied by a host of other problems, including mental health disorders. The Methods for the Epidemiology of Child and Adolescent Mental Disorders study (Kandel et al., 1997) demonstrated that the use of alcohol, cigarettes, and other illicit substances, even at relatively low doses, was significantly associated with anxiety, mood, and disruptive behavior disorders in young people, with gender differences essentially mirroring adult data. The likelihood that youth will engage in multiple co-occurring health-risk behaviors (i.e., not using seat belts, carrying weapons, smoking tobacco, substance abuse, risky sex) appears to increase with age. One nationally representative sample of adolescents (ages 12–21) demonstrated that while most young people did not engage in multiple risky behaviors, about one-third of those 14–17 did, as did about half of college youth. Males in all ages engaged in more risky behaviors than females. Young people not attending school in both the 14–17 and the 18–21 group engaged in more health-risk behaviors than those attending school (Brener & Collins, 1998). Longitudinal analyses (e.g., Tubman, Windle, & Windle, 1996) suggest that externalizing problems in children and adolescents are linked to increases in risky sexual behaviors and substance abuse. Two European studies showed little relationship between socioeconomic status and risky behaviors (Tuinstra, Groothoff, Van Den Jeuvel, & Post, 1998) and psychological well-being in young people (Bergman & Scott, 2001).

It is an oft-repeated axiom that health-risk behaviors are directly related to peer-group affiliation. At least one study demonstrated that the relationship between youth health-risk behaviors and peers may be more influential than that of the youth's parents (Beal, Ausiello, & Perrin, 2001). However, it may be that peer affiliation is more correlational than causal, whereas parents are likely to have greater direct influence over a youth's health-risk behavior in the long run. For example, in both cross sectional and prospective research with inner-city African-American youth, it was shown that parental monitoring of children's behavior was directly correlated with children's risky behaviors, including sex, drug use, drug trafficking, truancy, and violence (Xiaoming, Stanton, & Feigelman, 2000a, 2000b). It makes more sense to see peer affiliation as correlational (after all, it is only a matter of perspective when deciding which peer is the "bad influence"). Those young people considered "deviant" (i.e., "nonconformists," "stoners," and "burn-outs"), show the highest rates of risky behaviors. Once affiliated with troubled peer groups, they find it hard to extricate themselves (La Greca, Prinstein, & Fetter, 2001). Youths with disabilities (emotional, learning, and mobility) are significantly more likely than nondisabled youth to engage in risky behaviors such as sexual activity and substance abuse. Those with emotional disabilities were six times as likely to attempt suicide in the twelve months prior to the survey, and those with learning or mobility disabilities were three times as likely to attempt suicide (Blum, Kelly, & Ireland, 2001). Health-risk behaviors are also likely to be associated with higher rates of depression and anxiety, further complicating the clinical picture (D. A. Murphy et al., 2001). Increased emotional distress appears to be related to maladaptive coping, which may include drug and alcohol abuse (Arthur, 1998; O'Hare & Sherrer, 2000). Despite most stressors being in the mild to moderate range, some students suffer psychological problems severe enough to result in withdrawal from school (Weiner & Wiener, 1997).

Although cause-effect inferences should be made cautiously, more serious levels of behavioral risk factors seem to co-occur with a greater number of risky behaviors overall. For example, in addition to increased risk of sexually transmitted diseases (including HIV), the total number of sex partners a young person has correlates with risky behaviors that include substance abuse, carrying weapons, and violence in black and white males and females (Valois, Oeltmann, Waller, & Hussey, 1999). It has also become evident that bisexual and gay male and female adolescents share many of the same risks as their heterosexual counterparts, including those related to risky sex and substance abuse. Bisexual and gay adolescents appear more likely to have been sexually abused, however, and more likely to have engaged in sexual activity at a younger age (Saewyc, Bearinger, Heinz, Blum, & Resnick, 1998). In the same study, the data on bisexual and gay males demonstrated three to four times the rate of attempted suicide as their straight counterparts, as estimated from general population data. Young people present one of the more challenging yet potentially fruitful opportunities for secondary intervention.

Theories

Buckstein (1995) concisely reviews a number of prevalent theories to explain substance abuse in young people. These include parental genetic and social-learning influences; the development of alcohol expectancies (beliefs about the positive or negative effects of alcohol or other drug abuse); inadequate relationships with parents; early onset of a substance-abuse problem; academic problems; conduct disorder and other problems with aggression, interpersonal conflict, or other deviance; risky sexual behaviors; poor social bonds; other co-occurring psychopathology, such as depression, other mental illnesses, eating disorders; and living in stressful environments such as those marked by poverty and high levels of crime. It is understood that the interactions of these potential risk factors are complex, not well understood, and cumulative in the sense that more risk factors increase the chances of developing a serious substance-abuse problem.

Theories that explain the causes and maintenance of substance abuse and addiction in general are reviewed in greater detail in chapter 6. These theories need a developmental context in order to better understand the challenges facing young people, particularly in regard to psychosocial developmental influences. Developmental theories relevant to the behavior of adolescents and young adults have been applied to alcohol abuse (Schulenberg & Maggs, 2002; Schulenberg, Maggs, Steinmen, & Zucker, 2001). Developmental transitions are conceptualized as originating in the interaction of both distal and proximate influences on physical maturation, beliefs, expectancies and cultural context, family and other interpersonal experiences, personal values, and goals. These activities interact and are reciprocally influenced by the environment around the individual. Physiological changes (alcohol tolerance), peer relations, increased sexual activity and a new broadening of social relations, and new academic and occupational challenges, among other transitional/developmental events, present a whole range of opportunities for growth and adaptation or avoidance and psychosocial dysfunction. These developmental transitions include fundamental changes in pubertal and cognitive development; affiliative transitions with family, friends, and romantic relationships; achievement transitions; and identity transitions in self-definition and self-regulation. Schulenberg et al. identify overloaded coping abilities, an incongruity between developmental needs and circumstances, and the potentially growth-promoting aspects of risk-taking behavior as factors that may promote risky behaviors. A developmental perspective may inform prevention strategies by illuminating opportunities when prevention experts can interrupt and redirect certain risk behaviors, or alter interpersonal and contextual factors that could have an impact on existing risk factors. Prevention strategies may be more effective if they target young people's important life transitions during this time, use interventions that are salient to the young person's specific problems, and consider both freedom and the need to be accountable for one's behavior.

It has been long recognized that serious substance-abuse problems in youth tend to be part of a constellation of problem behaviors, and risk of future addiction appears to increase with multiple genetic, familial, social, and other environmental risk factors (Jessor & Jessor, 1977; Zucker & Fitzgerald, 1991; Buckstein, 1995). Nevertheless, even when multiple problems are present, long-term predictions regarding which individual is likely to continue developing a serious problem into adulthood are difficult at best, and most problems related to youthful drinking and drug use are transitory (K. Chen & Kandel, 1995; Fillmore, 1974, 1988). Thus, while long-term outcomes are always a concern, the focus of most theory on youthful substance abuse is on developmental influences and social-contextual factors related to drinking and acute negative consequences. Such theories emphasize the interaction of cognitive, behavioral, physiological, social, and environmental factors.

Social-cognitive models have dominated the literature on youthful drinking for some time, and have been shown to be useful by linking motivations for drinking, alcohol expectancies of drinking effects, stress, and social-contextual variables as reciprocal determinants of problem drinking (e.g., Abrams & Niaura, 1987; S. A. Brown et al., 1987; O'Hare, 1998a; M. L. Cooper, Russell, & George, 1988; Maisto, Carey, & Bradizza, 1999). This model has demonstrated that the interactions among physiological predisposition, beliefs, drinking behaviors, and preferred drinking contexts operate in complex ways. Cognitive, behavioral, and contextual factors are theoretically amenable to early-intervention strategies. Three major developments in recent years have contributed to a social-cognitive model of youthful drinking. These models include research on the structural-situational aspects of drinking (when, where, with whom), alcohol expectancy research, and research on high-risk drinking contexts.

The first area has demonstrated that college drinking is primarily a social affair done in same- and mixed-gender peer groups in an atmosphere of general conviviality (Harford & Grant, 1987; O'Hare, 1990b; Wechsler & McFadden, 1979). Older teens (twelfth graders) were shown to be more likely than younger adolescents to drink with peers, in large groups, and in someone else's home (Mayer, Forster, Murray, & Wagenaar, 1998). In a recent gender-comparison study of adult children of alcoholics in college, men appeared to be more inclined than women to drink in larger and same-sex groups, and convivial drinking appeared to be associated with better social adjustment (Senchak, Leonard, & Greene, 1998). The second area of research emphasizes important cognitive mediators of drinking known as alcohol expectancies, defined as beliefs in relatively specific types of reinforcement from drinking. Expectancy constructs as measured by the Alcohol Expectancy Questionnaire are correlated with drinking patterns, attitudes, and associated problems (S. A. Brown, 1985; S. A. Brown et al., 1980; S. A. Brown et al., 1987; Wall, Hinson, & McKee, 1998). The third theoretical area emphasizes high-risk drinking situations, including those associated with relapse during treatment and recovery (Marlatt & Gordon, 1985; Isenhart, 1993). Surveys of young people not in treatment have found consistently that, although most young people associate excessive drinking with convivial and celebratory experiences (Carey, 1993; O'Hare, 1997b), alcohol abuse is often used to cope with negative emotions such as anxiety, depression, and stress associated with interpersonal problems (Evans & Dunn, 1995; M. L. Cooper et al., 1988; O'Hare, 1998a).

How problem drinking is defined also depends on the perspective of the youthful drinker and that of others. For most young people, the only negative consequences of drinking at a party are being caught for vandalism, excessive noise, car accidents, urinating in public, and so forth. Young people who drink as part of dating and sexual encounters may find that alcohol facilitates positive encounters or that it results in negative consequences, such as unprotected sex or date rape (O'Hare, 1998a; J. Norris, 1994; M. L. Cooper, 2002; Abbey & Harnish, 1995). Those young people who drink as a way of coping with negative emotions are more likely to suffer from socioemotional problems related to drinking, and may be at greater risk for more serious drinking problems in the long run (Schuckit, 1998). A social-cognitive perspective informs secondary prevention efforts. Practitioners can help youthful drinkers improve situational awareness of risks, make better estimates about the potential for harm to themselves or others, and enhance their coping skills in reducing consumption and/or altering the context of use to reduce negative consequences.

Risky Sex as a Co-occurring Problem with Substance Abuse

Although the causal link between substance use and risky sexual behaviors is not thoroughly understood, it has become evident that the two are correlated. Young people account for a significant proportion of new AIDS cases (Leigh, 1999). Despite the plethora of messages about safe sex, young people do not use condoms consistently, and knowledge of HIV/AIDS risk does not reduce risky behaviors (J. E. Lewis, Malow, & Ireland, 1997; Staton et al., 1999; Koch, Palmer, Vicary, & Wood, 1999). Excessive drinking among young people increases the likelihood of high-risk sexual behavior, thereby increasing the possibility of both sexually transmitted diseases and sexual assault (A. O'Leary, Goodhart, Sweet Jemmott, & Boccher-Lattimore, 1992; Leigh & Schafer, 1993; Carroll & Carroll, 1995; M. L. Cooper & Orcutt, 1997; Abbey, McAuslan, & Ross, 1998). Although a disproportionate amount of the research on substance abuse and risky sex has been done with college students, similar findings with their noncollege cohorts have emerged. In a ten-year longitudinal study of an ethnically diverse (about half African-American) and environmentally high-risk group (about one-half residing in high-crime neighborhoods), Guo et al. (2002) demonstrated that binge drinking at an early age predicted a higher number of sex partners in adolescence, and marijuana use predicted increased likelihood of avoiding condom use. L. K. Brown and Lourie (2001) provide a brief overview of the theories and methods that have shown promise for understanding and reducing HIV health-risk behaviors: these include the theory of reasoned action, the health belief model, and social-cognitive theory (e.g., self-efficacy theory and transtheoretical model of change). Although there are some differences in these theories, they overlap considerably by emphasizing the interaction of cognitive factors, consequential behaviors, and situational variability. They also share implications for early intervention: providing new information, challenging existing dysfunctional cognitions, and enhancing self-efficacy and coping skills in at-risk situations.

Estimates from a number of studies suggest than more than half of college women report having been sexually assaulted. About 5% report that the assault ended in a completed rape. About one-half of the assaults appear to be alcohol related (often when both were drinking), and almost all of the assaults were committed by a man familiar to the woman (Abbey, 2002). The theoretical explanations regarding alcohol use and sexual assault are not straightforward and involve complex interactions among cognitive, situational, cultural and gender-based factors, among others (Leigh, 1999; M. L. Cooper, 2002; Abbey). Explanations for the theoretical linkage between risky sex and heavy drinking include general sensation seeking, impaired judgment, alcohol expectancies, and contextual factors related to sexual behaviors and drinking (Leigh; Steele & Josephs, 1990; Dermen & Cooper, 1994a, 1994b; O'Hare, 1998a; J. Norris, 1994; Schafer & Leigh, 1996).

Leigh (1990) demonstrated in a household survey that items related to the expectancy of sexual enhancement and disinhibition were associated with both the likelihood of drinking during a specific sexual situation and the amount of alcohol consumed during the respondent's most recent sexual encounter. Dermen and Cooper (1994a) conducted a survey with a more representative sample of over 900 adolescents (ages 13–19). They developed a scale that, in addition to sexual enhancement (S. A. Brown et al., 1980), included items relevant to disinhibition and specific risky sexual behaviors (e.g., unprotected sex). After validating the scale with confirmatory factor analysis, Dermen and Cooper (1994b) found that sex-specific expectancies were better than global alcohol expectancies in predicting specific sexual situations, but were equally or somewhat less useful than general global expectancies in predicting drinking at parties and on dates. Although men and women who drink in convivial and intimate circumstances both share increased expectancies of enhanced sexual relations, men are more likely to engage in risky sexual behaviors (Dermen, Cooper, & Agocha, 1998; Leigh & Aramburu, 1996; O'Hare, 1998b; M. L. Cooper & Orcutt, 1997), and these situations carry greater risks of harm for young women (Abbey et al., 1998).

Based on a considerable amount of survey research (A. O'Leary, 1992; J. Norris, 1994; M. L. Cooper, 1992; Abbey et al., 1998; Leigh, 1999; Abbey, 2002; O'Hare, 1998a, 2001b) a number of interrelated factors appear to increase the likelihood that rape will occur. These factors, both general and those related specifically to alcohol use, include

> male social-learning and personality disturbances, such as social-learning processes that present sexual aggressiveness in a positive light, other conduct- or impulse-disordered behaviors related to psychopathy, and antisocial personality;
>
> alcohol expectancies regarding sexual assertiveness or a belief in enhanced sexual experience through alcohol use;
>
> cultural and peer influences that encourage sexual aggressiveness and lack of consideration for a woman's prerogative to say no;
>
> the belief that if a woman is drinking she is sexually more available;
>
> the physiologically disinhibiting (and judgment-impairing) attributes of alcohol use; and

the use of alcohol intoxication as an excuse either for aggressive male sexual behavior or to hold a woman responsible for an assault (if she were drinking).

A multivariate model is emerging that outlines a useful assessment framework for early intervention. It includes, at a minimum, the following factors: person variables (i.e., gender, age, cultural background), alcohol expectancies, physiological gender differences, history of impulsivity and sensation-seeking related to drinking, patterns of excessive alcohol consumption, and situational factors that include both heavy drinking and sexual encounters. Although drinking and risky sex may be correlated, the relationship between them is complex, and explicit links between alcohol use and specific risky sexual behaviors have been difficult to demonstrate empirically (Abbey, 2002; M. L. Cooper, 2002).

Key Elements of Multidimensional/ Functional Assessment

Generally speaking, with the exception of substance abuse (see chapter 6), there are no formal "diagnostic criteria" for health-risk behaviors. At the more severe end of the spectrum, however, risky behaviors such as excessive drinking, drug use, and engaging in risky sexual behavior may be associated with other problems such as conduct disorder, APD, BPD, or another psychological or psychiatric disturbance. Even the substance abuse criteria in the *DSM-IV* provide only guidelines for determining whether a young person is diagnoseable or not, because there is no clear demarcation between what constitutes occasional misuse, problem use, or abuse. In addition, youthful substance abuse is typically transitory or context specific, and often does not meet the criteria of abuse and dependence. Thus the validity of employing *DSM* criteria for substance abuse with adolescents has been questioned (C. S. Martin & Winters, 1998). Nevertheless, the *DSM* guidelines for substance abuse and dependence are helpful to provide initial guidance for an assessment.

A motivational interviewing style (W. R. Miller & Rollnick, 1991; see chapter 6) is particularly well suited to working with young people. A strategy that shows respect for their personal experiences and encourages them to make their own judgments regarding the pros and cons of substance use and other risky behaviors is likely to elicit a more positive response than authoritative confrontation. Showing concern and interest in the other problems in their life, which may or may not be directly related to their substance use, will also be met with a more constructive level of engagement. If the young person is living at home, family interviews can be used conjointly, exclusively (for younger adolescents), or not at all, depending on the family situation. For more troubled teens, assessment and intervention guidelines for conduct disorder appear in chapter 13.

Assessment of substance abuse in young people demands an MDF approach similar to that use with adults (see chapter 6), with the understanding that there is likely to be a shorter substance-abuse history, and the points of concern are likely to focus on situational risks for negative consequences rather than a dependence syndrome (although that is a possibility that should always be checked). Signs of serious tolerance or withdrawal should be assessed, and a medical examination should check for drug use and sexually transmitted diseases (Buckstein, 1995). Type of substances used and careful estimates about the quantity and frequency of consumption are very important, but must be tied specifically to risks for acute health crises (e.g., alcohol poisoning) and other negative consequences, including psychological problems, interpersonal difficulties, academic and occupational deficits, general health concerns, and problems in the community. Since young people have problems that may be only co-incidentally associated with substance use, detailed functional assessment is needed to more closely tie their use to acute or chronic psychosocial problems.

Key questions guiding the functional assessment are the same as for adults: What types of substances? How much is used? How often? What are the psychological, emotional, interpersonal, occupational/academic consequences? The interviewer should be prepared to probe those areas that are most salient to youthful substance abuse and the individual's unique experiences. The use of alcohol and other drugs by the client is not a random event, and a detailed analysis of the drugs used, with whom, where, when, and under what circumstances will go a long way toward functionally tying substance use to key antecedents. These might include response to emotional distress, interpersonal problems, celebrations, and particular circumstances that may incur special risks, such as drinking or smoking pot while driving, on the job, during school hours, or as prelude to sexual encounters. A two-week charting of daily use patterns with special focus on problematic (excessive) use under risky circumstances will provide very helpful guidelines for early-intervention planning. Given that young people tend to underestimate the inherent risk in substance abuse, it may also be helpful to have them compare their average consumption level to established norms of their peers who may not consume as much as the student assumes (Read, Wood, Davidoff, McLacken, & Campbell, 2002). It also helps to explore psychological and emotional concerns, expectancies of alcohol's effects, and the specific circumstances within which a client abuses substances.

Instruments

A large number of alcohol screening, assessment, and diagnostic tools exist for adults (see chapter 6). Although some of them have been shown to have some utility for older adolescents (e.g., the AUDIT; Fleming, Barry, & MacDonald, 1991; O'Hare & Sherrer, 1999), many of them are not sensitive to the acute or contextually specific substance-use problems of young people. There are, however, a number of instruments designed for adolescents (see C. S. Martin & Winters, 1998 and Leccese & Waldron, 1994, for helpful reviews). Screens and assessment tools for adolescents tend to emphasize negative consequences of substance use associated with situational factors, rather than long-term indications of substance dependence. However, depression or interpersonal distress are not always reliable "proxy" indicators of substance abuse. Many young people, whether they drink or not, experience these problems. Thus, relying too heavily on co-occurring indicators may lead to a high level of false positives. Even first-hand accounts by significant others or "toxicology screens" can be misleading. Third parties may not be able to tell what substances were used, how much, or how often, and lab tests usually are not accurate indicators of quantity or frequency. Ultimately, there may be no adequate substitute for a thorough MDF assessment that is conducted in a comfortable environment where the young person can be open about substance use without fear of unreasonable reprisals.

Self-report instruments have been commonly used in survey research to detect and estimate the degree of negative consequences attributed to drinking (Wechsler et al., 1994; Wechsler et al., 2002). Although this approach may have some research utility, evidence of factorial validity or scale reliabilities are often not reported, and these data do not offer any validated taxonomy for categorizing different dimensions of problem drinking. Another instrument that addresses a range of psychosocial consequences associated with drinking, the Rutgers Alcohol Problem Inventory (H. R. White & Lebouvie, 1989), has been shown to correlate with various measures of abuse, but to have a relatively weak factor structure. Other instruments are available for more comprehensive substance-abuse assessment, but they often require a lengthy structured interview that is not practical where routine brief assessment tools are needed. Given the high prevalence of abusive drinking among young people, self-report screening devices that are brief, valid, and reliable are needed, so that practitioners can quickly evaluate and refer young people with drinking problems for further substance-abuse assessment and intervention.

The College Alcohol Problem Scale (CAPS) was developed and replicated with college students, mostly freshmen who were cited for breaking university drinking rules. Their age, their status as freshmen, and the fact that they got caught, suggest that this sample represents a group of young people at particular risk for problem drinking (O'Hare, 1997b; Maddock, Laforge, Rossi, & O'Hare, 2001). The original pool of twenty items was drawn from an array of instruments used in prominent college-drinking studies (e.g., O'Hare, 1990b; Wechsler & McFadden, 1979; Engs, 1977). Exploratory factor analysis was used with two separate samples to replicate the analysis of the same twenty items. Ten items were extracted for the original version of the scale, the CAPS. Chronbach alphas in both samples were comparable (socioemotional .88, .89; community .79, .76), and the CAPS demonstrated good concurrent validity with the quantity-frequency index, a version of the Michigan Alcoholism Screening Test (MAST), and peak drinking index from the AUDIT (O'Hare, 1997b; 1998b).

Using the same twenty items as in the original CAPS, Maddock et al. (2001) employed confirmatory factor analysis with a broader sample of university undergraduates to refine the original CAPS. The study resulted in an eight-item version, the CAPS-revised (CAPS-r) that defines two subscales similar to the original (instrument 16.1). One subscale is personal problems: feeling sad, blue, depressed; nervousness, irritability; feeling bad about oneself; and problems with appetite or sleeping. The other is social problems: engaged in unplanned sexual activity; drove under the influence; did not use protection when engaging in sex; and engaged in illegal activity associated with drug use. Internal consistency reliabilities were comparable to those of the original scale (personal problems alpha = .79, social problems alpha = .75).

The current eight-item version, printed here, requests that the respondent estimate the frequency with which they have experienced specific alcohol-related problems over the past year. Although there are no established norms, Mad-

---

INSTRUMENT 16.1   College Alcohol Problems Scale–Revised (CAPS-r)

Use the scale below to rate HOW OFTEN you have had any of the following problems over the past year <u>as a result of drinking alcoholic beverages</u>.

____1. Feeling sad, blue, or depressed
      1 Never   2 Yes, but not in the past year   3 1-2 times
      4 3-5 times   5 6-9 times   6 10 or more times

____2. Nervousness, irritability
      1 Never   2 Yes, but not in the past year   3 1-2 times
      4 3-5 times   5 6-9 times   6 10 or more times

____3. Caused you to feel bad about yourself
      1 Never   2 Yes, but not in the past year   3 1-2 times
      4 3-5 times   5 6-9 times   6 10 or more times

____4. Problems with appetite or sleeping
      1 Never   2 Yes, but not in the past year   3 1-2 times
      4 3-5 times   5 6-9 times   6 10 or more times

____5. Engaged in unplanned sexual activity
      1 Never   2 Yes, but not in the past year   3 1-2 times
      4 3-5 times   5 6-9 times   6 10 or more times

____6. Drove under the influence
      1 Never   2 Yes, but not in the past year   3 1-2 times
      4 3-5 times   5 6-9 times   6 10 or more times

____7. Did not use protection when engaging in sex
      1 Never   2 Yes, but not in the past year   3 1-2 times
      4 3-5 times   5 6-9 times   6 10 or more times

____8. Illegal activities associated with drug use
      1 Never   2 Yes, but not in the past year   3 1-2 times
      4 3-5 times   5 6-9 times   6 10 or more times

dock et al. surveyed over 700 undergraduates in a university in the northeast United States, and found the following mean scores: for personal problems, males 3.75, females 3.28; for social problems, males 3.47, females 4.93; and for total score, males 7.17, females 8.22. The CAPS-r can be used in an interview or as a self-report paper-and-pencil screen for identifying personal and social problems related to youthful drinking. Scores from individual items, subscales, and the global score (the sum of all eight items) can be used to establish baseline measures for assessment and to monitor and evaluate client response to early-intervention efforts (by changing the instructions from "past year" to "three months" or the start of treatment, etc., as needed). The CAPS-r takes about two to three minutes to administer, and requires only basic interviewing skills and knowledge of substance-abuse problems. The CAPS-r can be used use free of charge.

The Drinking Context Scale (DCS) was developed with college students (mostly freshmen of both sexes) cited their first time for breaking university drinking rules. Drinking context is defined here as a composite of social, emotional, and situational factors within which the respondent estimates the likelihood of drinking excessively (O'Hare, 1997a, 2001a). The DCS employs a continuous measurement scale, anchors respondents' view of alcohol use in their own drinking experience rather than their belief in drinking effects, and emphasizes the likelihood of drinking "excessively" (as defined subjectively by the respondent). Initial exploratory factor analysis resulted in three distinct subscales (convivial drinking, intimate drinking, drinking to cope with negative emotions, i.e., negative coping). The original scale accounted for 61.5% of the variance, and subscales demonstrated excellent internal reliabilities (.93, .89, and .90). These three subscales were moderately intercorrelated. Multiple analysis of variance demonstrated concurrent validity with the quantity-frequency index and a modified version of the MAST (O'Hare, 1997a). Later, a more rigorous assessment of the validity of the DCS (O'Hare, 2001a) was conducted with a similar population by employing confirmatory factor analysis with a much larger sample ($n = 505$) of participants in the same program. Results supported the validity and reliability of a nine-item version of the scale. Internal-consistency reliabilities were calculated for the three factor subscales of the DCS, and are convivial drinking, .82; intimate drinking, .81; and negative coping .85. These reliabilities are very good, considering the brevity of each subscale (longer scales tend to artificially inflate internal-consistency coefficients).

The DCS-9 (instrument 16.2) is a brief instrument that can be used as a screening device to identify at-risk drinking in young people, to augment assessment, or to monitor and evaluate early-intervention efforts. Identifying risky drinking contexts can provide an assessment/outcome framework for treatment planning and evaluation of coping-skills interventions that are described below. The individual items can be used as prompts within a qualitative interview to further explore excessive drinking within specific circumstances (e.g., when "partying," "before sex," when "angry" or "depressed"). The three subscales are easily summed, and a global measure of risky drinking can be obtained by sum-

INSTRUMENT 16.2   Drinking Context Scale (DCS)

Based on your <u>personal experience</u>, how would you RATE THE CHANCES that you might find yourself <u>drinking excessively</u> in the <u>following circumstances</u>? (Use the following scale to rate your responses.)

Extremely High	High	Moderate	Low	Extremely Low
5	4	3	2	1

Convivial drinking

When I'm at a party or similar other get-together	5	4	3	2	1
When I'm at a concert or other public event	5	4	3	2	1
When I'm celebrating something important to me	5	4	3	2	1

Intimate drinking

When I'm with my lover	5	4	3	2	1
When I'm on a date	5	4	3	2	1
Before having sex	5	4	3	2	1

Negative coping

When I've had a fight with someone close to me	5	4	3	2	1
When I'm feeling sad, depressed or discouraged	5	4	3	2	1
When I'm angry with myself or someone else	5	4	3	2	1

ming all nine items. No special training is required beyond basic interviewing skills and basic knowledge of alcohol problems in young people. Although no norms have been established, mean scores for 505 college students (O'Hare, 2001a) who were cited for underaged drinking are convivial drinking, 9.23; intimate drinking, 5.42; and negative coping, 4.30. Dividing each subscale total by three provides a relative mean that reflects the likelihood of drinking excessively within that context (4 = a "high" likelihood of drinking excessively). Dividing the total score for all items by nine also provides a relative mean reflecting the likelihood of drinking excessively. The DCS-9 is available for use at no charge.

SELECTING EFFECTIVE INTERVENTIONS

There is little compelling evidence that broad primary-prevention strategies targeted at reducing college drinking and associated problems have yielded substantively positive results (Moskowitz, 1989; Hanson & Engs, 1995; Werch, Pappas, & Castellon-Vogel, 1996; Wechsler et al., 2002; Clapp, Segars, & Voas, 2002; Walters, Bennett, & Noto, 2000). It may be more cost-effective in the long run to identify those young people who manifest problems with substance abuse, and offer them skill-based early-intervention programs. The link between substance abuse and risky sex also suggests that practitioners who work with young people incorporate good self-monitoring and coping skills to anticipate situations where sexual activity is likely, and work toward reducing negative consequences. This section reviews the evidence for effective early-intervention methods for adolescents and young adults who abuse alcohol and other drugs, and describes selected interventions.

As noted earlier in this chapter, most evidence-based early-intervention programs focus on harm reduction. This perspective is based on the assumption that many young people who experience psychosocial problems caused or exacerbated by substance use will benefit from modifying their use and developing better health-promoting coping skills (E. T. Miller, Turner, & Marlatt, 2001; Marlatt, 1996; Marlatt & Witkiewitz, 2002). Rather than mandating abstinence, an early-intervention approach with a goal of harm reduction addresses the relative risks associated with substance use and abuse, and targets problem and risk reduction along a continuum (which includes elective abstinence). A harm-reduction practitioner is less confrontational and emphasizes motivational engagement. The intervention follows a staged trajectory whereby the practitioner meets clients at their level of readiness to change, and collaboratively negotiates intervention goals through a guided process of weighing the pros and cons of altering substance-use patterns and related problem behaviors (Sobell et al., 1996).

Evidence-based early-intervention programs are overwhelmingly built upon social-cognitive theory and usually employ some combination of psychoeducation and cognitive-behavioral coping skills. Botvin and associates (e.g., Botvin, Baker, Dusenbury, Tortu, & Botvin 1990; Botvin, Griffin, Diaz, & Ifill-Williams, 2001) developed the Life Skills Training Program (LSTP), which has been shown in randomized trials to be effective at changing maladaptive cognitions linked to substance abuse. Although this program is technically a primary-prevention strategy, as it targets youths who have yet to evince a substance-use problem, it is included here as a good example of a more hands-on, skill-based, prevention effort similar to many current early-intervention models.

In describing the rationale for the program, Botvin et al. (1990) note the social-cognitive foundation for the curriculum, and emphasize the use of coping skills to help youths stop or avoid initiating drug use through a combination of psychoeducation, changing expectancies, and practicing drug-refusal skills. A three-year randomized controlled study was undertaken to test the efficacy of the LSTP. The goals of the program were to reduce cigarette smoking and use of alcohol and marijuana. Participants were educated about actual prevalence rates, (to provide norms to debunk the notion that "everybody's doing it"; examined the social acceptability and negative consequences of use; and practiced substance-refusal skills to improve self-efficacy in social situations. Fifty-six schools participated in the study, and pre- and posttest data were successfully collected from over 4,000 mostly white seventh graders. Students were randomly assigned to three conditions: (1) the LSTP (provided by a live trainer), (2) a videotaped version of the training, and (3) a no-treatment control group. The LSTP is designed to be implemented in twelve modules over fifteen class periods. Teaching techniques include lecture, demonstration, role-playing and performance feedback, reinforcement, and homework assignments. Student participants get "booster" sessions in the eighth and ninth grades to reinforce material learned in the seventh-grade training program. Teachers are trained in the LSTP in a one-day workshop, which includes the use of a program manual. Fidelity checks were regularly made of randomly selected classroom presentations of the program. Outcome measures included standard quantity and frequency measures for substance use, and standardized scales to assess changes in knowledge, assertiveness, and expectancies. Significantly less cigarette and marijuana smoking were found in both treatment conditions versus the control group, although overall mean differences were not substantive. In addition, no differences in alcohol consumption level was found between groups. Knowledge and attitudes toward substance use and the use of substance-refusal skills appeared to show a significant mediating effect for the active treatments versus the control group. Although results from the initial study appear to be modest, long-term follow-up data demonstrated some positive effects lasting until the end of high school (Botvin, Baker, Dusenbury, Botvin, & Diaz, 1995). For those students who received reasonably complete versions of the intervention, there were 44% and 66% fewer drug and polydrug users, respectively, in the treatment group.

Given that high school students who drink heavily tend to continue their drinking patterns into early adulthood, college freshmen may be the most likely to benefit from early-intervention methods (Marlatt & Witkiewitz, 2002). In one of the earlier CBT interventions for college students with mild to moderate drinking problems, Kivlahan, Marlatt, Fromme, Coppel, and Williams (1990) randomly assigned forty-three moderate problem drinkers (mean age twenty-three) to three conditions: a moderation-oriented CBT skills course, an alcohol information class, and an "assessment only" group. The CBT skills course (eight weeks) included models of addiction, consequences of alcohol abuse, estimating blood alcohol levels, moderate drinking skills, training in relaxation and nutrition coupled with encouragement to engage in aerobic exercise, monitoring and coping more assertively with risky drinking situations, challenging erroneous alcohol expectancies, and relapse-prevention skills to adhere better to one's self-imposed limits and rules concerning moderate drinking. The alcohol information class (also eight weeks long) consisted of a traditional medical-educational model that included films and lectures about the effects of alcohol and other drugs, family and legal aspects, and related topics. Several drinking measures, including self-monitoring charts, were employed with all three groups. Data were collected at baseline, and 4-, 8-, and 12-month follow-ups. Results showed no significant differences between the groups, but an encouraging trend toward less drinking in the CBT skills group.

A later replication of this skills approach (Baer et al., 1992) compared a six-week (ninty-minute) classroom training to individualized feedback based on motivational interviewing methods. Both treatment groups demonstrated comparable and substantive findings: an approximately 40% drop in alcohol consumption was maintained over a two-year period.

Marlatt et al. (1998) tested the effectiveness of a very brief motivational interview (see W. R. Miller & Rollnick, 1991; Heather, 1995) with individualized feedback for college freshmen who had filled out questionnaires regarding drinking and associated problems after they had been admitted to the university during their senior year of high school. Three hundred and forty-eight students were randomly assigned to either brief intervention or an assessment-only control group. Those assigned to brief treatment (which was provided in the winter of their freshman year) were also given self-monitoring cards and asked to track their drinking on a daily basis two weeks prior to the intervention. The motivational intervention was used to review the student's individual data, encourage students to compare their drinking with reported peer drinking norms, examine personal risk factors for problem drinking (e.g., family history of substance abuse), draw their own conclusions about their personal drinking habits and potential problems, and consider modifying their drinking to reduce negative consequences. In keeping with motivational enhancement principles, arguing with the student and direct confrontation were avoided.

In the second year of the study, students were mailed personalized feedback (comparing their data with college norms) based on data collected at baseline, and six- and twelve-month follow-ups. Those participants categorized as "high" and "extreme" risk were contacted for further motivational interviewing, and many accepted. Overall, outcomes revealed that those high-risk students demonstrated significantly greater reduction in problem drinking than students in the control group over a two-year follow-up period. Nevertheless, clinical significance of the changes was modest, and these high-risk students were still reporting more drinking and drinking-related consequences than the average college student. At the two-year follow-up, high-risk students who had received the motivational interview module were doing better than high-risk controls (L. J. Roberts, Neal, Kivlahan, Baer, & Marlatt, 2000), and the benefits continued to accrue over all four years of college (Baer, Kivlahan, Blume, Arthur, W. McKnight, & Marlatt, 2001). Overall, the intervention was considered by students to be "user friendly" and relevant to their everyday concerns. The program appeared to be useful as an initial prevention effort that, if unsuccessful, could be followed up with more intensive treatment as needed.

J. G. Murphy et al. (2001) and Borsari and Carey (2000) found similar results for brief intervention (motivational interview coupled with providing normative feedback) in randomized controlled trials. Overall, it appears that early-intervention methods using motivational engagement, CBT skills, and harm-reduction goals are the most promising approaches available for reducing substance use and related problems in adolescents and young adults (Larimer & Cronce, 2002).

Although early-intervention literature is disproportionately focused on college students, data on other groups are now forthcoming. In a controlled trial,

Monti et al. (1999) compared motivational interviewing (i.e., empathic listening, avoiding argument, highlighting discrepancies, engendering self-efficacy and self-determination) with standard care (brief admonitions against drinking and driving) offered in a busy urban hospital emergency room. Participants were ninety-four young adults, eighteen to nineteen years old, randomly assigned to each condition. Measures were taken on alcohol-use patterns, related problems, questions on drinking and driving, episodes of drinking and driving, and related indicators. Retrospective baseline was taken for the previous twelve months, with further measures taken at baseline and three- and six-month follow-up intervals. Results demonstrated that six months after their intial interview, the motivational interview group showed a significant reduction in drinking and driving and other social problems, and only half the number of alcohol-related injuries of the control group. Department of Motor Vehicle records showed significantly fewer moving violations for the motivational group versus the standard-care group. Monti et al. (2001), having reviewed the motivational enhancement literature with adolescents, concluded that motivational interviewing has shown harm-reduction benefits for alcohol and marijuana use for both older and younger adolescents, particularly with more resistant youths.

Exemplar Study: Generalizing Botvin et al.'s Work to Young People of Color.   Building on earlier work with the LSTP, Botvin et al. (2001) implemented a similar program in a randomized control trial (treatment versus standard New York City prevention curriculum) with predominantly African-American and Hispanic urban minority youth. The experimental program was like that described in Botvin et al. (1990), and was provided in fifteen sessions in the seventh grade, with ten booster sessions in the eighth grade. Standard indexes of alcohol consumption (including binge drinking), and drinking-related variables (e.g., knowledge, perceived benefits, normative expectations of peer use) were employed as outcome measures. Eighty percent of the participants completed pre- and posttest data at one year, although only 58% provided complete data in the second year of the program. As with the previous study, those who dropped out were also more likely to be heavier alcohol users, although rate of attrition did not differ between the two treatment conditions. The intervention resulted in a 57% decrease in binge drinking at both one- and two-year follow-ups as well as improvement in alcohol-related knowledge, attitudes, and peer drinking expectations. Thus, the study provides substantive evidence that skill-based large-scale prevention programs based on harm-reduction principles designed initially for white students can be implemented effectively with urban students of color.

Overall, while these studies show the potential effectiveness of such programs, consistent implementation and attrition remain a considerable challenge. In some cases, students with the greatest need for help may be those who are least likely to participate actively in such programs. For example, Moncher and Schinke (1994) implemented a similar CBT skill-based prevention approach to reduce smoking and smokeless tobacco use in Native American youth in grades six and seven, but showed few significant results. A. N. Weisz and Black (2001) conducted a small quasi-experimental study that demonstrated that a violence-prevention program could improve knowledge and attitudes regarding sexual assault and dating violence among African-American inner-city youths. Although results were promising, there remains a need for more controlled investigations of prevention and early-intervention research with multiproblem youths of color.

Descriptions of Effective Interventions

Early-intervention programs for youths engaged in risky behaviors share many elements. These approaches are typically given in a classroom or counseling setting, and include a combination of the following: education regarding alcohol and its effects (physical and psychological factors), cognitive modification (changing erroneous expectancies and perceived norms regarding others' drinking and drug-use habits), and coping-skills training (e.g., self-monitoring skills, setting and keeping targets for number of drinks, estimating blood alcohol level, drink-refusal practices, practicing safe sex). These programs emphasize psychoeducation and skills training to help young people survive this period of their lives by avoiding and negotiating high-risk situations to reduce negative consequences (harm to self or others), or achieve and maintain abstinence. Below, the key components of a well-regarded Alcohol Skills Training Program (ASTP) developed at the University of Washington are presented. These elements exemplify the state of the art of early-intervention programming for youth (relevant research was examined above). The main components of the program are outlined here (see E. T. Miller, Kilmer, et al., 2001).

1. Be flexible and approachable, and establish a good rapport with students. Clearly communicate the philosophy of ASTP, emphasizing informed choices versus prohibition, and showing respect for the choice of drinking goals that individuals make: moderation or abstinence. Confidentiality among the members is stressed.

2. Help students assess their own use by identifying and gauging discrepancies between their current drinking patterns (including reviewing the definition of a standard drink) and self-designed drinking goals. Help them compare their own drinking to actual drinking norms in the college community. Students who appear to have more serious problems and may be developing a dependence on alcohol or other drugs should be referred for primary substance-abuse intervention.

3. Provide an information-based lecture/discussion regarding basic pharmacology and physiological processes associated with drinking alcohol. This information should include absorption, metabolism, blood alcohol levels (BALs), tolerance, withdrawal, dependence, and cross-tolerance. (See chapter 6 and other relevant texts regarding these topics.)

4. Define and discuss BAL in more detail, along with psychophysiological effects of different BALs, and factors that influence BAL (e.g., rate and amount of drinking, gender, individual's weight).

5. Emphasize the psychological and behavioral effects associated with BAL and the "biphasic" response to alcohol (pleasing effects at lower levels, risks that occur at higher levels). Students should also generate and examine their own positive and negative beliefs and expectancies regarding drinking. Young people are encouraged to judge where the "point of diminishing returns" is likely to be for them, and to heed injunctions to avoid behaviors that are more likely to result in negative consequences at higher levels of consumption. Examine the role of tolerance as an indicator of a potentially serious problem, and examine the effects of alcohol when combined with other drugs.

6. Teach students to monitor their own drinking behavior. Now that the participants are more knowledgeable about drinking and its effects, they should put this knowledge into action. Although the exercises do not require or encourage students to drink, participants are taught to monitor their own consumption rate and the effects. Self-monitoring also emphasizes an analysis of the context of drinking: where they were, with whom, in what situation, in what frame of mind, and so forth.

7. Participants review their self-monitoring charts relative to their initial self-assessments and standard BAL chart. Assist them in reassessing how much they drank (including reviewing their heaviest drinking episode), help them evaluate how well they performed relative to their initial self-assessment, and relate these results to what they now know about alcohol metabolism and their own BAL estimates.

8. Help students review and debunk some of the erroneous beliefs they may hold regarding the positive effects of drinking. Help them gauge how much these effects are the result of alcohol versus their own behavior.

9. Reinforce the notion of moderation and not exceeding BALs above .05–.06. The emphasis at this point is to focus on skills to enhance moderate drinking and to reduce risks associated with heavier drinking. These skills include setting predetermined drinking limits, tracking the number of drink equivalents, spacing drinks over time, alternating drinks with nonalcoholic drinks, avoiding drinking games, using drink-refusal skills, and engaging in alternative nondrinking activities. Other skills include avoiding excessive drinking in situations where sexual activity is more likely, and planning for alternative transportation if needed.

10. At the final session, summarize key points about the program, keep the floor open to follow-up questions, and evaluate the program. Help students plan for the future should they consider changes in drinking habits down the road or require referrals for further help.

As with substance abuse, prevention research has repeatedly demonstrated that information provision alone is not associated with a reduction in risky sexual behaviors (Basen-Engquist, 1992; A. O'Leary, 1992; Raj, 1996). Growing evidence, however, has suggested that applying social-cognitive principles and skills (similar to those above) with at-risk young people can enhance self-efficacy and coping skills regarding drinking and safer sex (Darkes & Goldman, 1993; Sikkema, Winett, & Lombard, 1995). Programs that enhance a young person's skills in recognizing antecedent factors (i.e., thoughts, feelings, behaviors, and situations) and using skills that will reduce substance abuse and avoid unplanned/unprotected sex have been shown to be moderately effective.

IMPLEMENTING AND EVALUATING THE EVIDENCE-BASED INTERVENTION PLAN

CASE STUDY: ISABEL

Isabel, a nineteen-year old college freshman, arrived in the college health service to have a rash looked at. After a brief discussion and a couple of tests, the doctor told her that she had contracted syphilis. Upset and tearful, she was assured by the doctor that, at this stage of the disease, she would be easily cured with proper treatment. She also told Isabel that she should use more discretion in her choice of sexual partners, and insist that they use a condom. A nurse took a little more history, and queried her about her sexual activities in more depth. The discussion led to a screening for use of alcohol and other drugs. Isabel reported that she did like to party with her friends, and, on occasion, engaged in unplanned sex. She said she had been sexually active since she was fourteen, and thought she had learned to be careful. The nurse asked her if she had been intoxicated at the time of these encounters, and she reported that she probably wouldn't have slept with many of her partners unless she had

been. The nurse suggested Isabel make an appointment at the college counseling center to address these behaviors that appeared to be placing her at risk.

During her first visit with the social worker, Jen, Isabel discussed the conversation she had with the health-center nurse, and admitted that perhaps she took a few too many chances over the years. She felt fortunate that she had not contracted HIV. Jen queried her about the amount she consumed before engaging in these "spontaneous sexual adventures" (Isabel's phrase), and was told that usually smoked some pot and drank about six or seven drinks. She said she never drove a car during these times, but made sure she had a place to sleep. Often "it was some guy's place, so hanging out after the party was a good idea, and usually led to other stuff." How long had Isabel felt that she had been drinking too much? "Since I was in high school, about 15 or 16."

Multidimensional-Functional Assessment: Defining Problems and Goals

Jen said she wanted to get more background to understand better how this pattern of sexual activity and substance abuse evolved. Isabel told Jen that she came from Guatemala illegally with her mother when she was six years old to visit her aunt in Texas. She never knew her biological father. When she arrived, her mother told her that they were going to stay in the United States. After staying with her aunt for a little while, her mother met a man, Jim, and moved to the northeast United States. Jim was a bit older than her mother and was a long-haul truck driver, so he was gone for a week or so at a time. Isabel had the impression that her mother liked this man, and he seemed generally nice to both of them. Isabel eventually went to school, although by the time she started, she was a little older than the other children. Later, she found out that her mother had paid a lawyer to straighten out "paperwork" so they could stay in the United States. Her mother worked as a cleaning woman for companies that tended private homes, worked for catering companies, and did other related domestic-service work. The relationship with Jim seemed to work out over time. He wasn't around much, and Isabel recalls many times feeling like a "regular family." She eventually called Jim "Dad." Isabel learned to speak English very well, because she started school fairly young, and was an excellent student. She met other Guatemalans in her classes and other students of Hispanic background, so she kept up her Spanish as well.

When she was about twelve, Jim began to treat her a bit differently and began to show some interest in her sexually. Isabel was very uncomfortable with Jim when he pressed up against her. She remembers Jim saying that it was "all right, cause we're not really having sex. I just need you to sit on my lap for a few minutes." He was never rough, and treated her a little special after that, and she didn't want to upset her mother. Having heard about "stuff like this" in school, she knew it was wrong, but was afraid of the problems that would result if she told her mother or any of the teachers her "secret."

Jim's conduct continued intermittently for a while, usually when Isabel's mom was working late. After a couple of years, Isabel started dating other boys, and strangely, Jim didn't object much. She felt him pull away from her, but nothing more was said about it. Isabel didn't discuss it with anyone, and found herself more and more engaged with friends her own age. She was quite popular in high school, and had many friends and acquaintances. She continued to do very well in school, applied for college, was accepted at several schools, and decided to go to one out of state.

When Jen asked her how she felt about moving away, Isabel responded that she felt a little sad, but that she knew it was a good idea. She called her mother often, and said that her mother seemed to be pretty happy with her situation. Although she had generally enjoyed herself in high school, she now reported feeling "down in the dumps" at times. Spending time with friends seemed to help her, but she spent an increasing amount of time "getting high" with friends and drinking. She also found that she was very popular with the young men at school, and she developed an active sex life. She liked to please them, was told she was "good at it," and felt that she had an "edge" over the other girls. Despite some of the partying, she kept up her grades. School remained important to her. She felt it would be a way of avoiding having to work menial jobs as her mother did. She was appreciative of her mother's struggles, felt lucky about going to college, and took little for granted.

Jen asked her how often she felt depressed, and she responded that it seemed to be associated with some of the heavier partying. She would feel a bit lethargic for a day or so, and sometimes regretted her sexual encounters. But the feelings would usually dissipate, more or less. She sometimes wondered if this pattern were a problem, but given the amount of partying she witnessed around the dorm, she didn't feel all that different from the others. The social worker then queried her about why she came for counseling, if things weren't so bad. She responded that "getting syphilis scared me, and there's still the HIV thing. I'm afraid I'll get drunk, do something stupid, and get AIDS. I also have found that the work is harder in college, and I am afraid that I might fall behind. It's just that it is hard to say no when you are used to partying with people. I guess I could slow it down a bit, I'm just not sure how. I also don't know what to do about the sex thing. Sometimes I want to, sometimes I don't, but I often feel like it's expected of me. I've also never really had a steady boyfriend. That concerns me. Like 'what's wrong with me? Why am I different?' Sometimes it makes me feel lonely just having sex with these guys and forgetting about it," she laughed. Jen responded that there appeared to be pros and cons to the whole situation. Partying and being with friends was fun, and sex can be enjoyable too, but there appeared to be some drawbacks with her current repertoire. Jen reassured Isabel that no one was putting any pressure on her to change. She suggested that Isabel seemed to know that some "adjustments" were in order, and perhaps they could discuss how she would like to go about making them. Isabel expressed relief that she wasn't going to be "therapized to death" about her "issues," and agreed that the next step was up to her.

In the next session, Jen led a more detailed discussion about Isabel's moodiness, substance abuse, and casual sex. She asked Isabel to describe her "typical week" from one day to the next, and talk about her usual daily routine. According to Isabel, Mondays were a bit slow, but "who likes Mondays anyway?" The social worker asked her to elaborate. "I usually get some schoolwork done on Sundays, but not as much as I need to. I'm usually a little hung over, and I still feel the effects on Monday. I think it bothers my sleep." The social worker reflected: "So you start off with a deficit on Monday morning." She continued that Tuesdays and Wednesdays were pretty productive. Without partying, she got most of her work done. "I am actually feeling pretty good going into Thursday night. Then the partying starts." Isabel then described the next couple of days: dragging herself through her classes and then "partying bigtime" on Friday night. "That's when I usually get really messed up, hook up with someone, and wake up with some guy on Saturday morning. Saturdays are usually a lost day, and, sometimes, Saturday night I just go back to my dorm and hang out alone. Saturday night is more of a 'date night' for some of the girls, but that hasn't been my thing."

Together, Jen and Isabel tried to connect the dots. From Thursday evening until Sunday, it appears that Isabel was feeling regretful about compromising her ability to get things done, felt somewhat depressed due to the excessive drinking (six to eight "mixed drinks," she estimated), and marijuana use, and felt depressed and somewhat regretful and lonely in response to the casual sexual encounters. The social worker facetiously quipped, "So, from Thursdays to Sunday it's sex, drugs, and rock and roll . . . what's not to like?" Isabel responded, "Me. I don't like the way I am. I think I need to make some changes." They decided that next visit they would talk about what it was, specifically, that she would like to change.

During the following visit, they agreed that her moodiness, negative view of herself, mediocre academic performance, and risky sexual activities appeared to be related in some way. The rest of the discussion focused on which problem to address first, and how to approach each of these problems in a stepwise manner. It seemed that, perhaps, the excessive drinking and pot smoking were the immediate catalyst that usually "gets the ball rolling." Perhaps Isabel could try cutting down a bit, changing her drinking patterns, slowing down her consumption rate, and being more careful about what (and how much absolute alcohol) she was actually consuming.

Jen decided to summarize what they now knew about the problem before they discussed a list of treatment priorities. Isabel appeared to be drinking more than she realized. When they discussed quantity, it became apparent that she was usually consuming mixed drinks that either she or someone else poured. Since she preferred vodka-based drinks, she knew that the beverage was 80 proof (40% alcohol), but she didn't know how much she was actually drinking. She was under the impression that they were "strong" drinks because she could really taste the vodka. So Isabel was probably consuming considerably more than she thought, maybe ten to twelve drink equivalents rather than six or seven. In reviewing the consequences of consumption, she felt that her drinking was contributing to her mild to moderate depression, and increasing the chances of engaging in casual sex (which she only did when she was drunk). The casual sex was adding to her negative opinions about herself and "getting in the way" of her developing a different kind of relationship with men. Substance abuse was compromising the quality of her work, because she lacked the concentration and energy she needed for her studies. This sub-par performance was adding to her self-doubt and negative view of herself.

When they both discussed the context of drinking, it appeared that it was partly to join in and have fun, but it was also a "setup" for casual sex with an undetermined partner. Often she paid little heed to whether her partner was using protection. Although Isabel did not consider that she was deliberately using alcohol to cope with negative feelings, she considered the possibility that she had developed this pattern by drinking to cover up negative feelings about herself that she did not quite understand. They both agreed that the amount she drank needed to be assessed more carefully, and that it was very likely that cutting down would have a positive impact on her mood, her work, her choice of sex partners, and how she felt about herself.

Selecting and Designing the Intervention: Defining Strategies and Objectives

Isabel agreed to engage in a period of self-monitoring for a week to examine the exact amount of alcohol she was consuming, examine her thoughts and feelings in the specific "partying" circumstances she found herself in, and carefully consider the consequences. Jen suggested that she might consider cutting down or eliminating her marijuana use, and packing some condoms. They both designed a self-monitoring chart to record the day, the amount of alcohol consumed (she agreed to pour her own drinks), the situation, what she was thinking, how she was feeling, and what notable events occurred that evening. She also agreed to record any reflections the day after having had sexual relations. This period would take two weeks, and she agreed to keep her visit the following week to provide a progress report and troubleshoot any problems with the self-monitoring process.

After two weeks of self-assessment, they dicussed the results. The first week, Isabel measured her own drinks and realized that she had been consuming much more than she thought. When she measured her own, she was less intoxicated and, although she was attracted to one of the young men at the fraternity party, felt less inclined to "jump into bed" and able to better exercise discretion. She did not know if this was due to actually drinking less, or whether she was just paying more attention to the amount she was drinking and thinking about her choices. She also noticed on the second week that she drank a lot more, even though she was measuring her own drinks. She figured, "What the heck, I was good last week, I'm going to live it up this time." She did, and reported a negative experience with a young man who became somewhat aggressive. Being experienced in these matters, she was able to be very aggressive back, skillfully took advantage of an inherent vulnerability, and "successfully discouraged him." But she was shaken by the experience. She also recorded that the next day "I felt like crap about myself, and didn't get a thing done all day. That kind of sums up my situation, don't you think?" Jen responded, "Sounds to me like you've been sorting these things out for yourself."

Isabel seemed more than ready to make some "adjustments," so they agreed to get more specific about intervention objectives (table 16.1). They decided that the first objective would be to cut her alcohol consumption in half. They decided, that given her body weight, she could consume about four drinks over a six-hour evening. This change would help keep her blood alcohol level to a minimum, and would probably reduce her chances of making impulsive decisions. Jen suggested that she continue to pour and measure her own drinks (Isabel poured out one shot of vodka at her place to see what it looked like at the bottom of a plastic cup), and drink more slowly during the party, occasionally topping up the cup with just tonic water or fruit juice and seltzer. She also decided to replace every other drink with straight seltzer and a twist. The following two weeks she reported successfully cutting down her consumption by about half, and was feeling pretty good about getting more of her work done.

Her second objective was to avoid sleeping with anyone until she had a gone on a date with them at least one time. By the fourth visit, she also reported not "going home with anyone. But, I'm not sure how I feel about it." She had not yet agreed to date anyone, although she had been asked. She decided to wait on any decisions indefinitely. Considering this objective led to a more in-depth discussion about how she felt about men in general, and it became apparent that for much of her life she felt a mix of resentment and desire to please them and be liked in return. When Jen asked her to reflect on important relationships with men that she had in her life, she could only think of her "quasi-stepfather, Jim," who she felt some affection for, but also felt that he had betrayed her by "using me to get himself off." She decided that she might like to try a different type of arrangement with a male friend, but was not ready to try "dating" yet. That objective would remain on hold for a while.

Her third objective was to improve the quality of her schoolwork. She decided that, since she was drinking less, she could get up earlier on weekend mornings and put in some more time in the library. She decided that she would spend five hours working on her schoolwork every Saturday morning and five on Sunday in addition to the work she put in Monday through Wednesday. She felt this would double her productivity.

Her fourth objective was to start feeling better physically, to have more energy, and to feel better about her appearance. The social worker told her that if she stuck with it, the effects of exercise were sure to reduce stress, and symptoms of depression, and to improve her sleep and concentration. She decided to join a women's exercise class on campus where they combined aerobics with weight training. She saw herself as a physical person, but only intermittently had engaged in regular vigorous exercise. It would also give her the opportunity to meet some new women friends. Before the next session, she had already enrolled.

CBT skills training conducted within a motivational-enhancement/harm-reduction model seemed to be a promising approach to take, given Isabel's particular constellation of problems. Motivational engagement, psychoeducation, self-monitoring, drinking-moderation skills, cognitive therapy for depression, self-regulatory skills, and exercise for stress reduction seemed like a promising package that could be uniquely tailored for Isabel's needs. Jen's application of motivational interviewing helped Isabel to become quickly engaged in the process of weighing the pros and cons of her behaviors for herself, rather than feeling lectured or judged about them. She was already thinking about changing when she came in, and the social worker helped her move forward in a more purposeful and focused way. Jen also helped her experience a relationship with a female as collaborator, in a give-and-take helping relationship, something she had not had very often. She knew that she often kept her distance from other women, and preferred the company of men. Because her relationships with men were ephemeral, she often felt deeply alone. Self-monitoring helped her make tentative linkages among her current difficulties, and it even helped her obtain some insight into possible origins of problems that she had been experiencing for a long time. Cognitive methods helped her challenge her expectancies about drinking, which she erroneously thought was facilitating her encounters with men. An examination of the contextual aspects of her drinking also helped her understand what purpose it was serving—not just to have fun, but as a way of blocking out difficult feelings and fears she was having about encountering men in a more meaningful kind of relationship. Planned drink refusal and moderation skills helped her reduce the overall level of alcohol consumption, a change that had immediate positive effects on her behavior, mood, energy level, concentration, and academic performance. Regular vigorous exercise also helped her regulate stress, feel better about herself, and make friends with women who followed a more balanced and healthful lifestyle. As Isabel made progress over the following few weeks, she was also able to begin to talk about her loneliness, her anger and resentment at her stepfather, and her fears about encountering both men and women on a more honest and intimate level.

Selecting Scales and Creating Indexes to Monitor and Evaluate Client Progress

A uniquely designed self-monitoring chart served as an excellent assessment and evaluation tool; it provided Isabel with the opportunity to focus on and accurately record the actual number of drinks she was having (once she measured how much absolute alcohol she was really consuming), her daily mood (excellent, good, fair, poor), and the situational factors related to her thoughts, feelings, and behaviors (table 16.1). She was able to examine these changes over time,

TABLE 16.1   The client service plan for Isabel

Problems	Goals	Sample Objectives	Interventions	Assessment Tools
Excessive alcohol consumption (10–12 drinks during an evening once a week; less on one other evening); sometimes accompanied by marijuana use	Reduce alcohol consumption to a moderate level; cut down on pot use, ideally eliminate it	Develop self-monitoring chart with social worker; record thoughts, feelings, behaviors, and situational factors; count number of drinks; reduce number of measured drinks (1.5 oz. of absolute alcohol per drink) to 4 drinks over	Motivational interviewing, CBT moderation and self-regulation skills with harm-reduction goals; Self-monitoring and moderation skills, including blood alcohol estimating, moderation training (eat beforehand, skipping	AUDIT as a screening tool to provide feedback to client regarding level of drinking problem; Self-monitoring indexes and charting for measuring number of drinks, mood level, behaviors, consequences, and narrative reflections

Problems	Goals	Sample Objectives	Interventions	Assessment Tools
		the course of the evening Have at least one date with a person before sleeping with him; get to know him a bit	drinks, drinking more slowly, etc.); challenging alcohol expectancies, and examining drinking contexts and likely consequences	CAPS-r as assessment and monitoring tool to estimate self-anchored level of personal and social problems related to drinking
Unplanned and sometimes unprotected sex	Avoid spontaneous sexual activity; always insist on protection	Plan an activity with a woman friend on at least one occasion; plan a date with a male acquaintance	Cognitive therapy to focus on the quality of her relationships, her fears and inhibitions regarding intimacy, and experimenting with getting to know a male companion better before having sex	DCS as assessment and monitoring tool to examine context-specific excessive drinking
Lack of intimacy with others; no close female friends; little history of male intimate relationships	Develop better friendships and a "dating" relationship before having sex	Record and monitor mood as part of self-monitoring chart		
Moderate symptoms of depression; poor concentration, sleep disturbance, dysphoric mood; negative feelings about herself	Reduce symptoms of depression to a minimum: improve mood, sleep, concentration, etc.	Structure 5 hours on Saturday and Sunday mornings to work in the library	Examine female relationships, sense of distance with other women; explore female friendships as well	
Concerns about academic performance	Increase study time by 100%; grades are expected to improve as a result		Consider further examination of her feelings regarding having been molested by her stepfather, once drinking and risky sex are under control	
			Joined an exercise class on campus; would exercise vigorously twice per week	
			Discussed self-regulation skills: problem solving and time management to encourage consistency and plan rewards after each study session	

and using the chart gave her a personal and critical role in evaluating her own progress. The initial use of the AUDIT revealed that she was scoring above the cutoff score of eight (see chapter 6), and was well within the "problem drinking" range. The CAPS-r helped her identify that she was experiencing both personal (depression, feeling bad about herself) and social (risky sex activities) problems, in part as a result of drinking, and the DCS helped her identify the circumstances in which she was drinking excessively. When used repeatedly, every two weeks or so, the self-monitoring chart and these scales provided a helpful evaluative framework to judge her treatment progress.

SUMMARY

The excitement and adventure of adolescence and young adulthood also ushers in risks that, while not unique to young people, are considerably increased by inexperience and other psychosocial vulnerabilities associated with that time of life. Assessment for young people who abuse substances and engage in risky sexual behavior should emphasize a contextually defined functional analysis. Scales are available to help qualitatively probe for idiographic detail of the young person's risky behaviors, and to provide quantitative data to gauge problem severity and track changes over time. A combination of motivational interviewing; psychoeducation about drinking, drugs, and their effects; self-monitoring; and practicing moderation skills has been shown to be the most promising early-intervention method to date. More outcome research and program evaluation, however, must be conducted with noncollege youth and young people of color, many of whom are at greater risk due to socioeconomic factors.

AFTERWORD: THE FUTURE OF EVIDENCE-BASED PRACTICE IN SOCIAL WORK

Predicting the future is probably an effort best left for fools. Nevertheless, predict we must, or at least speculate in an informed way to the best of our ability. I am convinced that the drive toward evidence-based practice will continue into the foreseeable future for social work and the allied professions. I feel convinced of this because I cannot envision a viable future for social work if it does not pursue an evidence-based approach to providing human services. What would a "nonevidence-based" strategy look like, anyway?

For starters, there will unfortunately be no shortage of clients for some time to come. Social policies informed by the human sciences have a long way to go before the major problems-in-living in our society and elsewhere in the world are resolved. Problems not on the verge of extinction include serious mental illnesses, the effects of trauma on children and adults, domestic and community violence, the abuse and neglect of children, substance abuse and dependence, developmental disabilities, chronic and deadly diseases, homelessness and poverty, and the effects of war, dislocation, and terrorism. Readers know the list is much longer. Although clinical social workers focus on helping individuals, families, and small groups cope as best they can with the psychosocial consequences of these problems, scientific advances and major domestic and foreign policy improvements will have to evolve much further before these difficulties and disorders can be minimized.

One advance that I believe will occur is a greater degree of quality and uniformity in the conduct of evidence-based assessment across various fields of practice. Qualitative assessment protocol will become more and more structured, to ensure that key domains of human behavior and risk factors are reliably considered in routine practice. The adjunctive use of quantitative instruments will also increase as a way of measuring key elements of assessment and providing a basis for individual and program evaluation. Some fields of practice that do not currently have well-defined assessment protocol or adequate screening and assessment tools will require research to develop them.

Similar changes are ahead for social work interventions. Practices based on little more than theoretical or political musings, on references to uncontrolled studies, or solely on the practitioner's experience are not likely to survive. Although personal style and creativity will always have a place in practice, social workers will be increasingly expected to graduate from schools of social work with a firm foundation in evidence-based interventions. Further training, supervision, and consultation in evidence-based practice will be expected. Testing and credentialing will also need to reflect advances in sound human behavior theory, valid assessment protocol, evidence-based interventions, and research and evaluation methods. In the classroom, academic instructors will be challenged to balance "academic freedom" with ethical mandates to teach practices for which there is a substantive body of evidence from controlled research.

The future of research and evaluation also looms as a challenge. Most social workers (including me) did not apply to MSW schools because they wanted to become researchers. They applied because they wanted to help others. However, practitioners are now expected to be knowledgeable consumers of research in order to understand and critically interpret what makes for "best practices." In addition, an increasing number of MSW students will need more education to actively engage in research in order to advance knowledge of human behavior, develop assessment tools for social work clients and practitioners, and, especially, conduct outcome and evaluation research that tests the efficacy and effectiveness of social work practices. If the bulk of knowledge building is left to the allied helping professions, social work runs the risk of losing its unique character and mission.

I don't think that scenario will come to pass, however, and here are my reasons. Social work has always had a unique commitment to some of the more disenfranchised members of our society: the disabled, the poor, people of color, gays, and people otherwise out of the mainstream. Not only is that commitment an important part of our calling, it is also where the greatest opportunities are for further research in assessment intervention methods. Schools of social work that develop strong doctoral programs and cultivate a farm team of prospective Ph.D. students from their MSW programs can help move the profession forward at an aggressive pace. However, these programs will have to eschew political rhetoric and ideology as a substitute for rigorous training in research methods.

Whether the funds for helping social work clients originate in the private sector, the public sector, or (more likely) some combination of both, this financing will no longer flow without greatly improved forms of accountability. Practitioner-researchers who are more interested in conducting evaluation in the field rather than in controlled research settings should find the future of human service agencies somewhat exciting. One of the great needs in agencies is for practitioner-evaluators who can help management develop and implement evaluation systems that improve human service delivery and provide data for external reporting requirements. Such data bases can also provide a foundation for grant writing and research.

Despite some residual ambivalence, support for the adoption of evidence-based practices in social work and the allied professions is growing (G.T. Wilson,

1996; Howard & Jenson, 1999; Fortune & Proctor, 2001; E. Proctor, 2003). Evidence-based practices are being promoted by a wide range of influential professional and governmental bodies (Beutler, Clarkin, & Bongar, 2000; Mitchell, 2001), and thus the evolution and implementation of evidence-based practices in behavioral health and social services should be considered well under way. Refinement and integration of policy, academic research, practice, and evaluation will continue for the foreseeable future.

These trends are currently unfolding. Given that social workers provide the largest proportion of human services, we are poised to make extraordinary contributions to the future of several fields of practice. But those contributions, rooted in social workers' collective commitment to their clients, will go unacknowledged unless they are supported by published scientific evidence. In the near future, it is my hope that the qualifier "evidence-based" becomes superfluous when defining competent and caring social work practice. I hope we can simply call what we do "social work practice," with an implicit understanding that it is, in fact, evidence-based.

APPENDIXES

Rate your client's well-being **over the last 30 days** using the scale below. Score each of the following areas. Use everything you know about this client based on all sources of data. (If you provide treatment as part of a team, give a score based on team consensus.)

Poor	**Impaired**	**Marginal**	**Good**	**Excellent**
0	1	2	3	4

___ 1. **Mental status: cognitive functioning**: Consider the client's level of hallucinations, delusions, disorientation, bizarre behavior or speech, memory problems, serious confusion or other symptoms of serious cognitive impairment. How would you rate their overall mental status?

_____

_____

_____

___ 2. **Mental status: emotional state**: Consider the client's level of depression, anxiety, obsessional thinking and overall emotional state. How would you rate their overall emotional condition?

_____

_____

_____

___ 3. **Impulse control**: Think about your client's overall behavior. Consider things such as their ability to express themselves effectively, ability to work at things patiently, tendencies to verbally or physically lash out at others, run away, harm themselves or proneness to impulsive, criminal, or drug-abusing behavior. How would you rate their overall impulse control?

_____

_____

_____

___ 4. **Coping skills**: Think about your client's ability to cope with problems and everyday stresses. How would you rate their ability to assess problem situations, deal with "triggers," use stress reduction strategies, consider possible solutions to problems, perhaps reach out to others for help in order to deal effectively with their difficulties?

_____

_____

_____

___ 5. **Immediate social network** (close friends, spouse, family): Consider the quality of your client's relationships with those available friends, family, spouse (as applicable). How would you rate the quality of the interaction overall between your client and them with respect to closeness, intimacy, general interpersonal satisfaction, effective communications, conflict, level of hostility, aggression, abuse?

_____

_____

_____

___ 6. **Extended social relationships/network** (local community): Think about your client's relationships with persons outside their immediate family and social group. Consider their relationship to others in the community, their involvement in social groups, organizations, and general feeling of integration into the wider community in which they live. How would you rate their overall relationship with the community right now?

_____

_____

_____

___ 7. **Recreational activities**: Consider what the client does for fun (alone or social), hobbies, relaxation (reading, TV, video games, playing cards, etc.) and physical exercise (walking, jogging, biking, etc.). How would you rate the client's overall involvement in recreational activities?

_____

_____

_____

___ 8. **Living environment**: Think about your client's current or (if client is institutionalized) most recent living environment. Consider such things as adequacy of food, clothing, shelter, and safety. How would you rate their overall living environment?

_____

_____

_____

___ 9. **Use of alcohol and other drugs**: Consider the client's use of alcohol, illicit substances (cocaine, heroin, marijuana, PCP, hallucinogens, etc.) and illicit use of prescription medication. Consider the following: how often do they use them, in what quantity, and what are the psychological, physical, and social consequences associated with their use? How would you rate the client's overall functioning with regard to the use of alcohol and other drugs?

_____

_____

_____

___10. **Health**: Consider the client's overall health. Aside from normal, transient illnesses, think about health habits, chronic primary health disorders, their opinion of their own health, ability to engage in their usual activities relatively free from discomfort, overall energy level, hospitalizations and treatments for illness other than psychiatric ones. How would you rate their health overall?

_____

_____

_____

___11. **Independent living/self-care**: Consider how your client manages their household, takes care of personal hygiene, eats, sleeps and otherwise cares for themselves. How would you rate their performance in this area?

_____

_____

_____

___**12. Work (or role) satisfaction**: If the client works outside the home, is a homemaker or student, think for a moment about their work (or role) productivity. Considering the type of work or role in which they are engaged, how would you rate their overall work (role) productivity right now?

_____

_____

Psychological well-being subscale score: Sum items 1–4 = _____

Social well-being subscale score: Sum items 5–8 = _____

Total PSWS: Sum items 1–12 = _____

For relative severity scores on subscales

Psychological well-being relative severity score: Sum items 1–4 and divide by 4 =

_____

Social well-being relative severity score: Sum items 5–8 and divide by 4 = _____

Appendix B   Shortform Assessment for Children (SAC)

Date: _____/_____/_____   **Child's Name:** _____

Child's ID #: _____   **DOB:** _____/_____/_____   **Gender: M   F**

Use the behaviors listed below to describe this child as you know him or her.

Mark ⓪ if the behavior never occurs, ① if the behavior sometimes occurs, and ② if the behavior occurs often.

⓪ = Never   ① = Sometimes   ② Often

Behavior	Rating	Behavior	Rating
1. Has no respect for others	⓪ ① ②	25. Lacks self-confidence	⓪ ① ②
2. Doesn't follow rules	⓪ ① ②	26. Worries about health too much	⓪ ① ②
3. Is sad, unhappy, or feels down	⓪ ① ②	27. Attacks or hits others	⓪ ① ②
4. Is easily worried	⓪ ① ②	28. Hesitates to speak up in groups	⓪ ① ②
5. Is mean or cruel	⓪ ① ②	29. Yells or screams too much	⓪ ① ②
6. Steals from others	⓪ ① ②	30. Is quiet and doesn't share thoughts	⓪ ① ②
7. Fights a lot	⓪ ① ②	31. Is unsure of self or easily embarrassed	⓪ ① ②
8. Loses temper or throws tantrums	⓪ ① ②	32. Is aggressive	⓪ ① ②
9. Disobeys	⓪ ① ②	33. Has stomachaches without medical reason	⓪ ① ②
10. Curses or swears	⓪ ① ②	34. Stares into space or at nothing	⓪ ① ②
11. Is afraid he/she might do something bad	⓪ ① ②	35. Demands too much attention from others	⓪ ① ②
12. Is uncomfortable with attention from others	⓪ ① ②	36. Is irritable or stubborn	⓪ ① ②
13. Says he/she is not loved by anyone	⓪ ① ②	37. Has sudden mood swings	⓪ ① ②
14. Thinks he/she is worthless or second-rate	⓪ ① ②	38. Doesn't feel guilty about bad behavior	⓪ ① ②
15. Talks more than he/she should	⓪ ① ②	39. Is arrogant or over-bearing	⓪ ① ②
16. Hangs out with troublemakers	⓪ ① ②	40. Teases or provokes other children	⓪ ① ②
17. Has headaches without medical reason	⓪ ① ②	41. Destroys other people's things	⓪ ① ②
18. Cheats or lies	⓪ ① ②	42. Threatens or frightens others	⓪ ① ②
19. Is overly anxious or afraid	⓪ ① ②	43. Argues too much	⓪ ① ②
20. Blames him/herself too much	⓪ ① ②	44. Moves slowly or lacks energy	⓪ ① ②
21. Feels tired a lot	⓪ ① ②	45. Says he/she feels lonely	⓪ ① ②
22. Has pains without medical reason	⓪ ① ②	46. Is overly loud	⓪ ① ②
23. Keeps to him/herself a lot	⓪ ① ②	47. Is withdrawn and keeps apart from people	⓪ ① ②
24. Feels sick without medical reason	⓪ ① ②	48. Cries or appears tearful too much	⓪ ① ②

Comments:

Your Name: _____

Your relationship to the child is (mark only one):
① mother ② father ③ teacher ④ relative
⑤ foster parent ⑥ agency caregiver
⑦ other (describe): _____

Developed by: University of Tennessee
Children's Mental Health Services Research Center
with support from the National Institute of Mental Health

Before completing this scale, specify the number of client contacts this summary represents: _____

Using the scale below, score each item to estimate how often you actually use the following social work practice skill with this particular client. Under each item, describe more specifically the actual skill employed with this client.

Very often	Often	Moderately	Seldom	Never/almost never
4	3	2	1	0

Supportive/Facilitative Skills

___ 1. Provided emotional support for my client

___

___

___

___ 2. Endeavored to increase their self-confidence

___

___

___

___ 3. Helped my client to feel good about her/himself

___

___

___

___ 4. Tried to increase their confidence that I could really help them

___

___

___

Insight Facilitation Skills

___ 5. Helped them uncover troubling feelings

___

___

___

___ 6. Helped them learn from past experiences

___

___

___

___ 7. Explored how past relationships affect current problems

___

___

___

___ 8. Helped them learn from past attempts to solve problems

___

___

___

Therapeutic Coping Skills

___ 9. Taught them specific skills to deal with a certain problem

_____
_____
_____

___10. Taught them how to manage their own problem behaviors

_____
_____
_____

___11. Showed them how to reward themselves for progress with a problem

_____
_____
_____

___12. Taught them how to monitor their own behaviors

_____
_____
_____

___13. Collaborated with them on plans to cope with relapses of a problem

_____
_____
_____

Case Management Skills

___14. Assessed their level of material resources

_____
_____
_____

___15. Advocated on their behalf

_____
_____
_____

___16. Made referrals to other services

_____
_____
_____

___17. Gave them information about other services

_____
_____
_____

___18. Coordinated services for them with other agencies

_____
_____
_____

Please indicate to what degree you feel confident in employing the following knowledge and skills relevant to alcohol and other drug abuse interventions. Use the scale below and place your number answer in the space provided to the left of each question.

1 **Very low** confidence to no confidence in my knowledge/skills
2 **Low** confidence in my knowledge/skills
3 **Moderate** confidence in my knowledge/skills
4 **High** confidence in my knowledge/skills
5 **Very high** confidence in my knowledge/skills

How confident are you in . . .

Assessment/Treatment Planning.

___ 1. gathering data systematically from the client and other available collateral sources, using screening instruments and other methods that are sensitive to age, culture, and gender? At a minimum, data should include: current and historic substance use; health, mental health, and substance-related treatment history; mental status; and current social environmental, and/or economic constraints on the client's ability to follow through successfully with an action plan.

___ 2. determining the client's readiness for treatment/change and the needs of others involved in the current situation?

___ 3. reviewing the treatment options relevant to the client's needs, characteristics, and goals?

___ 4. constructing with the client and others, as appropriate, an initial action plan based on needs, preferences, and available resources?

___ 5. selecting and using comprehensive assessment instruments that are sensitive to age, gender, and culture?

___ 6. analyzing and interpreting the data to determine treatment recommendations?

___ 7. obtaining and interpreting all relevant assessment information?

___ 8. explaining assessment findings to the client and others potentially involved in treatment?

___ 9. screening for AOD [alcohol and other drugs] toxicity, withdrawal symptoms, aggression or danger to others, and potential for self-inflicted harm or suicide?

___10. identifying appropriate strategies for each outcome?

Case Management

___11. establishing and maintaining professional relations with civic groups, agencies, other professionals, governmental entities, and the community-at-large in order to ensure appropriate referrals, identify service gaps, expand community resources, and help address unmet needs?

1 = Very low   2 = Low   3 = Moderate   4 = High   5 = Very high

How confident are you in . . .

____12. continuously assessing and evaluating referral resources to determine their appropriateness?

____13. arranging referrals to other professionals, agencies community programs, or other appropriate resources to meet client needs?

____14. exchanging relevant information with the agency/professional to whom the referral is being made, in a manner consistent with confidentiality regulations and generally accepted professional standards of care?

____15. evaluating the outcome of the referral?

____16. initiating collaboration with referral sources?

Counseling—Individual

____17. establishing a helping relationship with the client characterized by warmth, respect, genuineness, concreteness, and empathy?

____18. facilitating the client's engagement in the treatment/recovery process?

____19. encouraging and reinforcing all client actions that are determined to be beneficial in progressing toward treatment goals?

____20. working appropriately with the client to recognize and discourage all behaviors inconsistent with progress toward treatment goals?

____21. recognizing how, when, and why to use the client's significant others to enhance or support the treatment plan?

____22. facilitating the development of basic and life skills associated with recovery?

____23. adapting counseling strategies to the individual characteristics of the client, including (but not limited to) disability, gender, sexual orientation, developmental level, acculturation, ethnicity, age, and health status?

Counseling—Group

____24. performing the actions necessary to start a group, including determining group type, purpose, size, and leadership; recruiting and selecting members; establishing group goals and clarifying behavioral ground rules for participating; identifying outcomes; and determining criteria and methods for termination or graduation from the group?

____25. facilitating the entry of new members and the transition of exiting members?

____26. facilitating group growth within the established ground rules, and precipitating movement toward group and individual goals by using methods consistent with group type?

____27. describing and summarizing client behavior within the group for the purpose of documenting the client's progress and identifying needs/issues that may require modification of the treatment plan?

1 = Very low   2 = Low   3 = Moderate   4 = High   5 = Very high

How confident are you in . . .

Ethics

____28. utilizing a range of supervisory options to process personal feelings and concerns about clients?

____29. conducting culturally appropriate self-evaluations of professional performance, applying ethical, legal, and professional standards to enhance self-awareness and performance?

____30. obtaining appropriate continuing professional education?

____31. assessing and participating in regular supervision and consultation sessions?

____32. developing and utilizing strategies to maintain physical and mental health?

Appendix E   Addiction Severity Index

Addiction Severity Index
Fifth Edition

SUMMARY OF PATIENT'S RATING SCALE

0 – Not at all
1 – Slightly
2 – Moderately
3 – Considerably
4 – Extremely

G1. I.D. NUMBER ▢▢▢▢

G2. LAST 4 DIGITS OF SSN ▢▢▢▢

G3. PROGRAM NUMBER ▢▢▢

G4. DATE OF
ADMISSION ▢▢▢▢▢▢
Mth. Day Year

G5. DATE OF
INTERVIEW ▢▢▢▢▢▢
Mth. Day Year

G6. TIME BEGUN ▢▢ : ▢▢

G7. TIME ENDED ▢▢ : ▢▢

G8. CLASS: ▢
1–Intake
2–Follow-up

G9. CONTACT CODE: ▢
1–In Person
2–Phone

G10. GENDER: ▢
1–Male
2–Female

G11. INTERVIEWER CODE ▢▢
NUMBER

G12. SPECIAL: ▢
1–Patient terminated
2–Patient refused
3–Patient unable to respond

GENERAL INFORMATION

NAME _____
CURRENT ADDRESS _____
_____

G13. GEOGRAPHIC CODE ▢▢▢
G14. How long have you lived
at this address? ▢▢ ▢▢
Yrs. Mths.
G15. Is this residence owned by
you or your family? ▢
G16. DATE OF
BIRTH ▢▢▢▢▢▢
Mth. Day Year
G17. RACE ▢
1–White (Not of Hispanic Origin)
2–Black (Not of Hispanic Origin)
3–American Indian
4–Alaskan Native
5–Asian of Pacific Islander
6–Hispanic–Mexican
7–Hispanic–Puerto Rican
8–Hispanic–Cuban
9–Other Hispanic
G18. RELIGIOUS PREFERENCE ▢
1–Protestant
2–Catholic
3–Jewish
4–Islamic
5–Other
6–None
G19. Have you been in a ▢
controlled environment
in the past 30 days?
1–No
2–Jail
3–Alcohol or Drug Treatment
4–Medical Treatment
5–Psychiatric Treatment
6–Other
G20. How many days? ▢▢

ADDITIONAL TEST RESULTS

G21. Shipley C.Q. ▢▢▢

G22. Shipley I.Q. ▢▢▢

G23. Beck Total Score ▢▢

G24. SCL-90 Total ▢▢▢

G25. MAST ▢▢

G26. _____ ▢▢▢

G27. _____ ▢▢▢

G28. _____ ▢▢▢

SEVERITY PROFILE

Problems	Medical	Employ/Support	Alcohol	Drug	Legal	Family/Social	Psychiatric
9							
8							
7							
6							
5							
4							
3							
2							
1							
0							

Page 1.

560

☐☐☐☐ I.D. NUMBER

MEDICAL STATUS

M1. How many times in your ☐☐
your life have you been
hospitalized for medical
problems? (Include o.d.'s, d.t.'s,
exclude detox.)

M2. How long ago was ☐☐ ☐☐
your last hospitaliza- Yrs. Mths.
tion for a physical
problem?

M3. Do you have any chronic ☐
medical problems which
continue to interfere with
your life?

M4. Are you taking any pre- ☐
scribed medication on a
regular basis for a physical
problem? 0-No 1-Yes

M5. Do you receive a pension for
a physical disability? (Exclude
psychiatric disability.)
0-No
1-Yes _____
Specify

M6. How many days have you ☐☐
experienced medical prob-
lems in the past 30 days?

*For questions M7 & M8 please
ask the patient to use the Patient's Rating Scale.*

M7. How troubled or bothered ☐
have you been by these
medical problems in the
past 30 days?

M8. How important to you ☐
now is treatment for these
medical problems?

Interviewer Severity Rating

M9. How would you rate the ☐
patient's need for medical
treatment?

Confidence Rating

Is the above information significantly distorted by:

M10. Patient's misrepresen- ☐
tation?
0-No 1-Yes

M11. Patient's inability to ☐
understand?
0-No 1-Yes

COMMENTS

EMPLOYMENT/SUPPORT STATUS

E1. Education completed ☐☐ ☐☐
Yrs. Mths.

E2. Training or technical ☐☐
education completed Mths.

E3. Do you have a profession, ☐
trade or skill?
0-No
1-Yes _____
Specify

E4. Do you have a valid ☐
driver's license?
0-No 1-Yes

E5. Do you have an automobile ☐
available for use? (Answer No
if no valid driver's license.)
0-No 1-Yes

E6. How long was your ☐☐ ☐☐
longest full-time job? Yrs. Mths.

E7. Usual (or last) occupation? ☐

_____
Specify in Detail

E8. Does someone contribute ☐
to your support in any way?

E9. (ONLY IF ITEM 8 IS YES) ☐
Does this constitute the
majority of your support?

E10. Usual employment ☐
pattern, past 3 years.
1-full time (40 hrs/wk)
2-part time (reg. Hrs)
3-part time (irreg., daywork)
4-student
5-service
6-retired/disability
7-unemployed
8-in controlled environment

E11. How many days were ☐☐
you paid for working in
the past 30? (include "under
the table" work.)

How much money did you receive
from the following sources in the
past 30 days?

E12. Employment ☐☐☐☐
(net income)

E13. Unemployment ☐☐☐☐
compensation

E14. DPA ☐☐☐☐

E15. Pension, benefits or ☐☐☐☐
social security

E16. Mate, family or friends ☐☐☐☐
(money for personal
expenses)

E17. Illegal ☐☐☐☐

E18. How many people depend ☐
on you for the majority of
their food, shelter, etc.?

E19. How many days have you ☐
experienced employment
problems in the past 30?

*For questions E20 & E21 please
ask the patient to use the Patient's Rating Scale.*

E20. How troubled or bothered ☐
have you been by these employment problems in the
past 30 days?

E21. How important to you ☐
now is counseling for these
employment problems?

Interviewer Severity Rating

E22. How would you rate the ☐
patient's need for employment counseling?

Confidence Rating

Is the above information significantly distorted by:

E23. Patient's misrepresentation? ☐

E24. Patient's inability to under- ☐
stand?

COMMENTS

▢▢▢▢ I.D. NUMBER

DRUG/ALCOHOL USE

	Past 30 Days	Life-time Years	Use Route Admin
D1. Alcohol-any use at all	▢▢	▢▢	▢
D2. Alcohol to intoxication	▢▢	▢▢	▢
D3. Heroin	▢▢	▢▢	▢
D4. Methadone	▢▢	▢▢	▢
D5. Other opiates/ analgesics	▢▢	▢▢	▢
D6. Barbiturates	▢▢	▢▢	▢
D7. Other seda- tives/hyp/ tranquilizers	▢▢	▢▢	▢
D8. Cocaine	▢▢	▢▢	▢
D9. Amphetamines	▢▢	▢▢	▢
D10. Cannabis	▢▢	▢▢	▢
D11. Hallucinogens	▢▢	▢▢	▢
D12. Inhalants	▢▢	▢▢	▢

D13. More than one substance per day (including alcohol)   ▢

Note: See manual for representa- tive examples for each drug class

Route of Administration: 1 = Oral, 2 = Nasal, 3 = Smoking, 4 = Non IV inj., 5 = IV inj.

D14. Which substance is the ▢▢ major problem? *Please code as above or* 00-No problem; 15-Alcohol & Drug (Dual addiction); 16-Polydrug; *when not clear, as patient.*

D15. How long was your last ▢▢ period of voluntary absti- nence from this major sub- stance? (00-never abstinent)

D16. How many months ago ▢▢ did this abstinence end? (00-still abstinent)

How many times have you:

D17. Had alcohol d.t.'s? ▢▢
D18. Overdosed on drugs? ▢▢

How many time in your life have you been treated for:

D19. Alcohol abuse? ▢▢
D20. Drug abuse? ▢▢

How many of these were detox only?

D21. Alcohol ▢▢
D22. Drug ▢▢

How many would you say you spent during the past 30 days on:

D23. Alcohol? ▢▢
D24. Drugs? ▢▢

D25. How many days have ▢▢ you been treated in an outpatient setting for alcohol or drugs in the past 30 days? (Include NA, AA).

How many days in the past 30 have you experienced:

D26. Alcohol problems? ▢▢
D27. Drug problems? ▢▢

For questions D28-D31 please ask the patient to use the Pa- tient's Rating Scale.

How troubled or bothered have you been in the past 30 days by these:

D28. Alcohol problems? ▢▢
D29. Drug problems? ▢▢

How important to you now is treatment for these:

D30. Alcohol problems? ▢
D31. Drug problems? ▢

Interviewer Severity Rating

How would you rate the patient's need for treatment for:

D32. Alcohol abuse? ▢
D33. Drug abuse? ▢

Confidence Rating

Is the above information signifi- cantly distorted by:

D34. Patient's misrepresen- ▢ tation? 0-No 1-Yes

D35. Patient's inability to ▢ understand? 0-No 1-Yes

COMMENTS

_____
_____
_____
_____
_____
_____
_____
_____
_____
_____
_____
_____

◻◻◻◻ I.D. NUMBER

LEGAL STATUS

L1. Was this admission prompted or suggested by the criminal justice system (judge, probation/parole officer, etc.)
0-No 1-Yes   ◻

L2. Are you on probation or parole?
0-No 1-Yes   ◻

How many times in your life have you been arrested and <u>charged</u> with the following:

L3. Shoplifting/vandalism   ◻◻
L4. Parole/probation violations   ◻◻
L5. Drug charges   ◻◻
L6. Forgery   ◻◻
L7. Weapons offense   ◻◻
L8. Burglary, larceny, B&E   ◻◻
L9. Robbery   ◻◻
L10. Assault   ◻◻
L11. Arson   ◻◻
L12. Rape   ◻◻
L13. Homicide, manslaughter   ◻◻
L14. Prostitution   ◻◻
L15. Contempt of court   ◻◻
L16. Other   ◻◻

L17. How many of these charges resulted in convictions?   ◻◻

How many time in your life have you been charged with the following:

L18. Disorderly conduct, vagrancy, public intoxication   ◻◻

L19. Driving while intoxicated   ◻◻

L20. Major driving violations (reckless driving, speeding, no license, etc.)   ◻◻

L21. How many months were you incarcerated in your life?   ◻◻ Mths.

L22. How long was your last incarceration?   ◻◻ Mths.

L23. What was it for? *(Use codes 3-16, 18-20. If multiple charges, code most severe.)*   ◻◻

L24. Are you presently awaiting charges, trial or sentence?
0-No 1-Yes   ◻

L25. What for? (If multiple charges, use most severe.)   ◻◻

L26. How many days in the past 30 were you detained or incarcerated?   ◻◻

L27. How many days in the past 30 have you engaged in illegal activities for profit?   ◻◻

*For questions L28 & L29 please ask the patient to use the **Patient's Rating Scale.***

L28. How serious do you feel your present legal problems are? (Exclude civil problems.)   ◻

L29. How important to you now is counseling or referral for these legal problems?   ◻

Interviewer Severity Rating

L30. How would you rate the patient's need for legal services or counseling?   ◻

Confidence Rating

L31. Patient's misrepresentation?   ◻

L32. Patient's inability to understand?   ◻

COMMENTS

_____

_____

_____

_____

FAMILY HISTORY

Have any of your relatives had what you call a significant drinking, drug use or psych problem—one that did or should have led to treatment?

	Mother's Side				Father's Side				Siblings		
	Alc	Drug	Psych		Alc	Drug	Psych		Alc	Drug	Psych
H1. Grandmother	◻	◻	◻	H6. Grandmother	◻	◻	◻	H11. Brother	◻	◻	◻
H2. Grandfather	◻	◻	◻	H7. Grandfather	◻	◻	◻	H12. Sister	◻	◻	◻
H3. Mother	◻	◻	◻	H8. Mother	◻	◻	◻				
H4. Aunt	◻	◻	◻	H9. Aunt	◻	◻	◻				
H5. Uncle	◻	◻	◻	H10. Uncle	◻	◻	◻				

Directions: Place "O" in relative category where the answer is clearly <u>no for all relatives in the category</u>; "1" where the answer is clearly <u>yes for any relative within the category</u>; "X" where the answer is <u>uncertain or "I don't know"</u>; and "N" where there <u>never was a relative from that category</u>. Code most problematic relative in cases of multiple members per category.   Page 4.

▢▢▢▢ I.D. NUMBER

F1. Marital Status ▢

1-Married   4-Separated
2-Remarried   5-Divorced
3-Widowed   6-Never Married

F2. How long have you ▢▢ ▢▢
been in this marital Yrs. Mths.
status? (*If never
married, since age 18.*)

F3. Are you satisfied with ▢
this situation?
0–No
1–Indifferent
2–Yes

F4. Usual living arrangements ▢
(past 3 yr.)
1-With sexual partner and children
2-With sexual partner alone
3-With children alone
4-With parents
5-With family
6-With friends
7-Alone
8-Controlled environment
9-No stable arrangements

F5. How long have you ▢▢ ▢▢
lived in those arrange- Yrs. Mths.
ments? (If with parents
or family, since age 18.)

F6. Are you satisfied with ▢
these living arrangements?
0–No
1–Indifferent
2–Yes

Do you live with anyone who:
0–No 1–Yes

F7. Has a current alcohol ▢
problem?

F8. Uses non-prescribed drugs? ▢

F9. With whom do you spend ▢
most of your free time:
1–Family
2–Friends
3–Alone

F10. Are you satisfied with ▢
spending your free time
this way?
0–No
1–Indifferent
2–Yes

F11. How many close friends ▢
do you have?

FAMILY/SOCIAL RELATIONSHIPS

Directions for F12-F26: Place "0" in relative category where the answer is clearly <u>no for all relatives in the category</u>; "1" where the answer is clearly <u>yes for any relative within the category</u>; "X" where the answer is <u>uncertain or "I don't know"</u>; and "N" where there <u>never was a relative from that category</u>.

Would you say you have had close, long lasting, personal relationships with any of the following people in your life?

F12. Mother   ▢
F13. Father   ▢
F14. Brothers/Sisters ▢
F16. Children   ▢
F17. Friends   ▢

Have you had significant periods in which you have experienced serious problems getting along with:

	Past 30 Days	In Your Life
F18. Mother	▢	▢
F19. Father	▢	▢
F20. Brothers/Sisters	▢	▢
F21. Sexual partner/ spouse	▢	▢
F22. Children	▢	▢
F23. Other significant family	▢	▢
F24. Close friends	▢	▢
F25. Neighbors	▢	▢
F26. Coworkers	▢	▢

Did any of these people (F18-F26) abuse you? 0 = No 1 = Yes

	Past 30 Days	In Your Life
F27. Emotionally (make you feel bad through harsh words)?	▢	▢
F28. Physically (caused you physical harm)?	▢	▢
F29. Sexually (forced sexual advances or sexual acts)?	▢	▢

How many days in the past 30 have you had serious conflicts:

F30. With your family? ▢▢

F31. With other people ▢▢
(excluding family)?

*For questions F32–F35 please ask the patient to use the **Patient's Rating Scale**.*

How troubled or bothered have you been in the past 30 days by these:

F32. Family problems?   ▢
F33. Social problems?   ▢

How important to you now is treatment or counseling for these:

F34. Family problems?   ▢
F35. Social problems?   ▢

Interviewer Severity Rating

F36. How would you rate the ▢
patient's need for family
and/or social counseling?

Confidence Rating

Is the above information significantly distorted by:

F37. Patient's misrepresen- ▢
tation?
0–No 1–Yes

F38. Patient's inability to ▢
understand?
0–No 1–Yes

COMMENTS

_____
_____
_____
_____
_____
_____
_____
_____
_____
_____
_____
_____
_____

☐☐☐☐ I.D. NUMBER

How many times have you been treated for any psychological or emotional problems?

P1. In a hospital   ☐☐

P2. As an outpatient or private   ☐☐
patient

P3. Do you receive a pension   ☐
for a psychiatric disability?
0-No 1-Yes

Have you had a significant period (that was not a direct result of drug/alcohol use) in which you have:

	Past 30 Days	In Your Life
P4. Experienced serious depression?	☐	☐
P5. Experienced serious anxiety or tension?	☐	☐
P6. Experienced hallucinations?	☐	☐
P7. Experienced trouble understanding, concentrating or remembering?	☐	☐
P8. Experienced trouble controlling violent behavior?	☐	☐
P9. Experienced serious thoughts of suicide?	☐	☐
P10. Attempted suicide?	☐	☐
P11. Been prescribed medication for any psychological emotional problem?	☐	☐

PSYCHIATRIC STATUS

P12. How many days in the   ☐☐
past 30 have you
experienced these
psychological or
emotional problems?

For questions P12 & P13 please ask the patient to use the Patient's Rating Scale.

P13. How many have you been   ☐
troubled or bothered by
these psychological or
emotional problems in the
past 30 days?

P14. How important to you   ☐
now is treatment for these
psychological problems?

THE FOLLOWING ITEMS ARE TO BE COMPLETED BY THE INTER-VIEWER

At the time of the interview, is patient:

0-No 1-Yes

P15. Obviously depressed/   ☐
withdrawn?

P16. Obviously hostile?   ☐

P17. Obviously anxious/   ☐
nervous?

P18. Having trouble with   ☐
reality testing, thought
disorders, paranoid thinking?

P19. Having trouble compre-   ☐
hending, concentrating,
remembering?

P20. Having suicidal thoughts?   ☐

P21. How would you rate the   ☐
patient's need for psychiatric/
psychological treatment?

Confidence Rating

Is the above information signifi-cantly distorted by:

P22. Patient's misrepresentation? ☐
0-No 1-Yes

P23. Patient's inability to under-   ☐
stand?
0-No 1-Yes

COMMENTS

_____
_____
_____
_____
_____
_____
_____
_____
_____
_____
_____
_____
_____

Interviewer: Date:

Client: Assessment no.:

Medication use:

4.4.A Regular use of alcohol:
4.5.A Regular use of soft drugs:
4.7.A Regular use of hard drugs:

1. Abandonment   **Notes:**
1.1   0 1 2 3 4 5 6 7 8 9 10   ....
1.2   0 1 2 3 4 5 6 7 8 9 10   ....
1.3   0 1 2 3 4 5 6 7 8 9 10   ....
1.4   0 1 2 3 4 5 6 7 8 9 10   ....
1.5   0 1 2 3 4 5 6 7 8 9 10   ....
1.6   0 1 2 3 4 5 6 7 8 9 10   ....
1.7   0 1 2 3 4 5 6 7 8 9 10   ....
                           Mean: _____

2. Interpersonal relationships
2.1   0 1 2 3 4 5 6 7 8 9 10   ....
2.2   0 1 2 3 4 5 6 7 8 9 10   ....
2.3   0 1 2 3 4 5 6 7 8 9 10   ....
2.4   0 1 2 3 4 5 6 7 8 9 10   ....
2.5   0 1 2 3 4 5 6 7 8 9 10   ....
2.6   0 1 2 3 4 5 6 7 8 9 10   ....
2.7   0 1 2 3 4 5 6 7 8 9 10   ....
2.8   0 1 2 3 4 5 6 7 8 9 10   ....
                           Mean: _____

3. Identity
3.1   0 1 2 3 4   ....
3.2   0 1 2 3 4   ....
3.3   0 1 2 3 4   ....
3.4   0 1 2 3 4   ....
3.5   0 1 2 3 4   ....
3.6   0 1 2 3 4   ....
3.7   0 1 2 3 4   ....
3.8   0 1 2 3 4   ....
                   Mean × 2.5 =   _____

4. Impulsivity
4.1   0 1 2 3 4 5 6 7 8 9 10   ....
4.2   0 1 2 3 4 5 6 7 8 9 10   ....
4.3   0 1 2 3 4 5 6 7 8 9 10   ....

4.4	0 1 2 3 4 5 6 7 8 9 10	....
4.5	0 1 2 3 4 5 6 7 8 9 10	....
4.6	0 1 2 3 4 5 6 7 8 9 10	....
4.7	0 1 2 3 4 5 6 7 8 9 10	....
4.8	0 1 2 3 4 5 6 7 8 9 10	....
4.9	0 1 2 3 4 5 6 7 8 9 10	....
4.10	0 1 2 3 4 5 6 7 8 9 10	....
4.11	0 1 2 3 4 5 6 7 8 9 10	....

Mean: _____

5. Parasuicidal behavior

5.1	0 1 2 3 4 5 6 7 8 9 10	....
5.2	0 1 2 3 4 5 6 7 8 9 10	....
5.3	0 1 2 3 4 5 6 7 8 9 10	....
5.4	0 1 2 3 4 5 6 7 8 9 10	....
5.5	0 1 2 3 4 5 6 7 8 9 10	....
5.6	0 1 2 3 4 5 6 7 8 9 10	....
5.7	0 1 2 3 4 5 6 7 8 9 10	....
5.8	0 1 2 3 4 5 6 7 8 9 10	....
5.9	0 1 2 3 4 5 6 7 8 9 10	....
5.10	0 1 2 3 4 5 6 7 8 9 10	....
5.11	0 1 2 3 4 5 6 7 8 9 10	....
5.12	0 1 2 3 4 5 6 7 8 9 10	....
5.13	0 1 2 3 4 5 6 7 8 9 10	....

Mean: _____

6. Affective instability

6.1	0 1 2 3 4 5 6 7 8 9 10	....
6.2	0 1 2 3 4 5 6 7 8 9 10	....
6.3	0 1 2 3 4 5 6 7 8 9 10	....
6.4	0 1 2 3 4 5 6 7 8 9 10	....
6.5	0 1 2 3 4 5 6 7 8 9 10	....

Mean: _____

7. Emptiness

7.1	0 1 2 3 4 5 6 7 8 9 10	....
7.2	0 1 2 3 4 5 6 7 8 9 10	....
7.3	0 1 2 3 4 5 6 7 8 9 10	....
7.4	0 1 2 3 4 5 6 7 8 9 10	....

Mean: _____

8. Outbursts of anger

8.1	0 1 2 3 4 5 6 7 8 9 10	....
8.2	0 1 2 3 4 5 6 7 8 9 10	....
8.3	0 1 2 3 4 5 6 7 8 9 10	....
8.4	0 1 2 3 4 5 6 7 8 9 10	....
8.5	0 1 2 3 4 5 6 7 8 9 10	....
8.6	0 1 2 3 4 5 6 7 8 9 10	....

Mean: _____

9. Dissociation and paranoid ideation

9.1   0 1 2 3 4 5 6 7 8 9 10   ....

9.2   0 1 2 3 4 5 6 7 8 9 10   ....

9.3   0 1 2 3 4 5 6 7 8 9 10   ....

9.4   0 1 2 3 4 5 6 7 8 9 10   ....

9.5   0 1 2 3 4 5 6 7 8 9 10   ....

9.6   0 1 2 3 4 5 6 7 8 9 10   ....

9.7   0 1 2 3 4 5 6 7 8 9 10   ....

9.8   0 1 2 3 4 5 6 7 8 9 10   ....

Mean: _____

Total sum of means: _____

Appendix G Scoring Worksheet for UCLA PTSD Index for DSM-IV, Revision 1: Child Version©

Subject ID# _____ **Age** _____ **Sex (circle): M   F**
# of days since traumatic event _____

CRITERION A-TRAUMATIC EVENT

Exposure to Traumatic Event
Questions 1–13: at least 1 "Yes" answer   YES   NO

Type of Traumatic Event rated as most
distressing (Question 14: write trauma
type in the blank)   _____

Criterion A1 met
Questions 15-21: at least 1 "Yes" answer   YES   NO

Criterion A2 met
Questions 22-26: at least 1 "Yes" answer   YES   NO

Criterion A met   YES   NO

Peritraumatic Dissociation   YES   NO
Question 27: answer "Yes"

PTSD SEVERITY: OVERALL SCORE

Question #/Score	Question #/Score
1._____	12._____
2._____	13._____
3._____	[Omit 14].
4._____	15._____
5._____	16._____
6._____	17._____
7._____	18._____
8._____	19._____
9._____	[Omit 20].
*10. or	
11._____	

(Sum the items from the above 2 columns, write sum below)

(Sum total   **PTSD SEVERITY**
of scores) = _____   **SCORE**

*Place the highest Score from either Question 10
or 11 in the blank above: Score Question 10.____/
Score Question 11.____

CRITERION B (REEXPERIENCING) SX.

Question #/DSM-IV Symptom	Score	
3. (B1) Intrusive recollections	_____	
5. (B2) Trauma/bad dreams	_____	
6. (B3) Flashbacks	_____	# of Criterion B
2. (B4) Cues: Psychological		Questions with
reactivity	_____	Score ≥ Symp-
18. (B5) Cues: Physiological		tom Cutoff:
reactivity	_____ _____	

CRITERION B SEVERITY
SCORE (Sum of above scores): = _____

DSM-IV CRITERION B MET:
(Diagnosis requires at least 1 "B" Symptom):   **YES   NO**

CRITERION C (AVOIDANCE) SX.

Question #/DSM-IV Symptom	Score	
9. (C1) Avoiding thoughts/feelings	_____	
17. (C2) Avoiding activities/people	_____	
15. (C3) Forgetting	_____	# of Criterion C
7. (C4) Diminished interest etc.	_____	Questions with
8. (C5) Detachment/estrangement	_____	Scores ≥ Symp-
*10. or 11. (C6) Affect restricted	_____	tom Cutoff:
		_____
19. (C7) Foreshort. future	_____	

[*Place the highest Score from either Question 10 or 11
in the blank above.]

CRITERION C SEVERITY
SCORE (Sum of above scores): = _____

DSM-IV CRITERION C MET:
(Diagnosis requires at least 3 "C" Symptoms): YES NO

CRITERION D (INCREASED AROUSAL) SX.

Question #/DSM-IV Symptom	Score	
13. (D1) Sleep problems	_____	
4. (D2) Irritability/anger	_____	
16. (D3) Concentration problems	_____	# of Criterion D
1. (D4) Hypervigilance	_____	Questions with
12. (D5) Exaggerated startle	_____	Score ≥ Symp-
		tom Cutoff:
		____

CRITERION D SEVERITY
SCORE (Sum of above scores): = _____

DSM-IV CRITERION D MET:
(Diagnosis requires at least 2 "D" Symptoms): YES NO

DSM-IV PTSD DIAGNOSTIC INFO.

DSM-IV FULL PTSD DIAGNOSIS LIKELY(Criteria A,
B, C, D all met) **YES NO**

PARTIAL PTSD LIKELY
[Criterion A met and:
Criteria (B + C) or (B + D) or (C + D)]   **YES NO**

Addiction Severity Index (ASI)
The ASI and training materials are available free of charge at www.tresearch.org.
Reprinted with permission of Thomas McLellan.

Agoraphobia Scale
Contact: Lars-Goran Ost at ost@psychology.su.sc.
Reprinted with permission from Ost, 1990.

Alcohol Use Disorders Identification Test (AUDIT)
Reprinted from USDHHS, 2003, pp. 311–314.

Borderline Personality Disorder Severity Index (BPDSI)
Contact: Josephine Giesen-Bloo, Department of Medical, Clinical, and Experimental
Psychology, University Maastricht, P.O. Box 616, NL-6200 MD Maastricht,
The Netherlands; e-mail: j.giesen@dep.unimaas.nl.
Reprinted with permission of Josephine Giesen-Bloo.

Brief Psychiatric Rating Scale–Anchored (BPRS-A)
Contact: David Lachar, Department of Psychiatry and Behavioral Sciences,
University of Texas, Houston Health Science Center, P.O. Box 20708, Houston, TX
77225; e-mail: david.lachar@uth.tmc.edu.
Reprinted with permission from Lachar et al., 2001.

Children's Depression Rating Scale–Revised Short Form (CDRS-r)
To obtain a copy, contact James Overholser, Department of Psychology, Case West-
ern Reserve University, Cleveland, OH 44106-7123; e-mail: overholser@po.cwru.edu.
Reprinted with permission from Overholser, Brinkman, Lehnert, & Ricciardi, 1995.

College Alcohol Problems Scale–Revised (CAPS-r)
Copies of CAPS-r are available free of charge from oharet@bc.edu.
Reprinted from USDHHS, 2003, pp. 340–342.

Drinking Context Scale (DCS-9)
Copies of DCS-9 are available free of charge from oharet@bc.edu.
Reprinted from USDHHS, 2003, pp. 359–362.

Drug Abuse Screening Test–10 (DAST-10)
To obtain a copy, contact Harvey Skinner, Department of Public Health Sciences,
Faculty of Medicine, University of Toronto, 12 Queen's Park Crescent West, Toronto,
Ontario M5S 1A8; e-mail: harvey.skinner@utoronto.ca.
Reprinted with permission of Skinner and the Centre for Addiction and Mental
Health, Toronto, Canada.

Eating Disorder Diagnostic Scale (EDDS)
A computerized scoring tool is available from Eric Stice at estice@ori.org.
Copyright 2000 by Eric Stice and Christy F. Telch. Reprinted with permission.

Geriatric Depression Scale (GDS)
The GDS is in the public domain.
Reprinted from Yesavage et al., 1983.

Hamilton Depression Rating Scale (HAM-D)
The HAM-D is in the public domain.
Reprinted from Hamilton, 1960.

Marital Disaffection Scale
Contact: e-mail: Kayserk@bc.edu.
Copyright 1990 by the National Council on Family Relations. Reprinted with permission.

New York Teacher Rating Scale (NYTRS)
Contact: Laurie Miller Brotman, New York University Child Study Center 577 First Ave., New York, NY 10016; email: millel02@med.nyu.edu.
Reprinted with permission of Laurie Miller Brotman.

Obsessive-Compulsive Inventory–Revised (OCI)
To obtain copies, contact Edna Foa, Center for the Treatment and Study of Anxiety, University of Pennsylvania, 3535 Market St., Suite 600N, Philadelphia, PA 19104; e-mail: foa@mail.med.upenn.edu.
Reprinted with permission of Edna B. Foa.

Post-Traumatic Stress Disorder Reaction Index (PTSD-RI)
The different formatted versions of the PTSD-RI, associated training materials, and scoring aids are available from the authors at rpynoos@mednet.ucla.edu.
Contact: Robert Pynoos, UCLA Trauma Psychiatry Service, 300 UCLA Medical Plaza, Suite 2232, Los Angeles, CA 90095-6968, (310) 206-8973.
Copyright 1998 Pynoos, Rodriguez, Steinberg, Stuber, & Frederick. Reprinted with permission of Robert Pynoos.

Practice Skills Inventory (PSI)
The PSI is available free of charge from oharet@bc.edu.
Copyright 1997 Tom O'Hare.

Psychosocial Well-Being Scale (PSWS)
The PSWS is available free of charge from oharet@bc.edu.
Copyright 2002 Tom O'Hare.

PTSD Symptom Scale Interview (PSS-I)
A manual is available from Nora Feeney and Edna Foa.
Contact: Edna B. Foa, Center for the Treatment and Study of Anxiety, University of Pennsylvania, 3535 Market St., Suite 600N, Philadelphia, PA 19104; e-mail; foa@mail.med.upenn.edu.
Reprinted with permission of Edna Foa.

Screen for Child Anxiety-Related Emotional Disorders (SCARED)
Contact: Boris Birmaher, Western Psychiatric Institute and Clinic,
Department of Child Psychiatry, 3811 O'Hara St., Pittsburgh, PA 15213;
e-mail: birmaherb@msx.upmc.edu.
Reprinted with permission of Boris Birmaher.

Shortform Assessment for Children (SAC)
The SAC scale and scoring software are available from Children's Mental Health
Services Research Center, Henson Hall, University of Tennessee, Knoxville, TN
37996-3332.
Reprinted with permission of University of Tennessee Children's Mental Health
Services Research Center.

Strengths and Weakness of ADHD Symptoms and Normal Behavior Scale (SWAN)
The SWAN extended version and related materials are available without charge at
www.ADHD.net.
Copyright James M. Swanson, University of California, Irvine. Reprinted with
permission.

Substance Abuse Treatment Self-Efficacy Scale (SATSES)
The SATSES is available free of charge from Katie Kranz, KSNAP@aol.com, or from
Tom O'Hare at oharet@bc.edu.
Copyright Katherine M. Kranz. Reprinted with permission.

REFERENCES

Abbey, A. (2002). Alcohol-related sexual assault: A common problem among college students. *Journal of Studies on Alcohol, 63,* 118-128.

Abbey, A., & Harnish, R. (1995). Perception of sexual intent: The role of gender, alcohol consumption, and rape supportive attitudes. *Sex Roles, 32,* 297-313.

Abbey, A., McAuslan, P., & Ross, L. T. (1998). Sexual assault perpetration by college men: The role of alcohol misperception of sexual intent, and sexual beliefs and experiences. *Journal of Social and Clinical Psychology, 17,* 167-195.

Abbott, P. J., Weller, S. B., Delaney, H. D., & Moore, B. A. (1998). Community reinforcement approach in the treatment of opiate addicts. *American Journal of Drug and Alcohol Abuse, 24,* 17-30.

Abel, E. M. (2000). Psychosocial treatments for battered women: A review of empirical research. *Research on Social Work Practice, 10,* 55-77.

Ablon, J. S., & Jones, E. E. (2002). Validity of controlled clinical trials of psychotherapy: Findings from the NIMH Treatment of Depression Collaborative Research Program. *American Journal of Psychiatry, 159,* 775-783.

Abramowitz, J. S., Brigidi, B. D., & Roche, K. R. (2001). Cognitive-behavioral therapy for obsessive compulsive disorder. *Research on Social Work Practice, 11,* 357-372.

Abrams, D. B., & Niaura, R. S. (1987). Social learning theory. In H. T. Blane & K. E. Leonard (Eds.), *Psychological theories of drinking and alcoholism* (pp. 131-178). New York: Guilford Press.

Abramson, L. Y., Seligman, M. E., & Teasdale, J. (1978). Learned helplessness in humans: Critique and reformulation. *Journal of Abnormal Psychology, 87,* 49-74.

Achenbach, T. M. (1991). *Manual for the Youth Self-Report and 1991 profile.* Burlington: University of Vermont Department of Psychiatry.

Achenbach, T. M. (1995). Empirically based assessment and taxonomy: Applications to clinical research. *Psychological Assessment, 7,* 261-274.

Acierno, R., Donohue, B., & Kogan, E. (1994). Psychological interventions for drug abuse: A critique and summation of controlled studies. *Clinical Psychology Review, 14,* 417-442.

Ackerman, N. W. (1966). *Treating the troubled family.* New York: Basic Books.

Ainsworth, M. D., Blehar, M. C., Waters, E., & Wall, E. (1978). *Patterns of attachment: A psychological study of the strange situation.* Hillsdale, NJ: Erlbaum.

Albert, M., Becker, T., McCrone, P., & Thornicroft, G. (1998). Social networks and mental health service utilization: A literature review. *International Journal of Social Psychiatry, 44,* 248-266.

Alcoholics Anonymous. (1981). *Twelve steps and twelve traditions*. New York: Alcoholics Anonymous World Services.

Alexander, J. F., Holtzworth-Munroe, A., & Jameson, P. B. (1994). The process and outcome of marital and family therapy: Research, review and evaluation. In A. E. Bergin & S. L. Garfield (Eds.), *The handbook of psychotherapy and behavior change* (4th ed., pp. 595-630). New York: Wiley.

Alexander, J. F., & Parsons, B. V. (1982). *Functional family therapy: Principles and procedures*. Carmel, CA: Brooks/Cole.

Alexander, J. F., Waldron, H. B., Newberry, A. M., & Liddle, N. (1988). Family approaches to treating delinquents. Newbury Park, CA: Sage.

Alford, B. A., & Correia, C. J. (1994). Cognitive therapy of schizophrenia: Theory and empirical status. *Behavior Therapy, 25,* 17-33.

Allen, J. P., & Mattson, M. E. (1993). Psychometric instruments to assist in alcoholism treatment planning. *Journal of Substance Abuse Treatment, 10,* 289-296.

Alter-Reid, K., Gibbs, M. S., Lachenmeyer, J. R., Sigal, J., & Massoth, N. A. (1986). Sexual abuse of children: A review of the empirical findings. *Clinical Psychology Review, 6,* 249-266.

Amaro, H. (1995). Love, sex and power. *American Psychologist, 50,* 437-447.

Amaya-Jackson, L., & March, J. S. (1995). Posttraumatic stress disorder. In J. S. March (Ed.), *Anxiety disorders in children and adolescents* (pp. 276-317). New York: Guilford Press.

Ambrogne, J. A. (2002). Reduced-risk drinking as a treatment goal: What clinicians need to know. *Journal of Substance Abuse Treatment, 22,* 45-53.

American Academy of Child and Adolescent Psychiatry. (1990). *Guidelines for clinical evaluation of child sexual abuse*. Washington, DC: Author.

American Academy of Child and Adolescent Psychiatry. (1997a). Practice parameters for the forensic evaluation of children and adolescents who may have been physically or sexually abused. *Journal of the American Academy of Child and Adolescent Psychiatry, 36,* 423-442.

American Academy of Child and Adolescent Psychiatry. (1997b). Summary of the practice parameters for the assessment and treatment of children, adolescents, and adults with ADHD. *Journal of the American Academy of Child and Adolescent Psychiatry, 36,* 1311-1317.

American Academy of Child and Adolescent Psychiatry. (2001a). Practice parameter for the assessment and treatment of children and adolescents with suicidal behavior. *Journal of the Academy of Child and Adolescent Psychiatry, 40*(Suppl.), 24s-51s.

American Academy of Child and Adolescent Psychiatry. (2001b). Summary of the practice parameters for the use of stimulant medications in the treatment of children, adolescents, and adults. *Journal of the American Academy of Child and Adolescent Psychiatry, 40,* 1352-1355.

American Academy of Pediatrics. (1991). Guidelines for the evaluation of the sexual abuse of children. *Pediatrics, 87,* 254-260.

American Professional Society on the Abuse of Children. (1990). *Guidelines for psychosocial evaluation of suspected sexual abuse in young children*. Chicago: Author.

American Psychiatric Association. (2000). *Diagnostic and statistical manual of mental disorders* (4th ed., text revision). Washington, DC: American Psychiatric Association.

American Psychological Association. (1994). Guidelines for child custody evaluations in divorce proceedings. *American Psychologist, 49,* 677-680.

Ammerman, R. T., Cassisi, J. E., Hersen, M., & Van Hasselt, V. B. (1986). Consequences of physical abuse and neglect in children. *Clinical Psychology Review, 6,* 291-310.

Amodeo, M., & Jones, L. K. (1997). Viewing alcohol and other drug use cross culturally: A cultural framework for clinical practice. *Families in Society, 78,* 240-254.

Anastopoulos, A. D. (1998). A training program for parents of children with attention-deficit/hyperactivity disorder. In J. M. Briesmeister & C. E. Schaefer (Eds.), *Handbook of parent training: Parents as co-therapists for children's behavior problems* (pp. 27-60). New York: Wiley.

Anastoulos, A. D., Smith, J. M., & Wien, E. E. (1998). Counseling and training parents. In R. A. Barkley (Ed.), *Attention-deficit hyperactivity disorder: A handbook for diagnosis and treatment* (pp. 373-393). New York: Guilford Press.

Anderson, I. M. (2000). Selective serotonin reuptake inhibitors versus tricyclic antidepressants: A meta-analysis of efficacy and tolerability. *Journal of Affective Disorders, 58,* 19-36.

Anderson, J., Moeschberger, M., Chen, M. S., Junn, P., Wewers, M. E., & Guthrie, R. (1993). An acculturation scale for Southeast Asians. *Social Psychiatry and Psychiatric Epidemiology, 28,* 134-141.

Anderson, S. A. (2001). Clinical evaluation of violence in couples: The role of assessment instruments. *Journal of Family Psychotherapy, 12,* 1-18.

Anderson, S. A., & Cramer-Benjamin, D. B. (1999). The impact of couple violence on parenting and children: An overview and clinical implications. *American Journal of Family Therapy, 27,* 1-19.

Angermeyer, M. C., Kuhn, L., & Goldstein, J. M. (1990). Gender and the course of schizophrenia: Differences in treated outcomes. *Schizophrenia Bulletin, 16,* 293-307.

Annis, H. M. (1982). *Inventory of Drinking Situations.* Toronto: Addiction Research Foundation.

Annis, H. M., & Davis, C. S. (1991). Relapse prevention. *Alcohol Health and Research World, 15,* 3, 204-212.

Anthony, W. A., & Blanch, A. (1989). Research on community support services: What have we learned? *Psychosocial Rehabilitation Journal, 12,* 55-81.

Antony, M. M., & Swinson, R. P. (2000). *Phobic disorders and panic in adults: A guide to assessment and treatment.* Washington, DC: American Psychological Association.

Appel, A. E., & Holden, G. W. (1998). The co-occurrence of spouse and physical child abuse: A review and appraisal. *Journal of Family Psychology, 12,* 578-599.

Appelbaum, P. S. (1996). Law and psychiatry: Jaffee vs. Redmond: Psychotherapist-patient privilege in the federal courts. *Psychiatric Services, 47,* 1033-1052.

Appelbaum, P. S. (2001). Thinking carefully about out-patient civil commitment. *Psychiatric Services, 52,* 347-350.

Armstrong, C., & Hill, M. (2001). Support services for vulnerable families with young children. *Child and Family Social Work, 6,* 351-358.

Arnold, L. E., Abikoff, H. B., Cantwell, D. P., Conners, C. K., Elliott, G., Greenhill, L. L., et al. (1997). National Institute of Mental Health collaborative multimodal treatment study of children with ADHD (MTA): Design challenges and choices. *Archives of General Psychiatry, 54,* 865-870.

Arntz, A., van den Hoorn, M., Cornelis, J., Verheul, R., van den Bosch, W., & de Bie, A. (2003). Reliability and validity of the Borderline Personality Disorder Severity Index. *Journal of Personality Disorders, 17*, 45-59.

Arriaza, C. A., & Mann, T. (2001). Ethnic differences in eating disorder symptoms among college students: The confounding role of body mass index. *Journal of American College Health, 49*, 309-315.

Arroyo, J. A., Westerberg, V. S., & Tonigan, J. S. (1998). Comparison of treatment utilization and outcome for Hispanics and non-Hispanic whites. *Journal of Studies on Alcohol, 59*, 286-291.

Arthur, N. (1998). The effects of stress, depression, and anxiety on postsecondary students' coping strategies. *Journal of College Student Development, 39*, 11-22.

Asarnow, J. R., Scott, C. V., & Mintz, J. (2002). A combined cognitive-behavioral family education intervention for depression in children: A treatment development study. *Cognitive Therapy and Research, 26*, 221-229.

Ashford, J. B., Sales, B. D., & Reid, W. H. (2001). Political, legal, and professional challenges to treating offenders with special needs. In J. B. Ashford, B. D. Sales, & W. H. Reid (Eds.), *Treating adult and juvenile offenders with special needs* (pp. 31-49). Washington, DC: American Psychological Association.

Ashley, O., Marsden, M., & Brady, T. (2003). Effectiveness of substance abuse treatment programming for women: A review. *American Journal of Drug and Alcohol Abuse, 29*, 19-53.

AuClaire, P., & Schwartz, I. (1986). *An evaluation of the effectiveness of intensive home-based services as an alternative to placement for adolescents and their families.* Minneapolis: University of Minnesota, Hubert H. Humphrey Institute of Public Affairs.

Austin, S. B. (2000). Prevention research in eating disorders: Theory and new directions. *Psychological Medicine, 30*, 1249-1262.

Avison, W. R., & Gotlib, I. H. (1994). Introduction and overview. In W. R. Avison & I. H. Gotlib (Eds.), *Stress and mental health: Contemporary issues and prospects for the future* (pp. 3-12). New York: Plenum Press.

Axelson, D. A., & Birmaher, B. (2001). Relation between anxiety and depressive disorders in childhood and adolescence. *Depression and Anxiety, 14*, 67-78.

Azar, S. T., Povilaitis, T. Y., Lauretti, A. F., & Pouquette, C. L. (1998). The current status of etiological theories in intrafamilial child maltreatment. In J. R. Lutzker (Ed.), *Handbook of child abuse research and treatment* (pp. 3-30). New York: Plenum Press.

Azrin, N. H. (1976). Improvements in the community reinforcement approach to alcoholism. *Behaviour Research and Therapy, 14*, 339-348.

Azrin, N. H., Sisson, R. W., Meyers, R., & Godley, M. (1982). Alcoholism treatment by disulfiram and community reinforcement therapy. *Journal of Behavior Therapy and Experimental Psychiatry, 13*, 105-112.

Azzi-Lessing, L., & Olsen, L. J. (1996). Substance abuse-affected familes in the child welfare system: New challenges, alliances. *Social Work, 41*, 15-23.

Babor, T. F., & Grant, M. (1989). From clinical research to secondary prevention: International collaboration in the development of the Alcohol Use Disorders Identification Test (AUDIT). *Alcohol Health and Research World, 13*, 371-374.

Babor, T. F., Kranzler, H. R., & Lauerman, R. J. (1989). Early detection of harmful alcohol consumption: Comparison of clinical, laboratory, and self-report screening procedures. *Addictive Behaviors, 13*, 139-157.

Babor, T. F., Stephens, R., & Marlatt, G. A. (1987). Verbal report methods in clinical research on alcoholism: Response bias and its minimization. *Journal of Studies on Alcohol, 48*, 410-424.

Baer, J. S., Kivlahan, D. R., Blume, A. W., Arthur, W., McKnight, P., & Marlatt, G. A. (2001). Brief intervention for heavy-drinking college students: 4-year follow-up and natural history. *American Journal of Public Health, 91*, 1310-1316.

Baer, J. S., Marlatt, G. A., Kivlahan, D. R., Fromme, K., Larimer, M. E., & Williams, E. (1992). An experimental test of three methods of alcohol risk reduction with young adults. *Journal of Consulting and Clinical Psychology, 60*, 974-979.

Bailley, S., Lachar, D., Rhoades, H. M., Diefenbach, G., Espadas, A., & Varner, R. V. (2004). Quantifying symptomatic change during acute psychiatric hospitalization using new subscales for the anchored Brief Psychiatric Rating Scale. *Psychological Services, 1*, 68-82.

Baily, V. (1998). Conduct disorders in young children. In P. Graham (Ed.), *Cognitive-behaviour therapy for children and families* (pp. 95-109). New York: Cambridge University Press.

Baker, H. S., & Baker, M. N. (1987). Heinz Kohut's self-psychology: An overview. *American Journal of Psychiatry, 144*, 1-9.

Bandura, A. (1977). *Social learning theory*. Englewood Cliffs, NJ: Prentice Hall.

Bandura, A. (1986). *Social foundations of thought and action: A social cognitive theory*. Englewood Cliffs, NJ: Prentice Hall.

Bandura, A. (1999). A sociocognitive analysis of substance abuse: An agentic perspective. *Psychological Science, 10*, 214-217.

Barber, J. G., & Gilbertson, R. (1996). An experimental study of brief unilateral intervention for partners of heavy drinkers. *Research on Social Work Practice, 6*, 325-336.

Barber, J. G., & Gilbertson, R. (1997). Unilateral interventions for women living with heavy drinkers. *Social Work, 42*, 69-78.

Barkley, R. A. (1987). *Defiant children: A clinician's manual for parent training*. New York: Guilford Press.

Barkley, R. A. (1995). *Taking charge of ADHD: The complete authoritative guide for parents*. New York: Guilford Press.

Barkley, R. A. (1997a). Attention-deficit/hyperactivity disorder. In E. J. Mash & L. G. Terdal (Eds.), *Assessment of childhood disorders* (pp. 71-129). New York: Guilford Press.

Barkley, R. A. (1997b). Behavioral inhibition, sustained attention, and executive functions constructing a unifying theory of ADHD. *Psychological Bulletin, 121*, 65-94.

Barkley, R. A. (2002). Psychosocial treatments for attention deficit/hyperactivity disorder in children. *Journal of Clinical Psychiatry, 63*, 36-43.

Barkley, R. A., & Edwards, G. (1998). Diagnostic interview, behavior rating scales, and the medical examination. In R. A. Barkley (Ed.), *Attention-deficit hyperactivity disorder: A handbook for diagnosis and treatment* (pp. 263-293). New York: Guilford Press.

Barkley, R. A., Edwards, G., Laneri, M., Fletcher, K., & Meevia, L. (2001). The efficacy of problem-solving communication training alone, behavior management training alone, and their combination for parent-adolescent conflict in teenagers with ADHD and ODD. *Journal of Consulting and Clinical Psychology, 69*, 926-941.

Barkley, R. A., Shelton, T. L., Crosswait, C., Moorehouse, M., Fletcher, K., Barrett, S., et al. (2000). Multimethod psychoeducational intervention for preschool children with disruptive behavior: Preliminary results at post-treatment. *Journal of Child Psychology and Psychiatry, 41*, 319-332.

Barletta, J., Beamish, P., Patrick, M., Andersen, K., & Pappas, N. (1996). Obsessive-compulsive disorder: Emerging standard of care. *Psychotherapy in Private Practice, 15*, 19-31.

Barlow, D. H. (1988). *Anxiety and its disorders: The nature and treatment of anxiety and panic.* New York: Guilford Press.

Barlow, D. H. (1997). Cognitive-behavioral therapy for panic disorder: Current status. *Journal of Clinical Psychiatry, 58*(suppl. 2), 32-35.

Barnes, M. F. (1995). Sex therapy in the couples context: therapy issues of victims of sexual trauma. *American Journal of Family Therapy, 23*, 351-360.

Barrett, P. M. (1998). Evaluation of cognitive-behavioral group treatments for childhood anxiety disorders. *Journal of Clinical Child Psychology, 27*, 459-468.

Barrett, P. M., Dadds, M. R., & Rapee, R. M. (1996). Family treatment of childhood anxiety: A controlled trial. *Journal of Consulting and Clinical Psychology, 64*, 333-342.

Barrett, P. M., Duffy, A. L., Dadds, M. R., & Rapee, R. M. (2001). Cognitive-behavioral treatment of anxiety disorders in children: Long-term (6-year) follow-up. *Journal of Consulting and Clinical Psychology, 69*, 135-141.

Barrios, B. A., & Hartmann, D. P. (1997). In E. J. Mash & L. G. Terdal (Eds.), *Assessment of childhood disorders* (3rd ed., pp. 230-327). New York: Guilford Press.

Basen-Engquist, K. (1992). Psychosocial predictors of "safer sex" behavior in young adults. *AIDS Education and Prevention, 4*, 120-134.

Basic Behavioral Science Task Force. (1996). Basic behavioral science research for mental health: Sociocultural and environmental processes. *American Psychologist, 51*, 722-731.

Bateman, A., & Fonagy, P. (1999). Effectiveness of partial hospitalization in the treatment of borderline personality disorder: A randomized controlled trial. *American Journal of Psychiatry, 156*, 1563-1569.

Baucom, D. H., & Epstein, N. (1990). *Cognitive-behavioral marital therapy.* New York: Brunner/Mazel.

Baucom, D. H., Epstein, N., & Rankin, L. A. (1995). Cognitive aspects of cognitive behavioral marital therapy. In N. S. Jacobson & A. S. Gurman (Eds.), *Clinical handbook of couple therapy* (pp. 65-90). New York: Guilford Press.

Baucom, D. H., Mueser, K. T., Shoham, V., Daiuto, A. D., & Stickle, T. R. (1998). Empirically supported couple and family interventions for marital distress and adult mental health problems. *Journal of Consulting and Clinical Psychology, 66*, 53-88.

Baum, C. G. (1989). Conduct disorders. In T. H. Ollendick & M. Hersen (Eds.), *Handbook of childhood psychopathology* (2nd ed., pp. 171-196). New York: Plenum Press.

Beach, S. R., & O'Leary, K. D. (1992). Treating depression in the context of marital discord: Outcome and predictors of response for marital therapy vs. cognitive therapy. *Behavior Therapy, 23*, 507-528.

Beal, A. C., Ausiello, J., & Perrin, J. M. (2001). Social influences on health-risk behaviors among minority school students. *Journal of Adolescent Health, 28*, 474-480.

Beauvais, F. (1998). American Indians and alcohol. *Alcohol Health and Research World, 22*, 253-259.

Bebout, R., Drake, R., Haiyi, X., McHugo, G., & Harris, M. (1997). Housing status among formerly homeless dually diagnosed adults. *Psychiatric Services, 48*, 936-941.

Beck, A. T. (1976). *Cognitive therapy and the emotional disorders.* New York: New American Library.

Beck, A. T. (1996). Beyond belief: A theory of modes, personality and psychopathology. In P. M. Salkovskis (Ed.), *Frontiers of cognitive therapy* (pp. 1-25). New York: Guilford Press.

Beck, A. T., & Emery, G. (with Greenberg, R.L.). (1985). *Anxiety and phobias: A cognitive perspective.* New York: Basic Books.

Beck, A.T., Rush, A. J., Shaw, B. F., & Emery, G. (1979). *Cognitive therapy of depression.* New York: Guilford Press.

Beck, A. T., Steer, R. A., & Garbin, M. G. (1988). Psychometric properties of the Beck Depression Inventory: Twenty-five years of evaluation. *Clinical Psychology Review, 8,* 77-100.

Beck, A.T., Ward, C. H., Mendelson, M., Mock, J., & Erbaugh, J. (1961). An inventory for measuring depression. *Archives of General Psychiatry, 4,* 561-571.

Becker, J. V., & Johnson, B. R. (2001). Treating juvenile sex offenders. In J. B. Ashford, B. D. Sales, & W. H. Reid (Eds.), *Treating adult and juvenile offenders with special needs* (pp. 273-289). Washington, DC: American Psychological Association.

Beckerman, N. L., Letteney, S., & Lorber, K. (2000). Key emotional issues for couples of mixed HIV status. *Social Work in Health Care, 31,* 25-41.

Beckett, J. O., & Dungee-Anderson, D. (2000). Older persons of color: Asian-Pacific Islander Americans, African Americans, Hispanic Americans and American Indians. In R. L. Schneider, N. P. Kropf, & A. J. Kisor (Eds.), *Gerontological social work* (pp. 257-301). Belmont, CA: Wadsworth.

Beckman, L. J. (1994). Treatment needs of women with alcohol problems. *Alcohol Health and Research World, 18,* 206-211.

Bedell, J. R., Hunter, R. H., & Corrigan, P. W. (1997). Current approaches to assessment and treatment of persons with serious mental illness. *Professional Psychology: Research and Practice, 28,* 217-228.

Beekman, A., de Beurs, E., van Balkom, A., Deeg, D., van Dyck, R., & van Tilburg, W. (2000). Anxiety and depression in later life: Co-occurrence and communality of risk factors. *American Journal of Psychiatry, 157,* 89-95.

Behroozi, C. S. (1992). A model for social work with involuntary applicants in groups. *Social Work with Groups, 15,* 223-238.

Beidel, D. C., & Morris, T. L. (1995). Social phobia. In J. S. March (Ed.), *Anxiety disorders in children and adolescents* (pp. 181-211). New York: Guilford Press.

Bellack, A. S., & DiClemente, C. C. (1999). Treating substance abuse among patients with schizophrenia. *Psychiatric Services, 50,* 75-80.

Bellack, A. S., Mueser, K. T., Gingerich, S., & Agresta, J. (1997). *Social skills training for schizophrenia: A step-by-step guide.* New York: Guilford Press.

Belsky, J. (1993). Etiology of child maltreatment: A developmental-ecological analysis. *Psychological Bulletin, 114,* 413-434.

Benbenishty, R. (1996). Integrating research and practice: Time for a new agenda. *Research on Social Work Practice, 6,* 77-82.

Bennett, L. A., Janca, A., Grant, B. F., & Sartorius, N. (1993). Boundaries between normal and pathological drinking. *Alcohol Health and Research World, 17*, 190-195.

Bennett, L. W. (1995). Substance abuse and the domestic assault of women. *Social Work, 40*, 760-771.

Bennett, M. E., McCrady, B. S., Johnson, V., & Pandina, R. J. (1999). Problem drinking from young adulthood to adulthood: Patterns, predictors and outcomes. *Journal of Studies on Alcohol, 60*, 605-614.

Benson, H. (1975). *The relaxation response.* New York: Avon.

Bentley, K. J. (1998). Psychopharmacological treatment of schizophrenia: What social workers need to know. *Research on Social Work Practice, 8*, 384-405.

Bergman, M. M., & Scott, J. (2001). Young adolescents' wellbeing and health-risk behaviours: Gender and socio-economic differences. *Journal of Adolescence, 24*, 183-197.

Berry, J. W. (1986). The acculturation process and refugee behavior. In C. L. Williams & J. Westermeyer (Eds.), *Refugee mental health in resettlement countries* (pp. 25-36). New York: Hemisphere.

Beutler, L. E. (1999). Manualizing flexibility: The training of eclectic therapists. *Journal of Clinical Psychology, 55*, 399-404.

Beutler, L. E., & Clarkin, J. F. (1990). Systematic treatment selection: Toward targeted therapeutic interventions. New York: Brunner/Mazel.

Beutler, L. E., Clarkin, J. F., & Bongar, B. (2000). *Guidelines for the systematic treatment of the depressed patient.* New York: Oxford University Press.

Bezirganian, S., Cohen, P., & Brook, J. S. (1993). The impact of mother-child interaction on the development of borderline personality disorder. *American Journal of Psychiatry, 150*, 1836-1842.

Bibb, J. L., & Chambless, D. L. (1986). Alcohol use and abuse among diagnosed agoraphobics. *Behavior Research and Therapy, 24*, 49-58.

Biederman, J., Rosenbaum, J. F., Chaloff, J., & Kagan, J. (1995). Behavioral inhibition as a risk factor. In J. S. March (Ed.), *Anxiety disorders in children and adolescents* (pp. 61-81). New York: Guilford Press.

Birleson, P. (1981). The validity of depressive disorder in childhood and the development of a self-rating scale: A research report. *Journal of Child Psychology and Psychiatry, 22*, 73-88.

Birleson, P., Hudson, I., Buchanan, D. G., & Wolff, S. (1987). Clinical evaluation of a self-rating scale for depressive disorder in childhood (Depression Self-Rating Scale). *Journal of Child Psychology and Psychiatry, 28*, 43-60.

Birmaher, B., Brent, D. A., Chiappetta, L., Bridge, J., Monga, S., & Baugher, M. (1999). Psychometic properties of the Screen for Child Anxiety-Related Emotional Disorders (SCARED): A replication study. *Journal of the American Academy of Child and Adolescent Psychiatry, 38*, 1230-1236.

Birmaher, B., Brent, D. A., Kolko, D. J., Baugher, M., Bridge, J., Holder, D., et al. (2000). Clinical outcome after short-term psychotherapy for adolescents with major depressive disorder. *Archives of General Psychiatry, 57*, 29-36.

Birmaher, B., Khetarpal, S., Brent, D., Cully, M., Balach, L., Kaufman, J., et al. (1997). The Screen for Child Anxiety-Related Emotional Disorders (SCARED): Scale construction and psychometric characteristics. *Journal of the American Academy of Child and Adolescent Psychiatry, 36*, 545-553.

Birmaher, B., Ryan, N. D., Williamson, D. E., Brent, D. A., & Kaufman, J. (1996). Childhood and adolescent depression: A review of the past 10 years. Part 2. *Journal of the American Academy of Child and Adolescent Psychiatry, 35*, 1575-1583.

Bisson, J. I., & Shepherd, J. P. (1995). Psychological reactions of victims of violent crime. *British Journal of Psychiatry, 167*, 718-720.

Black, B. (1995). Separation anxiety disorder and panic disorder. In J. S. March (Ed.), *Anxiety disorders in children and adolescents* (pp. 212-234). New York: Guilford Press.

Black, D. W., Monahan, P., Baumgard, C. H., & Bell, S. E. (1997). Predictors of long-term outcome in 45 men with antisocial personality disorder. *Annals of Clinical Psychiatry, 9*, 211-217.

Blake, D. D., & Sonnenberg, R. T. (1998). Outcome research on behavioral and cognitive-behavioral treatments for trauma survivors. In V. M. Follette, J. I. Ruzek, & F. R. Abueg (Eds.), *Cognitive-behavioral therapies for trauma* (pp. 15-47). New York: Guilford Press.

Blake, D. D., Weathers, F. W., Nagy, L. M., Kaloupek, D. G., Gusman, F. D., Charney, D. S., et al. (1995). The development of a clinician-administered PTSD scale. *Journal of Traumatic Stress, 8*, 75-90.

Blake, D. D., Weathers, F. W., Nagy, L. M., Kaloupek, D. G., Klauminzer, G., Charney, D. S., et al. (1990). A clinician rating scale for assessing current and lifetime PTSD: The CAPS-1. *Behavior Therapist, 13*, 187-188.

Blanchard, E. B. (1994). Behavioral medicine and health psychology. In A. E. Bergin & S. L. Garfield (Eds.), *The handbook of psychotherapy and behavior change* (4th ed., pp. 701-733). New York: Wiley.

Blankertz, L. E., & Cnaan, R. A. (1994, December). Assessing the impact of two residential programs for dually diagnosed homeless individuals. *Social Service Review*, 536-560.

Blechman, E. A., & Brownell, K. D. (1998). *Behavioral medicine and women: A comprehensive handbook*. New York: Guilford Press.

Blechman, E. A., & Vryan, K. D. (2000). Prosocial family therapy: A manualized preventive intervention for juvenile offenders. *Aggression and Violent Behavior, 5*, 343-378.

Bloom, M., Fischer, J., & Orme, J. G. (1999). *Evaluating practice: Guidelines for the accountable professional* (2nd ed.). Boston: Allyn and Bacon.

Blum, R. W., Kelly, A., & Ireland, M. (2001). Health-risk behaviors and protective factors among adolescents with mobility impairments and learning and emotional disabilities. *Journal of Adolescent Health, 28*, 481-490.

Blumenthal, S. J. (1994). Women and depression. *Journal of Women's Health, 3*, 467-479.

Bodholdt, R. H., Richards, H. R., & Gacono, C. B. (2000). Assessing psychopathy in adults: The Psychopathy Checklist-Revised and screening version. In C. B. Gacono (Ed.), *The clinical and forensic assessment of psychopathy: A practitioner's guide* (pp. 55-86). Mahwah, NJ: Erlbaum.

Bogerts, B. (1993). Recent advances in the neuropathology of schizophrenia. *Schizophrenia Bulletin, 19*, 431-445.

Bograd, M., & Mederos, F. (1999). Battering and couples therapy: Universal screening and selection of treatment and modality. *Journal of Marital and Family Therapy, 25*, 291-312.

Bohn, M. J., Babor, T. F., & Kranzler, H. R. (1995). Alcohol Use Disorders Identification Test (AUDIT): Validation of a screening instrument for use in medical settings. *Journal of Studies on Alcohol, 56*, 423-432.

Bolton, D., Luckie, M., & Steinberg, D. (1995). Long-term course of obsessive-compulsive disorder treated in adolescence. *Journal of the American Academy of Child and Adolescent Psychiatry, 34*, 1441-1450.

Bond, G. R., Becker, D. R., Drake, R. E., Rapp, C. A., Meisler, N., Lehman, A. F., et al. (2001). Implementing supported employment as an evidence-based practice. *Psychiatric Services, 52*, 313-322.

Bond, G. R., Drake, R. E., Mueser, K. T., & Becker, D. R. (1997). An update on supported employment for people with severe mental illness. *Psychiatric Services, 48*, 335-346.

Bongar, B., Maris, R. W., Berman, A. L., & Litman, R. E. (1992). Outpatient standards of care and the suicidal patient. *Suicide and Life-Threatening Behavior, 22*, 453-477.

Borduin, C. M, Henggeler, S. W., Blaske, D. M., & Stein, R. (1990). Multisystemic treatment of adolescent sexual offenders. *International Journal of Offender Therapy and Comparative Criminology, 35*, 105-114.

Borduin, C. M., Mann, B. J., Cone, L. T., Henggeler, S. W., Fucci, B. R., & Blaske, D. M., et al. (1995). Multisystemic treatment of serious juvenile offenders: Long-term prevention of criminality and violence. *Journal of Consulting and Clinical Psychology, 63*, 569-578.

Borsari, B., & Carey, K. B. (2000). Effects of brief motivational intervention with college student drinkers. *Journal of Consulting and Clinical Psychology, 68*, 728-733.

Botvin, G. J., Baker, E., Dusenbury, L. D., Botvin, E. M., & Diaz, T. (1995). Long-term follow-up results of a randomized drug abuse prevention trial in a white middle-class population. *Journal of the American Medical Association, 273*, 1106-1112.

Botvin, G. J., Baker, E., Dusenbury, L., Tortu, S., & Botvin, E. M. (1990). Preventing adolescent drug abuse through a multimodal cognitive-behavioral approach: Results of a 3-year study. *Journal of Consulting and Clinical Psychology, 58*, 437-446.

Botvin, G. J., Griffin, K. W., Diaz, T., & Ifill-Williams, M. (2001). Preventing binge drinking during early adolescence: One- and two-year follow-up of a school-based prevention intervention. *Psychology of Addictive Behaviors, 15*, 360-365.

Bourke, M. L., & Donohue, B. (1996). Assessment and treatment of juvenile sex offenders: An empirical review. *Journal of Child Sexual Abuse, 5*, 47-70.

Bouton, M. E. (2000). A learning theory perspective on lapse, relapse and the maintenance of behavior change. *Health Psychology, 19*, 57-63.

Bowers, W. A., Evans, K., & van Cleve, L. (1996). Treatment of adolescent eating disorders. In M. A. Reinecke, F. M. Dattilio, & A. Freeman (Eds.), *Cognitive therapy with children and adolescents: A case book for clinical practice* (pp. 227-250). New York: Guilford Press.

Bowlby, J. (1969). *Attachment and loss: Vol. 1. Attachment.* New York: Basic Books.

Bowlby, J. (1980). *Attachment and loss: Vol. 3. Loss, sadness and depression.* New York: Basic Books.

Bowman, M. L. (1999). Individual difference in posttraumatic distress: Problems with the *DSM-IV* model. *Canadian Journal of Psychiatry, 44*, 21-33.

Bradshaw, W. (1996). Structured group work in individuals with schizophrenia: A coping skills approach. *Research on Social Work Practice, 6*, 139-153.

Bramblett, R., Wodarski, J. S., & Thyer, B. A. (1991). Social work practice with antisocial children: A review of current issues. *Journal of Applied Social Sciences, 15*, 169-182.

Brandell, J. R., & Perlman, F. T. (1997). Psychoanalytic theory. In J. R. Brandell (Ed.), *Theory and practice in clinical social work* (pp. 38-82). New York: Free Press.

Brandt, J. R., Kennedy, W. A., Patrick, C. J., & Curtin, J. J. (1997). Assessment of psychopathy in a population of incarcerated adolescent offenders. *Psychological Assessment, 9*, 429-435.

Brannen, S. J., & Rubin, A. (1996). Comparing the effectiveness of gender-specific and couples groups in a court-mandated spouse abuse treatment program. *Research on Social Work Practice, 6*, 405-424.

Braswell, L., & Bloomquist, M. L. (1991). *Cognitive-behavioral therapy with ADHD children: Child, family, and school interventions.* New York: Guilford Press.

Brems, C., & Johnson, M. E. (1997). Clinical implications of the co-occurrence of substance use and other psychiatric disorders. *Professional Psychology Research and Practice, 28*, 437-447.

Brener, N. D., & Collins, J. L. (1998). Co-occurrence of health-risk behaviors among adolescents in the United States. *Journal of Adolescent Health, 22*, 209-213.

Brennan, P. L., & Moos, R. H. (1996). Late-life drinking behavior. *Alcohol Health and Research World, 20*, 197-204.

Brent, D. A., Holder, D., Kolko, D., Birmaher, B., Baugher, M., Roth, C., et al. (1997). A clinical psychotherapy trial for adolescent depression comparing cognitive, family and supportive therapy. *Archives of General Psychiatry, 54*, 877-885.

Brent, D. A., Kolko, D. J., Birmaher, B., Baugher, M., & Bridge, J. (1999). A clinical trial for adolescent depression: Predictors of additional treatment in the acute and follow-up phases of the trial. *Journal of the Academy of Child and Adolescent Psychiatry, 38*, 263-270.

Brent, D. A., Kolko. D. J., Birmaher, B., Baugher, M., Bridge, J., Roth, C., et al. (1998). Predictors of treatment efficacy in a clinical trial of three psychosocial treatments for adolescent depression. *Journal of the American Academy of Child and Adolescent Psychiatry, 37*, 906-914.

Breslau, N., Davis, G., Andreski, P., Federman, B., & Anthony, J. C. (1998). Epidemiological findings on post traumatic stress disorder and co-morbid disorders in the general population. In B. P. Dohrenwend (Ed.), *Adversity, stress and psychopathology* (pp. 319-330). New York: Oxford University Press.

Breslau, N., Davis, G., Andreski, P., & Peterson, E. (1991). Traumatic events and post-traumatic stress disorder in an urban population of young adults. *Archives of General Psychiatry, 48*, 216-222.

Brestan, E. V., & Eyberg, S. (1998). Effective psychosocial treatments of conduct-disordered children and adolescents: 29 years, 82 studies, and 5, 272 kids. *Journal of Clinical Child Psychology, 27*, 180-189.

Bride, B. E. (2001). Single-gender treatment of substance abuse: Effect on treatment retention and completion. *Social Work Research, 25*, 223-232.

Briere, J. (1992). *Child abuse trauma: Theory and treatment of lasting effects.* Newbury Park, CA: Sage.

Briere, J. (1996). *Trauma Symptom Checklist for Children* (TSCC). Odessa, FL: Psychological Assessment Resources.

Brown, G. W. (1998). Loss and depressive disorders. In B. P. Dohrenwend (Ed.), *Adversity, stress and psychopathology* (pp. 358-370). New York: Oxford University Press.

Brown, J., Cohen, P., Johnson, J. G., & Salzinger, S. (1998). A longtitudinal analysis of risk factors for child maltreatment: Findings of a 17-year prospective study of officially recorded and self-reported child abuse and neglect. *Child Abuse and Neglect, 22*, 1065-1078.

Brown, L. K., & Lourie, K. J. (2001). Motivational interviewing and the prevention of HIV among adolescents. In P. M. Monti, S. M. Colby, & T. A. O'Leary (Eds.), *Adolescents, alcohol and substance abuse: Reaching teens through brief interventions.* New York: Guilford Press.

Brown, R. A., Evans, D. M., Miller, I. W., Burgess, E. S., & Mueller, T. I. (1997). Cognitive-behavioral treatment for depression in alcoholism. *Journal of Consulting and Clinical Psychology, 65*, 715-726.

Brown, S. A. (1985). Expectancies vs. background in the prediction of college drinking patterns. *Journal of Consulting and Clinical Psychology, 53*, 123-130.

Brown, S. A., Christiansen, B. A., & Goldman, M. S. (1987). The Alcohol Expectancy Questionnaire: An instrument for the assessment of adolescent and adult alcohol expectancies. *Journal of Studies on Alcohol, 48*, 483-491.

Brown, S. A., Goldman, M., Inn, A., & Anderson, L. (1980). Expectancies of reinforcement from alcohol: Their domain and relation to drinking patterns. *Journal of Consulting and Clinical Psychology, 48*, 419-426.

Brown, T. G., Werk, A., Caplan, T., & Seraganian, P. (1999). Violent substance abusers in domestic violence treatment. *Violence and Victims, 14*, 179-190.

Brown, V. B., Ridgely, M. S., Pepper, B., Levine, I. S., & Ryglewicz, H. (1989). The dual crisis: Mental illness and substance abuse: Present and future directions. *American Psychologist, 44*, 565-569.

Brownell, K. D., Marlatt, G. A., Lichtenstein, E., & Wilson, G. T. (1986). Understanding and preventing relapse. *American Psychologist, 41*, 765-782.

Brunk, M., Henggeler, S. W., & Whelan, J. P. (1987). Comparison of multisystemic therapy and parent training in the brief treatment of child abuse and neglect. *Journal of Consulting and Clinical Psychology, 55*, 171-178.

Buchanan, R. W. (1995). Clozapine efficacy and safety. *Schizophrenia Bulletin, 21*, 579-591.

Buckstein, O. G. (1995). *Adolescent substance abuse: Assessment, prevention and treatment.* New York: Wiley.

Buckstein, O. G., Brent, D. A., & Kaminer, Y. (1989). Comorbidity of substance abuse and other psychiatric disorders in adolescents. *American Journal of Psychiatry, 146*, 1131-1141.

Budd, K. S., Felix, E. D., Poindexter, L. M., Naik-Polan, A. T., & Sloss, C. F. (2002). Clinical assessment of children in child protection cases: An empirical analysis. *Professional Psychology: Research and Practice, 33*, 3-12.

Budd, K. S., Poindexter, L. M., Felix, E. D., & Naik-Polan, A. T. (2001). Clinical assessment of parents in child protection cases: An empirical analysis. *Law and Human Behavior, 25*, 93-108.

Budman, S. H., & Gurman, A. S. (1988). *The theory and practice of brief therapy.* New York: Guilford Press.

Burnette, D. (1998). Grandparents rearing grandchildren: A school-based small group intervention. *Research on Social Work Practice, 8*, 10-27.

Burnette, M. F., & Drake, R. E. (1997). Gender differences in patients with schizophrenia and substance abuse. *Comprehensive Psychiatry, 38*, 109-116.

Burns, B., & Santos, A. B. (1995). Assertive community treatment: An update of randomized trials. *Psychiatric Services, 46*, 669-675.

Burns, G. L., & Patterson, D. R. (1990). Conduct problem behaviors in a stratified random sample of children and adolescents: New standardization data on the Eyberg Child Behavior Inventory. *Psychological Assessment: A Journal of Consulting and Clinical Psychology, 2*, 391-397.

Burns, G. L., & Patterson, D. R. (2000). Factor structure of the Eyberg Child Behavior Inventory: A parent rating scale of oppositional defiant behavior toward adults, inattentive behavior, and conduct problem behavior. *Journal of Clinical Child Psychology, 29*, 569-577.

Burns, G. L., Patterson, D. R., Nussbaum, B. R., & Parker, C. M. (1991). Disruptive behaviors in an outpatient pediatric population: Additional standardization data on the Eyberg Child Behavior Inventory. *Psychological Assessment: A Journal of Consulting and Clinical Psychology, 3*, 202-207.

Busby, D. M., Christensen, C., Crane, D. R., & Larson, J. H. (1995). A revision of the dyadic adjustment scale for use with distressed and nondistressed couples: Construct hierarchy and multidimensional scales. *Journal of Marital and Family Therapy, 21*, 289-308.

Bystritsky, A., Munford, P. R., Rosen, R. M., Martin, K. M., Vapnik, T., Gorbis, E. E., et al. (1996). A preliminary study of partial hospital management of severe obsessive-compulsive disorder. *Psychiatric Services, 47*, 170-174.

Cadoret, R., & Cain, C. (1980). Sex differences in predictors of antisocial behavior in adoptees. *Archives of General Psychiatry, 37*, 1171-1175.

Caetano, R. (1993). Ethnic minority groups and Alcoholics Anonymous: A review. In B. S. McCrady & W. R. Miller (Eds.), *Research on Alcoholics Anonymous: Opporunities and alternatives* (pp. 209-232). New Brunswick, NJ: Rutgers Center of Alcohol Studies.

Caetano, R., & Clark, C. L. (1998). Trends in alcohol consumption patterns among whites, blacks and Hispanics: 1984 and 1995. *Journal of Studies on Alcohol, 59*, 659-668.

Caetano, R., Clark, C. L., & Tam, T. (1998). Alcohol consumption among racial/ethnic minorities. *Alcohol Health and Research World, 22*, 233-241.

Cahill, S., Carrigan, M., & Frueh, B. (1999). Does EMDR work? And if so, why? A critical review of the controlled outcome and dismantling research. *Journal of Anxiety Disorders, 13*, 5-33.

Callaway, J. T. (1998). Psychopharmacological treatment of dementia. *Research on Social Work Practice, 8*, 452-474.

Camasso, M. J., & Jagannathan, R. (2000). Modeling the reliability and predictive validity of risk assessment in child protective services. *Children and Youth Services Review, 22*, 873-896.

Campbell, D., & Stanley, J. (1963). *Experimental and quasi-experimental designs for research*. Chicago: Rand McNally.

Carey, K. B. (1993). Situational determinants of heavy drinking among college students. *Journal of Counseling Psychology, 40*, 217-220.

Carey, K. B. (1996a). Substance use reduction in the context of outpatient psychiatric treatment: A collaborative, motivational, harm reduction approach. *Community Mental Health Journal, 32,* 291-306.

Carey, K. B. (1996b). Treatment of co-occurring substance abuse and major mental illness. *New Directions for Mental Health Services, 70,* 19-31.

Carey, K. B., Cocco, K. M., & Simons, J. S. (1996). Concurrent validity of clinicians' ratings of substance abuse among psychiatric outpatients. *Psychiatric Services, 47,* 842-847.

Carey, K. B., & Teitelbaum, L. M. (1996). Goals and methods of alcohol assessment. *Professional Psychology Research and Practice, 27,* 460-466.

Carey, M. P., Carey, K. B., & Kalichman, S. C. (1997). Risk for human immunodeficiency virus (HIV) infection among persons with severe mental illnesses. *Clinical Psychology Review, 17,* 271-291.

Carlson, B. E., & Russer-Hogan, R. (1991). Trauma experiences, stress, dissociation and depression in Cambodian refugees. *American Journal of Psychiatry, 148,* 1548-1551.

Carlson, G. A., & Cantwell, D. P. (1980). A survey of depressive symptoms, syndrome and disorder in a child psychiatric population. *Journal of Child Psychology and Psychiatry, 21,* 19-25.

Carroll, J. L., & Carroll, L. M. (1995). Alcohol use and risky sex among college students. *Psychological Reports, 76,* 723-726.

Carten, A. J. (1996). Mothers in recovery: Rebuilding families in the aftermath of addiction. *Social Work, 41,* 215-223.

Carter, J. D., Joyce, P. R., Mulder, R. T., Sullivan, P. F., & Luty, S. E. (1999). Gender differences in the frequency of personality disorders in depressed outpatients. *Journal of Personality Disorders, 13,* 67-74.

Carter, R. T. (1995). *The influence of race and racial identity in psychotherapy: Toward a racially inclusive model.* New York: Wiley.

Castellanos, F. X. (1998). Tic disorders and obsessive-compulsive disorder. In B. T. Walsh (Ed.), *Child psychopharmacology* (pp. 1-28). Washington, DC: American Psychiatric Press.

Cattell, R. B. (1965). *The scientific analysis of personality.* Chicago: Aldine.

Cautela, J. R. (1993). Insight in behavior therapy. *Journal of Behavior Therapy and Experimental Psychiatry, 24,* 155-159.

Celio, A. A., Winzelberg, A. J., Eppstein-Herald, D., Wilfley, D., Springer, E. A., Dev, P., & Taylor, C. B. (2000). Reducing risk factors for eating disorders: Comparison of an Internet-based and classroom-delivered psychoeducational program. *Journal of Consulting and Clinical Psychology, 68,* 650-657.

Chaffin, M., & Shultz, S. K. (2001). Psychometric evaluation of the Children's Impact of Traumatic Events Scale-Revised. *Child Abuse and Neglect, 25,* 401-411.

Chamberlain, P., & Rosicky, J. G. (1995). The effectiveness of family therapy in the treatment of adolescents with conduct disorders and delinquency. *Journal of Marital and Family Therapy, 21,* 441-459.

Chambless, D. L., & Gillis, M. M. (1996). Cognitive therapy of anxiety disorders. In K. S. Dobson & D. Craig (Eds.), *Advances in cognitive-behavioral therapy* (pp. 116-144). Newbury Park, CA: Sage.

Chambless, D. L., & Hollon, S. D. (1998). Defining empirically supported therapies. *Journal of Consulting and Clinical Psychology, 66,* 7-18.

Chemtob, C. M., Tolin, D. F., Van der Kolk, B. A., & Pitman, R. K. (2000). Eye movement desensitization and reprocessing. In E. B. Foa, T. M. Keane, & M. J. Friedman (Eds.), *Effective treatments for PTSD: Practice guidelines from the International Society for Traumatic Stress Studies* (pp. 139-154). New York: Guilford Press.

Chen, K., & Kandel, D. (1995). The natural history of drug use from adolescents to the mid-thirties in a general population sample. *American Journal of Public Health, 85,* 41-47.

Chen, L., Eaton, W., Gallo, J., Nestadt, G., & Crum, R. (2000). Empirical examination of current depression categories in a population-based study: Symptoms, course and risk factors. *American Journal of Psychiatry, 157,* 573-580.

Chen, W. J., Faraone, S. V., Biederman, J., & Tsuang, M. T. (1994). Diagnostic accuracy of the Child Behavior Checklist Scales for Attention-Deficit Hyperactivity Disorder: A receiver operating characteristics analysis. *Journal of Consulting and Clinical Psychology, 62,* 1017-1025.

Cheung, Y. W. (1991). Ethnicity and alcohol/drug use revisited: A framework for future research. *International Journal of the Addictions, 25,* 581-605.

Christensen, A., Jacobson, N. S., & Babcock, J. C. (1995). In N. S. Jacobson, & A. S. Gurman (Eds.), *Clinical handbook of couple therapy* (pp. 31-64). New York: Guilford Press.

Christophersen, E. R., & Finney, J. W. (1999). Oppositional defiant disorder. In R. T. Ammerman, M. Hersen, & C. G. Last (Eds.), *Handbook of prescriptive treatments for children and adolescents* (2nd ed., pp. 102-113). Boston: Allyn and Bacon.

Cicchetti, D., Rogosch, A., & Toth, S. L. (1994). A developmental psychopathology perspective on depression in children and adolescents. In W. M. Reynolds & H. F. Johnston (Eds.), *Handbook of depression in children and adolescents* (pp. 123-141). New York: Plenum Press.

Clapp, J. D., Segars, L., & Voas, R. (2002). A conceptual model of the alcohol environment of college students. *Journal of Human Behavior in the Social Environment, 5,* 73-90.

Clark, D. A., & Beck, A. T. (with Alford, B. A.). (1999). *Scientific foundations of cognitive theory and therapy of depression.* New York: Wiley.

Clark, R. E. (2001). Family support and substance use outcomes for persons with mental illness and substance use disorders. *Schizophrenia Bulletin, 27,* 93-101.

Clark, R. E., Ricketts, S. K., & McHugo, G. J. (1999). Legal system involvement and costs for persons in the treatment for severe mental illness and substance abuse disorders. *Psychiatric Services, 50,* 641-647.

Cleckley, H. (1941). *The mask of sanity.* St. Louis, MO: Mosby.

Clum, G. A., Broyles, S., Borden, J., & Watkins, P. L. (1990). Validity and reliability of the Panic Attack Symptoms and Cognitions Questionnaires. *Journal of Psychopathology and Behavioral Assessment, 12,* 233-245.

Coatsworth, J. D., Pantin, H., McBride, C., Briones, E., Kurtines, W., & Szapocznik, J. (2002). Ecodevelopmental correlates of behavior problems in young Hispanic females. *Applied Developmental Science, 6,* 126-143.

Cocco, K. M., & Carey, K. B. (1998). Psychometric properties of the Drug Abuse Screening Test in psychiatric outpatients. *Psychological Assessment, 10,* 408-414.

Coffey, S. F., Dansky, B. S., Falsetti, S. A., Saladin, M. E., & Brady, K. T. (1998). Screening for PTSD in a substance abuse sample: Psychometric properties of a modified version of the PTSD Symptom Scale self-report. *Journal of Traumatic Stress, 11,* 393-399.

Coleman, H., Unrau, Y. A., & Manyfingers, B. (2001). Revamping family preservation services for native families. *Journal of Ethnic and Cultural Diversity in Social Work, 10,* 49-68.

Collett, B. R., Ohan, J. L., & Myers, K. M. (2003). Ten-year review of scales: Part 6. Scales assessing externalizing behaviors. *Journal of the American Academy of Child and Adolescent Psychiatry, 42,* 1143-1170.

Combs-Orme, T., & Thomas, K. H. (1997). Assessment of troubled families. *Social Work Research, 21,* 261-269.

Compas, B. E. (1997). Depression in children and adolescents. In E. J. Mash & L. G. Terdal (Eds.), *Assessment of childhood disorders* (3rd ed., pp. 197-229). New York: Guilford Press.

Compton, B. R., & Gallaway, B. (1999). *Social work processes* (6th ed.). Pacific Grove, CA: Brooks/Cole.

Compton, S. N., Burns, B. J., Egger, H. L., & Robertson, E. (2002). Review of the evidence base for treatment of childhood psychopathology: Internalizing disorders. *Journal of Consulting and Clinical Psychology, 70,* 1240-1266.

Compton, W. M., Cottler, L. B., Abdallah, A. B., Phelps, D. L., Spitznagel, E. L., & Horton, J. C. (2000). Substance dependence and other psychiatric disorders among drug dependent subjects: Race and gender correlates. *American Journal on Addictions, 9,* 113-125.

Conners, C. K. (1997). *Conners' rating scales-revised technical manual.* North Tonawanda, NY: Multi-Health Systems.

Conners, C. K., Epstein, J., & March, J. (2001). Multimodal treatment of ADHD(MTA): An alternative outcome analysis. *Journal of the American Academy of Child and Adolescent Psychiatry, 40,* 159-167.

Conte, H. R., Plutchik, R., Karasu, T. B., & Jerrett, I. (1980). A self-report borderline scale: Discriminative validity and preliminary norms. *Journal of Nervous and Mental Disease, 168,* 428-435.

Conte, J. (1984, May-June). Progress in treating the sexual abuse of children. *Social Work,* 258-263.

Conte, J., & Schuerman, J. (1987). The effects of sexual abuse on chidren: A multidimensional view. *Journal of Interpersonal Violence, 2,* 380-390.

Cooke, D. J., & Michie, C. (1997). An item response theory analysis of the Hare Psychopathy Checklist-revised. *Psychological Assessment, 9,* 3-14.

Cooper, M. L. (1992). Alcohol and increased behavioral risk for AIDS. *Alcohol Health and Research World, 16,* 64-72.

Cooper, M. L. (2002). Alcohol use and risky sexual behavior among college students and youth: Evaluating the evidence. *Journal of Studies on Alcohol, 63,* 101-117.

Cooper, M. L., & Orcutt, H. K. (1997). Drinking and sexual experience on first dates among adolescents. *Journal of Abnormal Psychology, 106,* 191-202.

Cooper, M. L., Russell, M., & George, W. H. (1988). Coping, expectancies and alcohol abuse: A test of social learning theory formulations. *Journal of Abnormal Psychology, 97,* 218-230.

Cooper, Z., & Fairburn, C. (1987). The eating disorder examination: A semi-structured interview for the assessment of the specific psychopathology of eating disorders. *International Journal of Eating Disorders, 6,* 1-8.

Corcoran, J. (2000). Family interventions with child physical abuse and neglect: A critical review. *Children and Youth Services Review, 22,* 563-591.

Corcoran, K., & Gingerich, W. J. (1994). Practice evaluation in the context of managed care. *Research on Social Work Practice, 4,* 326-337.

Corcoran, K., Gingerich, W. J., & Briggs, H. E. (2001). Practice evaluation: Setting goals and monitoring change. In H. E. Briggs & K. Corcoran (Eds.), *Social work practice: Treating common client problems* (pp. 66-84). Chicago: Lyceum Books.

Corcoran, K., & Vandiver, V. (1996). *Maneuvering the maze of managed care: Skills for mental health practitioners.* New York: Free Press.

Corrigan, E. (1985). Gender differences in alcohol and other drug use. *Addictive Behaviors, 10,* 313-317.

Corrigan, P. (1997). Behavior therapy empowers persons with severe mental illness. *Behavior Modification, 21,* 45-61.

Corwin, M. (1996, January). Early intervention strategies with borderline clients. *Families in Society: The Journal of Contemporary Human Services,* 40-49.

Costanzo, P., Miller-Johnson, S., & Wencel, H. (1995). Social development. In J. S. March (Ed.), *Anxiety disorders in children and adolescents* (pp. 82-108). New York: Guilford Press.

Costello, E. J., & Angold, A. (1988). Scales to assess child and adolescent depression: Checklists, screens, and nets. *Journal of the American Academy of Child and Adolescent Psychiatry, 27,* 726-737.

Cournos, F., & McKinnon, K. (1997). HIV seroprevalence among people with severe mental illness in the United States: A critical review. *Clinical Psychology Review, 17,* 259-269.

Craighead, L. W., Craighead, W. E., Kazdin, A. P., & Mahoney, M. J. (Eds.). (1994). *Cognitive and behavioral interventions: An empirical approach to mental health problems.* Boston: Allyn and Bacon.

Craighead, W. E., Smucker, M. R., Craighead, L. W., & Ilardi, S. S. (1998). Factor analysis of the Children's Depression Inventory in a community sample. *Psychological Assessment, 10,* 156-165.

Crane, D. R., Middleton, K. C., & Bean, R. A. (2000). Establishing criterion scores for the Kansas Marital Satisfaction Scale and the Revised Dyadic Adjustment Scale. *American Journal of Family Therapy, 28,* 53-60.

Craske, M. G. (1996a). Cognitive-behavioral approaches to panic and agoraphobia. In K. S. Dobson & K. D. Craig (Eds.), *Advances in cognitive-behavioral therapy* (pp. 145-173). Thousand Oaks, CA: Sage.

Craske, M. G. (1996b). An integrated treatment approach to panic disorder. *Bulletin of the Menninger Clinic, 60,* A87-A104.

Craske, M. G. (1997). Fear and anxiety in children and adolescents. *Bulletin of the Menninger Clinic, 61,* A4-A36.

Craske, M. G. (1999). *Anxiety disorders: Psychological approaches to theory and treatment.* Boulder, CO: Westview Press.

Craske, M. G., & Zoeller, L. A. (1995). Anxiety disorders: The role of marital therapy. In N. S. Jacobson, & A. S. Gurman (Eds.), *Clinical handbook of couple therapy* (pp. 394-410). New York: Guilford Press.

Critchlow, B. (1986). The powers of John Barleycorn. *American Psychologist, 41,* 751-764.

Crits-Christoph, P. (1998). Psychosocial treatment for personality disorders. In P. E. Nathan & J. M. Gorman (Eds.), *A guide to treatments that work* (pp. 544-553). New York: Oxford University Press.

Crouch, J. L., Smith, D. W., Ezzell, C. E., & Saunders, B. E. (1999). Measuring reactions to sexual trauma among children: Comparing the Children's Impact of Traumatic Events Scale and the Trauma Symptom Checklist for Children. *Child Maltreatment, 4*, 255-263.

Culp, R. E., Heide, J., & Richardson, M. T. (1987). Maltreated children's developmental scores: Treatment versus nontreatment. *Child Abuse and Neglect, 11*, 29-34.

Culp, R. E., Richardson, M. T., & Heide, J. S. (1987). Differential developmental progress of maltreated children in day treatment. *Social Work, 32*, 497-499.

Cummings, S. M. (2003). The efficacy of an integrated group treatment program for depressed assisted living residents. *Research on Social Work Practice, 13*, 608-621.

Cunningham, J. A., Sobell, L. C., Sobell, M. B., & Kapur, G. (1995). Resolution from alcohol problems with and without treatment: Reasons for change. *Journal of Substance Abuse, 7*, 365-372.

Cunningham, M. D., & Reidy, T. J. (1998). Antisocial personality disorder and psychopathy: Diagnostic dilemmas in classifying patterns of antisocial behavior in sentencing evaluations. *Behavioral Sciences and the Law, 16*, 333-351.

Cunningham, M. D., & Reidy, T. J. (1999). Don't confuse me with the facts: Common errors in violence risk assessment at capital sentencing. *Criminal Justice and Behavior, 26*, 20-43.

Curry, J. F. (2001). Specific psychotherapies for childhood and adolescent depression. *Biological Psychiatry, 49*, 1091-1100.

Cutchen, M. A., & Simpson, R. G. (1993). Interrater reliability among teachers and mental health professionals when using the Revised Behavior Problem Checklist. *Journal of Psychoeducational Assessment, 11*, 4-11.

Daghestani, A. N., Dinwiddie, S. H., & Hardy, D. W. (2001). Antosocial personality disorders in and out of correctional and forensic settings. *Psychiatric Annals, 31*, 441-446.

Dahl, A. A. (1995). Commentary on borderline personality disorder. In J. Livesley (Ed.), *The DSM-IV personality disorders* (pp. 158-164). New York: Guilford Press.

Daiuto, A. D., Baucom, D. H., Epstein, N., & Dutton, S. S. (1998). The application of behavioral couples therapy to the assessment and treatment of agoraphobia: Implications of empirical research. *Clinical Psychology Review, 18*, 663-687.

Daley, D. (1987). Relapse prevention with substance abusers. *Social Work, 32*, 159-163.

Dare, C., & Eisler, I. (2002). Family therapy and eating disorders. In C. G. Fairburn & K. D. Brownell (Eds.), *Eating disorders and obesity: A comprehensive handbook* (2nd ed., pp. 314-319). New York: Guilford Press.

Darkes, J., & Goldman, M. S. (1993). Expectancy challenge and drinking reduction: Experimental evidence for a mediational process. *Journal of Consulting and Clinical Psychology, 61*, 344-353.

Davidson, P. R., & Parker, K. C. (2001). Eye movement desensitization and reprocessing (EMDR): A meta-analysis. *Journal of Consulting and Clinical Psychology, 69*, 305-316.

Dawes, R. M. (1989). *House of cards: Psychology and psychotherapy built on myth.* New York: Free Press.

De Bonis, M., De Boeck, P., Lida-Pulik, H., Hourtane, M., & Feline, A. (1998). Self-concept and mood: A comparative study between depressed patients with and without borderline personality disorder. *Journal of Affective Disorders, 48*, 191-197.

Deckel, A. W., Hesselbrock, V., & Bauer, L. (1996). Antisocial personality disorder, childhood delinquency, and frontal brain functioning: EEG and neuropsychological findings. *Journal of Clinical Psychology, 52,* 639-650.

Dees, S. M., Dansereau, D. F., & Simpson, D. D. (1994). A visual representation system for drug abuse counselors. *Journal of Substance Abuse Treatment, 11,* 517-523.

DePanfilis, D., & Zuravin, S. J. (1999). Predicting child maltreatment recurrences during treatment. *Child Abuse and Neglect, 8,* 729-743.

DePanfilis, D., & Zuravin, S. J. (2001). Assessing risk to determine the need for services. *Children and Youth Services Review, 23,* 3-20.

Dermen, K. H., & Cooper, M. L. (1994a). Sex-related alcohol expectancies among adolescents: Part 1. Scale development. *Psychology of Addictive Behaviors, 8,* 152-160.

Dermen, K. H., & Cooper, M. L. (1994b). Sex-related alcohol expectancies among adolescents: Part 2. Prediction of drinking in social and sexual situations. *Psychology of Addictive Behaviors, 8,* 161-168.

Dermen, K. H., Cooper, M. L., & Agocha, V. B. (1998). Sex-related expectancies as moderators of the relationship between alcohol use and risky sex in adolescents. *Journal of Studies on Alcohol, 59,* 71-77.

Derogatis, L. R., & Melisaratos, N. (1983). The Brief Symptom Inventory: An introductory report. *Psychological Medicine, 13,* 595-605.

DeShazer, S. (1985). *Keys to solution in brief therapy.* New York: Norton.

Dessaulles, A., Johnson, S. M., & Denton, W. H. (2003). Emotion-focused therapy for couples in the treatment of depression: A pilot study. *American Journal of Family Therapy, 31,* 345-353.

DeVellis, R. F. (2000). *Scale development: Theory and applications,* Thousand Oaks, CA: Sage.

Devilly, G., & Spence, S. (1999). The relative efficacy and treatment distress of EMDR and a cognitive behavioral trauma treatment protocol in the amelioration of post-traumatic stress disorder. *Journal of Anxiety Disorders, 13,* 131-157.

Dick, L. P., & Gallagher-Thompson, D. (1996). Late-life depression. In M. Hersen & V. B. Van Hasselt (Eds.), *Psychological treatment of older adults: An introductory text* (pp. 181-208). New York: Plenum Press.

Dickerson, F. B. (1997). Assessing clinical outcomes: The community functioning of persons with serious mental illness. *Psychiatric Services, 48,* 897-902.

DiClemente, C. C., Bellino, L. E., & Neavins, T. M. (1999). Motivation for change and alcoholism treatment. *Alcohol Research and Health, 23,* 86-92.

DiClemente, C. C., Carbonari, J. P., Montgomery, R. P. G., & Hughes, S. O. (1994). The Alcohol Abstinence Self-Efficacy Scale. *Journal of Studies on Alcohol, 55,* 141-148.

DiClemente, C. C., & Hughes, S. O. (1990). Stages of change profiles in outpatient alcoholism treatment. *Journal of Substance Abuse, 2,* 217-235.

Disney, E. R., Elkins, I. J., McGue, M., & Iacono, W. G. (1999). Effects of ADHD, conduct disorder, and gender on substance use and abuse in adolescence. *American Journal of Psychiatry, 156,* 1515-1521.

Dixon, L. B., Adams, C., & Lucksted, A. (2000). Update on family psychoeducation for schizophrenia. *Schizophrenia Bulletin, 26,* 5-20.

Dixon, L. B., & Lehman, A. F. (1995). Family interventions for schizophrenia. *Schizophrenia Bulletin, 21,* 631-643.

Dixon, L. B., Lehman, A. F., & Levine, J. (1995). Conventional antipsychotic medications for schizophrenia. *Schizophrenia Bulletin, 21,* 567-577.

Dixon, L. B., McFarlane, W. R., Lefley, H., Lucksted, A., Cohen, M., Falloon, I., et al. (2001). Evidence-based practices for services to families of people with psychiatric disabilities. *Psychiatric Services, 52*, 903-910.

Dobson, K. S. (1989). A meta-analysis of the efficacy of cognitive therapy for depression. *Journal of Consulting and Clinical Psychology, 57*, 414-419.

Dobson, K. S., & Craig, K. D. (Eds.). (1996). *Advances in cognitive-behavioral therapy*. Thousand Oaks, CA: Sage.

Dobson, K. S., & Jackman-Cram, S. (1996). Common change processes in cognitive-behavioral processes for depression. In K. S. Dobson & K. D. Craig (Eds.), *Advances in cognitive-behavioral therapy* (pp. 63-82). Thousand Oaks, CA: Sage.

Dohrenwend, B. P. (1998). Overview of evidence for the importance of adverse environmental conditions in causing psychiatric disorders. In B. P. Dohrenwend (Ed.), *Adversity, stress and psychopathology* (pp. 523-538). New York: Oxford University Press.

Dohrenwend, B. P., & Dohrenwend, B. S. (1974). Social and cultural influences on psychopathology. *Annual Review of Psychology, 25*, 417-452.

Dohrenwend, B. P., Levav, I., Shrout, P. E., Schwartz, S., Naveh, G., Link, B. G., et al. (1998). Ethnicity, socioeconomic status, and psychiatric disorders: A test of the social causation-social selection issue. In B. P. Dohrenwend (Ed.), *Adversity, stress and psychopathology* (pp. 285-318). New York: Oxford University Press.

Donabedian, A. (1980). *Explorations in quality assessment and monitoring: Vol. 1. The definition of quality and approaches to its assessment*. Ann Arbor, MI: Health Administration Press.

Donovan, D. (1999). Assessment strategies and measures in addictive behaviors. In B. S. McCrady & E. S. Epstein (Eds), *Addictions: A comprehensive guidebook* (pp. 187-215). New York: Oxford University Press.

Dore, M. M. (1999). Emotionally and behaviorally disturbed children in the child welfare system: Points of preventive intervention. *Children and Youth Services Review, 21*, 7-29.

Dore, M. M., Kauffman, E., Nelson-Zlupko, L., & Granfort, E. (1996, December). Psychosocial functioning and treatment needs of latency-age children from drug-involved families. *Families in Society: The Journal of Contemporary Human Services*, 595-603.

Dorfman, R. A., Lubben, J. E., Mayer-Oakes, A., Atchison, K., Schweitzer, S. O., DeJong, F. J., et al. (1995). Screening for depression among a well elderly population. *Social Work, 40*, 295-304.

Downey, G., Feldman, S., Khuri, J., & Friedman, S. (1994). Maltreatment and childhood depression. In W. M. Reynolds & H. F. Johnston (Eds.), *Handbook of depression in children and adolescents* (pp. 481-508). New York: Plenum Press.

Dozois, D. J., Dobson, K. S., & Ahnberg, J. L. (1998). A psychometric evaluation of the Beck Depression Inventory-II. *Psychological Assessment, 10*, 83-89.

Draine, J. (1997). A critical review of randomized field trials of case management for individuals with serious and persistent mental illness. *Research on Social Work Practice, 7*, 32-51.

Drake, R. E. (1998). Brief history, current status, and future place of assertive community treatment. *American Journal of Orthopsychiatry, 68*, 172-175.

Drake, R. E., Alterman, A. I., & Rosenberg, S. R. (1993). Detection of substance use disorders in severely mentally ill patients. *Community Mental Health Journal, 29*, 175-192.

Drake, R. E., Green, A. I., Mueser, K. T., & Goldman, H. H. (2003). The history of community mental health treatment and rehabilitation for persons with severe mental illness. *Community Mental Health Journal, 39*, 427-440.

Drake, R. E., McHugo, G. J., Clark, R. E., Teague, G. B., Xie, H., Miles, K., et al. (1998). Assertive community treatment for patients with co-occurring severe mental illness and substance use disorder: A clinical trial. *American Journal of Orthopsychiatry, 68*, 201-215.

Drake, R. E., Mercer-McFadden, C., Mueser, K. T., Hugo, G. J., & Bond, G. R. (1998). Review of integrated mental health and substance abuse treatment for patients with dual disorders. *Schizophrenia Bulletin, 24*, 589-608.

Drake, R. E., & Mueser, K. T. (1996). Alcohol-use disorder and severe mental illness. *Alcohol Health and Research World, 2*, 87-93.

Drake, R. E., & Mueser, K. T. (2000). Psychosocial approaches to dual diagnosis. *Schizophrenia Bulletin, 26*, 105-118.

Drake, R. E., & Mueser, K. T. (2002). Co-occurring alcohol use disorder and schizophrenia. *Alcohol and Health, 26*, 99-102.

Drake, R. E., Mueser, K. M., Clark, R. E., & Wallach, M. A. (1996). The course, treatment, and outcome of substance disorder in persons with severe mental illness. *American Journal of Orthopsychiatry, 66*, 42-51.

Drake, R. E., Osher, F. C., & Wallach, M. A. (1989). Alcohol use and abuse in schizophrenia: A prospective community study. *Journal of Nervous and Mental Disease, 177*, 408-414.

Drake, R. E., Rosenberg, S. D., & Mueser, K. T. (1996). Assessing substance use disorder in persons with severe mental illness. *New Directions for Mental Health Services, 70*, 3-17.

Drake, R. E., & Wallach, M. A. (2000). Dual diagnosis: 15 years of progress. *Psychiatric Services, 51*, 1126-1129.

Drake, R. E., Yovetich, N. A., Bebout, R. R., Harris, M., & McHugo, G. J. (1997). Integrated treatment for dually diagnosed homeless adults. *Journal of Nervous and Mental Disease, 180*, 298-305.

Duan, C., & Hill, C. E. (1996). The current state of empathy research. *Journal of Counseling Psychology, 43*, 261-274.

Duggal, S., Carlson, E. A., Sroufe, L. A., & Egeland, B. (2001). Depressive symptomatology in childhood and adolescence. *Development and Psychopathology, 13*, 143-164.

Dumaine, M. L. (2003). Meta-analysis of interventions with co-occurring disorders of severe mental illness and substance abuse: Implications for social work practice. *Research on Social Work Practice, 13*, 142-165.

Dutton, D. G., Bodnarchuk, M., Kropp, R., Hart, S. D., & Ogloff, J. P. (1997). Client personality disorders affecting wife assault post-treatment recidivism. *Violence and Victims, 12*, 37-50.

Dutton, D. G., Starzomski, A., & Ryan, L. (1996). Antecedents of abusive personality and abusive behavior in wife assaulters. *Journal of Family Violence, 11*, 113-132.

Dzieglielewski, S. F., & Leon, A. M. (1998). Pharmacological treatment of major depression. *Research on Social Work Practice, 8*, 475-490.

Dziegielewski, S. F., Resncik, C., Nelson-Gardell, D., & Harrison, D. F. (1998). Treatment of sexual dysfunctions: What social workers need to know. *Research on Social Work Practice, 8*, 685-697.

D'Zurilla, T. J., & Goldfried, M. R. (1971). Problem solving and behavior modification. *Journal of Abnormal Psychology, 78*, 107-126.

Eckert, P. A. (1993). Acceleration of change: Catalysts in brief therapy. *Clinical Psychology Review, 13*, 241-253.

Edelstein, B., Staats, N., Kalish, K. D., & Northrop, L. E. (1996). Assessment of older adults. In M. Hersen & V. B. Van Hasselt (Eds.), *Psychological treatment of older adults: An introductory text* (pp. 35-68). New York: Plenum Press.

Edmond, T., Rubin, A., & Wambach, K. G. (1999). The effectiveness of EMDR with adult female survivors of childhood sexual abuse. *Social Work Research, 23*, 103-116.

Eisen, M. L., & Goodman, G. S. (1998). Trauma, memory, and suggestibility in children. *Development and Psychopathology, 10*, 717-738.

Eisen, S. V., Dill, D. L., & Grob, M. C. (1994). Reliability and validity of a brief patient-report instrument for psychiatric outcome evaluation. *Hospital and Community Psychiatry, 45*, 242-247.

Eisler, I., Dare, C., Russell, G. F., Szmukler, G., le Grange, D., & Dodge, E. (1997). Family and individual therapy in anorexia nervosa: A 5-year follow-up. *Family and Individual Therapy in Anorexia Nervosa, 54*, 1025-1030.

El-Bassel, N., Ivanoff, A., Schilling, R. F., Gilbert, L., Borne, D., & Chen, D. (1995). Preventing HIV/AIDS in drug-abusing incarcerated women through skills building and social support enhancement. *Social Work Research, 19*, 131-141.

Elbogen, E. B., & Tomkins, A. J. (2000). From the psychiatric hospital to the community: Integrating conditional release and contingency management. *Behavioral Sciences and the Law, 18*, 427-444.

Elkin, I. (1994). The NIMH treatment of depression collaborative research program: Where we began and where we are. In A. E. Bergin & S. L. Garfield (Eds.), *The handbook of psychotherapy and behavior change* (4th ed., pp. 114-142). New York: Wiley.

Elkin, I., Parloff, M. B., Hadley, S. W., & Autry, J. H. (1985). NIMH treatment of depression collaborative research program: Background and research plan. *Archives of General Psychiatry, 42*, 305-316.

Elkin, I., Shea, M. T., Watkins, J. T., Imber, S. D., Sotsky, S. M., Collins, J. F., et al. (1989). National Institute of Mental Health Treatment of Depression Collaborative Program: General effectiveness of treatments. *Archives of General Psychiatry, 46*, 971-982.

Emmelkamp, P. M. G. (1994). Behavior therapy with adults. In A. E. Bergin & S. L. Garfield (Eds.), *The handbook of psychotherapy and behavior change* (4th ed., pp. 379-427). New York: Wiley.

Emrick, C. (1974). A review of psychologically oriented treatment of alcoholism: Part 1. The use and interrelationships of outcome criteria and drinking behavior following treatment. *Quarterly Journal of Studies on Alcohol, 35*, 523-549.

Emrick, C. (1982). Evaluation of alcoholism psychotherapy methods. In E. M. Pattison & E. Kauffman (Eds.), *The Encyclopedic handbook of alcoholism* (pp. 41-78). New York: Gardener Press.

Emrick, C. (1993). Alcoholics Anonymous: What is currently known? In B. S. McCrady & W. R. Miller (Eds.), *Research on Alcoholics Anonymous: Opportunities and alternatives* (pp. 41-78). New Brunswick, NJ: Rutgers Center of Alcohol Studies.

Endicott, J., Spitzer, R. L., Fleiss, J. L., & Cohen, J. (1976). The Global Assessment Scale: A procedure for measuring overall severity of psychiatric disturbance. *Archives of General Psychiatry, 33*, 766-771.

English, D. J., & Graham, J. C. (2000). An examination of relationships between children's protective services social worker assessment of risk and independent LONGSCAN measures of risk constructs. *Children and Youth Services Review, 22*, 897-933.

Engs, R. C. (1977). Drinking patterns and drinking problems of college students. *Journal of Studies on Alcohol, 38*, 2144-2156.

Epstein, N. H., Baucom, D. H., & Daiuto, A. (1997). Cognitive-behavioural couples therapy. In W. K. Halford & H. J. Markham (Eds.), *Clinical handbook of marriage and couples intervention* (pp. 415-449). New York: Wiley.

Erikson, E. H. (1950). *Childhood and society*. New York: Norton.

Erlenmeyer-Kimling, L. (1996). A look at the evolution of developmental models of schizophrenia. In S. Matthysse, D. L. Levy, J. Kagan & F. M. Benes (Eds.), *Psychopathology: The evolving science of mental disorder* (pp. 229-252). Cambridge: Cambridge University Press.

Eronen, M., Angermeyer, M. C., & Schulze, B. (1998). The psychiatric epidemiology of violent behavior. *Social Psychiatry and Psychiatric Epidemiology, 33*, s13-s23.

Essock, S. M., Frisman, L. K., & Kontos, N. J. (1998). Cost-effectiveness of assertive community treatment teams. *American Journal of Orthopsychiatry, 68*, 179-190.

Estrada, A. U., & Pinsoff, W. M. (1995). The effectiveness of family therapies for selected behavioral disorder of childhood. *Journal of Marital and Family Therapy, 21*, 403-440.

Evans, D. M., & Dunn, N. J. (1995). Alcohol expectancies, coping responses and self-efficacy judgments: A replication and extension of Cooper et al's 1988 study in a college sample. *Journal of Studies on Alcohol, 56*, 186-193.

Everson, M. D., & Boat, B. W. (1994). Putting the anatomical doll controversy in perspective: An examination of the major uses and criticisms of the dolls in child sexual abuse evaluations. *Child Abuse and Neglect, 18*, 113-129.

Eyberg, S. M., & Robinson, E. A. (1983). Conduct problem behavior: Standardization of a behavioral rating scale with adolescents. *Journal of Clinical Child Psychology, 12*, 347-357.

Eyberg, S. M., & Ross, A. W. (1978). Assessment of child behavior problems: The validation of a new inventory. *Journal of Clinical Child Psychology, 7*, 113-116.

Eysenck, H. J. (1952). The effects of psychotherapy: An evaluation. *Journal of Consulting Psychology, 16*, 319-324.

Eysenck, H. J. (1960). *The structure of human personality*. London: Routledge and Kegan Paul.

Fairburn, C. G. (1993). Interpersonal psychotherapy for bulimia nervosa. In G. L. Klerman & M. M. Weissman (Eds.), *New applications of interpersonal psychotherapy* (pp. 353-378). Washington, DC: American Psychiatric Association.

Fairburn, C. G. (1997). Eating disorders. In D. M. Clark & C. G. Fairburn (Eds.), *Science and practice of cognitive behaviour therapy* (pp. 209-241). New York: Oxford University Press.

Fairburn, C. G., & Beglin, S. J. (1990). Studies of the epidemiology of bulimia nervosa. *American Journal of Psychiatry, 147*, 401-408.

Fairburn, C. G., & Beglin, S. J. (1994). Assessment of eating disorders: Interview or self-report questionnaire? *International Journal of Eating Disorders, 16*, 363-370.

Fairburn, C. G., Cooper, Z., Doll, H. A., Norman, P., & O'Connor, M. (2000). The natural course of bulimia nervosa and binge eating disorder in young women. *Archives of General Psychiatry, 57*, 659-665.

Fairburn, C. G., Jones, R., Peveler, R. C., Carr, S. J., Solomon, R. A., O'Connor, M. E., et al. (1991). Three psychological treatments for bulimia nervosa. *Archives of General Psychiatry, 48*, 463-469.

Fairburn, C. G., Jones, R., Peveler, R. C., Hope, R. A., & O'Connor, M. (1993). Psychotherapy and bulimia nervosa: Longer-term effects of interpersonal psychotherapy, behavior therapy, and cognitive behavior therapy. *Archives of General Psychiatry, 50*, 419-428.

Fairburn, C. G., Marcus, M. D., & Wilson, G. T. (1993). Cognitive-behavior therapy for binge eating and bulimia nervosa: A comprehensive treatment manual. In C. G. Fairburn & G. T. Wilson (Eds.), *Binge eating: Nature, assessment and treatment* (pp. 361-404). New York: Guilford Press.

Fairburn, C. G., Norman, P. A., Welch, S. L., O'Connor, M. E., Doll, H. A., & Peveler, R. C. (1995). A prospective study of outcome in bulimia nervosa and the long-term effects of three psychological treatments. *Archives of General Psychiatry, 52*, 304-312.

Fairburn, C. G., & Wilson, G. T. (Eds.). (1993). *Binge eating: Nature, assessment and treatment*. New York: Guilford Press.

Falloon, R. H., & Coverdale, J. H. (1994). Cognitive-behavioural family interventions for major mental disorders. *Behaviour Change, 11*, 213-222.

Falloon, R. H., Roncone, R., Malm, U., & Coverdale, J. H. (1998). Effective and efficient treatment strategies to enhance recovery from schizophrenia: How much longer will people have to wait before we provide them? *Psychiatric Rehabilitation Skills, 2*, 107-127.

Fals-Stewart, W., O'Farrell, T., & Birchler, G. (1997). Behavioral couples therapy for male substance-abusing patients: A cost outcomes analysis. *Journal of Consulting and Clinical Psychology, 65*, 789-802.

Fantuzzo, J. W., Jurecic, L., Stovall, A., Hightower, A. D., Goins, C., & Schachtel, D. (1988). Effects of adult and peer social initiations on the social behavior of withdrawn, maltreated preschool children. *Journal of Consulting and Clinical Psychology, 56*, 34-39.

Fantuzzo, J. W., & Mohr, W. K. (1999). Prevalence and effects of child exposure to domestic violence. *Future of Children, 9*, 21-32.

Faraone, S. V., Biederman, J., Jetton, J. G., & Tsuang, M. T. (1997). Attention deficit disorder and conduct disorder: Longitudinal evidence for a familial subtype. *Psychological Medicine, 27*, 291-300.

Farmer, E. M. Z., Compton, S. N., Burns, B. J., & Robertson, E. (2002). Review of the evidence base for treatment of childhood psychopathology externalizing disorders. *Journal of Consulting and Clinical Psychology, 70*, 1267-1302.

Farrell, S. P., Hains, A. A., & Davies, W. H. (1998). Cognitive behavioral interventions for sexually abused children exhibiting PTSD symptomatology. *Behavior Therapy, 29*, 241-255.

Farrington, D. P. (2000). Psychosocial predictors of adult antisocial personality and adult convictions. *Behavioral Sciences and the Law, 18*, 605-622.

Fava, G. A., Rafanelli, C., Grandi, S., Canestrari, R., & Morphy, M. A. (1998). Six-year outcome for cognitive behavioral treatment of residual symptoms in major depression. *American Journal of Psychiatry, 155*, 1443-1445.

Fava, M., Rankin, M.A., Wright, E. C., Alpert, J. E., Nierenberg, A.A., Pava, J., et al. (2000). Anxiety disorders in major depression. *Comprehensive Psychiatry, 41*, 97-102.

Feit, M. D., & Cuevas-Feit, N. M. (1996). An overview of social work practice with the elderly. In M. J. Holosko & M. D. Feit (Eds.), *Social work practice with the elderly* (2nd ed., pp. 3-20). Toronto: Canadian Scholar's Press.

Fergusson, D. M., & Mullen, P. E. (1999). *Childhood sexual abuse: An evidence-based perspective.* Developmental Clinical Psychology and Psychiatry Series (#40). Thousand Oaks, CA: Sage.

Fillmore, K. M. (1974). Drinking and problem drinking in early adulthood and middle age: An exploratory 20-year follow-up study. *Quarterly Journal of Studies on Alcohol, 35*, 819-840.

Fillmore, K. M. (1988). *Alcohol use across the life course.* Toronto: Addiction Research Foundation.

Fine, S., Forth, A., Gilbert, M., & Haley, G. (1991). Group therapy for adolescent depressive disorder: A comparison of social skills and therapeutic support. *Journal of the American Academy of Child and Adolescent Psychiatry, 30*, 79-85.

Finkelhor, D. (1988). The trauma of child sexual abuse: Two models. *Journal of Interpersonal Violence, 2*, 348-366.

Finkelhor, D., & Berliner, L. (1995). Research on the treatment of sexually abused children: A review and recommendations. *Journal of the American Academy of Child and Adolescent Psychiatry, 34*, 1408-1423.

Finkelhor, D., & Browne, A. (1985). The traumatic impact of sexual abuse: A conceptualization. *American Journal of Orthopsychiatry, 55*, 530-541.

Finkelhor, D., & Dziuba-Leatherman, J. (1994). Children as victims of violence: A national survey. *Pediatrics, 94*, 413-420.

Finkelhor, D., Hotaling, G., Lewis, I.A., & Smith, C. (1990). Sexual abuse in a national survey of adult men and women: Prevalence, characteristics, and risk factors. *Child Abuse and Neglect, 14*, 19-28.

Finley, L. (1998). The cultural context: Families coping with severe mental illness. *Psychiatric Rehabilitation Journal, 21*, 230-240.

Finney, J.W., & Moos, R. H. (1991). The long-term course of treated alcoholism: Part 1. Mortality, relapse and remission rates and comparisons with community controls. *Journal of Studies on Alcohol, 51*, 44-54.

Finney, J.W., Moos, R. H., & Timko, C. (1999). The course of treated and untreated substance use disorders: Remission and resolution, relapse and mortality. In B. S. McCrady & E. E. Epstein (Eds.), *Addictions: A comprehensive guidebook* (pp. 30-49). New York: Oxford University Press.

Finn-Stevenson, M., Desimone, L., & Chung, A. (1998). Linking child care and support services with the school: Pilot evaluation of the school of the 21st century. *Children and Youth Services Review, 20*, 177-205.

Fischer, D. J., Himle, J. A., & Hanna, G. L. (1998). Group behavioral therapy for adolescents with obsessive-compulsive disorder: Preliminary outcomes. *Research on Social Work Practice, 8*, 629-636.

Fischer, J. (1973). Is casework effective? A review. *Social Work, 18*, 5-20.

Fischer, J. (1981). The social work revolution. *Social Work, 26*, 199-207.

Fischer, M., Barkley, R.A., Smallish, L., & Fletcher, K. (2002). Young adult follow-up of hyperactive children: Self-reported psychiatric disorders, comorbidity, and the role of childhood conduct problems and teen CD. *Journal of Abnormal Child Psychology, 30*, 463-475.

Fishbein, D. H. (2000). Introduction. In D. H. Fishbein (Ed.), *The science, treatment, and prevention of antisocial behaviors:Application to the criminal justice system* (pp. 1-8). Kingston, NJ: Civic Research Institute.

Fisher, W. H., Packer, I. K., Grisso, T., McDermeit, M., & Brown, J. K. (2000). From case management to court clinic: Examining forensic system involvement of persons with severe mental illness. *Mental Health Services Research, 2*, 41-49.

Fitzpatrick, T. R. (1998). Bereavement events among elderly men: The effects of stress and health. *Journal of Applied Gerontology, 17*, 204-228.

Fleming, M. F., Barry, K. L., & MacDonald, R. (1991). The Alcohol Use Disorders Identification Test (AUDIT) in a college sample. *International Journal of the Addictions, 26*, 1173-1185.

Fletcher, B. W., Tims, F. M., & Brown, B. S. (1997). Drug Abuse Treatment Outcome Study (DATOS): Treatment evaluation research in the United States. *Psychology of Addictive Behaviors, 11*, 216-229.

Floyd, A. S., Monahan, S. C., Finney, J. W., & Morley, J. A. (1996). Alcoholism treatment outcome studies, 1980-1992: The nature of the research. *Addictive Behaviors, 21*, 413-428.

Floyd, F. J., Haynes, S. N., & Kelly, S. (1997). Marital assessment: A dynamic functional-analytic approach. In W. K. Halford & H. J. Markham (Eds.), *Clinical handbook of marriage and couples intervention* (pp. 349-377). New York: Wiley.

Foa, E. B., Dancu, C. V., Hembree, E. A., Joycox, L. H., Meadows, E. A., & Street, G. P. (1999). A comparison of exposure therapy, stress inoculation training, and their combination for reducing posttraumatic stress disorder in female assault victims. *Journal of Consulting and Clinical Psychology, 67*, 194-200.

Foa, E. B., Huppert, J. D., Leiberg, S., Langner, R., Kichic, R., Hajcak, G., & Salkovskis, P. (2002). The Obsessive-Compulsive Inventory: Development and validation of a short version. *Psychological Assessment, 10*, 206-214.

Foa, E. B., & Kozak, M. J. (1996). Obsessive compulsive disorder. In C. Lindemann (Ed.), *Handbook of the treatment of the anxiety disorders* (pp. 137-171). Northvale, NJ: Aronson.

Foa, E. B., & Kozak, M. J. (1998). Clinical applications of bioinformational theory: Understanding anxiety and its treatment. *Behavior Therapy, 29*, 675-690.

Foa, E. B., Kozak, M. J., Salkovskis, P. M., Coles, M. E., & Amir, N. (1998). The validation of a new obsessive-compulsive disorder scale: The Obsessive-Compulsive Inventory. *Psychological Assessment, 10*, 206-214.

Foa, E. B., & Meadows, E. A. (1997). Psychosocial treatments for posttraumatic stress disorder: A critical review. *Annual Review of Psychology, 48*, 449-480.

Foa, E. B., Riggs, D. S., Dancu, C. V., & Rothbaum, B. O. (1993). Reliability and validity of a brief instrument for assessing post-traumatic stress disorder. *Journal of Traumatic Stress, 6*, 459-473.

Foa, E. B., & Rothbaum, B. O. (1998). *Treating the trauma of rape: Cognitive-behavioral therapy for PTSD*. New York: Guilford Press.

Foa, E. B., Rothbaum, B. O., Riggs, D. S., & Murdock, T. B. (1991). Treatment of posttraumatic stress disorder in rape victims: A comparison between cognitive-behavioral procedures and counseling. *Journal of Consulting and Clinical Psychology, 59*, 715-723.

Foa, E. B., & Tolin, D. F. (2000). Comparison of the PTSD Symptom Scale-Interview version and the Clinician Administered PTSD Scale. *Journal of Traumatic Stress, 13*, 181-191.

Fokias, D., & Tyler, P. (1995). Social support and agoraphobia: A review. *Clinical Psychology Review, 15*, 347-366.

Follette, V. M., Ruzek, J. I., & Abueg, F. R. (1998). A contextual analysis of trauma: Assessment and treatment. In V. M. Follette, J. I. Ruzek, & F. R. Abueg (Eds.), *Cognitive-behavioral therapies for trauma* (pp. 3-14). New York: Guilford Press.

Folstein, M. F., Folstein, S., & McHugh, P. R. (1975). Mini-Mental State: A practical method for grading the cognitive state of patients for the clinician. *Journal of Psychiatric Research, 12*, 189-198.

Fonagy, P., Steele, M., Steele, H., Leigh, T., Kennedy, R., Mattoon, G., et al. (1996). The relation of attachment status, psychiatric classification, and response to psychotherapy. *Journal of Consulting and Clinical Psychology, 64*, 22-31.

Fonagy, P., Target, M., & Gergely, G. (2000). Attachment and borderline personality disorder: A theory and some evidence. *Psychiatric Clinics of North America, 23*, 103-122.

Fonseca, A. C., & Perrin, S. (2001). Clinical phenomenology, classification and assessment of anxiety disorders in children and adolescents. In W. K. Silverman & P. D. A. Treffers (Eds.), *Anxiety disorders in children and adolescents: Research, assessment and intervention* (pp. 126-158). New York: Cambridge University Press.

Forehand, R. L., & McMahon, R. J. (1981). *Helping the non-compliant child: A clinician's guide to parent training.* New York: Guilford Press.

Foreyt, J. P., & Mikhail, C. (1997). Anorexia nervosa and bulimia nervosa. In E. J. Mash & L. G. Terdal (Eds.), *Assessment of childhood disorders* (3rd ed., pp. 683-716). New York: Guilford Press.

Forth, A. E., Hart, S. D., & Hare, R. D. (1990). Assessment of psychopathy in male young offenders. *Psychological Assessment: A Journal of Consulting and Clinical Psychology, 2*, 342-344.

Fortune, A. E., & Proctor, E. K. (2001). Research on social work interventions. *Social Work Research, 25*, 67-69.

Foster, S. L. (1994). Assessing and treating parent-adolescent conflict. In M. Hersen, R. Eisler, & P. Miller (Eds.), *Progress in behavior modification, Vol. 29* (pp. 53-72). New York: Academic Press.

Foster, S. L., & Robin, A. L. (1997). Family conflict and communication in adolescence. In E. J. Mash & L. G. Terdal (Eds.), *Assessment of childhood disorders* (3rd ed., pp. 627-682). New York: Guilford Press.

Fraenkel, P. (1997). Systems approaches to couple therapy. In W. K. Halford & H. J. Markham (Eds.), *Clinical handbook of marriage and couples intervention* (pp. 379-413). New York: Wiley.

Frances, R. J., & Miller, S. I. (Eds.). (1998). *Clinical textbook of addictive disorders.* New York: Guilford Press.

Franklin, C., & Jordan, C. (2003). An integrative skills assessment approach. In C. Jordan & C. Franklin (Eds.), *Clinical assessment for social workers: Quantitative and qualitative methods* (2nd ed., pp. 1-52). Chicago: Lyceum Books.

Franklin, C., Streeter, C., & Springer, D. (2001). Validity of the FACES IV family assessment measure. *Research on Social Work Practice, 11*, 576-596.

Franklin, M. E., Abramowitz, J. S., Kozak, M. J., Levitt, J. T., & Foa, E. B. (2000). Effectiveness of exposure and ritual prevention for obsessive-compulsive disorder: Randomized compared with non-randomized samples. *Journal of Consulting and Clinical Psychology, 68*, 594-602.

Franz, D., & Gross, A. M. (1998). Assessment of child behavior problems: Externalizing disorders. In A. S. Bellack & M. Hersen (Eds.), *Behavioral assessment: A practical handbook* (4th ed., pp. 361-377). Boston: Allyn and Bacon.

Fraser, J. A., Armstrong, K. L., Morris, J. P., & Dadds, M. R. (2000). Home visiting intervention for vulnerable families with newborns: Follow-up results of a randomized controlled trial. *Child Abuse and Neglect, 11*, 1399-1429.

Fraser, M. (1996, January). Cognitive problem solving and aggressive behavior among children. *Families in Society: The Journal of Contemporary Human Services*, 19-31.

Fraser, M. W., Day, S. H., Galinsky, M. J., Hodges, V. G., & Smokowski, P. R. (2004). Conduct problems and peer rejection in childhood: A randomized trial of the Making Choices and Strong Families programs. *Research on Social Work Practice, 14*, 313-324.

Frederick, C. J. (1985). Selected foci on the spectrum of posttraumatic stress disorders. In J. Laube & S. A. Murphy (Eds.), *Perspectives on disaster recovery* (pp. 110-130). East Norwalk, CT: Appleton-Century-Crofts.

Fredman, N., & Sherman, R. (1987). *Handbook of measurements for marriage and family therapy*. New York: Brunner/Mazel.

Freedman, D. (2001). False prediction of future dangerousness: Error rates and Psychopathy Checklist-Revised. *Journal of the American Academy of Psychiatry and the Law, 29*, 89-95.

Freeman, E. M. (1991). Addictive behaviors: State of the art issues in social work treatment. In E. M. Freeman (Ed.), *The addiction process: Effective social work approaches* (pp. 1-9). New York: Longman.

Freeston, M. H., Ladouceur, R., Gagnon, F., Thibodeau, N., Rheaume, J., Letarte, H., et al. (1997). Cognitive-behavioral treatment of obsessive thoughts: A controlled study. *Journal of Consulting and Clinical Psychology, 65*, 405-413.

Freud, A. (1946). *The ego and the mechanisms of defense*. New York: International Universities Press.

Freud, S. (1923). *The ego and the id*. London: Hogarth.

Freud, S. (1938). *The basic writings of Sigmund Freud*. New York: Random House.

Freud, S. (1966). *Introductory lectures on psychoanalysis*. New York: Norton. (Original work published 1922.)

Friedman, L. H. (1991). Evaluating the impact of intensive family preservation services in New Jersey. In K. Wells & D. Biegel (Eds.), *Family preservation services: Research and evaluation* (pp. 47-71). Newbury Park, CA: Sage.

Friedman, M. (1997). Posttraumatic stress disorder. *Journal of Clinical Psychiatry, 58*(suppl. 9), 33-36.

Friedrich, W. N. (1993). Sexual victimization and sexual behavior in children: A review of recent literature. *Child Abuse and Neglect, 17*, 59-66.

Fritzler, B. K., Hecker, J. E., & Losee, M. C. (1997). Self-directed treatment with minimal therapist contact: Preliminary findings for obsessive-compulsive disorder. *Behaviour Research and Therapy, 35*, 627-631.

Frueh, B. C., Brady, K. L., & de Arellano, M. A. (1998). Racial differences in combat-related PTSD: Empirical findings and conceptual issues. *Clinical Psychology Review, 18*, 287-305.

Frye, M. A., Altshuler, L. L., McElroy, S. L., Suppes, T., Keck, P. E., Denicoff, K., et al. (2003). Gender differences in prevalence, risk, and clinical correlates of alcoholism comorbidity in bipolar disorder. *American Journal of Psychiatry, 160*, 883-889.

Fuller, R. K., & Hiller-Sturmhofel, S. (1999). Alcoholism treatment in the United States: An overview. *Alcohol Research and Health, 23,* 69-77.

Fulwiler, C., & Ruthazer, R. (1999). Premorbid risk factors for violence in adult mental illness. *Comprehensive Psychiatry, 40,* 96-100.

Furby, L., Weinrott, M. R., & Blackshaw, L. (1989). Sex offender recidivism: A review. *Psychological Bulletin, 105,* 3-30.

Furman, W., & Flanagan, A. S. (1997). The influence of earlier relationships on marriage: An attachment prespective. In W. K. Halford & H. J. Markham (Eds.), *Clinical handbook of marriage and couples intervention* (pp. 179-202). New York: Wiley.

Gacono, C. B., Nieberding, R. J., Owen, A., Rubel, J., & Bodholdt, R. (2001). Treating conduct disorder, antisocial, and psychopathic personalities. In J. B. Ashford, B. D. Sales, & W. H. Reid (Eds.), *Treating adult and juvenile offenders with special needs* (pp. 99-129). Washington, DC: American Psychological Association.

Galvan, F. H., & Caetano, R. (2003). Alcohol use and related problems among ethnic minorities in the United States. *Alcohol Research and Health, 27,* 87-94.

Gambrill, E. (1990). *Critical thinking in clinical practice.* San Francisco: Jossey-Bass.

Gambrill, E. (1995). Less marketing and more scholarship. *Social Work Research, 19,* 38-47.

Gambrill, E. (2001). Social work: An authority-based profession. *Research on Social Work Practice, 11,* 166-175.

Gambrill, E. (2004). Contributions of critical thinking and evidence-based practice to the fulfillment of the ethical obligations of professionals. In H. E. Briggs & T. L. Rzepnicki (Eds.), *Using evidence in social work practice: Behavioral perspectives* (pp. 3-19). Chicago: Lyceum Books.

Garbarino, J. (1977, November). The human ecology of child maltreatment: A conceptual model of research. *Journal of Marriage and the Family,* 721-735.

Garbarino, J. (1997). The role of economic deprivation in the social context of child maltreatment. In M. E. Helfer, R. S. Kempe, & R. D. Krugman (Eds.), *The battered child* (5th ed., pp. 49-60). Chicago: University of Chicago Press.

Garbarino, J., & Kostelny, K. (1992). Child maltreatment as a community problem. *Child Abuse and Neglect, 16,* 455-464.

Garber, J., Little, S., Hilsman, R., & Weaver, K. R. (1998). Family predictors of suicidal symptoms in young adolescents. *Journal of Adolescence, 21,* 445-457.

Garfield, S. L. (1996). Some problems associated with "validated" forms of psychotherapy. *Clinical Psychology: Science and Practice, 3,* 218-229.

Garmezy, N. (1991). Resilience in children's adaptation to negative life events and stressed environments. *Pediatric Annals, 20,* 459-466.

Garner, D. M., Olmsted, M. P., & Policy, J. (1983). Development and validation of a multidimensional Eating Disorder Inventory for anorexia nervosa and bulimia. *International Journal of Eating Disorders, 2,* 15-34.

Gaudin, J. M. (1993). Effective intervention with neglectful families. *Criminal Justice and Behavior, 20,* 66-89.

Geismar, L., & Wood, K. (1986). *Family and delinquency: Resocializing the young offender.* New York: Human Sciences Press.

Geller, J. (1995). A biopsychosocial rationale for coerced community treatment in the management of schizophrenia. *Psychiatric Quarterly, 66,* 219-235.

Gelles, R. J. (1997). *Intimate violence in families* (3rd ed.). Thousand Oaks, CA: Sage.

Gelles, R. J., & Cornell, C. P. (1990). *Intimate violence in families* (2nd ed.). Thousand Oaks, CA: Sage.

Gelles, R. J., & Straus, M. A. (1987). Is violence toward children increasing? A comparison of 1975 and 1985 national survey rates. *Journal of Interpersonal Violence, 2,* 212-222.

Gendreau, P. (1996a). Offender rehabilitation: What we know and what needs to be done. *Criminal Justice and Behavior, 23,* 144-161.

Gendreau, P. (1996b). The principles of effective intervention with offenders. In A. T. Harland (Ed.), *Choosing correctional options that work: Defining demand and evaluating the supply* (pp. 117-130). Thousand Oaks, CA: Sage.

Gerbasi, J.B., Bonnie, R.J., & Binder, R.L. (2000). Resource document on mandatory outpatient treatment. *Journal of the American Academy of Psychiatry and the Law, 28,* 127-144.

Gershater-Molko, R.M., Lutzker, J.R., & Sherman, J.A. (2002). Intervention in child neglect: An applied behavioral perspective. *Aggression and Violent Behavior, 7,* 103-124.

Gfoerer, J. C., Greenblatt, J. C., & Wright, D. A. (1997). Substance use in the U.S. college-age population: Differences according to educational status and living arrangement. *American Journal of Public Health, 87,* 62-65.

Gibbs, L. E. (2003). *Evidence-based practice for the helping professions: A practical guide with integrated multimedia.* Pacific Grove, CA: Brooks/Cole.

Gibbs, L. E., & Gambrill, E. (2002). Evidence-based practice: Counterarguments to objections. *Research on Social Work Practice, 12,* 452-476.

Gingerich, K. J., Turnock, P., Litfin, J. K., & Rosen, L. E. (1998). Diversity and attention deficit hyperactivity disorder. *Journal of Clinical Psychology, 54,* 415-426.

Gleason, W. J. (1997). Psychological and social dysfunctions in battering men: A review. *Aggression and Violent Behavior, 2,* 43-52.

Glisson, C., Hemmelgarn, A. L., & Post, J.A. (2002). The Shortform Assessment for Children: An assessment and outcome measure for child welfare and juvenile justice. *Research on Social Work Practice, 12,* 82-106.

Gloria, A. M., & Peregoy, J. J. (1996). Counseling Latino alcohol and other substance users/abusers. *Journal of Substance Abuse Treatment, 13,* 119-126.

Gmel, G., & Rehm, J. (2003). Harmful alcohol use. *Alcohol Research and Health, 27,* 39-51.

Godley, S. H., Finch, M., Dougan, L., McDonnell, M., McDermeit, M., & Carey, A. (2000). Case management for dually diagnosed individuals involved in the criminal justice system. *Journal of Substance Abuse Treatment, 18,* 137-148.

Gold, M. (1994). Neurobiology of addiction and recovery: The brain, the drive for the drug, and the 12-step fellowship. *Journal of Substance Abuse Treatment, 11,* 93-97.

Goldberg, L. R. (1993). The structure of phenotypical personality traits. *American Psychologist, 48,* 26-34.

Goldfried, M. R. (1980). Toward the delineation of therapeutic change principles. *American Psychologist, 35,* 991-999.

Goldfried, M. R. (1995). *From cognitive-behavior therapy to psychotherapy integration.* New York: Springer.

Goldman, A., & Greenberg, L. (1992). Comparison of integrated systemic and emotionally focused approaches to couples therapy. *Journal of Consulting and Clinical Psychology, 60,* 962-969.

Goldman, S. J., D'Angelo, E. J., & DeMaso, D. R. (1993). Psychopathology in the families of children and adolescents with borderline personality disorder. *American Journal of Psychiatry, 150*, 1832-1835.

Goldstein, H. (1986). A cognitive-humanistic approach to the court-ordered vs. voluntary hard-to-reach client. *Social Casework, 67*, 27-36.

Goldstein, J. M., & Tsuang, M. T. (1990). Gender and schizophrenia: An introduction and synthesis of findings. *Schizophrenia Bulletin, 16*, 179-183.

Goldstein, M. J., & Miklowitz, D. J. (1995). The effectiveness of psychoeducational family therapy in the treatment of schizophrenic disorders. *Journal of Marital and Family Therapy, 21*, 361-376.

Gomberg, E. S. L. (1994). Risk factors for drinking over a woman's life span. *Alcohol Health and Research World, 18*, 220-227.

Gomberg. E. S. L. (1999). Women. In B. S. McCrady & E. S. Epstein (Eds.), *Addictions: A comprehensive guidebook* (pp. 527-541). New York: Oxford University Press.

Goodman, G., Bottoms, B., Shaver, P. R., & Qin, J. (1995, April). *Factors affecting children's susceptibility versus resistance to false memory*. Paper presented at the biennial meeting of the Society for Research in Child Development, Indianapolis, IN.

Goodman, L. A., Salyers, M. P., Mueser, K. T., Rosenberg, S. D., Swartz, M., Essock, S. M., et al. (2001). Recent victimization in women and men with severe mental illness: Prevalence and correlates. *Journal of Traumatic Stress, 14*, 615-632.

Goodman, S. H., Sewell, D. R., Cooley, E. L., & Leavitt, N. (1993). Assessing levels of adaptive functioning: The Role Functioning Scale. *Community Mental Health Journal, 29*, 119-131.

Goodman, W., Price, L., Rasmussen, S., Mazure, C., Fleischmann, R. L., Hill, C. L., et al. (1989). The Yale-Brown Obsessive Compulsive Scale. *Archives of General Psychiatry, 46*, 1006-1011.

Goodyer, I. M. (1995). Life events and difficulties: Their nature and effects. In I. M. Goodyer (Ed.), *The depressed child and adolescent: Developmental and clinical perspectives* (pp. 171-193). New York: Cambridge University Press.

Gopaul-McNichol, G. N., & Brice-Baker, J. (1998). *Cross-cultural practice: Assessment, treatment and training*. New York: Wiley.

Gorman-Smith, D., & Tolan, P. (1998). The role of exposure to community violence and developmental problems among inner-city youth. *Development and Psychopathology, 10*, 101-116.

Gortner, E. T., Gollan, J. K., Dobson, K. S., & Jacobson, N. S. (1998). Cognitive-behavioral treatment for depression: Relapse prevention. *Journal of Consulting and Clinical Psychology, 66*, 377-384.

Gottman, J. M. (1993a). The roles of conflict engagement, escalation, and avoidance in marital interaction: A longitudinal view of five types of couples. *Journal of Consulting and Clinical Psychology, 61*, 6-15.

Gottman, J. M. (1993b). A theory of marital dissolution and stability. *Journal of Family Psychology, 7*, 57-75.

Gottman, J. M. (1998). On the etiology of marital decay and its consequences: Comments from a clinical psychologist. In T. N. Bradbury (Ed.), *The developmental course of marital dysfunction* (pp. 423-426). New York: Cambridge University Press.

Graham, H. L., Maslin, J., Copello, A., Birchwood, M., Mueser, K., McGovern, D., et al. (2001). Drug and alcohol problems amongst individuals with severe mental health problems in an inner city area of the UK. *Social Psychiatry and Psychiatry of Epidemiology, 36*, 448-455.

Grant, B. F., & Dawson, D. A. (1999). Alcohol and drug use, abuse and dependence: Classification, prevalence and comorbidity. In B. S. McCrady & E. E. Epstein (Eds.), *Addictions: A comprehensive guidebook* (pp. 9-29). New York: Oxford University Press.

Grant, B. F., & Harford, T. C. (1995). Comorbidity between *DSM-IV* alcohol use disorders and major depression: Results of a national survey. *Drug and Alcohol Dependence, 39*, 197-206.

Grant, B. F., Harford, T. C., Dawson, D. A., Chou, P., Dufour, M., & Pickering, R. (1994). NIAAA's Epidemiologic Bulletin No. 35: Prevalence of *DSM-IV* alcohol abuse and dependence: United States, 1992. *Alcohol Health and Research World, 18*, 243-248.

Grant, B. F., & Pickering, R. P. (1996). Comorbidity between *DSM-IV* alcohol and drug use disorders: Results from the National Longitudinal Alcohol Epidemiologic Survey. *Alcohol Health and Research World, 20*, 67-72.

Granvold, D. K. (1996, June). Constructivist psychotherapy. *Families in Society: The Journal of Contemporary Human Services*, 345-357.

Greenfield, T. K., & Rogers, J. D. (1999). Who drinks most of the alcohol in the U.S.? The policy implications. *Journal of Studies on Alcohol, 60*, 78-89.

Greenhill, L. L. (1998). Child attention deficit hyperactivity disorder. In B. T. Walsh (Ed.), *Child psychopharmacology* (pp. 91-109). Washington, DC: American Psychiatric Association Press.

Greenhill, L. L., Pine, D., March, J., Birmaher, B., & Riddle, M. (1998). Assessment measures in anxiety disorders research. *Psychopharmacology Bulletin, 34*, 155-164.

Greenhill, L. L., & Waslick, B. (1997). Management of suicidal behavior in children and adolescents. *The Psychiatric Clinics of North America, 20*, 641-666.

Grencavage, L. M., & Norcross, J. C. (1990). Where are the commonalities among the therapeutic common factors? *Professional Psychology: Research and Practice, 21*, 372-378.

Griffin, R. (1991, February). Assessing the drug-involved client. *Families in Society: The Journal of Contemporary Human Services*, 87-94.

Grilo, C. M., Masheb, R. M., & Wilson, G. T. (2001). A comparison of different methods for assessing the features of eating disorders in patients with binge eating disorder. *Journal of Consulting and Clinical Psychology, 69*, 317-322.

Grilo, C. M., Sanislow, C., Fehon, D. C., Martino, S., & McGlashan, T. H. (1999). Psychological and behavioral functioning in adolescent psychiatric inpatients who report histories of childhood abuse. *American Journal of Psychiatry, 156*, 538-543.

Grogan-Kaylor, A. (2000). Who goes into kinship care? The relationship of child and family characteristics to placement into kinship foster care. *Social Work Research, 24*, 132-141.

Gruber, K. J., Fleetwood, T. W., & Herring, M. W. (2001). In-home continuing care services for substance-affected families: The Bridges Program. *Social Work, 46*, 267-277.

Grych, J. H., & Fincham, F. D. (1990). Marital conflict and children's adjustment: A cognitive contextual framework. *Psychological Bulletin, 108*, 267-290.

Guarnaccia, P. J. (1997). A cross cultural perspective on anxiety disorders. In S. Friedman (Ed.), *Cultural issues in the treatment of anxiety* (pp. 1-20). New York: Guilford Press.

Guarnaccia, P. J., & Parra, P. (1996). Ethnicity, social status, and families' experiences of caring for a mentally ill family member. *Community Mental Health Journal, 32*, 243-260.

Gumley, A., O'Grady, M., McNay, L., Reilly, J., Power, K., & Norrie, J. (2003). Early intervention for relapse in schizophrenia: Results of a 12-month randomized controlled trial of cognitive behavioural therapy. *Psychological Medicine, 33*, 419-431.

Gunderson, J. G. (1984). *Borderline personality disorder.* Washington, DC: American Psychiatric Association.

Gunderson, J. G., Ronningstam, E., & Smith, L. E. (1995). Narcissitic personality disorder. In J. Livesley (Ed.), *The DSM-IV personality disorders* (pp. 201-212). New York: Guilford Press.

Gunderson, J. G., Zanarini, M. C., & Kisiel, C. L. (1995). Borderline personality disorder. In J. Livesley (Ed.), *The DSM-IV personality disorders* (pp. 141-157). New York: Guilford Press.

Guntrip, H. (1969). *Schizoid phenomena, object relations and the self.* New York: International Universities Press.

Guo, J., Chung, I., Hill, K. G., Hawkins, J. D., Catalano, R. F., & Abbott, R. D. (2002). Developmental relationships between adolescent substance use and risky sexual behavior in young adulthood. *Journal of Adolescent Health, 31*, 354-362.

Gupta, R. (2000). Treatment of depression in an elderly Asian Indian male: A cognitive behavioral approach. *Clinical Gerontologist, 22*, 87-90.

Gurman, A. S., Kniskern, D. P., & Pinsof, W. M. (1986). Research on marital and family therapies. In S. L. Garfield & A. E. Bergin (Eds.), *Handbook of psychotherapy and behavior change* (3rd ed., pp. 565-626). New York: Wiley.

Gutierrez, L. M. (1990). Working with women of color: An empowerment perspective. *Social Work, 35*, 149-153.

Haas, S. M., & Stafford, L. (1998). An initial examination of maintenance behaviors in gay and lesbian relationships. *Journal of Social and Personal Relationships, 15*, 846-855.

Hahlweg, K., & Markman, H. J. (1988). Effectiveness of behavioral marital therapy: Empirical status of behavioral techniques in preventing and alleviating marital distress. *Journal of Consulting and Clinical Psychology, 56*, 440-447.

Haley, J. (1976). *Problem solving therapy.* San Francisco: Jossey-Bass.

Halford, W. K. (1998). The ongoing evolution of behavioral couples therapy: Retrospect and prospect. *Clinical Psychology Review, 18*, 613-633.

Halford, W. K., & Bouma, R. (1997). Individual psychopathology and marital distress. In W. K. Halford & H. J. Markham (Eds.), *Clinical handbook of marriage and couples intervention* (pp. 291-322). New York: Wiley.

Halford, W. K., Hahlweg, K., & Dunne, M. (1990). The cross-cultural consistency of marital communication associated with marital distress. *Journal of Marriage and the Family, 52*, 487-500.

Hall, G. C. (1995). Sexual offender recidivism revisited: A meta-analysis of recent treatment studies. *Journal of Consulting and Clinical Psychology, 63,* 802-809.

Hamberger, L. K., & Hastings, J. E. (1991). Personality correlates of men who batter and nonviolent men: Some continuities and discontinuities. *Journal of Family Violence, 6,* 131-147.

Hamilton, M. (1960). A rating scale for depression. *Journal of Neurology, Neurosurgery and Mental Science, 105,* 985-987.

Hanf, C. (1970). *Shaping mothers to shape their children's behavior.* Portland: University of Oregon Medical School.

Hankin, B., Abramson, L. Y., Moffitt, T. E., Silva, P. A., McGee, R., & Angell, K. (1998). Development of depression from preadolescence to young adulthood: Emerging gender differences in a 10-year longitudinal study. *Journal of Abnormal Psychology, 107,* 128-140.

Hanson, D. J., & Engs, R. C. (1995). Collegiate drinking: Adminstrator perceptions, campus policies and student behaviors. *National Association of Student Personnel Administrators, 32,* 106-115.

Hare, R. D. (1991). *The Hare Psychopathy Checklist-Revised manual.* Toronto: Multi-Health Systems.

Hare, R. D. (1999). Psychopathy as a risk factor for violence. *Psychiatric Quarterly, 70,* 181-197.

Hare, R. D., Harpur, T. J., Hakstian, A. R., Forth, A. E., & Hart, S. D. (1990). The psychopathy checklist: Reliability and factor structure. *Psychological Assessment: A Journal of Consulting and Clinical Psychology, 2,* 338-341.

Hare, R. D., & Hart, S. D. (1995). Commentary on antisocial personality disorder: The *DSM-IV* field trial. In J. Livesley (Ed.), *The DSM-IV personality disorders* (pp. 127-134). New York: Guilford Press.

Hare, R. D., McPherson, L. M., & Forth, A. E. (1988). Male psychopaths and their criminal careers. *Journal of Consulting and Clinical Psychology, 56,* 710-714.

Harford, T., & Grant, B. F. (1987). Psychosocial factors in adolescent drinking contexts. *Journal of Studies on Alcohol, 48,* 551-557.

Hargreaves, W. A., Shumway, M., Hu, T.-W., & Cuffel, B. (1998). *Cost-outcome methods for mental health.* San Diego, CA: Academic Press.

Harnish, L. D., Tolan, P. H., & Guerra, N. G. (1996). Treatment of oppositional defiant disorder. In M. A. Reineke, F. M. Dattilio, & A. Freeman (Eds.), *Cognitive therapy with children and adolescents: A casebook for clinical practice* (pp. 62-78). New York: Guilford Press.

Harpur, T. J., Hakstian, A. R., & Hare, R. D. (1988). Factor structure of the Psychopathy Checklist. *Journal of Consulting and Clinical Psychology, 56,* 741-747.

Harpur, T. J., Hare, R. D., & Hakstian, A. R. (1989). Two-factor conceptualization of psychopathy: Construct validity and assessment implications. *Psychological Assessment: A Journal of Consulting and Clinical Psychology, 1,* 6-17.

Harrington, R. (1995). *Depressive disorder in childhood and adolescence.* New York: Wiley.

Harrington, R., Whittaker, J., & Shoebridge, P. (1998). Psychological treatment of depression in children and adolescents: A review of treatment research. *British Journal of Psychiatry, 173,* 291-298.

Harrington, R., Wood, A., & Verduyn, C. (1998). Clinically depressed adolescents. In P. Graham (Ed.), *Cognitive-behaviour therapy for children and families* (pp. 156-193). New York: Cambridge University Press.

Harris, M. (1996). Treating sexual abuse trauma with dually diagnosed women. *Community Mental Health Journal, 32*, 371-385.

Hart, S. D., & Hare, R. D. (1989). Discriminant validity of the Psychopathy Checklist in a forensic psychiatric population. *Psychological Assessment: A Journal of Consulting and Clinical Psychology, 1*, 211-218.

Hart, S. D., Kropp, P. R., & Hare, R. D. (1988). Performance of male psychopaths following conditional release from prison. *Journal of Consulting and Clinical Psychology, 56*, 227-232.

Hartman, C. R., & Burgess, A. W. (1990). Sexual abuse of children: Causes and consequences. In D. Ciccetti & V. Carlson (Eds.), *Child maltreatment: Theory and research on the causes and consequences of child abuse and neglect* (pp. 95-128). New York: Cambridge University Press.

Hartmann, D. P., Roper, B. L., & Bradford, D. C. (1979). Some relationships between behavioral and traditional assessment. *Journal of Behavioral Assessment, 1*, 3-21.

Hasin, D. S. (1991). Diagnostic interviews for assessment: Background, reliability, validity. *Alcohol Health and Research World, 15*, 293-301.

Haskett, M. E., Miller, J. W., Whitworth, J. M., & Huffman, J. M. (1992, October). Intervention with cocaine-abusing mothers. *Families in Society: The Journal of Contemporary Human Services*, 451-461.

Hastings, J. E., & Hamberger, L. K. (1988). Personality characteristics of spouse abusers: A controlled comparison. *Violence and Victims, 3*, 31-47.

Hawkins, K. A., & Sinha, R. (1998). Can line clinicians master the conceptual complexities of dialectical behavior therapy? An evaluation of a state department of mental health training program. *Journal of Psychiatric Research, 32*, 379-384.

Hayashida, M. (1998). An overview of outpatient and inpatient detoxification. *Alcohol Health and Research World, 22*, 44-46.

Hayes, R. L., Halford, W. K., & Varghese, F. T. (1995). Social skills training with chronic schizophrenic patients: Effects on negative symptoms and community functioning. *Behavior Therapy, 26*, 433-449.

Haynes, S. N. (1998). The changing nature of behavioral assessment. In A. S. Bellack & M. Hersen (Eds.), *Behavioral assessment: A practical handbook*. Boston: Allyn and Bacon.

Hazelrigg, M. D., Cooper, H. M., & Borduin, C. M. (1987). Evaluating the effectiveness of family therapies: An integrative review and analysis. *Psychological Bulletin, 101*, 428-442.

Heath, A. C. (1995). Genetic influences on alcoholism risk: A review of adoption and twin studies. *Alcohol Health and Research World, 19*, 166-171.

Heath, D. B. (1991). Uses and misuses of the concept of ethnicity in alcohol studies: An essay on deconstruction. *International Journal of the Addictions, 25*, 607-628.

Heather, N. (1995). Brief intervention strategies. In R. K. Hester & W. R. Miller (Eds.), *Handbook of alcoholism treatment approaches: Effective alternatives* (2nd ed., pp. 105-122). Boston: Allyn and Bacon.

Heineman-Pieper, M. (1985). The future of social work research. *Social Work Research and Abstracts, 21*, 3-11.

Heinssen, R. K., Levendusky, P. G., & Hunter, R. H. (1995). Client as colleague: Therapeutic contracting with the seriously mentally ill. *American Psychologist, 50*, 522-532.

Helsel, W. J., & Matson, J. L. (1984). The assessment of depression in children: The internal structure of the Child Depression Inventory (CDI). *Behaviour Research and Therapy, 22,* 289-298.

Helzer, J. E., & Pryzbeck, T. R. (1988). The co-occurrence of alcoholism with other psychiatric disorders in the general population and its impact on treatment. *Journal of Studies on Alcohol, 49,* 219-224.

Hemmelgarn, A. L., Glisson, C., & Sharp, S. R. (2003). The validity of the Shortform Assessment for Children (SAC). *Research on Social Work Practice, 13,* 510-530.

Hemsley, D. R. (1996). Schizophrenia: A cognitive model and its implications for psychological intervention. *Behavior Modification, 20,* 139-169.

Hendrick, S. (1981). Self-disclosure and marital satisfaction. *Journal of Personality and Social Psychology, 40,* 1150-1159.

Hendrick, S. (1988). A generic measure of relationship satisfaction. *Journal of Marital and Family Therapy, 50,* 93-98.

Hendrick, S. S., Dicke, A., & Hendrick, C. (1998). The Relationship Assessment Scale. *Journal of Social and Personal Relationships, 15,* 137-142.

Henggeler, S. W., Melton, G. B., & Smith, L. A. (1992). Family preservation using multisystemic therapy: An effective alternative to incarcerating serious juvenile offenders. *Journal of Consulting and Clinical Psychology, 60,* 953-961.

Henggeler, S. W., Melton, G. B., Smith, L. A., Schoenwald, S. K., & Hanley, J. H. (1993). Family preservation using multisystemic treatment: Long-term follow-up to a clinical trial with serious juvenile offenders. *Journal of Child and Family Studies, 2,* 283-293.

Henggeler, S. W., Rodick, J. D., Borduin, C. M., Hanson, C. L., Watson, S. M., & Urey, J. R. (1986). Multisystemic treatment of juvenile offenders: Effects on adolescent behavior and family interactions. *Developmental Psychology, 22,* 132-141.

Henggeler, S. W., Schoenwald, S. K., Borduin, C. M., Rowland, M. D., & Cunningham, P. B. (1998). *Multisystemic treatment of antisocial behavior in children and adolescents.* New York: Guilford Press.

Henggeler, S. W., & Sheidow, A. J. (2003). Conduct disorder and delinquency. *Journal of Marital and Family Therapy, 29,* 505-522.

Henry, W. P. (1996). Structural analysis of social behavior as a common metric for programmatic psychopathology and psychotherapy research. *Journal of Consulting and Clinical Psychology, 64,* 1263-1275.

Henry, W. P., Strupp, H. H., Schacht, T. E., & Gaston, L. (1994). Psychodynamic approaches. In A. E. Bergin & S. L. Garfield (Eds.), *The handbook of psychotherapy and behavior change* (4th ed., 105-108). New York: Wiley.

Hepworth, D. H., Rooney, R. H., & Larsen, J. A. (1997). *Direct social work practice: Theories and skills* (5th ed.). Pacific Grove, CA: Brooks/Cole.

Herbert, M. (1998). Adolescent conduct disorders. In P. Graham (Ed.), *Cognitive-behaviour therapy for children and families* (pp. 194-216). New York: Cambridge University Press.

Herman, D. B., Susser, E. S., & Struening, E. L. (1998). Homelessness, stress and psychopathology. In B. P. Dohrenwend (Ed.), *Adversity and psychopathology* (pp. 132-141). New York: Oxford University Press.

Herman, J. (1992). *Trauma and recovery.* New York: Basic Books.

Herman, S. E., Frank, K. A., Mowbray, C. T., Ribisl, K. M., Davidson, W. S., Bootsmiller, B., et al. (2000). Longitudinal effects of integrated treatment on alcohol use for persons with serious mental illness and substance abuse disorders. *Journal of Behavioral Health Services and Research, 27*, 286-302.

Herpertz-Dahlmann, B., Muller, B., Herpertz, S., Heussen, N., Hebebrand, J., & Remschmidt, H. (2001). Prospective 10-year follow-up in adolescent anorexia nervosa: Course, outcome, psychiatric comorbidity, and psychosocial adaptation. *Journal of Child Psychology and Psychiatry, 42*, 603-612.

Hersen, M. (1985). Single-case experimental designs. In A. S. Bellack, M. Hersen, & A. E. Kazdin (Eds.), *International handbook of behavior modification and therapy* (pp. 85-124). New York: Plenum Press.

Hesselbrock, M. N., Babor, T. F., Hesselbrock, V., Meyer, R. E., & Workman, K. (1983). "Never believe an alcoholic"? On the validity of self-report measures of alcohol dependence and related constructs. *International Journal of the Addictions, 18*, 593-609.

Hesselbrock, M. N., Hesselbrock, V. M., & Epstein, E. E. (1999). Theories of etiology of alcohol and other drug use disorders. In B. S. McCrady & E. E. Epstein (Eds.), *Addictions: A comprehensive guidebook* (pp. 50-74). New York: Oxford University Press.

Hiday, V. A., Swanson, J. W., Swartz, M. S., Borum, R., & Wagner, H. R. (2001). Victimization: A link between mental illness and violence? *International Journal of Law and Psychiatry, 24*, 559-572.

Higgins, D. J., & McCabe, M. P. (2001). Multiple forms of child abuse and neglect: Adult retrospective reports. *Aggression and Violent Behavior, 6*, 547-578.

Higgins, S. T., Budney, A. J., Bickel, W. K., Foerg, F. E., Donham, R., & Badger, G. J. (1994). Incentives improve outcome in outpatient behavioral treatment of cocaine dependence. *Archives of General Psychiatry, 51*, 568-576.

Higgins, S. T., Budney, A. J., Bickel, W. K., Hughes, J. R., Foerg, F., & Badger, G. (1993). Achieving cocaine abstinence with a behavioral approach. *American Journal of Psychiatry, 150*, 763-769.

Higgins, S. T., & Petry, N. M. (1999). Contingency management. *Alcohol Research and Health, 23*, 122-127.

Higgins, S. T., Sigmon, S., Wong, C., Heil, S., Badger, G., Donham, R., et al. (2003). Community reinforcement for cocaine-dependent outpatients. *Archives of General Psychiatry, 60*, 1043-1052.

Higgins, S. T., Wong, C., Badger, G., Ogden, D., & Dantona, R. (2000). Contingent reinforcement increases cocaine abstinence during outpatient treatment and 1 year follow-up. *Journal of Consulting and Clinical Psychology, 68*, 64-72.

Hilarski, C., & Wodarski, J. S. (2001). Comorbid substance abuse and mental illness: Diagnosis and treatment. *Journal of Social Work Practice in the Addictions, 1*, 105-119.

Hill, C. E., Nutt, E. A., & Jackson, S. (1994). Trends in psychotherapy process research: Samples, measures, researchers, and classic publications. *Journal of Counseling and Psychology, 4*, 364-377.

Hingson, R., & Winter, M. (2003). Epidemiology and consequences of drinking and driving. *Alcohol Research and Health, 27*, 63-78.

Hinshaw, S. P., Klein, R. G., & Abikoff, H. (1998). Childhood attention deficit hyperactivity disorder: Nonpharmacological and combination treatments. In P. E. Nathan & J. M. Gorman (Eds.), *A guide to treatments that work* (pp. 26-41). New York: Oxford University Press.

Hoagwood, K., Kelleher, K. J., Feil, M., & Comer, D. M. (2000). Treatment services for children with ADHD: A national perspective. *Journal of the American Academy of Child and Adolescent Psychiatry, 39*, 198-206.

Hochhausen, N. M., Lorenz, A. R., & Newman, J. P. (2002). Specifying the impulsivity of female inmates with borderline personality disorder. *Journal of Abnormal Psychology, 111*, 495-505.

Hoffman, K. J., & Sasaki, J. E. (1997). Comorbidity of substance abuse and PTSD. In C. S. Fullerton & R. J. Ursano (Eds.), *Post-traumatic stress disorder: Acute and long-term responses to trauma and disaster* (pp. 159-174). Washington, DC: American Psychiatric Press.

Hogarty, G. E. (2002). *Personal therapy for schizophrenia and related disorders.* New York: Guilford Press.

Hogarty, G. E., Kornblith, S. J., Greenwald, D., DiBarry, A. L., Cooley, S., Flesher, S., et al. (1995). Personal therapy: A disorder-relevant psychotherapy for schizophrenia. *Schizophrenia Bulletin, 21*, 379-393.

Holahan, C. J., & Moos, R. H. (1994). Life stressors and mental health. In W. R. Avison & I. H. Gotlib (Eds.), *Stress and mental health: Contemporary issues and prospects for the future* (pp. 213-238). New York: Plenum Press.

Holden, G., Cuzzi, L., Rutter, S., Rosenberg, G., & Chernack, P. (1996). The Hospital Social Work Self-Efficacy Scale: Initial development. *Research on Social Work Practice, 6*, 353-365.

Holder, H., Longabaugh, R., Miller, W. R., & Rubonis, A. V. (1991). The cost effectiveness of treatment for alcoholism: A first approximation. *Journal of Studies on Alcohol, 52*, 517-540.

Hollon, S. D., & Beck, A. T. (1994). Cognitive and cognitive-behavioral therapies. In A. E. Bergin & S. L. Garfield (Eds.), *The handbook of psychotherapy and behavior change* (4th ed., pp. 428-466). New York: Wiley.

Hollon, S. D., & Carter, M. (1994). Depression in adults. In L. Craighead, W. Craighead, A. Kazdin, & M. Mahoney (Eds.), *Cognitive and behavioral interventions: An empirical approach to mental health problems* (pp. 89-104). Needham Heights, MA: Allyn and Bacon.

Hollon, S. D., Derubeis, R. J., Evans, M. D., Wiemer, M. J., Garvey, M. J., Grove, W. M., et al. (1992). Cognitive therapy and pharmacotherapy for depression. *Archives of General Psychiatry, 49*, 774-781.

Hollon, S. D., Shelton, R. C., & Davis, D. D. (1993). Cognitive therapy for depression: Conceptual issues and clinical efficacy. *Journal of Consulting and Clinical Psychology, 61*, 270-275.

Hollon, S. D., Shelton, R. C., & Loosen, P. T. (1991). Cognitive therapy and pharmacotherapy for depression. *Journal of Consulting and Clinical Psychology, 59*, 88-99.

Holtzworth-Munroe, A., Bates, L., Smutzler, N., & Sandin, E. (1997). A brief review of the research on husband violence: Part 1. Maritally violent versus nonviolent men. *Aggression and Violent Behavior, 2*, 65-99.

Holtzworth-Munroe, A., Smutzler, N., & Bates, L. (1997). A brief review of the research on husband violence: Part 3: Sociodemographic factors, relationship factors, and differing consequences of husband and wife violence. *Aggression and Violent Behavior, 2*, 285-307.

Holtzworth-Munroe, A., Smutzler, N., & Sandin, E. (1997). A brief review of the research on husband violence: Part 2: The psychological effects of husband violence on battered women and their children. *Aggression and Violent Behavior, 2*, 179-213.

Hooper, S. R., & March, J. S. (1995). Neuropsychology. In J. S. March (Ed.), *Anxiety disorders in children and adolescents* (pp. 35-60). New York: Guilford Press.

Hopko, D. R., Lachar, D., Bailley, S. E., & Varner, R. V. (2001). Assessing predictive factors for extended hospitalization at acute psychiatric admission. *Psychiatric Services, 52*, 1367-1373.

Hopps, J. G., Pinderhughes, E., & Shankar, R. (1995). *The power to care: Clinical practice effectiveness with overwhelmed clients.* New York: Free Press.

Horan, S., Kang, G., Levine, M., Duax, C., Luntz, B., & Tasa, C. (1993). Empirical studies on foster care: Review and assessment. *Journal of Sociology and Social Welfare, 20*, 131-154.

Horne, A. M., Glaser, B. A., & Calhoun, G. B. (1999). Conduct disorders. In R. T. Ammerman, M. Hersen, & C. G. Last (Eds.), *Handbook of prescriptive treatments for children and adolescents* (2nd ed., pp. 84-101). Boston: Allyn and Bacon.

Horowitz, M. J. (1997). *Stress response syndromes: PTSD, grief and adjustment disorders* (3rd ed.). Northvale, NJ: Aronson.

Horvath, A. O., & Greenberg, L. S. (1989). Development and validation of the working alliance inventory. *Journal of Counseling Psychology, 36*, 223-233.

Horvath, E., & Weissman, M. M. (1997). Epidemiology of anxiety disorders across cultural groups. In S. Friedman (Ed.), *Cultural issues in the treatment of anxiety* (pp. 21-29). New York: Guilford Press.

Hotaling, G. T., & Sugarman, D. B. (1986). An analysis of risk markers in husband to wife violence: The current state of knowledge. *Violence and Victims, 1*, 101-124.

Hotopf, M., Sharp, D., & Lewis, G. (1998). What's in a name? A comparison of four psychiatric assessments. *Social Psychiatry and Psychiatric Epidemiology, 33*, 27-31.

Houston-Vega, M. K., Nuehring, E. M., & Daguio, E. R. (1997). *Prudent practice: A guide for managing malpractice risk.* Washington, DC: NASW Press.

Howard, M. O., & Jenson, J. M. (1999). Clinical practice guidelines: Should social work develop them? *Research on Social Work Practice, 9*, 283-301.

Howard, M. O., McMillen, C. J., & Pollio, D. E. (2003). Teaching evidence-based practice: Toward a new paradigm for social work education. *Research on Social Work Practice, 13*, 234-259.

Howells, K., & Day, A. (2002). Grasping the nettle: Treating and rehabilitating the violent offender. *Australian Psychologist, 37*, 222-228.

Hser, Y., Maglione, M., Polinsky, M. L., & Anglin, M. D. (1998). Predicting drug treatment entry among treatment-seeking individuals. *Journal of Substance Abuse Treatment, 15*, 213-220.

Hubbard, R. L., Craddock, S. G., Flynn, P. M., Anderson, J., & Etheridge, R. M. (1997). Overview of 1-year follow-up outcomes in the Drug Abuse Treatment Outcome Study (DATOS). *Psychology of Addictive Behaviors, 11*, 261-278.

Hudson, W. (1982). Scientific imperatives in social work research and practice. *Social Service Review, 56*, 246-258.

Hudson, W. W., & McMurty, S. L. (1997). Comprehensive assessment in social work practice: The Multi-problem Screening Inventory. *Research on Social Work Practice, 7*, 79-98.

Humphreys, K. (1999). Professional interventions that facilitate 12-step self-help group involvement. *Alcohol Research and Health, 23*, 93-98.

Hurley, D. (1991). Women, alcohol and incest: An analytical review. *Journal of Studies on Alcohol, 52*, 253-268.

Huss, M. T., & Langhinrichsen-Rohling, J. (2000). Identification of the psychopathic batterer: The clinical, legal and policy implications. *Aggression and Violent Behavior, 5*, 403-422.

Hutchings, J., Appelton, P., Smith, M., Lane, E., & Nash, S. (2002). Evaluation of two treatments for children with severe behaviour problems: Child behaviour and maternal mental health outcomes. *Behavioural and Cognitive Psychotherapy, 30*, 279-295.

Huxley, N. A., Rendall, M., & Sederer, L. (2000). Psychosocial treatments in schizophrenia: A review of the past 20 years. *Journal of Nervous and Mental Disease, 188*, 187-201.

Hyler, S., Skodol, A., Kellman, H., Oldham, J., & Rosnick, L. (1990). Validity of the Personality Diagnostic Questionnaire–Revised: Comparison with two structured interviews. *American Journal of Psychiatry, 147*, 1043-1048.

Inciardi, J. A., Martin, S. S., Butzin, C. A., Hooper, R. M., & Harrison, L. D. (1997). An effective model of prison-based treatment for drug-involved offenders. *Journal of Drug Issues, 27*, 261-278.

Ironson, G., Freund, B., Strauss, J., & Williams, J. (2002). Comparison of two treatments for traumatic stress: A community-based study of EMDR and Prolonged Exposure. *Journal of Clinical Psychology, 58*, 113-128.

Isenhart, C. E. (1993). Psychometric evaluation of a short form of the Inventory of Drinking Situations. *Journal of Studies on Alcohol, 54*, 345-349.

Ivanoff, A., Blythe, B. J., & Briar, S. (1987). The empirical practice debate. *Social Casework: The Journal of Contemporary Social Work, 68*, 290-298.

Ivarsson, T., & Gillberg, C. (1997). Depressive symptoms in Swedish adolescents: Normative data using the Birleson Depression Self-rating Scale (DSRS). *Journal of Affective Disorders, 42*, 59-68.

Jacobsen, E. (1938). *Progressive muscle relaxation.* Chicago: University of Chicago Press.

Jacobson, N. S. (1991). Behavioral vs. insight-oriented marital therapy: Labels can be misleading. *Journal of Consulting and Clinical Psychology, 59*, 142-145.

Jacobson, N. S., & Addis, M. E. (1993). Research on couples and couple therapy: What do we know? Where are we going? *Journal of Consulting and Clinical Psychology, 61*, 85-93.

Jacobson, N. S., Christensen, A., Prince, S. E., Cordova, J., & Eldridge, K. (2000). Integrative behavioral couple therapy: An acceptance-based promising new treatment for couple discord. *Journal of Consulting and Clinical Psychology, 68*, 351-355.

Jacobson, N. S., Dobson, K. S., Truax, P. A., Addis, M. E., Koerner, K., Gollan, J. K., et al. (1996). A component analysis of cognitive-behavioral treatment for depression. *Journal of Consulting and Clinical Psychology, 64*, 295-304.

Jacobson, N. S., Holzworth-Munroe, A., & Schmaling, K. B. (1989). Marital therapy and spouse involvement in the treatment of depression, agoraphobia and alcoholism. *Journal of Consulting and Clinical Psychology, 57*, 5-10.

Jacobson, N. S., & Margolin, G. (1979). *Marital therapy: Strategies based on social learning and behaviour exchange principles.* New York: Guilford Press.

Jager, A. D. (1999). Forensic psychiatry. *International Medical Journal, 6*, 249-253.

James, P. S. (1991). Effects of a communication training component added to an emotionally focused couples therapy. *Journal of Marital and Family Therapy, 17*, 263-275.

Jansson, L., & Ost, L. (1982). Behavioral treatments for agoraphobia: An evaluative review. *Clinical Psychology Review, 2*, 311-336.

Jensen, C. (1994). Psychosocial treatment of depression in women: Nine single-subject evaluations. *Research on Social Work Practice, 4*, 267-282.

Jerrell, J. M., & Ridgely, M. S. (1995). Comparative effectiveness of three approaches to serving people with severe mental illness and substance abuse disorders. *Journal of Nervous and Mental Disease, 183*, 566-576.

Jessor, R., & Jessor, S. L. (1977). *Problem behavior and psychosocial development: A longitudinal study of youth*. New York: Academic Press.

Johnson, D. L. (1997). Overview of severe mental illness. *Clinical Psychology Review, 17*, 247-257.

Johnson, J. L., Sher, K. J., & Rolf, J. E. (1991). Models of vulnerability to psychopathology in children of alcholics. *Alcohol Health and Research World, 15*, 33-42.

Johnson, P. L., & O'Leary, D. K. (1996). Behavioral components of marital satisfaction: An individualized assessment approach. *Journal of Consulting and Clinical Psychology, 64*, 417-423.

Johnson, R. M., Kotch, J. B., Catellier, D. J., Dufort, V., Junter, W., & Amaya-Jackson, L. (2002). Adverse behavioral and emotional outcomes from child abuse and witnessed violence. *Child Maltreatment, 7*, 179-186.

Johnson, S. M. (2003). The revolution in couple therapy: A practitioner-scientist perspective. *Journal of Marital and Family Therapy, 29*, 365-384.

Johnson, S. M., & Greenberg, L. S. (1985a). Differential effects of experiential and problem solving interventions in resolving marital conflict. *Journal of Consulting and Clinical Psychology, 53*, 175-184.

Johnson, S. M., & Greenberg, L. S. (1985b). Emotionally focused couples therapy: An outcome study. *Journal of Marital and Family Therapy, 11*, 313-317.

Johnson, S. M., & Greenberg, L. S. (1988). *Emotionally-focused therapy for couples*. New York: Guilford Press.

Johnson, S. M., & Greenberg, L. S. (1995). The emotionally focused approach to problems in adult attachment. In N. S. Jacobson & A. S. Gurman (Eds.), *Clinical handbook of couple therapy* (pp. 121-141). New York: Guilford Press.

Johnson. V. W. (1973). *I'll quit tomorrow*. New York: Harper and Row.

Johnson, W. G., Tsoh, J. Y., & Varnado, P. J. (1996). Eating disorders: Efficacy of pharmacological and psychological interventions. *Clinical Psychology Review, 16*, 457-478.

Johnston, C. W., & Alozie, N. O. (2001). The effect of age on criminal processing: Is there an advantage in being "older"? *Journal of Gerontological Social Work, 34*, 65-82.

Johnston, L. D., O'Malley, P. M., & Bachman, J. G. (1996). *National survey results on drug use: Monitoring the future study (1975-1994): Vol. 2. College students and young adults*. Rockville, MD: National Institute for Alcohol Abuse and Alcoholism..

Joint Commission on the Accreditation of Healthcare Organizations. (2004). *Comprehensive accreditation manual for behavioral healthcare, 2004-2005*. Oakbrook Terrace, IL: Author.

Jones, A. C., & Chao, C. M. (1997). Racial, ethnic and cultural issues in couples therapy. In W. K. Halford & H. J. Markham (Eds.), *Clinical handbook of marriage and couples intervention* (pp. 157-178). New York: Wiley.

Jones, E. E., & Pulos, S. M. (1993). Comparing the process in psychodynamic and cognitive-behavioral therapies. *Journal of Consulting and Clinical Psychology, 61,* 306-316.

Jordan, C. E., & Walker, R. (1994). Guidelines for handling domestic violence cases in community mental health centers. *Psychiatric Services, 45,* 147-151.

Joseph, S., Williams, R., & Yule, W. (1997). *Understanding post-traumatic stress: A psychosocial perspective on PTSD and treatment.* New York: Wiley.

Kadden, R. M. (1994). Cognitive-behavioral approaches to alcoholism treatment. *Alcohol Health and Research World, 18,* 279-286.

Kagan, J. (1989). Temperamental contributions to social behavior. *American Psychologist, 44,* 668-674.

Kagan, J. (1997). Conceptualizing psychopathology: The importance of developmental profiles. *Development and Psychopathology, 9,* 321-334.

Kahn, J. S., Kehle, T. J., Jenson, W. R., & Clark, E. (1990). Comparison of cognitive-behavioral, relaxation and self-modeling interventions for depression among middle school students. *School Psychology Review, 19,* 196-211.

Kandel, D. B., Johnson, J. G., Bird, H. R., Canino, G., Goodman, S. H., Lahey, B. B., et al. (1997). Psychiatric disorders associated with substance use among children and adolescents: Findings from the Methods for the Epidemiology of Child and Adolescent Mental Disorders (MECA) study. *Journal of Abnormal Child Psychology, 25,* 121-132.

Kandel, D. B., Johnson, J., Bird, H., Weissman, M., Goodman, S., Lahey, B., et al. (1999). Psychiatric comorbidity among adolescents with substance use disorders: Findings from the MECA study. *Journal of the American Academy of Child and Adolescent Psychiatry, 35,* 743-751.

Kanfer, F. H. (1970). Self-monitoring: Methodological limitations and clinical applications. *Journal of Consulting and Clinical Psychology, 35,* 148-152.

Kaplan, H. I., & Saddock, B. J. (1998). *Synopsis of psychiatry* (8th ed.). Baltimore: Williams and Wilkins.

Kaplan, S. J., Pelcovitz, D., & Labruna, V. (1999). Child and adolescent abuse and neglect research: A review of the past 10 years: Part 1. Physical and emotional abuse and neglect. *Journal of the American Academy of Child and Adolescent Psychiatry, 38,* 1214-1222.

Karls, J. M., & Wandrei, K. E. (Eds.). (1994). *The PIE classification system for social functioning problems.* Washington, DC: NASW Press.

Karney, B. R., & Bradbury, T. N. (1995). The longitudinal course of marital quality and stability: A review of theory, method and research. *Psychological Bulletin, 11,* 3-34.

Karno, M., Golding, J. M., Sorenson, S. B., & Burnam, M. A. (1988). The epidemiology of obsessive-compulsive disorder in five U.S. communities. *Archives of General Psychiatry, 45,* 1094-1099.

Kashubeck-West, S., & Mintz, L. B. (2001). Eating disorders in women: Etiology, assessment, and treatment. *The Counseling Psychologist, 29,* 627-634.

Kashubeck-West, S., Mintz, L. B., & Saunders, K. J. (2001). Assessment of eating disorders in women. *The Counseling Psychologist, 29,* 662-694.

Kaslow, N. J., & Thompson, M. P. (1998). Applying the criteria for empirically supported treatment to studies of psychosocial interventions for child and adolescent depression. *Journal of Clinical Child Psychology, 27*, 146-155.

Kayser, K. (1996). The Marital Disaffection Scale: An inventory for assessing emotional estrangement in marriage. *American Journal of Family Therapy, 24*, 83-88.

Kayser, K. (1997). Couples therapy. In J. R. Brandell (Ed.), *Theory and practice in clinical social work* (pp. 254-287). New York: Free Press.

Kazdin, A. E. (1978). Methodological and interpretive problems of single-case experimental designs. *Journal of Consulting and Clinical Psychology, 46*, 629-642.

Kazdin, A. E. (1994a). Methodology, design and evaluation in psychotherapy research. In A. E. Bergin & S. L. Garfield (Eds.), *The handbook of psychotherapy and behavior change* (4th ed., pp. 19-71). New York: Wiley.

Kazdin, A. E. (1994b). Psychotherapy for children and adolescents. In A. E. Bergin & S. L. Garfield (Eds.), *The handbook of psychotherapy and behavior change* (4th ed., pp. 543-594). New York: Wiley.

Kazdin, A. E. (1997). Practitioner review: Psychosocial treatments for conduct disorder in children. *Journal of Child Psychology and Psychiatry, 38*, 161-178.

Kazdin, A. E. (1998). *Research design in clinical psychology* (3rd ed.). Boston: Allyn and Bacon.

Kazdin, A. E., Bass, D., Siegel, T., & Thomas, C. (1989). Cognitive-behavioral therapy and relationship therapy in the treatment of children referred for antisocial behavior. *Journal of Consulting and Clinical Psychology, 57*, 522-535.

Kazdin, A. E., & Kendall, P. C. (1998). Current progress and future plans for developing effective treatments: Comments and perspectives. *Journal of Clinical Child Psychology, 27*, 217-226.

Kazdin, A. E., & Weisz, J. R. (1998). Identifying and developing empirically supported child and adolescent treatments. *Journal of Consulting and Clinical Psychology, 66*, 19-36.

Kazdin, A. E., & Wilson, G. T. (1980). *The evaluation of behavior therapy: Issues, evidence and research strategies.* Lincoln: University of Nebraska Press.

Keane, T. M. (1998). Psychological effects of military combat. In B. P. Dohrenwend (Ed.), *Adversity, stress and psychopathology* (pp. 52-65). New York: Oxford University Press.

Keane, T. M., Caddell, J., & Taylor, K. (1988). Mississippi Scale for Combat-Related Posttraumatic Stress Disorder: Three studies in reliability and validity. *Journal of Consulting and Clinical Psychology, 56*, 85-90.

Kelly, J. L., & Petry, N. M. (2000). HIV risk behaviors in male substance abusers with and without antisocial personality disorder. *Journal of Substance Abuse Treatment, 19*, 59-66.

Kempe, C. H., Silverman, F. N., Steele, B. F., Droegemueller, W., & Silver, H. K. (1962). The battered child syndrome. *Journal of the American Medical Association, 181*, 17-24.

Kendall, P. C. (1992). *Anxiety disorders in youth: Cognitive behavioral interventions.* Boston: Allyn and Bacon.

Kendall, P. C. (1993). Cognitive-behavioral therapies with youth: Guiding theory, current status, and emerging developments. *Journal of Consulting and Clinical Psychology, 61*, 235-247.

Kendall, P. C. (1994).Treating anxiety disorders in children: Results of a randomized clinical trial. *Journal of Consulting and Clinical Psychology, 62,* 100-110.

Kendall, P. C., Flannery-Schroeder, E., Panichelli-Mindel, S. M., Southam-Gerow, M., Henin, A., & Warman, M. (1997).Therapy for youths with anxiety disorders: A second randomized clinical trial. *Journal of Consulting and Clinical Psychology, 65,* 366-380.

Kendall, P. C., Korlander, E., Chansky, T. E., & Brady, E. U. (1992). Comorbidity of anxiety and depression in youth: Treatment implications. *Journal of Consulting and Clinical Psychology, 60,* 869-880.

Kendall, P. C., & Southam-Gerow, M. A. (1996). Long-term follow-up of a cognitive-behavioral therapy for anxiety-disordered youth. *Journal of Consulting and Clinical Psychology, 64,* 724-730.

Kendall-Tackett, K. A., Williams, L. M., & Finkelhor, D. (1993). Impact of sexual abuse on children: A review and synthesis of recent empirical studies. *Psychological Bulletin, 113,* 164-180.

Kennedy, G. J., Metz, H., & Lowinger, R. (1996). Epidemiology and inferences regarding the etiology of late-life suicide. In G. J. Kennedy (Ed.), *Suicide and depression in late life* (pp. 3-22). New York: Wiley.

Kernberg, O. F. (1975). *Borderline conditions and pathological narcissism.* New York: Aronson.

Kernberg, O. F. (1976). *Object relations theory and clinical psychoanalysis.* New York: Aronson.

Kernberg, O. F. (1999).The psychotherapeutic treatment of borderline patients. In J. Derksen, C. Maffei, & H. Groen (Eds.), *Treatment of personality disorders* (pp. 167-182). New York: Kluwer Academic/Plenum Press.

Kersten, K. (1990). The process of marital disaffection: Interventions at various stages. *Family Relations, 39,* 257-265.

Kertzman, S. G., Treves, I. A., Treves, T. A., Vainder, M., & Korczyn, A. D. (2002). Hamilton Depression Scale in dementia. *International Journal of Psychiatry in Clinical Practice, 6,* 91-94.

Kessler, R. C., McGonagle, K., Zhao, S., Nelson, C., Hughes, M., Eshleman, S., et al. (1994). Lifetime and 12-month prevalence of *DSM-III-R* psychiatric disorders in the United States. *Archives of General Psychiatry, 51,* 8-19.

Kessler, R. C., Nelson, C. B., McGonagle, K., Edlund, M. J., Frank, R. G., & Leaf, P. (1996). The epidemiology of co-occurring addictive and mental disorders: Implications for prevention and service utilization. *American Journal of Orthopsychiatry, 66,* 17-31.

Kessler, R. C., Sonnega, A., Bromet, E., Hughes, M., & Nelson, C. B. (1995). Posttraumatic stress disorder in the National Comorbidity Survey. *Archives of General Psychiatry, 52,* 1048-1060.

Kettlewell, P. W., Mizes, J. S., & Wasylyshyn, N. A. (1992). A cognitive-behavioral group treatment of bulimia. *Behavior Therapy, 23,* 657-670.

Kety, S. S. (1996). Genetic and environmental factors in the etiology of schizophrenia. In S. Matthysse, D. L. Levy, J. Kagan, & F. M. Benes (Eds.), *Psychopathology: The evolving science of mental disorder* (pp. 477-487). New York: Cambridge University Press.

Kilpatrick, D. G., & Resnick, H. S. (1993). Post traumatic stress disorder associated with exposure to criminal victimization in clinical and community populations.

In R. J. McNally, J. R. Davidson, & E. B. Foa (Eds.), *Post traumatic stress disorder: DSM-IV and beyond* (pp. 113-146). Washington, DC: American Psychiatric Press.

Kilpatrick, D. G., Resnick, H. S., Saunders, B. E., & Best, C. L. (1998). Rape, other violence against women, and posttraumatic stress disorder. In B. P. Dohrenwend (Ed.), *Adversity, stress and psychopathology* (pp. 161-176). New York: Oxford University Press.

Kilpatrick, D. G., Saunders, B. E., Amick-McMullan, A., Best, C. L., Veronen, L. J., & Resnick, H. S. (1989). Victim and crime factors associated with the development of crime-related post-traumatic stress disorder. *Behavior Therapy, 20,* 199-214.

Kilpatrick, D. G., Saunders, B. E., Veronen, L. J., Best, C. L., & Von, J. M. (1987). Criminal victimization: Lifetime prevalence, reporting to police, and psychological impact. *Crime and Delinquency, 33,* 479-489.

King, C. A., Ghaziuddin, N., McGovern, L., Brand, E., Hill, E., & Naylor, M. (1996). Predictors of comorbid alcohol and substance abuse in depressed adolescents. *Journal of the Academy of Child and Adolescent Psychiatry, 35,* 743-751.

King, D. W., Leskin, G. A., King, L. A., & Weathers, F. W. (1998). Confirmatory factor analysis of the Clinician-Administered PTSD Scale: Evidence for the dimensionality of posttraumatic stress disorder. *Psychological Assessment, 10,* 90-96.

King, N. J., Hamilton, D. I., & Ollendick, T. H. (1988). *Children's phobias: A behavioural perspective.* Chichester, United Kingdom: Wiley.

King, N. J., Tonge, B. J., Mullen, P., Myerson, N., Heyne, D., Rollings, S., et al. (2000). Treating sexually abused children with posttraumatic stress symptoms: A randomized controlled trial. *Journal of the American Academy of Child and Adolescent Psychiatry, 39,* 1347-1355.

Kingdon, D. G., & Turkington, D. (1991). The use of cognitive behavior therapy with a normalizing rationale in schizophrenia. *Journal of Nervous and Mental Disease, 179,* 207-211.

Kinney, J., Haapala, D. A., & Booth, C. (1991). *Keeping families together: The Homebuilders model.* New York: Aldine de Gruyter.

Kinney, J., Madsen, B., Fleming, T., & Haapala, D. A. (1977). Homebuilders: Keeping families together. *Journal of Consulting and Clinical Psychology, 45,* 667-673.

Kinzie, J. D., Manson, S. M., Do, T. V., Nguyen, T. T. L., Bui, A., & Than, N. P. (1982). Development and validation of a Vietnamese-language depression rating scale. *American Journal of Psychiatry, 139,* 1276-1280.

Kirisci, L., Moss, H. B., & Tarter, R. E. (1996). Psychometric evaluation of the Situational Confidence Questionnaire in adolescents: Fitting a graded item response model. *Addictive Behaviors, 21,* 303-317.

Kirk, S. A. (1999). Good intentions are not enough: Practice guidelines for social work. *Research on Social Work Practice, 9,* 302-310.

Kitano, H. H. (1989). Alcohol and Asian-Americans. In T. D. Watts & R. Wright (Eds.), *Alcoholism in minority populations* (pp. 143-156). Springfield, IL: Charles C. Thomas.

Kivlahan, D. R., Marlatt, G. A., Fromme, K., Coppel, D. B., & Williams, E. (1990). Secondary prevention with college drinkers: Evaluation of an alcohol skills training program. *Journal of Consulting and Clinical Psychology, 58,* 805-810.

Klee, L., Schmidt, C., & Ames, G. (1991). Indicators of women's alcohol problems: What women themselves report. *International Journal of the Addictions, 26,* 879-895.

Klein, W. C., & Bloom, M. (1995). Practice wisdom. *Social Work, 40,* 799–807.

Klerman, G. L., & Weissman, M. M. (1993). *New applications of interpersonal psychotherapy.* Washington, DC: American Psychiatric Association.

Klerman, G. L., Weissman, M. M., Rounsaville, B. J., & Chevron, E. S. (1984). *Interpersonal psychotherapy of depression.* New York: Basic Books.

Klinkenberg, W. D., & Calsyn, R. J. (1998). Gender differences in the receipt of aftercare and psychiatric hospitalization among adults with severe mental illness. *Comprehensive Psychiatry, 39,* 137–142.

Klosko, J. S., & Sanderson, W. C. (1999). *Cognitive-behavioral treatment of depression.* Northvale, NJ: Aronson.

Knapp, S., & VandeCreek, L. (2000). Recovered memories of childhood abuse: Is there an underlying professional consensus? *Professional Psychology: Research and Practice, 31,* 365–371.

Knight, K., Hiller, M. L., & Simpson, D. D. (1999). Evaluating corrections-based treatment for the drug-abusing criminal offender. *Journal of Psychoactive Drugs, 31,* 299–304.

Kobak, K. A., Greist, J. H., Jefferson, J. W., Katzelnick, D. J., & Henk, H. J. (1998). Behavioral versus pharmacological treatments of obsessive compulsive disorder: A meta-analysis. *Psychopharmacology, 136,* 205–216.

Koch, P. B., Palmer, R. F., Vicary, J. R., & Wood, J. M. (1999). Mixing sex and alcohol in college: Female-male HIV risk model. *Journal of Sex Education and Therapy, 24,* 99–108.

Kohn, R., Dohrenwend, B. P., & Mirotznik, J. (1998). Epidemiological findings on selected psychiatric disorders in the general population. In B. P. Dohrenwend (Ed.), *Adversity, stress and psychopathology* (pp. 235–284). New York: Oxford University Press.

Kolko, D. J., Brent, D. A., Baugher, M., Bridge, J., & Birmaher, B. (2000). Cognitive and family therapies for adolescent depression treatment specificity, mediation, and moderation. *Journal of Consulting and Clinical Psychology, 68,* 603–614.

Kopelowicz, A. (1997). Social skill training: The moderating influence of culture in the treatment of Latinos with schiophrenia. *Journal of Psychopathology and Behavioral Assessment, 19,* 101–108.

Kornstein, S. (1997). Gender differences in depression: Implications for treatment. *Journal of Clinical Psychiatry, 58,* 12–18.

Koss, M. (1993). Detecting the scope of rape: A review of prevalence research methods. *Journal of Interpersonal Violence, 8,* 198–222.

Koss, M. P., & Butcher, J. N. (1986). Research on brief therapy. In S. L. Garfield & A. E. Bergin (Eds.), *Handbook of psychotherapy and behavior change* (3rd ed., pp. 627–670). New York: Wiley.

Koss, M. P., & Shiang, J. (1994). Research on brief psychotherapy. In A. E. Bergin & S. L. Garfield (Eds.), *The handbook of psychotherapy and behavior change* (4th ed., pp. 664–700). New York: Wiley.

Koss-Chioino, J. (1999). Depression among Puerto Rican women: Culture, etiology and diagnosis. *Hispanic Journal of Behavioral Sciences, 21,* 330–350.

Kotler, L. A., Cohen, P., Davies, M., Pine, D. S., & Walsh, B. T. (2001). Longitudinal relationships between childhood, adolescent, and adult eating disorders. *Journal of the American Academy of Child and Adolescent Psychiatry, 40,* 1434–1440.

Kovacs, M. (1985). The Children's Depression Inventory (CDI). *Psychopharmacology Bulletin, 21,* 995–998.

Kovacs, M., & Bastiaens, L. J. (1995). The psychotherapeutic management of major depressive and dysthymic disorders in childhood and adolescence: Issues and prospects. In I. M. Goodyer (Ed.), *The depressed child and adolescent: Developmental and clinical perspectives* (pp. 281–310). New York: Cambridge University Press.

Kovacs, M., Rush, A. J., Beck, A. T., & Hollon, S. D. (1981). Depressed outpatients treated with cognitive therapy or pharmacotherapy: A one-year follow-up. *Archives of General Psychiatry, 38,* 34–39.

Kranz, K. (2003). Development of the Alcohol and Other Drug Self-Efficacy Scale. *Research on Social Work Practice, 13,* 724–741.

Kranz, K., & O'Hare, T. (in press). The Substance Abuse Treatment Self-Efficacy Scale: A confirmatory factor analysis. *Journal of Social Service Research.*

Kudler, H. S., Blank, A. S., & Krupnick, J. L. (2000). Psychodynamic therapy. In E. B. Foa, T. M. Keane, & M. J. Friedman (Eds.), *Effective treatments for PTSD: Practice guidelines from the International Society for Traumatic Stress Studies* (pp. 176–198). New York: Guilford Press.

Kuehnle, K. (1996). *Assessing allegations of child sexual abuse.* Sarasota, FL: Professional Resource Press.

Kulka, R. A., Schlenger, W. E., Fairbank, J. A., Hough, R. L., Jordan, B. K., Marmar, C. R., et al. (1988). *National Vietnam Veterans Readjustment Study (NVVRS): Description, current status, and initial PTSD prevalence estimates.* Research Triangle Park, NC: Research Triangle Institute.

Kuno, E., Rothbard, A. B., Averyt, J., & Culhane, D. (2000). Homelessness among persons with serious mental illness in an enhanced communty-based mental health system. *Psychiatric Services, 51,* 1012–1016.

Kurdek, L. A. (1998). Relationship outcomes and their predictors: Longitudinal evidence from heterosexual married, gay cohabiting, and lesbian cohabitating couples. *Journal of Marriage and the Family, 60,* 553–568.

Kutchins, H., & Kirk, S. A. (1988). The business of diagnosis: *DSM-III* and clinical social work. *Social Work, 33,* 215–220.

Kutchins, H., & Kirk, S. A. (1997). *Making us crazy: The psychiatric bible and the creation of mental disorders.* New York: Free Press.

Lachar, D., Bailley, S. E., Rhoades, H. M., Espadas, A., Aponte, M., Cowan, K. A., et al. (2001). New subscales for an anchored version of the Brief Psychiatric Rating Scale: Construction, reliability, and validity in acute psychiatric admissions. *Psychological Assessment, 13,* 384–395.

La Greca, A. M., Prinstein, M. J., & Fetter, M. D. (2001). Adolescent peer crown affiliation: Linkages with health-risk behaviors and close friendships. *Journal of Pediatric Psychology, 26,* 131–143.

Lahey, B. B., Gordon, R. A., Loeber, R., Stouthamer-Loeber, M., & Farrington, D. P. (1999). Boys who join gangs: A prospective study of predictors of first gang entry. *Journal of Abnormal Child Psychology, 27,* 261–276.

Lamb, H. R., & Weinberger, L. E. (1998). Persons with severe mental illness in jails and prisons: A review. *Psychiatric Services, 49,* 483–492.

Lamb, M. (1994). *The investigation of child sexual abuse: An interdisciplinary consensus statement.* Bethesda, MD: National Instititute of Child Health and Human Development.

Lambert, M. J., & Bergin, A. E. (1994). The effectiveness of psychotherapy. In A. E. Bergin & S. L. Garfield (Eds.), *The handbook of psychotherapy and behavior change* (4th ed., pp. 143–189). New York: Wiley.

Lambert, M. J., Shapiro, D. A., & Bergin, A. E. (1986). The effectiveness of psychotherapy. In S. L. Garfield & A. E. Bergin (Eds.), *The handbook of psychotherapy and behavior change* (3rd ed., pp. 157-187). New York: Wiley.

Lane, S. D., & Cherek, D. R. (2000). Biological and behavioral investigation of aggression and impulsivity. In D. H. Fishbein (Ed.), *The science, treatment, and prevention of antisocial behaviors: Application to the criminal justice system* (pp. 5-21). Kingston, NJ: Civic Research Institute.

Larimer, M. E., & Cronce, J. M. (2002). Identification, prevention and treatment: A review of individual-focused strategies to reduce problematic alcohol consumption by college students. *Journal of Studies on Alcohol, 63*, 148-163.

Larimer, M. E., Palmer, R. S., & Marlatt, G. A. (1999). Relapse prevention: An overview of Marlatt's cognitive-behavioral model. *Alcohol Research and Health, 23*, 151-159.

Last, C. G. (1989). Anxiety disorders. In T. H. Ollendick & M. Hersen (Eds.), *Handbook of childhood psychopathology* (2nd ed., pp. 219-227). New York: Plenum Press.

Last, C. G., Hansen, C., & Franco, N. (1998). Cognitive-behavioral treatment of school phobia. *Journal of the American Academy of Child and Adolescent Psychiatry, 37*, 404-411.

Lawrence, E., & Bradbury, T. N. (2001). Physical aggression and marital dysfunction: A longitudinal analysis. *Journal of Family Psychology, 15*, 135-154.

Lawrence, E., Eldridge, K. A., & Christensen, A. (1998). The enhancement of traditional behavioral couples therapy: Consideration of individual factors and dyadic development. *Clinical Psychology Review, 18*, 745-764.

Layne, C. M., Saltzman, W. R., Savjak, N., Popovic, T., Music, M., Djapo, N., et al. (2001). Trauma/grief focused group psychotherapy: School-based postwar intervention with traumatized Bosnian adolescents. *Group Dynamics: Theory, Research and Practice, 5*, 277-290.

Lazarus, A. A. (1981). *The practice of multimodal therapy.* New York: McGraw-Hill.

Lazarus, A. A. (1997). *Brief but comprehensive psychotherapy: The multimodal way.* New York: Springer.

Lazarus, R. S., & Folkman, S. (1984). *Stress, appraisal and coping.* New York: Springer.

Lebow, J. (2000). What does the research tell us about couples and family therapies? *Psychotherapy in Practice, 56*, 1083-1094.

Lebow, J., & Gurman, A. S. (1995). Research assessing couple and family therapy. *Annual Review of Psychology, 46*, 27-57.

Leccese, M., & Waldron, H. B. (1994). Assessing adolescent substance use: A critique of current measurement instruments. *Journal of Substance Abuse Treatment, 11*, 553-563.

Leda, C., & Rosenheck, R. (1995). Race in the treatment of homeless mentally ill veterans. *Journal of Nervous and Mental Disease, 183*, 529-537.

Lee, C., Gavriel, H., Drummond, P., Richards, J., & Greenwald, R. (2002). Treatment of PTSD: Stress inoculation training with prolonged exposure compared to EMDR. *Journal of Clinical Psychology, 58*, 1071-1089.

Lefley, H. P. (1992). Expressed emotion: Conceptual, clinical and social policy issues. *Hospital and Community Psychiatry, 43*, 591-598.

Lehman, A. F. (1988). A quality of life interview for the chronically mentally ill. *Evaluation and Program Planning, 11*, 51-62.

Lehman, A. F. (1995). Vocational rehabilitation in schizophrenia. *Schizophrenia Bulletin, 21*, 645-656.

Lehman, A. F., McNary, S. W., & O'Grady, K. E. (1997). Measuring subjective life satisfaction in persons with severe and persistent mental illness: A measurement quality and structural model analysis. *Psychological Assessment, 9*, 503-507.

Lehman, A. F., Steinwachs, D. M., & Co-Investigators of the PORT Project (1998). At issue: Translating research into practice: The schizophrenia patient outcomes research team (PORT) recommendations. *Schizophrenia Bulletin, 24*, 1-10.

Lehman, C., Brown, T. A., & Barlow, D. H. (1998). Effects of cognitive-behavioral treatment for panic disorder with agoraphobia on concurrent alcohol abuse. *Behavior Therapy, 29*, 423-433.

Leichsenring, F. (1999). Development and first results of the borderline personality inventory: A self-report instrument for assessing borderline personality organization. *Journal of Personality Assessment, 73*, 45-63.

Leigh, B. C. (1990). The relationship of sex-related alcohol expectancies to alcohol consumption and sexual behavior. *British Journal of the Addictions, 85*, 919-928.

Leigh, B. C. (1999). The risks of drinking among young adults: Peril, chance, adventure: Concepts of risk, alcohol use and risky behavior in young adults. *Addiction, 94*, 371-383.

Leigh, B. C., & Aramburu, B. (1996). The role of alcohol and gender in choices and judgments about hypothetical sexual encounters. *Journal of Applied Social Psychology, 26*, 20-30.

Leigh, B. C., & Schafer, J. C. (1993). Heavy drinking occasions and the occurrence of sexual activity. *Psychology of Addictive Behaviors, 7*, 197-200.

Leventhal, J. M. (1996). Twenty years later: We do know how to prevent child abuse and neglect. *Child Abuse and Neglect, 20*, 647-653.

Levine, M. P., & Piran, N. (2001). The prevention of eating disorders: Toward a participatory ecology of knowledge, action, and advocacy. In R. H. Striegel-Moore & L. Smolak (Eds.), *Eating disorders: Innovative directions in research and practice* (pp. 233-253). Washington, DC: American Psychological Association.

Levinger, G. (1976). A social psychological perspective on marital dissolution. *Journal of Social Issues, 32*, 21-47.

Lewis, J. E., Malow, R. M., & Ireland, S. J. (1997). HIV/AIDS risk in heterosexual college students: A review of a decade of literature. *Journal of American College Health, 45*, 147-158.

Lewis, R. E., Walton, E., & Fraser, M. W. (1995). Examining family reunification services: A process analysis of a successful experiment. *Research on Social Work Practice, 5*, 259-282.

Lewisohn, P. M. (1974). A behavioral approach to depression. In R. J. Freidman & M. M. Katz (Eds.), *The psychology of depression: Contemporary theory and research* (pp. 157-178). Washington, DC: Winston/Wiley.

Lewisohn, P. M., Clarke, G. N., Hops, H., & Andrews, J. (1990). Cognitive-behavioral treatment for depressed adolescents. *Behavior Therapy, 21*, 385-401.

Lewisohn, P. M., Rohde, P., Seeley, J. R., Klein, D. N., & Gotlib, I. (2000). Natural course of adolescent major depressive disorder in a community sample: Predictors of recurrence in young adults. *American Journal of Psychiatry, 157*, 1584-1591.

Lex, B. (1994). Alcohol and other drug abuse among women. *Alcohol Health and Research World, 18*, 212-219.

Liberman, R. P., Kopelowicz, A., & Young, A. S. (1994). Biobehavioral treatment and rehabilitation of schizophrenia. *Behavior Therapy, 25,* 89-107.

Liberto, J. G., Oslin, D. W., & Ruskin, P. E. (1992). Alcoholism in older persons: A review of the literature. *Hospital and Community Psychiatry, 43,* 975-984.

Liberto, J. G., Oslin, D. W., & Ruskin, P. E. (1996). Alcoholism in older populations. In L. L. Carstensen, B. A. Edelstein, & L. Dornbrand (Eds.), *The practical handbook of clinical gerontology* (pp. 324-348). Thousand Oaks, CA: Sage.

Liddle, H. A., & Dakof, G. A. (1995). Efficacy of family therapy for drug abuse: Promising but not definitive. *Journal of Marital and Family Therapy, 21,* 511-543.

Liddle, H. A., & Hogue, A. (2000). A family-based, developmental-ecological preventive intervention for high-risk adolescents. *Journal of Marital and Family Therapy, 26,* 265-279.

Liepman, M. R. (1993). Using family influence to motivate alcoholics to enter treatment: The Hohson Institute Intervention Approach. In T. J. O'Farrell, (Ed.), *Treating alcohol problems: Marital and family interventions* (pp. 54-77). New York: Guilford Press.

Lindahl, K. M., Clements, M., & Markman, H. (1998). Development of marriage: A 9-year perspective. In T. N. Bradbury (Ed.), *The developmental course of marital dysfunction* (pp. 205-236). New York: Cambridge University Press.

Lindahl, K. M., Malik, N. M., & Bradbury, T. N. (1997). The developmental course of couples' relationships. In W. K. Halford & H. J. Markham (Eds.), *Clinical handbook of marriage and couples intervention* (pp. 203-224). New York: Wiley.

Linehan, M. M. (1993a). *Cognitive-behavioral treatment of borderline personality disorder.* New York: Guilford Press.

Linehan, M. M. (1993b). *Skills training manual for treating borderline personality disorder.* New York: Guilford Press.

Linehan, M. M., Armstrong, H. E., Suarez, A., Allmon, D., & Heard, H. L. (1991). Cognitive-behavioral treatment of chronically parasuicidal borderline patients. *Archives of General Psychiatry, 48,* 1060-1064.

Linehan, M. M., Heard, H. L., & Armstrong, H. E. (1993). Naturalistic follow-up of a beahavioral treatment for chronically parasuicidal borderline patients. *Archives of General Psychiatry, 50,* 971-974.

Linehan, M. M., Kanter, J. W., & Comtois, K. A. (1999). Dialectical behavior therapy for borderline personality disorder. In D. S. Janowsky (Ed.), *Psychotherapy indications and outcomes* (pp. 93-118). Washington, DC: American Psychiatric Press.

Linehan, M. M., Tutek, D. A., Heard, H. L., & Armstrong, H. E. (1994). Interpersonal outcome of cognitive behavioral treatment for chronically suicidal borderline patients. *American Journal of Psychiatry, 151,* 1771-1776.

Lipsey, M. W., & Wilson, D. B. (1993). The efficacy of psychological, educational, and behavioral treatment: Confirmation from meta-analysis. *American Psychologist, 48,* 1181-1209.

Litten, R. Z., & Allen, J. P. (1999). Medications for alcohol, illicit drug, and tobacco dependence: An update of research findings. *Journal of Substance Abuse Treatment, 16,* 105-112.

Locke, H., & Wallace, K. (1959). Short marital adjustment and prediction tests: Their reliability and validity. *Marriage and Family Living, 2,* 251-255.

Loevinger, J. (1976). *Ego development: Conceptions and theories.* San Francisco: Jossey-Bass.

Loftus, E. F. (1993). The reality of repressed memories. *American Psychologist, 48,* 518-537.

Loftus, E. F. (1994). The repressed memory controversy. *American Psychologist, 49,* 443-445.

Lohr, J., Lilienfeld, S., Tolin, D., & Herbert, J. (1999). Eye movement desensitization and reprocessing: An analysis of specific versus nonspecific treatment factors. *Journal of Anxiety Disorders, 13,* 185-207.

Longabaugh, R., & Morgenstern, J. (1999). Cognitive-behavioral coping-skills therapy for alcohol dependence: Current status and future directions. *Alcohol Research and Health, 23,* 78-85.

LoPiccolo, J. (1994). Sexual dysfunction. In L. W. Craighead, W. E. Craighead, A. E. Kazdin, & M. J. Mahoney (Eds.), *Cognitive and behavioral interventions: An empirical approach to mental health problems* (pp. 183-196). Boston: Allyn and Bacon.

Lordan, E. J., Kelley, J. M., Peters, C. P., & Siegfried, R. J. (1997). Treatment placement decisions: How substance abuse professionals assess and place clients. *Evaluation and Program Planning, 20,* 137-149.

Lowe, L.A. (1998). Using the Child Behavior Checklist in assessing conduct disorder: Issues of reliability and validity. *Research on Social Work Practice, 8,* 286-301.

Luborsky, L., Singer, B., & Luborsky, L. (1975). Comparative studies of psychotherapies: Is it true that "Everyone has won and all must have prizes"? *Archives of General Psychiatry, 32,* 995-1008.

Lutzker, J. R., Bigelow, K. M., Doctor, R. M., Gershater, R. M., & Greene, B. F. (1998). An ecobehavioral model for the prevention and treatment of child abuse and neglect: History and applications. In J. R. Lutzker (Ed.), *Handbook of child abuse research and treatment* (pp. 239-266). New York: Plenum Press.

Lutzker, J. R., Bigelow, K. M., Doctor, R. M., & Kessler, M. L. (1998). Safety, health care, and bonding within an ecobehavioral approach to treating and preventing child abuse and neglect. *Journal of Family Violence, 13,* 163-185.

Lutzker, J. R., & Rice, J. M. (1984). Project 12-Ways: Measuring outcome of a large in-home service for treatment and prevention of child abuse and neglect. *Child Abuse and Neglect, 8,* 519-524.

Lutzker, J. R., & Rice, J. M. (1987). Using recidivism data to evaluate Project 12-Ways: An ecobehavioral approach to the treatment and prevention of child abuse and neglect. *Journal of Family Violence, 2,* 283-289.

Lutzker, J. R., Van Hasselt, V. B., Bigelow, K. M., Greene, B. F., & Kessler, M. L. (1998). Child abuse and neglect: Behavioral research, treatment and theory. *Aggression and violent behavior, 3,* 181-196.

Lyons, J. S., Howard, K. I., O'Mahoney, M. T., & Lish, J. D. (1997). *The measurement and management of clinical outcomes in mental health.* New York: Wiley.

Lyons, P., Doueck, H. J., & Wodarski, J. S. (1996). Risk assessment for child protective services: A review of the empirical literature on instrument performance. *Social Work Research, 20,* 143-155.

MacDonald, B. J. (1998). Issues in therapy with gay and lesbian couples. *Journal of Sex and Marital Therapy, 24,* 165-190.

MacDonald, G., Sheldon, B., & Gillespie, J. (1992). Contemporary studies of the effectiveness of social work. *British Journal of Social Work, 22,* 615-643.

Mackey, R.A., & O'Brien, B.A. (1998). Marital conflict management: Gender and ethnic differences. *Social Work, 43,* 128-140.

MacLeod, J., & Nelson, G. (2000). Programs for the promotion of family wellness and the prevention of child maltreatment: A meta-analytic review. *Child Abuse and Neglect, 24,* 1127-1149.

MacMillan, H. L., MacMillan, J. H., Offord, D. R., Griffith, L., & MacMillan, A. (1994a). Primary prevention of child physical abuse: A critical review: Part 1. *Journal of Child Psychology and Psychiatry, 35,* 835-856.

MacMillan, H. L., MacMillan, J. H., Offord, D. R., Griffith, L., & MacMillan, A. (1994b). Primary prevention of child sexual abuse: A critical review: Part 2. *Journal of Child Psychology and Psychiatry, 35,* 857-876.

Madanes, C. (1981). *Strategic family therapy*. San Francisco: Jossey-Bass.

Maddock, J. E., Laforge, R. G., Rossi, J. S., & O'Hare, T. (2001). The College Alcohol Problem Scale. *Addictive Behaviors, 26,* 385-398.

Magee, W. J., Eaton, W., Wittchen, H., McGonagle, K., & Kessler, R. (1996). Agoraphobia, simple phobia, and social phobia in the national comorbidity survey. *Archives of General Psychiatry, 53,* 159-168.

Mahler, M. M. (1968). *On human symbiosis and vicissitudes of individuation*. New York: International Universities Press.

Mahoney, M. J. (1977). Reflections on the cognitive-learning trend in psychotherapy. *American Psychologist, 32,* 5-13.

Maisto, S. A., Carey, K., & Bradizza, C. (1999). Social learning theory. In K. E. Leonard & H. T. Blane (Eds.), *Psychological theories of drinking and alcoholism* (pp. 106-163). New York: Guilford Press.

Maisto, S. A., Carey, M. P., Carey, K. B., Gordon, C. M., & Gleason, J. R. (2000). Use of the AUDIT and the DAST-10 to identify alcohol and drug use disorders among adults with severe and persistent mental illness. *Psychological Assessment, 12,* 186-192.

Maletzky, B. M., & Steinhauser, C. (2002). A 25-year follow-up of cognitive/behavioral therapy with 7, 275 sexual offenders. *Behavior Modification, 26,* 123-147.

Malow, R. M., McMahon, R., Cremer, D. J., Lewis, J. E., & Alferi, S. M. (1997). Psychosocial predictors of HIV risk among adolescent offenders who abuse drugs. *Psychiatric Services, 48,* 185-187.

Manassis, K. (2000). Childhood anxiety disorders: Lessons from the literature. *Canadian Journal of Psychiatry, 45,* 724-730.

Manassis, K. (2001). Child-parent relations: Attachment and anxiety disorders. In W. K. Silverman & P. D. A. Treffers (Eds.), *Anxiety disorders in children and adolescents: Research, assessment and intervention* (pp. 255-272). New York: Cambridge University Press.

Mann, B. J., & Borduin, C. M. (1991). A critical review of psychotherapy outcome studies with adolescents, 1978-1988. *Adolescence, 26,* 505-541.

Manoleas, P. (Ed.). (1996). *The cross-cultural practice of clinical case management in mental health*. New York: Haworth Press.

March, J. S. (1995). Cognitive-behavioral psychotherapy for children and adolescents with OCD: A review and recommendations for treatment. *Journal of the Academy of Child and Adolescent Psychiatry, 34,* 7-18.

March, J. S., & Leonard, H. L. (1996). Obsessive-compulsive disorder in children and adolescents: A review of the past 10 years. *Journal of the American Academy of Child and Adolescent Psychiatry, 35,* 1265-1273.

March, J. S., Leonard, H. L., & Swedo, S. E. (1995). Obsessive-compulsive disorder. In J. S. March (Ed.), *Anxiety disorders in children and adolescents* (pp. 251-275). New York: Guilford Press.

Marcus, R. F., & Swett, B. (2002). Violence and intimacy in close relationships. *Journal of Interpersonal Violence, 17*, 570-586.

Marino, R., Stuart, G. W., & Minas, I. H. (2000). Acculturation of values and behavior: A study of Vietnamese immigrants. *Measurement and Evaluation in Counseling and Development, 33*, 21-41.

Markowitz, J. C. (1999). Developments in interpersonal psychotherapy. *Canadian Journal of Psychiatry, 44*, 556-561.

Marks, I. M. (1987). *Fears, phobias and rituals: Panic, anxiety and their disorders.* New York: Oxford University Press.

Marlatt, G. A. (1996). Harm reduction: Come as you are. *Addictive Behaviors, 21*, 779-788.

Marlatt, G. A., Baer, J. S., Kivlahan, D. R., Dimeff, L. A., Larimer, M. E., Quigley, L. A., et al. (1998). Screening and brief intervention for high-risk college student drinkers: Results from a 2-year follow-up assessment. *Journal of Consulting and Clinical Psychology, 66*, 604-615.

Marlatt, G. A., & George, W. (1984). Relapse prevention: Introduction and overview of the model. *British Journal of the Mental Health Problems and Alcohol Abuse Addictions, 79*, 261-273.

Marlatt, G. A., & Gordon, J. R. (1985). *Relapse prevention: Maintenance strategies in the treatment of addictive behaviors.* New York: Guilford Press.

Marlatt, G. A., & Witkiewitz, K. (2002). Harm reduction approaches to alcohol use: Health promotion, prevention, and treatment. *Addictive Behaviors, 27*, 867-886.

Marlowe, M. J., O'Neill-Byrne, K., Lowe-Ponsford, F., & Watson, J. P. (1996). The Borderline Syndrome Index: A validation study using the Personality Assessment Schedule. *British Journal of Psychiatry, 168*, 72-75.

Marsella, A. J., Friedman, M. J., & Spain, E. H. (1996). Ethnocultural aspects of PTSD: An overview of issues and research directions. In A. J. Marsella, M. J. Friedman, E. T. Gerrity, & R. M. Scurfield (Eds.), *Ethnocultural aspects of post-traumatic stress disorder* (pp. 105-130). Washington, DC: American Psychological Association.

Marshall, C., & Rossman, G. B. (1995). *Designing qualitative research* (2nd ed.). Thousand Oaks, CA: Sage.

Marshall, W. L. (1996). Assessment, treatment and theorizing about sex offenders: Developments during the past twenty years and future directions. *Criminal Justice and Behavior, 23*, 162-199.

Martens, W. H. (2000). Antisocial and psychopathic personality disorders: Causes, course, and remission: A review article. *International Journal of Offender Therapy and Comparative Criminology, 44*, 406-430.

Martin, C. S., & Winters, K. C. (1998). Diagnosis and assessment of alcohol use disorders among adolescents. *Alcohol Health and Research World, 22*, 95-106.

Martin, S. S., Butzin, C. A., & Inciardi, J. A. (1995). Assessment of a multistage therapeutic community for drug involved offenders. *Journal of Psychoactive Drugs, 27*, 109-116.

Masters, W., & Johnson, V. (1970). *Human sexual inadequacy.* Boston: Little Brown.

Masterson, J. F. (1981). *The narcissistic and borderline personality disorders: An integrated developmental approach.* New York: Brunner/Mazel.

Mather, J. H., & Lager, P. B. (2000). *Child welfare: A unifying model of practice.* Belmont, CA: Brooks/Cole.

Mattaini, M. A. (1996). The abuse and neglect of single-case designs. *Research on Social Work Practice, 6*, 83-91.

Mattaini, M. A., McGowan, B. G., & Williams, G. (1996). Child maltreatment. In M. A. Mattaini & B. A. Thyer (Eds.), *Finding solutions to social problems: Behavioral strategies for change* (pp. 223-266). Washington DC: American Psychological Association.

Mattson, M. E. (1994). Patient-treatment matching: Rationale and results. *Alcohol Health and Research World, 18,* 287-295.

Mattson, M. E., Allen, J., Longabaugh, R., Nickless, C., Connors, G. J., & Kadden, R. M. (1994). A chronological review of empirical studies matching alcoholic clients to treatment. *Journal of Studies on Alcohol, 55,* 16-29.

Maxfield, L., & Hyer, L. (2002). The relationship between efficacy and methodology in studies investigating EMDR treatment of PTSD. *Journal of Clinical Psychology, 58,* 23-41.

Mayer, R. R., Forster, J. L., Murray, D. M., & Wagenaar, A. C. (1998). Social settings and situations of underage drinking. *Journal of Studies on Alcohol, 59,* 207-215.

Mazure, C. M., Halmi, K. A., Sunday, S. R., Romano, S. J., & Einhorn, A. M. (1994). The Yale-Brown-Cornell Eating Disorder Scale: Development, use, reliability and validity. *Journal of Psychiatric Research, 28,* 425-445.

McAlpine, C., Marshall, C. C., & Doran, N. H. (2001). Combining child welfare and substance abuse services: A blended model of intervention. *Child Welfare, 80,* 129-149.

McConnaughy, E. A., DiClemente, C. C., Prochaska, J. O., & Velicer, W. F. (1989). Stages of change in psychotherapy: A follow-up report. *Psychotherapy, 26,* 494-503.

McCrady, B. S., & Epstein, E. E. (Eds.). (1999). *Addictions: A comprehensive guidebook.* New York: Oxford University Press.

McCrady, B. S., Noel, N. E., Abrams, D. B., Stout, R. L., Nelson, H. F., & Hay, W. M. (1986). Comparative effectiveness of three types of spouse involvement in outpatient behavioral alcoholism treatment. *Journal of Studies on Alcohol, 47,* 459-467.

McDonald and Associates, Inc. (1990). *Evaluation of AB1562 in home care demonstration projects: Vol. 1. Final Report.* Sacramento, CA: Author.

McDonald, L., Billingham, S., Conrad, T., Morgan, A., O., N., & Payton, E. (1997, March–April). Families and schools together (FAST): Integrating community development with clinical strategies. *Families in Society: The Journal of Contemporary Human Services,* 140-155.

McDonald, T., & Marks, J. (1991, March). A review of risk factors assessed in child protective services. *Social Service Review,* 112-132.

McDonough, M., & Kennedy, N. (2002). Pharmacological management of obsessive-compulsive disorder: A review for clinicians. *Harvard Review of Psychiatry, 10,* 127-137.

McFarlane, A. C., & Girolamo, G. D. (1996). The nature of traumatic stressors and the epidemiology of posttraumatic reactions. In B. A. Van der Kolk, A. C. McFarlane, & L. Weisaeth (Eds.), *Traumatic stress: The effects of overwhelming experience on mind, body and society* (pp. 129-154). New York: Guilford Press.

McFarlane, A. C., & Yehuda, R. (1996). Resilience, vulnerability, and the course of post traumatic reactions. In B. A. Van der Kolk, A. C. McFarlane, & L. Weisaeth (Eds.), *Traumatic stress: The effects of overwhelming experience on mind, body and society* (pp. 155-181). New York: Guilford Press.

McFarlane, W. R., Lukens, E., Link, B., Dushay, R., Deakins, S. A., Newmark, M., et al. (1995). Multiple-family groups and psychoeducation in the treatment of schizophrenia. *Archives of General Psychiatry, 52,* 679-687.

McGleughlin, J., Meyer, S., & Baker, J. (1999). Assessing sexual abuse allegations in divorce, custody, and visitation disputes. In R. M. Galatzer-Levy & L. Kraus (Eds.), *The scientific basis of child custody decisions* (pp. 357-388). New York: Wiley.

McGloin, J. M., & Widom, C. S. (2001). Resilience among abused and neglected children grown up. *Development and Psychopathology, 13,* 1021-1038.

McGlynn, F. D., & Rose, M. P. (1998). Assessment of fear and anxiety. In A. S. Bellack & M. Hersen (Eds.), *Behavioral assessment: A practical handbook* (pp. 179-189). Boston: Allyn and Bacon.

McGuire, J., & Hatcher, R. (2001). Offense-focused problem solving: Preliminary evaluation of a cognitive skills program. *Criminal Justice and Behavior, 28,* 564-587.

McHugo, G. J., Drake, R. E., Burton, H. L., & Ackerson, T. H. (1995). A scale for assessing the stage of substance abuse treatment in persons with severe mental illness. *Journal of Nervous and Mental Disease, 183,* 762-767.

McHugo, G. J., Hargreaves, W., Drake, R. E., Clark, R. E., Xie, H., Bond, G. R., et al. (1998). Methodological issues in assertive community treatment studies. *American Journal of Orthopsychiatry, 68,* 246-260.

McIntosh, V. V., Bulik, C. M., McKenzie, J. M., Luty, S. E., & Jordan, J. (2000). Interpersonal psychotherapy for anorexia nervosa. *International Journal of Eating Disorders, 27,* 125-139.

McLellan, A. T., Luborsky, L., O'Brien, C. P., & Woody, G. E. (1980). An improved diagnostic instrument of substance abuse patients: The Addiction Severity Index. *Journal of Nervous and Mental Disease, 168,* 26-33.

McLellan, A. T., Luborsky, L., Woody, G. E., & O'Brien, C. P. (1983). Predicting response to alcohol and drug abuse treatment: The role of psychiatric severity. *Archives of General Psychiatry, 40,* 620-625.

McMahon, R. J., & Estes, A. M. (1997). Conduct problems. In E. J. Mash & L. G. Terdal (Eds.), *Assessment of childhood disorders* (3rd ed., pp. 130-193). New York: Guilford Press.

McMahon, R. J., & Forehand, R. (1984). Parent training for the non-compliant child: Treatment outcome, generalization, and adjunctive therapy procedures. In R. F. Dangel & R. A. Polster (Eds.), *Parent training: Foundations of research and practice* (pp. 298-328). New York: Guilford Press.

Mechanic, D. (1996). Emerging issues in international mental health services research. *Psychiatric Services, 47,* 371-375.

Meezan, W., & O'Keefe, M. (1998). Evaluating the effectiveness of multifamily group therapy in child abuse and neglect. *Research on Social Work Practice, 8,* 330-353.

Meichenbaum, D. (1974). *Cognitive behavior modification.* Morristown, NJ: General Learning Press.

Meichenbaum, D., & Turk, D. (1987). *Facilitating treatment adherence: A practitioner's guidebook.* New York: Plenum Press.

Meissner, W. W. (1978). The conceptualization of marriage and family dynamics from a psychoanalytic perspective. In T. J. Paolino & B. S. McCrady (Eds.), *Marriage and family therapy* (pp. 25-88). New York: Brunner/Mazel.

Mercer, C. C., Mueser, K. T., & Drake, R. E. (1998). Organizational guidelines for dual disorders programs. *Psychiatric Quarterly, 69,* 145-168.

Meston, C. M., Heiman, J. R., Trapnell, P. D., & Carlin, A. S. (1999). Ethnicity, desireable responding, and self-reports of abuse: A comparison of European- and Asian-ancestry undergraduates. *Journal of Consulting and Clinical Psychology, 67,* 139-144.

Meyers, R. J., & Smith, J. E. (1995). *Clinical guide to alcohol treatment: The community reinforcement approach.* New York: Guilford Press.

Milgram, N. A. (1989). Children under stress. In T. H. Ollendick & M. Hersen (Eds.), *Handbook of childhood psychopathology* (2nd ed., pp. 399-415). New York: Plenum Press.

Miller, B. C. (1995). Characteristics of effective day treatment programming for persons with borderline personality disorder. *Psychiatric Services, 46,* 605-608.

Miller, C. (2001). Childhood animal cruelty and interpersonal violence. *Clinical Psychology Review, 21,* 735-749.

Miller, E. T., Kilmer, J. R., Kim, E. L., Weingardt, K. R., & Marlatt, G. A. (2001). Alcohol skills training for college students. In P. M. Monti, S. M. Colby, & T. A. O'Leary (Eds.), *Adolescents, alcohol and substance abuse: Reaching teens through brief interventions* (pp. 183-215). New York: Guilford Press.

Miller, E. T., Turner, A. P., & Marlatt, G. A. (2001). The harm reduction approach to the secondary prevention of alcohol problems in adolescents and young adults: Considerations across a developmental spectrum. In P. M. Monti, S. M. Colby, & T. A. O'Leary (Eds.), *Adolescents, alcohol and substance abuse: Reaching teens through brief interventions* (pp. 58-79). New York: Guilford Press.

Miller, L. S., & Kamboukos, D. (2000). Symptom-specific measures for disorders usually first diagnosed in infancy, childhood, or adolescence. In J. A. Rush, Jr. (Ed.), *Handbook of psychiatric measures: Task force for the handbook of psychiatric measures* (pp. 325-356). Washington, DC: American Psychiatric Association.

Miller, L. S., Klein, R. G., Piacentini, J., Abikoff, H., Shah, M. R., Samoilov, A., et al. (1995). The New York Teacher Rating Scale for disruptive and anti-social behavior. *Journal of the American Academy of Child and Adolescent Psychiatry, 34,* 359-370.

Miller, W. R. (1992). Effectiveness of treatment for substance abuse. *Journal of Substance Abuse Treatment, 9,* 93-102.

Miller, W. R., & Hester, R. K. (1986). Inpatient alcoholism treatment: Who benefits? *American Psychologist, 41,* 794-805.

Miller, W. R., & Kurtz, E. (1994). Models of alcoholism used in treatment: Contrasting AA and other perspectives with which it is often confused. *Journal of Studies on Alcohol, 55,* 159-166.

Miller, W. R., Meyers, R. J., & Hiller-Sturmhofel, S. (1999). The community-reinforcement approach. *Alcohol Research and Health, 23,* 116-120.

Miller, W. R., Meyers, R. J., & Tonigan, J. (1999). Engaging the unmotivated in treatment for alcohol problems: A comparison of three strategies for intervention through family members. *Journal of Consulting and Clinical Psychology, 67,* 688-697.

Miller, W. R., & Rollnick, S. (1991). Dealing with resistance. In W. R. Miller & S. Rollnick (Eds.), *Motivational interviewing: Preparing people for change* (pp. 100-112). New York: Guilford Press.

Millon, T., & Davis, R. (1995). Conceptions of personality disorders: Historical perspectives, the DSMS, and future directions. In J. Livesley (Ed.), *The DSM-IV personality disorders* (pp. 3-28). New York: Guilford Press.

Milner, J. S. (1994). Assessing physical child abuse risk: The child abuse potential inventory. *Clinical Psychology Review, 14,* 547-583.

Milner, J. S., Gold, R. G., & Wimberley, R. C. (1986). Prediction and explanation of child abuse: Cross-validation of the child abuse potential inventory. *Journal of Consulting and Clinical Psychology, 54,* 865-866.

Milner, J. S., Murphy, W. D., Valle, L. A., & Tolliver, R. M. (1998). Assessment issues in child abuse evaluations. In J. R. Lutzker (Ed.), *Handbook of child abuse research and treatment* (pp. 75-115). New York: Plenum Press.

Minkoff, K. (2000). *Dual diagnosis: An integrated model for the treatment of people with co-occurring psychiatric and substance disorders in managed care systems.* (Videotaped lecture produced by the Mental Illness Education Project, Inc., P.O. Box 470813, Brookline Village, MA 02447.)

Mitchell, C. G. (1999). Treating anxiety in a managed care setting: A controlled comparison of medication alone versus medication plus cognitive-behavioral group therapy. *Research on Social Work Practice, 9*, 188-200.

Mitchell, C. G. (2001). Patient satisfaction with manualized versus standard interventions in a managed care context. *Research on Social Work Practice, 11*, 473-484.

Moffitt, T. E., Caspi, A., Dickson, N., Silva, P., & Stanton, W. (1996). Childhood-onset versus adolescent-onset antisocial conduct problems in males: Natural history from ages 3 to 18 years. *Development and Psychopathology, 8*, 399-424.

Moisan, P. A., Sanders-Phillips, K., & Moisan, P. M. (1997). Ethnic differences in circumstances of abuse and symptoms of depression and anger among sexually abused black and Latino boys. *Child Abuse and Neglect, 21*, 473-488.

Molina, B. S. G., Smith, B. H., & Pelham, W. E. (1999). Interactive effects of attention deficit hyperactivity disorder and conduct disorder in early adolescent substance abuse. *Psychology of Addictive Behaviors, 13*, 348-358.

Mollica, R. F., Poole, C., & Tor, S. (1998). Symptoms, functioning, and health problems in a massively traumatized population: The legacy of the Cambodian tragedy. In B. P. Dohrenwend (Ed.), *Adversity, stress and psychopathology* (pp. 34-51). New York: Oxford University Press.

Mollica, R. F., Wyshak, G., de Marneffe, D., Khuon, F., & Lavelle, J. (1987). Indochinese versions of the Hopkins Symptom Checklist-25: A screening instrument for the psychiatric care of the refugees. *American Journal of Psychiatry, 144*, 497-500.

Monahan, J. (1996). Violence prediction: The past twenty and the next twenty years. *Criminal Justice and Behavior, 23*, 107-120.

Moncher, M., & Schinke, S. (1994). Group intervention to prevent tobacco use among Native American youth. *Research on Social Work Practice, 4*, 160-171.

Monga, S., Birmaher, B., Chiappetta, L., Brent, D., Kaufman, J., Bridge, J., et al. (2000). Screen for Child Anxiety-Related Emotional Disorders (SCARED): Convergent and divergent validity. *Depression and Anxiety, 12*, 85-91.

Monti, P. M., Barnett, N. P., O'Leary, T. A., & Colby, S. M. (2001). Motivational enhancement for alcohol-involved adolescents. In P. M. Monti, S. M. Colby, & T. A. O'Leary (Eds.), *Adolescents, alcohol and substance abuse: Reaching teens through brief interventions* (pp. 145-182). New York: Guilford Press.

Monti, P. M., Colby, S. M., Barnett, N. P., Spirito, A., Rohsenow, D. J., Myers, M., et al. (1999). Brief intervention for harm reduction with alcohol-positive older adolescents in a hospital emergency department. *Journal of Consulting and Clinical Psychology, 67*, 989-994.

Monti, P. M., & Rohsenow, D. J. (1999). Coping-skills training and cue-exposure therapy in the treatment of alcoholism. *Alcohol Research and Health, 23*, 107-115.

Mooney, J. F., Kline, P. M., & Davoren, J. C. (1999). Collaborative interventions: Promoting psychosocial competence and academic achievement. In R. W. C. Tourse &

J. F. Mooney (Eds.), *Collaborative practice: School and human service partnerships* (pp. 105-135). Westport, CT: Praeger.

Moore, D. R., & Arthur, J. L. (1989). Juvenile delinquency. In T. H. Ollendick & M. Hersen (Eds.), *Handbook of childhood psychopathology* (2nd ed., pp. 197-217). New York: Plenum Press.

Moorey, S. (1989). Drug abusers. In J. Scott, J. Williams, & A. T. Beck (Eds.), *Cognitive therapy in clinical practice: An illustrative casebook* (pp. 157-182). London: Routledge.

Moos, R. H., & Moos, B. S. (1992). *Life Stressors and Social Resources Inventory: Adult form manual.* Palo Alto, CA: Center for Health Care Evaluation, Department of Veterans Affairs and Stanford University Medical Centers.

Moos, R. H., & Moos, B. S. (1998). The staff workplace and the quality and outcome of substance abuse treatment. *Journal of Studies on Alcohol, 59*, 43-51.

Morgenstern, J., Labouvie, E., McCrady, B., Kahler, C., & Frey, R. (1997). Affiliation with Alcoholics Anonymous after treatment: A study of its therapeutic effects and mechanisms of action. *Journal of Consulting and Clinical Psychology, 65*, 768-777.

Morrow-Howell, N., Becker-Kemppainen, S., & Lee, J. (1998). Evaluating an intervention for the elderly at increased risk of suicide. *Research on Social Work Practice, 8*, 28-46.

Morse, G. A., Calsyn, R. J., Klinkenberg, W. D., Trusty, M. L., Gerber, F., Smith, R., Temelhoff, B., et al. (1997). An experimental comparison of three types of case management for homeless mentally ill persons. *Psychiatric Services, 48*, 497-503.

Moskowitz, J. M. (1989). The primary prevention of alcohol problems: A critical review of the research literature. *Journal of Studies on Alcohol, 50*, 54-88.

Mowbray, C. T., Oyserman, D., Bybee, D., McFarlane, P., & Rueda-Riedle, A. (2001). Life circumstances of mothers with serious mental illness. *Psychiatric Rehabilitation Journal, 25*, 114-123.

Mowrer, O. A. (1960). *Learning theory and behavior.* New York: Wiley.

Mueser, K. T., Bond, G. R., Drake, R. E., & Resnick, S. G. (1998). Models of community care for severe mental illness: A review of research on case management. *Schizophrenia Bulletin, 24*, 37-74.

Mueser, K. T., Drake, R. E., & Bond, G. R. (1997). Recent advances in psychiatric rehabilitation for patients with severe mental illness. *Harvard Review of Psychiatry, 5*, 123-137.

Mueser, K. T., & Glynn, S. M. (1999). *Behavioral family therapy for psychiatric disorders* (2nd ed.). Oakland, CA: New Harbinger.

Mueser, K. T., Noordsy, D. L., Drake, R. E., & Fox, L. (2003). *Integrated treatment for dual disorders: A guide to effective practice.* New York: Guilford Press.

Mueser, K. T., Rosenberg, S. D., Drake, R. E., Miles, K. M., Wolford, G., Vidaver, R., et al. (1999). Conduct disorder, antisocial personality disorder and substance use disorders in schizophrenia and major affective disorders. *Journal of Studies on Alcohol, 60*, 278-284.

Mullen, E. J. (1995). Pursuing knowledge through qualitative research. *Social Work Research, 19*, 29-32.

Mullholland, A. M., & Mintz, L. B. (2001). Prevalence of eating disorders among African American women. *Journal of Counseling Psychology, 48*, 111-116.

Murphy, D. A., Durako, S. J., Moscicki, A., Vermund, S. H., Ma, Y., Schwarz, D. F., et al. (2001). No change in health risk behaviors over time among HIV infected adolescents in care: Role of psychological distress. *Journal of Adolescent Health, 29s*, 57-63.

Murphy, J. G., Duchnick, J. J., Vuchinich, R. E., Davison, J. W., Karg, R. S., Olson, A. M., et al. (2001). Relative efficacy of a brief motivational intervention for college student drinkers. *Psychology of Addictive Behaviors, 15*, 373-379.

Myers, K., & Winters, N. C. (2002). Ten-year review of scales: Part 2. Scales for internalizing disorders. *Journal of the American Academy of Child and Adolescent Psychiatry, 41*, 634-659.

Myric, H., & Anton, R. F. (1998). Treatment of alcohol withdrawal. *Alcohol Health and Research World, 22*, 38-46.

Nader, K. O. (1997). Assessing traumatic experiences in children. In J. P. Wilson & T. M. Keane (Eds.), *Assessing psychological trauma and PTSD* (pp. 191-214). New York: Guilford Press.

Nader, K. O., (2001). Treatment methods for childhood trauma. In J. P. Wilson, M. J. Friedman, & J. D. Lindy (Eds.), *Treating psychological trauma and PTSD* (pp. 278-334). New York: Guilford Press.

Nader, K. O., Pynoos, R. S., Fairbanks, L. A., & Frederick, C. (1990). Children's PTSD reactions one year after a sniper attack at their school. *American Journal of Psychiatry, 147*, 1526-1530.

Najavits, L. M., Weiss, R. D., & Liese, B. S. (1996). Group cognitive-behavioral therapy for women with PTSD and substance use disorder. *Journal of Substance Abuse Treatment, 13*, 13-22.

Naleppa, M. J., & Reid, W. J. (1998). Task-centered case management for the elderly: Developing a practice model. *Research on Social Work Practice, 8*, 63-85.

Nathan, P. E., & Gorman, J. M. (Eds.). (1998). *A guide to treatments that work*. New York: Oxford University Press.

Nathan, P. E., & McCrady, B. S. (1987). Bases for the use of abstinence as a goal in the behavioral treatment of alcohol abusers. *Drugs and Society, 1*, 109-131.

Naugle, A. E., & Follette, W. C. (1998). A functional analysis of trauma symptoms. In V. M. Follette, J. I. Ruzek, & F. R. Abueg (Eds.), *Cognitive-behavioral therapies for trauma* (pp. 48-76). New York: Guilford Press.

Negy, C., & Snyder, D. K. (1997). Ethnicity and acculturation: Assessing Mexican American couples' relationships using the Marital Satisfaction Inventory-revised. *Psychological Assessment, 9*, 414-421.

Nelson-Zlupko, L., Dore, M. M., Kauffman, E., & Kaltenbach, K. (1996). Women in recovery: Their perceptions of treatment effectiveness. *Journal of Subtance Abuse Treatment, 13*, 51-59.

Newman, F. L., Howard, K. I., Windle, C. D., & Hohmann, A. A. (1994). Introduction to the special section on seeking new methods in mental health services research. *Journal of Consulting and Clinical Psychology, 62*, 667-669.

Ngo, D., Tran, T. V., Gibbons, J. L., & Oliver, J. M. (2001). Acculturation, premigration traumatic experiences and depression among Vietnamese Americans. *Journal of Human Behavior in the Social Environment, 3*, 225-242.

Nicassio, P. M. (1983). Psychosocial correlates of alienation: Study of a sample of Indochinese refugees. *Journal of Cross-Cultural Psychology, 14*, 337-351.

Nichols, M. P., & Schwartz, R. C. (1995). *Family therapy: Concepts and methods* (3rd ed.). Boston: Allyn and Bacon.

Nieuwenhuizen, C., Schene, A. H., Boevink, W. A., & Wolf, J. R. L. M. (1997). Measuring the quality of life of clients with severe mental illness: A review of instruments. *Psychiatric Rehabilitation Journal, 20,* 33-41.

Noel, N. E., & McCrady, B. S. (1993). Alcohol focused spouse involvement with behavioral martial therapy. In T. J. O'Farrell (Ed.), *Treating alcohol problems: Marital and family interventions* (pp. 210-235). New York: Guilford Press.

Nordstrom, G., & Burglund, M. A. (1987). A prospective study of successful long-term adjustment in alcohol dependence: Social drinking versus abstinence. *Journal of Studies on Alcohol, 48,* 95-103.

Norris, F. H. (1990). Screening for traumatic stress: A scale for use in the general population. *Journal of Applied Social Psychology, 20,* 1704-1718.

Norris, F. H. (1992). Epidemiology of trauma: Frequency and impact of different potentially traumatic events on different demographic groups. *Journal of Consulting and Clinical Psychology, 60,* 409-418.

Norris, F. H., & Riad, J. K. (1997). Standardized self-report measures of civilian trauma and post traumatic stress disorder. In J. P. Wilson & T. M. Keane (Eds.), *Assessing psychological trauma and PTSD* (pp. 7-42). New York: Guilford Press.

Norris, J. (1994). Alcohol and female sexuality: A look at expectancies and risks. *Alcohol Health and Research World, 18,* 197-201.

Northey, W. F., Wells, K. C., Silverman, W. K., & Bailey, C. E. (2003). Childhood behavioral and emotional disorders. *Journal of Marital and Family Therapy, 29,* 523-545.

Nowinski, J. (1999). Self-help groups for addictions. In B. S. McCrady & E. E. Epstein (Eds.), *Addictions: A comprehensive guidebook* (pp. 328-346). New York: Oxford University Press.

Nunes-Dinis, M., & Barth, R. P. (1993). Cocaine treatment and outcome. *Social Work, 38,* 611-617.

Nurius, P. S., & Gibson, J. W. (1990). Clinical observation, inference, reasoning and judgment in social work: An update. *Social Work Research and Abstracts, 26,* 18-25.

Nygaard, R. L. (2000). The dawn of therapeutic justice. In D. H. Fishbein (Ed.), *The science, treatment, and prevention of antisocial behaviors: Application to the criminal justice system* (pp. 1-18). Kingston, NJ: Civic Research Institute.

O'Brien, K., & Vincent, N. K. (2003). Psychiatric comorbidity in anorexia and bulimia nervosa: Nature, prevalence, and causal relationships. *Clinical Psychology Review, 23,* 57-74.

Odiah, C., & Wright, D. (2000). Forensic practice in the helping professions: Advocate and adversary roles as a threat to therapeutic alliances and fiduciary relations. *Journal of Offender Rehabilitation, 31,* 57-68.

O'Donnell, C. R., Wilson, K. K., & Tharp, R. G. (2002). The cross-cultural context: Lessons from community development projects. In G. B. Melton, R. A. Thompson, & M. A. Small (Eds.), *Toward a child-centered neighborhood-based child protection system: A report of the consortium on children, families and the law* (pp. 104-114). Westport, CT: Praeger.

O'Donohue, W., & Fanetti, M. (1996). Assessing the occurrence of child sexual abuse: An information processing, hypothesis testing approach. *Aggression and Violent Behavior, 1,* 269-281.

O'Donohue, W., Fanetti, M., & Elliott, A. (1998). Trauma in children. In V. M. Follette, J. I. Ruzek, & F. R. Abueg (Eds.), *Cognitive-behavioral therapies for trauma* (pp. 355-382). New York: Guilford Press.

Oei, T. P. S., & Shuttlewood, G. J. (1996). Specific and nonspecific factors in psychotherapy: A case of cognitive therapy for depression. *Clinical Psychology Review, 16*, 83-103.

O'Farrell, T. J., Choquette, K. A., & Cutter, H. S. (1998). Couples relapse prevention sessions after behavioral marital therapy for male alcoholics: Outcomes during the three years after starting treatment. *Journal of Studies on Alcohol, 59*, 357-370.

O'Farrell, T. J., Choquette, K. A., Cutter, H. S. G., Brown, E. D., & McCourt, W. F. (1993). Behavioral marital therapy with and without additional couples relapse prevention sessions for alcoholics and their wives. *Journal of Studies on Alcohol, 54*, 652-666.

O'Farrell, T. J., & Fals-Stewart, W. (1999). Treatment models and methods: Family models. In B. S. McCrady & E. E. Epstein (Eds.), *Addictions: A comprehensive guidebook* (pp. 287-305). New York: Oxford University Press.

O'Farrell, T J., & Fals-Stewart, W. (2000). Behavioral couples therapy for alcoholism and drug abuse. *Journal of Substance Abuse Treatment, 18*, 51-54.

O'Farrell, T. J., & Fals-Stewart, W. (2003). Alcohol abuse. *Journal of Marital and Family Therapy, 29*, 121-146.

Ogborne, A. C., Wild, T. C., Braun, K., & Newton-Taylor, B. (1998). Measuring treatment process beliefs among staff of specialized addiction treatment services. *Journal of Substance Abuse Treatment, 15*, 301-312.

Oggins, J., Leber, D., & Veroff, J. (1993). Race and gender differences in black and white newlyweds' perceptions of sexual and marital relations. *Journal of Sex Research, 30*, 152-160.

O'Hare, T. (1990a). Alcohol expectancies and social anxiety in male and female undergraduates. *Addictive Behaviors, 15*, 561-566.

O'Hare, T. (1990b). Drinking in college: Consumption patterns, problems, sex differences and legal drinking age. *Journal of Studies on Alcohol, 51*, 536-541.

O'Hare, T. (1991). Integrating research and practice: A framework for implementation. *Social Work, 36*, 3, 220-223.

O'Hare, T. (1993). Alcohol consumption and presenting problems in an out-patient mental health clinic, *Addictive Behaviors, 18*, 57-65.

O'Hare, T. (1995a). Differences in Asian and white drinking: Consumption level, drinking contexts and expectancies. *Addictive Behaviors, 20*, 261-266.

O'Hare, T. (1995b). Mental health problems and alcohol abuse: Co-occurrence and gender differences. *Health and Social Work, 20*, 207-214.

O'Hare, T. (1996a). Court-ordered vs. voluntary clients: Problem differences and readiness for change. *Social Work, 41*, 417-422.

O'Hare, T. (1996b). Readiness for change: Variation by intensity and domain of client distress. *Social Work Research, 20*, 13-17.

O'Hare, T. (1997a). Measuring excessive alcohol use in college drinking contexts: The Drinking Context Scale. *Addictive Behaviors, 22*, 469-477.

O'Hare, T. (1997b). Measuring problem drinking in first time offenders: Development and validation of the College Alcohol Problem Scale. *Journal of Substance Abuse Treatment, 14*, 383-387.

O'Hare, T. (1998a). Alcohol expectancies and excessive drinking contexts in young adults. *Social Work Research, 22*, 44-50.

O'Hare, T. (1998b). Replicating the College Alcohol Problem Scale with college first offenders. *Journal of Alcohol and Drug Education, 43,* 75-82.

O'Hare, T. (2001a). The Drinking Context Scale: A confirmatory analysis. *Journal of Substance Abuse Treatment, 20,* 129-136.

O'Hare, T. (2001b). Substance abuse and risky sex in young people: Validating the risky sex scale. *Journal of Primary Prevention, 22,* 89-101.

O'Hare, T. (2002). Evidence-based social work practice with mentally ill persons who abuse alcohol and other drugs. *Social Work in Mental Health, 1,* 43-62.

O'Hare, T., & Collins, P. (1997). Development and validation of a scale for measuring social work practice skills. *Research on Social Work Practice, 7,* 228-238.

O'Hare, T., Collins, P., & Walsh, T. (1998). Validating the practice skills inventory with experienced clinical social workers. *Research on Social Work Practice, 8,* 552-563.

O'Hare, T., & Sherrer, M. (1999). Validating the Alcohol Use Disorder Identification Test with college first offenders. *Journal of Substance Abuse Treatment, 17,* 113-119.

O'Hare, T., & Sherrer, M. (2000). Co-occurring stress and substance abuse in college first offenders. *Journal of Human Behavior in the Social Environment, 3,* 29-44.

O'Hare, T., Sherrer, M., Connery, H., Thornton, J., LaButti, A., & Emrick, K. (2003). Further validation of the Psycho-Social Wellbeing Scale. *Community Mental Health Journal, 39,* 115-129.

O'Hare, T., Sherrer, M., Cutler, J., McCall, T., Dominique, K., & Garlick, K. (2002). Validating the psychosocial well being scale among mentally ill clients with substance abuse problems. *Social Work in Mental Health, 1,* 15-30.

O'Hare, T., Sherrer, M. V., LaButti, A., & Emrick, K. (2004). Validating the Alcohol Use Disorders Identification Test with persons who have serious mental illness. *Research on Social Work Practice, 14,* 36-42.

O'Hare, T., & Tran, T. V. (1997). Predicting problem drinking in college students: Gender differences and the CAGE questionnaire. *Addictive Behaviors, 22,* 13-21.

O'Hare, T., & Tran, T. V. (1998). Substance abuse among Southeast Asians in the U.S.: Implications for practice and research. *Social Work in Health Care, 26,* 69-80.

O'Hare, T., Tran, T. V., & Collins, P. (2002). Validating the Practice Skills Inventory: A confirmatory factor analysis. *Research on Social Work Practice, 12,* 653-668.

O'Keane, V. (2000). Evolving model of depression as an expression of multiple interacting risk factors. *British Journal of Psychiatry, 177,* 482-483.

O'Laughlin, E. M., & Murphy, M. J. (2000). Use of computerized continuous performance tasks for assessment of ADHD: A guide for practitioners. *Independent Practitioner, 20,* 282-287.

O'Leary, A. (1992). Self-efficacy and health: Behavioral and stress-physiological mediation. *Cognitive Therapy and Research, 16,* 229-245.

O'Leary, A., Goodhart, F., Sweet Jemmott, L., & Boccher-Lattimore, D. (1992). Predictors of safer sex on the college campus: A social cognitive theory analysis. *Journal of American College Health, 40,* 254-263.

O'Leary, K. D., Barling, J., Arias, I., Rosenbaum, A., Malone, J., & Tyree, A. (1989). Prevalence and stability of physical aggression between spouses: A longitudinal analysis. *Journal of Consulting and Clinical Psychology, 57,* 263-268.

O'Leary, K. D., & Beach, S. R. (1990). Marital therapy: A viable treatment for depression and marital discord. *American Journal of Psychiatry, 147*, 183-186.

O'Leary, K. D., Malone, J., & Tyree, A. (1994). Physical aggression in early marriage: Prerelationship and relationship effects. *Journal of Consulting and Clinical Psychology, 62*, 594-602.

Ollendick, T. H. (1983). Reliability and validity of the Revised Fear Survey Schedule for Children (FSSC-R). *Behaviour Research and Therapy, 21*, 685-692.

Ollendick, T. H., & Hirshfeld-Becker, D. R. (2002). The developmental psychopathology of social anxiety disorder. *Biological Psychiatry, 1*, 44-58.

Ollendick, T. H., & King, N. J. (1994a). Diagnosis, assessment and treatment of internalizing problems in children: The role of longitudinal data. *Journal of Consulting and Clinical Psychology, 62*, 918-927.

Ollendick, T. H., & King, N. J. (1994b). Fears and their level of interference in adolescents. *Behaviour Research and Therapy, 32*, 635-638.

Ollendick, T. H., & King, N. J. (1998). Empirically supported treatments for children with phobic and anxiety disorders: Current status. *Journal of Child Psychology, 27*, 156-167.

Ollendick, T. H., Mattis, S. G., & King, N. J. (1993). Panic in children and adolescents: A review. *Journal of Child Psychology and Psychiatry, 35*, 113-134.

Olsen, D. H., Russell, C., & Sprenkel, D. (1989). *FACES III manual.* St. Paul: University of Minnesota.

O'Malley, P. M., & Johnston, L. D. (2002). Epidemiology of alcohol and other drug use among American college students. *Journal of Studies on Alcohol, 63*, 23-39.

O'Neill, S. E. Parra, G. R., & Sher, K. J. (2001). Clinical relevance of heavy drinking during the college years: Cross-sectional and prospective perspectives. *Psychology of Addictive Behaviors, 15*, 350-359.

Oosterlaan, J. (2001). Behavioural inhibition and the development of childhood anxiety disorders. In W. K. Silverman & P. D. A. Treffers (Eds.), *Anxiety disorders in children and adolescents: Research, assessment and intervention* (pp. 45-71). New York: Cambridge University Press.

Orford, J. (1990). Alcohol and the family. In L. T. Kozlowski, H. Annis, H. D. Cappell (Eds.), *Research advances in alcohol and drug problems* (pp. 81-155). New York: Plenum Press.

Orlinsky, D. E., Grawe, K., & Parks, B. K. (1994). Process and outcome in psychotherapy: Noch einmal. In A. E. Bergin & S. L. Garfield (Eds.), *The handbook of psychotherapy and behavior change* (4th ed., pp. 270-376). New York: Wiley.

Orlinsky. D. E., & Howard, K. I. (1986). Process and outcome in psychotherapy. In S. L. Garfield & A. E. Bergin (Eds.), *The handbook of psychotherapy and behavior change* (pp. 311-384). New York: Wiley.

Osborn, D. P. J. (2001). The poor physical health of people with mental illness. *Western Journal of Medicine, 175*(5), 329-332.

Osher, F. C., & Kofoed, L. (1989). Treatment of patients with psychiatric and psychoactive substance abuse disorders, *Hospital and Community Psychiatry, 40*, 1025-1030.

Ossana, S. M. (2000). Relationship and couples counseling. In R. M. Perez, K. A. DeBord, & K. J. Bieschke (Eds.), *Handbook of counseling and psychotherapy with lesbian, gay, and bisexual clients* (pp. 275-302). Washington, DC: American Psychiatric Association.

Ost, L. (1990). The Agoraphobia Scale: An evaluation of its reliability and validity. *Behaviour Research and Therapy, 28*, 323-329.

Ost, L., & Treffers, P. D. A. (2001). Onset, course, and outcome for anxiety disorders in children. In W. K. Silverman & P. D. A. Treffers (Eds.), *Anxiety disorders in children and adolescents: Research, assessment and intervention* (pp. 293-312). New York: Cambridge University Press.

Otto-Salaj, L. L., Heckman, T. G., Stevenson, L. Y., & Kelly, J. A. (1998). Patterns, predictors and gender differences in HIV risk among severely mentally ill men and women. *Community Mental Health Journal, 34*, 175-190.

Overall, J. E., & Gorham, D. R. (1962). The Brief Psychiatric Rating Scale. *Psychological Reports, 10*, 799-812.

Overholser, J. C., Brinkman, D. C., Lehnert, K. L., & Ricciardi, A. M. (1995). Children's Depression Rating Scale-revised: Development of a short form. *Journal of Clinical Child Psychology, 24*, 443-452.

Pagelow, M. D. (1992). Adult victims of domestic violence: Battered women. *Journal of Interpersonal Violence, 7*, 87-120.

Palmer, T. (1996). Programmatic and nonprogrammatic aspects of successful intervention. In A. T. Harland (Ed.), *Choosing correctional options that work: Defining the demand and evaluating the supply* (pp. 131-182). Thousand Oaks, CA: Sage.

Pandina, R. J., & Johnson, V. (1990). Serious alcohol and drug problems among adolescents with a family history of alcoholism. *Journal of Studies on Alcohol, 51*, 278-282.

Paris, J. (1995). Commentary on narcissistic personality disorder. In J. Livesley (Ed.), *The DSM-IV personality disorders* (pp. 213-217). New York: Guilford Press.

Paris, J. (1997a). Antisocial and borderline personality disorders: Two separate diagnoses or two aspects of the same psychopathology? *Comprehensive Psychiatry, 38*, 237-242.

Paris, J. (1997b). Childhood trauma as an etiological factor in the personality disorders. *Journal of Personality Disorders, 11*, 34-49.

Pasch, L. A., & Bradbury, T. N. (1998). Social support, conflict, and the development of marital dysfunction. *Journal of Consulting and Clinical Psychology, 66*, 219-230.

Patrick, J., Links, P., Reekum, R. V., & Mitton, M. J. (1995). Using the PDQ-R scale as a brief screening measure in the differential diagnosis of personality disorder. *Journal of Personality Disorders, 9*, 266-274.

Patterson, G. R. (1982). *Coercive family process.* Eugene, OR: Castalia Press.

Pattison, E. M., Sobell, M. B., & Sobell, L. C. (1977). *Emerging concepts of alcohol dependence.* New York: Springer.

Pecora, P. J., Whittaker, J. K., Maluccio, A. N., & Barth, R. P. (2000). *The child welfare challenge: Policy, practice, and research* (2nd ed.). New York: Aldine de Gruyter.

Peele, S. (1989). *The diseasing of America: Addiction treatment out of control.* Lexington, MA: Lexington Books.

Pelham, W. E., Wheeler, T., & Chronis, A. (1998). Empirically supported psychosocial treatments for attention deficit hyperactivity disorder. *Journal of Clinical Child Psychology, 27*, 190-205.

Penn, D. L., & Mueser, K. T. (1996). Research update on the psychosocial treatment of schizophrenia. *American Journal of Psychiatry, 153*, 607-617.

Perkins, W. (2002). Surveying the damage: A review of research on consequences of alcohol misuse in college populations. *Journal of Studies on Alcohol, 63*, 91-100.

Persons, J. B., & Fresco, D. M. (1998). Assessment of depression. In A. S. Bellack & M. Hersen (Eds.), *Behavioral assessment: A practical handbook* (pp. 210-231). Boston: Allyn and Bacon.

Peruzzi, N., & Bongar, B. (1999). Assessing risk for completed suicide in patients with major depression: Psychologists' views of critical factors. *Professional Psychology Research and Practice, 30*, 576-580.

Petrakis, I., Gonzalez, G., Rosenheck, R., & Krystal, J. (2002). Comorbidity of alcoholism and psychiatric disorders. *Alcohol Research and Health, 26*, 81-89.

Petry, N., Martin, B., Cooney, J., & Kranzler, H. (2000). Give them prizes, and they will come: Contingency management treatment of alcohol dependence. *Journal of Consulting and Clinical Psychology, 68*, 250-257.

Petti, T. A. (1989). Depression. In T. H. Ollendick & M. Hersen (Eds.), *Handbook of childhood psychopathology* (2nd ed., pp. 229-246). New York: Plenum Press.

Pfiffner, L., & Barkley, R. A. (1998). Treatment of ADHD in school settings. In R. A. Barkley (Ed.), *Attention-deficit hyperactivity disorder: A handbook for diagnosis and treatment* (pp. 458-490). New York: Guilford Press.

Piacentini, J., & Bergman, R. L. (2000). Obsessive-compulsive disorder in children. *Psychiatric Clinics of North America, 23*, 519-533.

Pickens, R. W., & Svikis, D. S. (1991). Genetic contributions to alcoholism diagnosis. *Alcohol Health and Research World, 15*, 272-277.

Pike, K. M., Dohm, F. A., Striegel-Moore, R. H., Wilfley, D., & Fairburn, C. G. (2001). A comparison of black and white women with binge eating disorder. *American Journal of Psychiatry, 158*, 1455-1460.

Pilling, S., Bebbington, P., Kuipers, E., Garety, P., Geddes, J., Martindale, B., et al. (2002). Psychological treatments in schizophrenia: Part 2. Meta-analyses of randomized controlled trials of social skills training and cognitive remediation. *Psychological Medicine, 32*, 783-791.

Pilling, S., Bebbington, P., Kuipers, E., Garety, P., Geddes, J., Orbach, G., et al. (2002). Psychological treatments in schizophrenia: Part 1. Meta-analysis of family intervention and cognitive behaviour therapy. *Psychological Medicine, 32*, 763-782.

Pinderhughes, E. (1989). *Understanding race, ethnicity and power: The key to efficacy in clinical practice.* New York: Free Press.

Pine, D. S., & Grun, J. (1998). Anxiety disorders. In B. T. Walsh (Ed.), *Child psychopharmacology* (pp. 115-148). Washington, DC: American Psychiatric Press.

Pomeroy, E. C., Kiam, R., & Abel, E. M. (1999). The effectiveness of a psychoeducational group for HIV-infected/affected incarcerated women. *Research on Social Work Practice, 9*, 171-187.

Pottick, K. J., Hansell. S., & Barber, C. C. (1998). An inpatient measure of adolescent and child psychosocial services and treatment. *Social Work Research, 22*, 217-231.

Poznanski, E. O., Cook, S. C., & Carroll, B. J. (1979). A depression rating scale for children. *Pediatrics, 64*, 442-450.

Poznanski, E. O., Grossman, J. A., Buchsbaum, Y., Banegas, M., Freeman, L., & Gibbons, R. (1984). Preliminary studies of the reliability and validity of the Children's Depression Rating Scale. *Journal of the American Academy of Child Psychiatry, 23*, 191-197.

Pratt, H. D., Phillips, E. L., Greydanus, D. E., & Patel, D. R. (2003). Eating disorders in the adolescent population: Future directions. *Journal of Adolescent Research, 18*, 297-317.

Prendergast, M. L., Anglin, M. D., & Wellisch, J. (1995). Treatment for drug-abusing offenders under community supervision. *Federal Probation, 59*, 66-75.

Prins, P. J. M. (2001). Affective and cognitive processes and the development and maintenance of anxiety and its disorders. In W. K. Silverman & P. D. A. Treffers (Eds.), *Anxiety disorders in children and adolescents: Research, assessment and intervention* (pp. 23-44). New York: Cambridge University Press.

Prochaska, J. O., & DiClemente, C. C. (1984). *The transtheoretical approach: Crossing the traditional boundaries of therapy*. Homewood, IL: Irwin.

Prochaska, J. O., DiClemente, C. C., & Norcross, J. C. (1992). In search of how people change: Applications to addictive behaviors. *American Psychologist, 47*, 1102-1114.

Prochaska, J. O., Velicier, W. F., Rossi, J. S., & Goldstein, M. G. (1994). Stages of change and decisional balance for 12 problem behaviors. *Health Psychology, 13*, 39-46.

Proctor, E. (2003). Research to inform the development of social work interventions. *Social Work Research, 27*, 3-5.

Project Match Research Group. (1997). Matching alcoholism treatments to client heterogeneity: Project MATCH post treatment drinking outcomes. *Journal of Studies on Alcohol, 58*, 7-29.

Project Worth. (1997). Current approaches to drug treatment for women offenders. *Journal of Substance Abuse Treatment, 15*, 151-163.

Putnam, F. W. (2003). Ten-year research update review: Child sexual abuse. *Journal of the American Academy of Child and Adolescent Psychiatry, 42*, 269-278.

Pynoos, R. S., Frederick, C., Nader, K., Arroyo, W., Eth, S., Nunez, W., et al. (1987). Life threat and posttraumatic stress in school-age children. *Archives of General Psychiatry, 44*, 1057-1063.

Pynoos, R. S., Goenjian, A., Tashjian, M., Karakashian, M., Manjikian, R., Manoukian, G., et al. (1993). Posttraumatic stress reactions in children after the 1988 Armenian earthquake. *British Journal of Psychiatry, 163*, 239-244.

Quay, H. C. (1983). A dimensional approach to behavior disorder: The Revised Behavior Problem Checklist. *School Psychology Review, 12*, 244-249.

Quigley, L. A., & Marlatt, G. A. (1996). Drinking among young adults: Prevalence, patterns and consequences. *Alcohol Health and Research World, 20*, 185-196.

Quinsey, V. L., Harris, G. T., Rice, M. E., & Lalumiere, M. L. (1993). Assessing treatment efficacy in outcome studies of sex offenders. *Journal of Interpersonal Violence, 8*, 512-523.

RachBeisel, J., Scott, J., & Dixon, L. (1999). Co-occurring severe mental illness and substance use disorders: A review of recent research. *Psychiatric Services, 50*, 1427-1434.

Rachman, S. (1980). Emotional processing. *Behaviour Research and Therapy, 18*, 51-60.

Raj, A. (1996). Identification of social cognitive variables as predictors of safer sex behavior and intent in heterosexual college students. *Journal of Sex and Marital Therapy, 22*, 247-259.

Ran, M., Xiang, M., Chan, C., Leff, J., Simpson, P., Huang, M., et al. (2003). Effectiveness of psychoeducational intervention for rural Chinese families experiencing schizophrenia. *Social Psychiatry and Psychiatric Epidemiology, 38*, 69-75.

Randolf, F. L., Ridgway, P., & Carling, P. J. (1991). Residential programs for persons with severe mental illness: A nationwide survey of state-affiliated agencies. *Hospital and Community Psychiatry, 42*, 1111-1115.

Rapoport, J. L., Swedo, S. E, & Leonard, H. L. (1992). Childhood obsessive-compulsive disorder. *Journal of Clinical Psychiatry, 53*, 11-16.

Rapport, M. D. (Ed.). (1992). Treatment of children with attention-deficit hyperactivity disorder (ADHD). *Behavior Modification, 16*(special series), 155-163.

Raskin, N. J., & Rogers, C. R. (1995). Person-centered therapy. In R. J. Corsini & D. Wedding (Eds.), *Current Psychotherapies* (4th ed., pp. 128-161). Itasca, IL: Peacock.

Ray, O., & Ksir, C. (1999). *Drugs, society and human behavior* (8th ed.). New York: McGraw-Hill.

Raytek, H. S., McCrady, B. S., Epstein, E. E., & Hirsch, L. S. (1999). Therapeutic alliance and the retention of couples in conjoint alcoholism treament. *Addictive Behaviors, 24*, 317-330.

Read, J. P., Wood, M. D., Davidoff, O. J., McLacken, J., & Campbell, J. F. (2002). Making the transition from high school to college: The role of alcohol-related social influence factors in students' drinking. *Substance Abuse, 23*, 53-65.

Reamer, F. (1995). Malpractice claims against social workers: First facts. *Social Work, 40*, 595-601.

Rector, N., Seeman, M., & Segal, Z. (2003). Cognitive therapy for schizophrenia: A preliminary randomized controlled trial. *Schizophrenia Research, 63*, 1-11.

Regier, D. A., Farmer, M. E., Rae, D. S ., Locke, B. Z., Keith, S. J., Judd, L. L., et al. (1990). Comorbidity of mental disorders with alcohol and other drug abuse. *Journal of the American Medical Association, 264*, 2511-2518.

Rehm, J., Gmel, G., Sempos, C., & Trevisan, M. (2003). Alcohol-related morbidity and mortality. *Alcohol Research and Health, 27*, 39-51.

Rehm, L. P. (1977). A self-control model of depression. *Behavior Therapy, 8*, 787-804.

Reichert, S. K. (1992). Medical evaluation of the sexually abused child. In M. E. Helfer, R. S. Kempe, & R. D. Krugman (Eds.), *The battered child* (5th ed., pp. 313-328). Chicago: University of Chicago Press.

Reid, W. J. (1997a). Evaluating the dodo's verdict: Do all interventions have equivalent outcomes? *Social Work Research, 21*, 5-18.

Reid, W. J. (1997b, June). The future of clinical social work. *Social Service Review*, 200-213.

Reid, W. J., & Hanrahan, P. (1982). Recent evaluations of social work: Grounds for optimism. *Social Work, 27*, 328-340.

Remschmidt, H., & Schulz, E. (1995). Psychopharmacology of depressive states in childhood and adolescence. In I. M. Goodyer (Ed.), *The depressed child and adolescent: Developmental and clinical perspectives* (pp. 253-279). New York: Cambridge University Press.

Renaud, J., Brent, D. A., Baugher, M., Birmaher, B., Kolko, D. J., & Bridge, J. (1998). Rapid response to psychosocial treatment for adolescent depression: A two-year follow-up. *Journal of the American Academy of Child and Adolescent Psychiatry, 37*, 1184-1190.

Resnick, H. S., Kilpatrick, D. G., Dansky, B. S., Saunders, B. E., & Best, C. L. (1993). Prevalence of civilian trauma and post traumatic stress disorder in a representative national sample of women. *Journal of Consulting and Clinical Psychology, 61*, 984-991.

Reynolds, C. F., Frank, E., Perel, J. M., Imber, S. D., Cornes, C., Miller, M. D., et al. (1999). Nortriptyline and interpersonal psychotherapy as maintenance therapies for recurrent major depression: A randomized controlled trial in patients older than 59 years. *Journal of the American Medical Association, 281*, 39-45.

Reynolds, W. M. (1992). Depression in children and adolescents. In W. M. Reynolds (Ed.), *Internalizing disorders in children and adolescents* (pp. 149-253). New York: Wiley.

Reynolds, W. M. (1994). Assessment of depression in children and adolescents by self-report questionnaires. In W. M. Reynolds & H. F. Johnston (Eds.), *Handbook of depression in children and adolescents* (pp. 209-234). New York: Plenum Press.

Reynolds, W. M., & Coats, K. I. (1986). A comparison of cognitive-behavioral therapy and relaxation training for the treatment of depression in adolescents. *Journal of Consulting and Clinical Psychology, 54*, 653-660.

Rice, L. N., & Greenberg, L. S. (1984). The new research paradigm. In L. N. Rice & L. S. Greenberg (Eds.), *Patterns of change: Intensive analysis of psychotherapy process* (pp. 7-25). New York: Guilford Press.

Rice, M. (1997). Violent offender research and implications for the criminal justice system. *American Psychologist, 52*, 414-423.

Rice, M., & Harris, G. (1995). Violent recidivism: Assessing predictive validity. *Journal of Consulting and Clinical Psychology, 63*, 737-748.

Richey, C. A. (1994). Social support training. In D. K. Granvold (Ed.), *Cognitive and behavioral treatment: Methods and applications* (pp. 299-338). Pacific Grove, CA: Brooks/Cole.

Richters, J. E., Arnold, L. E., Jensen, P. S., Abikoff, H., Conners, C. K., Greenhill, L. I., et al. (1995). *NIMH collaborative multisite multimodal treatment study of children with ADHD: Part 1. Background and rationale. Journal of the American Academy of Child and Adolescent Psychiatry, 34*, 987-1000.

Rife, J. C., & Belcher, J. R. (1994). Assisting unemployed older workers to become reemployed: An experimental evaluation. *Research on Social Work Practice, 4*, 3-13.

Riggs, D. S., & Foa, E. B. (1993). Obsessive compulsive disorder. In D. H. Barlow (Ed.), *Clinical handbook of psychological disorders: A step-by-step manual* (pp. 189-239). New York: Guilford Press.

Riggs, P. D., Baker, S., Mikulich, S. K., Young, S. E., & Crowley, T. J. (1995). Depression in substance-dependent delinquents. *Journal of the American Academy of Child and Adolescent Psychiatry, 34*, 764-771.

Roberts, A. R., & Brownell, P. (1999). A century of forensic social work: Bridging the past to the present. *Social Work, 44*, 359-369.

Roberts, I., Kramer, M. S., & Suissa, S. (1996). Does home visiting prevent childhood injury? A systematic review of randomised controlled trials. *British Medical Journal, 312*, 29-33.

Roberts, L. J., Neal, D. J., Kivlahan, D. R., Baer, J. S., & Marlatt, G. A. (2000). Individual drinking changes following a brief intervention among college students: Clinical significance in an indicated preventive context. *Journal of Consulting and Clinical Psychology, 68*, 500-505.

Roberts, L. J., Shaner, A., & Eckman, T. A. (1999). *Overcoming addictions: Skills training for people with schizophrenia.* New York: Norton.

Robin, A. L. (1998a). *ADHD in adolescents: Diagnosis and treatment*. New York: Guilford Press.

Robin, A. L. (1998b). Training families with ADHD adolescents. In R. A. Barkley (Ed.), *Attention-deficit hyperactivity disorder: A handbook for diagnosis and treatment* (pp. 413-457). New York: Guilford Press.

Robins, C. J., & Hayes, A. M. (1993). An appraisal of cognitive therapy. *Journal of Consulting and Clinical Psychology, 61*, 205-214.

Robins, L. N. (1966). *Deviant children grown up*. Baltimore: Williams and Wilkins.

Rock, M. (2001). Emerging issues with mentally ill offenders: Causes and social consequences. *Administration and Policy in Mental Health, 28*, 165-180.

Rodgers, B., Korten, A., Jorm, A., Jacomb, P., Christensen, H., & Henderson, A. (2000). Non-linear relationships in associations of depression and anxiety with alcohol use. *Psychological Medicine, 30*, 421-432.

Rogers, C. (1951). *Client-centered therapy*. Boston: Houghton Mifflin.

Rogers, S., & Silver, S. (2002). Is EMDR an exposure therapy? A review of trauma protocols. *Journal of Clinical Psychology, 58*, 43-59.

Rogers, S., Silver, S., Goss, J., Obenchain, J., Willis, A., & Whitney, R. (1999). A single session, group study of exposure and eye movement desensitization and reprocessing in treating posttraumatic stress disorder among Vietnam War veterans: Preliminary data. *Journal of Anxiety Disorders, 13*, 119-130.

Ronan, K. R., & Deane, F. P. (1998). Anxiety disorders. In P. Graham (Ed.), *Cognitive-behaviour therapy for children and families* (pp. 74-94). New York: Cambridge University Press.

Rooney, R. H. (1992). *Strategies for working with involuntary clients*. New York: Columbia University Press.

Rooney, R. H., & Bibus, A. A. (2001). Clinical practice with involuntary clients in community settings. In H. E. Briggs & K. Corcoran (Eds.), *Social work practice: Treating common client problems* (pp. 391-406). Chicago: Lyceum Books.

Root, R. W., & Resnick, R. J. (2003). An update on the diagnosis and treatment of attention-deficit/hyperactivity disorder in children. *Professional Psychology: Research and Practice, 34*, 34-41.

Rosen, A. (2003). Evidence-based social work practice: Challenges and promise. *Social Work Research, 27*, 197-208.

Rosen, R. C., & Leiblum, S. R. (1995). Treatment of sexual disorders in the 1990s: An integrated approach. *Journal of Consulting and Clinical Psychology, 63*, 877-890.

Rosenberg, H., & Davis, L. (1994). Acceptance of moderate drinking by alcohol treatment services in the United States. *Journal of Studies on Alcohol, 55*, 167-172.

Rosenberg, S. D., Drake, R. E., Wolford, G. L., Mueser, K. T., Oxman, T. E., Vidaver, R. M., et al. (1998). Dartmouth Assessment of Lifestyle Instrument (DALI): A substance use disorder screen for people with severe mental illness. *American Journal of Psychiatry, 155*, 232-238.

Rosenheck, R., & Fontana, A. (1996). Ethnocultural variations in service use among veterans suffering from PTSD. In A. J. Marsella, M. J. Friedman, E. T. Gerrity, & R. M. Scurfield (Eds.), *Ethnocultural aspects of post-traumatic stress disorder* (pp. 483-504). Washington, DC: American Psychological Association.

Rossi, P. H., & Freeman, H. E. (1993). *Evaluation: A systematic approach*. Thousand Oaks, CA: Sage.

Rossi, P. H., Schuerman, J., & Budd, S. (1999). Understanding decisions about child maltreatment. *Evaluation Review, 23*, 579-598.

Rothbaum, B. O., Foa, E. B., Riggs, D. S., Murdock, T., & Walsh, W. (1992). A prospective examination of post-traumatic stress disorder in rape victims. *Journal of Traumatic Stress, 5*, 455-475.

Rothbaum, B. O., Meadows, E. A., Resick, P., & Foy, D. W. (2000). Cognitive-behavioral therapy. In E. B. Foa, T. M. Keane, & M. J. Friedman (Eds.), *Effective treatments for PTSD: Practice guidelines from the International Society for Traumatic Stress Studies* (pp. 60-83). New York: Guilford Press.

Rothman, J. (1991). A model of case management: Toward empirically based practice. *Social Work, 36*, 520-528.

Rounsaville, B. J., Dolinsky, Z. S., Babor, T. F., & Meyer, R. E. (1987). Psychopathology as a predictor of treatment outcome in alcoholics, *Archives of General Psychiatry, 44*, 505-513.

Roy-Byrne, P., Dafadakis, C., Ries, R., Decker, K., Jones, R., Bolte, M. A., et al. (1995). A psychiatrist-rated battery of measures for assessing the clinical status of psychiatric inpatients. *Psychiatric Services, 46*, 347-352.

Roy-Byrne, P., Dafadakis, C., Unutzer, J., & Ries, R. (1996). Evidence for limited validity of the revised Global Assessment of Functioning Scale. *Psychiatric Services, 47*, 864-866.

Royse, D., & Thyer, B. A. (1996). *Program evaluation: An introduction.* Chicago: Nelson-Hall.

Royse, D., Thyer, B. A., Padgett, D. K., & Logan, T. K. (2001). *Program evaluation: An introduction* (3rd ed.). Pacific Grove, CA: Brooks/Cole.

Rubin, A. (1985). Practice effectiveness: More grounds for optimism, *Social Work, 30*, 469-476.

Rubin, A. (1991). The effectiveness of outreach counseling and support groups for battered women: A preliminary evaluation. *Research on Social Work Practice, 1*, 332-357.

Rubin, A. (1992). Is case management effective for people with serious mental illness? A research review. *Health and Social Work, 17*, 138-150.

Rubin, A., Cardenas, J., Warren, K., Pike, C. K., & Wambach, K. (1998). Outdated practitioner views about family culpability and severe mental disorders. *Social Work, 43*, 412-422.

Ruef, A. M., Litz, B. T., & Schlenger, W. E. (2000). Hispanic ethnicity and risk for combat-related posttraumatic stress disorder. *Cultural Diversity and Ethnic Minority Psychology, 6*, 235-251.

Russell, D. E. H. (1983). The incidence and prevalence of intrafamilial and extrafamilial sexual abuse of female children. *Child Abuse and Neglect, 7*, 133-146.

Russell, D. E. H. (1984). The prevalence and seriousness of incestuous abuse: Stepfathers vs. biological fathers. *Child Abuse and Neglect, 8*, 15-22.

Rutter, M. (1997). Nature-nurture integration: The example of anti-social behavior. *American Psychologist, 52*, 390-398.

Rutter, M., & Rutter, M. (1993). *Developing minds: Challenge and continuity across the life span.* New York: Basic Books.

Ryan, C. S., Sherman, P. S., & Judd, C. M. (1994). Accounting for case manager effects in the evaluation of mental health services. *Journal of Consulting and Clinical Psychology, 62*, 965-974.

Ryan, T. (1998). Perceived risks associated with mental illness: Beyond homicide and suicide. *Social Science Medicine, 46,* 287-297.

Ryle, A. (1997). The structure and development of borderline personality disorder: A proposed model. *British Journal of Psychiatry, 170,* 82-89.

Ryle, A., & Golynkina, K. (2000). Effectiveness of time-limited cognitive analytic therapy of borderline personality disorder: Factors associated with outcome. *British Journal of Medical Psychology, 73,* 197-210.

Sabo, A. (1997). Etiological significance of associations between childhood trauma and borderline personality disorder: Conceptual and clinical implications. *Journal of Personality Disorders, 11,* 50-70.

Sadowski, C. M., & Friedrich, W. N. (2000). Psychometric properties of the Trauma Symptom Checklist for Children (TSCC) with psychiatrically hospitalized adolescents. *Child Maltreatment, 5,* 364-372.

Saewyc, E. M., Bearinger, L. H., Heinz, P. A., Blum, R. W., & Resnick, M. D. (1998). Gender differences in health and risk behaviors among bisexual and homosexual adolescents. *Journal of Adolescent Health, 23,* 181-188.

Safford, F. (1997). Differential assessment of dementia and depression in elderly people. In F. Safford & G. Krell (Eds.), *Gerontology for health professionals: A practice guide* (2nd ed., pp. 56-73). Washington DC: NASW Press.

Safran, J. D. (Ed). (1998). *The widening scope of cognitive therapy: The therapeutic relationship, emotion, and the process of change.* Northvale, NJ: Aronson.

Safren, S. A., Gonzalez, R. E., Horner, K. J., Leung, A. W., Heimberg, R. G., & Juster, H. R. (2000). Anxiety in ethnic minority youth: Methodological and conceptual issues and review of the literature. *Behavior Modification, 24,* 147-183.

Saleeby, D. (1996). Strengths perspective in social work practice: Extensions and cautions. *Social Work, 41,* 296-305.

Salkovskis, P. M. (1985). Obsessional-compulsive problems: A cognitive-behavioural analysis. *Behaviour Research and Therapy, 23,* 571-583.

Salkovskis, P. M. (1989). Cognitive-behavioural factors and the persistence of intrusive thoughts in obsessional problems. *Behaviour Research and Therapy, 27,* 677-682.

Sallee, F. R., & Greenawald, J. (1995). Neurobiology. In J. S. March (Ed.), *Anxiety disorders in children and adolescents* (pp. 3-34). New York: Guilford Press.

Sallee, F. R., & March, J. S. (2001). Neuropsychiatry of paediatric anxiety disorders. In W. K. Silverman & P. D. A. Treffers (Eds.), *Anxiety disorders in children and adolescents: Research, assessment and intervention* (pp. 90-125). New York: Cambridge University Press.

Salmon, P. (2001). Effects of physical exercise on anxiety, depression, and sensitivity to stress: A unifying theory. *Clinical Psychology Review, 21,* 33-61.

Salzer, M. S., Nixon, C. T., Schut, L. J. A., Karver, M. S., & Bickman, L. (1997). Validating quality indicators: Quality as relationship between structure, process and outcome. *Evaluation Review, 21,* 292-309.

Sanchez-Craig, M. (1980). Random assignment to abstinence or controlled drinking in a cognitive-behavioral program: Short-term effects on drinking behavior. *Addictive Behaviors, 5,* 35-39.

Sanchez-Craig, M., & Lei, H. (1986). Disadvantages of imposing the goal of abstinence on problem drinkers: An empirical study. *British Journal of Addiction, 81,* 505-512.

Sanders, M. R., Markie-Dadds, C., & Nicholson, J. M. (1997). Concurrent interventions for marital and children's problems. In W. K. Halford & H. J. Markham (Eds.), *Clinical handbook of marriage and couples intervention* (pp. 509-535). New York: Wiley.

Sanders, M. R., Nicholson, J. M., & Floyd, F. J. (1997). Couples' relationships and children. In W. K. Halford & H. J. Markham (Eds.), *Clinical handbook of marriage and couples intervention* (pp. 225-253). New York: Wiley.

Sanjuan, P., & Langenbucher, J. (1999). Age-limited populations: Youth, adolescents and older adults. In B. S. McCrady & E. E. Epstein (Eds.), *Addictions: A comprehensive guidebook* (pp. 477-498). New York: Oxford University Press.

Santisteban, D. A., Coatsworth, D., Perez-Vidal, A., Mitrani, V., Jean-Gilles, M., & Szapocznik, J. (1997). Brief structural/strategic family therapy with African-American and Hispanic high-risk youth. *Journal of Community Psychology, 25*, 453-471.

Santisteban, D. A., Szapocznik, J., Perez-Vidal, A., Kurtines, W. M., Murray, E. J., & LaPeriere, A. (1996). Efficacy of interventions for engaging youth/familes into treatment and some factors that may contribute to differential effectiveness. *Journal of Family Psychology, 10*, 35-44.

Sarason, I. G., Pierce, G. R., & Sarason, B. R. (1994). General and specific perceptions of social support. In W. R. Avison & I. H. Gotlib (Eds.), *Stress and mental health: Contemporary issues and prospects for the future* (pp. 151-177). New York: Springer.

Sarwer, D. B., & Durlak, J. A. (1997). A field trial of the effectiveness of behavioral treatment for sexual dysfunctions. *Journal of Sex and Marital Therapy, 23*, 87-97.

Saunders, J. B., Aasland, O. G., Amundsen, A., & Grant, M. (1993). Alcohol consumption and related problems among primary health care patients: WHO collaborative project on early detection of persons with harmful alcohol consumption: Part 1. *Addiction, 88*, 349-362.

Saunders, J. B., Aasland, O. G., Babor, T. F., de la Fuente, J. R., & Grant, M. (1993). Development of the Alcohol Use Disorders Identification test (AUDIT): WHO collaborative project on early detection of persons with harmful alcohol consumption: Part 2. *Addiction, 88*, 791-804.

Saxon, A. J., Wells, E. A., Fleming, C., Jackson, T. R., & Calsyn, D. A. (1996). Pre-treatment characteristics, program philosophy and level of ancillary services as predictors of methadon maintenance treatment outcome. *Addiction, 91*, 1197-1209.

Sayers, S. L., & Sarwer, D. B. (1998). Assessment of marital dysfunction. In A. S. Bellack & M. Hersen (Eds.), *Behavioral assessment: A practical handbook* (pp. 293-314). Boston: Allyn and Bacon.

Saywitz, K. J., Goodman, G. S., & Lyon, T. D. (2002). Interviewing children in and out of court: Current research and practice implications. In J. E. B. Meyers, L. Berliner, J. Briere, C. T. Hendrix, C. Jenny, & T. A. Reid (Eds.), *The APSAC handbook on child maltreatment* (2nd ed., pp. 349-377). Thousand Oaks, CA: Sage.

Saywitz, K. J., Mannarino, A. P., Berliner, L., & Cohen, J. A. (2000). Treatment for sexually abused children and adolescents. *American Psychologist, 55*, 1040-1049.

Scaturo, D. J. (2001). The evolution of psychotherapy and the concept of manualization: An integrative perspective. *Professional Psychology: Research and Practice, 32*, 522-530.

Schafer, J., & Leigh, B. C. (1996). A comparison of the factor structures of adolescent and adult alcohol effect expectancies. *Addictive Behaviors, 21*, 403-408.

Scharff, J. S. (1995). Psychoanalytic marital therapy. In N. S. Jacobson & A. S. Gurman (Eds.), *Clinical handbook of couple therapy* (pp. 164-196). New York: Guilford Press.

Scherer, M. W., & Nakamura, C. Y. (1968). A fear survey schedule for children (FSS-C): A factor analytic comparison with manifest anxiety (CMAS). *Behaviour Research and Therapy, 6*, 173-182.

Schilling, R. F., El-Bassel, N., Hadden, B., & Gilbert, L. (1995). Skills-training groups to reduce HIV transmission and drug use among methadone patients. *Social Work, 40*, 91-101.

Schinke, S. P., Schilling, R. F., Kirkham, M. A., Gilchrist, L. D., Barth, R. P., & Blythe, B. J. (1986). Stress management skills for parents. *Journal of Child and Adolescent Psychotherapy, 3*, 293-298.

Schliebner, C. T. (1994). Gender-sensitive therapy: An alternative for women in substance abuse treatment. *Journal of Substance Abuse Treatment, 11*, 511-515.

Schmidt, N. B., & Koselka, M. (2000). Gender differences in patients with panic disorder: Evaluating cognitive mdiation of phobic avoidance. *Cognitive Therapy and Research, 24*, 533-550.

Schmidt, U. (1998). Eating disorders and obesity. In P. Graham (Ed.), *Cognitive-behaviour therapy for children and families* (pp. 262-281). New York: Cambridge University Press.

Schniering, C. A., Hudson, J. L., & Rapee, R. (2000). Issues in the diagnosis and assessment of anxiety disorders in children and adolescents. *Clinical Psychology Review, 20*, 453-478.

Schuckit, M. (1998). Biological, psychological and environmental predictors of the alcoholism risk: A longitudinal study. *Journal of Studies on Alcohol, 59*, 485-494.

Schulenberg, J. E., & Maggs, J. L. (2002). A developmental perspective on alcohol use and heavy drinking during adolescence and the transition to young adulthood. *Journal of Studies on Alcohol, 63*, 54-70.

Schulenberg, J. E., Maggs, J. L., Steinman, K. J., & Zucker, R. A. (2001). Development matters: Taking the long view on substance abuse etiology and intervention during adolescence. In P. M. Monti, S. M. Colby, & T. A. O'Leary (Eds.), *Adolescents, alcohol and substance abuse: Reaching teens through brief interventions* (pp. 19-57). New York: Guilford Press.

Schwartz, A., & Schwartz, R. M. (1993). *Depression: Theories and treatment.* New York: Columbia University Press.

Schwartz, J. (1998). Neuroanatomical aspects of cognitive-behavioural therapy response in obsessive-compulsive disorder: An evolving perspective on brain and behaviour. *British Journal of Psychiatry, 173*(Suppl. 35), 38-44.

Scogin, F., & McElreath, L. (1994). Efficacy of psychosocial treatments for geriatric depression: A quantitative review. *Journal of Consulting and Clinical Psychology, 62*, 69-74.

Scott, J. E., & Dixon, L. B. (1995). Assertive community treatment and case management for schizophrenia. *Schizophrenia Bulletin, 21*, 657-668.

Seligman, M. E. (1975). *Helplessness: On depression, development and death.* San Francisco: Freeman.

Seltzer, M. (1971). The Michigan Alcoholism Screening Test: The quest for a new diagnostic instrument. *American Journal of Psychiatry, 127*, 1653-1658.

Semidei, J., Radel, L. F., & Nolan, C. (2001). Substance abuse and child welfare: Clear linkages and promising responses. *Child Welfare, 80*, 109-128.

Senchak, M., Leonard, K. E., & Greene, B. W. (1998). Alcohol use among college students as a function of their typical social drinking context. *Psychology of Addictive Behaviors, 12*, 62-70.

Serin, R. C., & Brown, S. L. (2000). The clinical use of the Hare Psychopathy Checklist–Revised in contemporary risk assessment. In C. B. Gacono (Ed.), *The clinical and forensic assessment of psychopathy: A practitioner's guide* (pp. 251-268). Mahwah, NJ: Erlbaum.

Serin, R. C., & Preston, D. L. (2001). Managing and treating violent offenders. In J. B. Ashford, B. D. Sales, & W. H. Reid (Eds.), *Treating adult and juvenile offenders with special needs* (pp. 249-271). Washington, DC: American Psychological Association.

Shadish, W. R., Montgomery, L. M., Wilson, P., Wilson, M. R., Bright, I., & Okwumabua, T. (1993). Effects of family and marital psychotherapies: A meta-analysis. *Journal of Consulting and Clinical Psychology, 61*, 992-1002.

Shafran, R. (1998). Childhood obsessive-compulsive disorder. In P. Graham (Ed.), *Cognitive-behaviour therapy for children and families* (pp. 45-73). New York: Cambridge University Press.

Shalev, A. Y. (1996). Stress versus traumatic stress: From acute homeostatic reactions to chronic psychopathology. In B. A. Van der Kolk, A. C. McFarlane, & L. Weisaeth, (Eds.), *Traumatic stress: The effects of overwhelming experience on mind, body and society* (pp. 77-101). New York: Guilford Press.

Shalev, A. Y., Bonne, O., & Eth, S. (1996). Treatment of posttraumatic stress disorder: A review. *Psychosomatic Medicine, 58*, 165-182.

Shapiro, F. (1996). Eye movement desensitization and reprocessing (EMDR): Evaluation of controlled PTSD research. *Journal of Behavioral and Experimental Psychiatry, 27*, 209-218.

Shapiro, F. (2002). EMDR 12 years after its introduction: Past and future research. *Journal of Clinical Psychology, 58*, 1-22.

Shea, M. T., Elkin, I., Imber, S. D., Sotsky, S. M., Watkins, J. T., Pilkonis, P. A., et al. (1992). Course of depressive symptoms over follow-up: Findings from the National Institute of Mental Health Treatment of Depression Collaborative Program. *Archives of General Psychiatry, 49*, 782-787.

Sheehan, T., & Owen, P. (1999). The disease model. In B. S. McCrady & E. E. Epstein (Eds.), *Addictions: A comprehensive guidebook* (pp. 268-286). New York: Oxford University Press.

Shekter-Wolfson, L. F., Woodside, D. B., & Lackstrom, J. (1997). Social work treatment of anorexia and bulimia: Guidelines for practice. *Research on Social Work Practice, 7*, 5-31.

Shelton, T. L., Barkley, R. A., Crosswait, C., Moorehouse, M., Fletcher, K., Barrett, S., et al. (2000). Multimethod psychoeducational intervention for preschool children with disruptive behavior: Two-year post-treatment follow-up. *Journal of Abnormal Child Psychology, 28*, 253-266.

Shenton, M. E. (1996). Temporal lobe structural abnormalities in schizophrenia: A selective review and presentation of new magnetic resonance findings. In S. Matthysse, D. L. Levy, J. Kagan, & F. M. Benes (Eds.), *Psychopathology: The evolving science of mental disorder* (pp. 51-99). New York: Cambridge University Press.

Sher, K. (1987). Stress dampening response. In H. Blane & K. Leonard (Eds.), *Psychological theories of drinking and alcoholism* (pp. 227-271). New York: Guilford Press.

Sher, K. (1997). Psychological characteristics of children of alcoholics. *Alcohol Health and Research World, 21*, 247-254.

Shoevers, R. A., Beekman, A., Deeg, D., Geerlings, M., Jonker, C., & Van Tilburg, W. (2000). Risk factors for depression in later life: Results of a prospective community based study (AMSTEL). *Journal of Affective Disorders, 59*, 127-137.

Shulman, L. (1992). *The skills of helping: Individuals, families and groups*. Itasca, IL: Peacock.

Siegel, D. (1984). Defining empirically based practice. *Social Work, 29*, 325-331.

Sigvardsson, S., Cloninger, R., Bohman, M., & von Knorring, A. (1982). Predisposition to petty criminality in Swedish adoptees. *Archives of General Psychiatry, 39*, 1248-1253.

Sikkema, K. J., Winett, R. A., & Lombard, D. N. (1995). Development and evaluation of an HIV-risk reduction program for female college students. *AIDS Education and Prevention, 7*, 145-159.

Silberg, J., Pickles, A., Rutter, M., Hewitt, J., Simonoff, E., Maes, H., et al. (1999). The influence of genetic factors and life stress on depression among adolescent girls. *Archives of General Psychiatry, 56*, 225-232.

Silverman, W. K., & Berman, S. L. (2001). Psychosocial interventions for anxiety disorders in children: Status and future directions. In W. K. Silverman & P. D. A. Treffers (Eds.), *Anxiety disorders in children and adolescents: Research, assessment and intervention* (pp. 313-334). New York: Cambridge University Press.

Silverman, W. K., Kurtines, W. M., Ginsburg, G. S., Weems, C. F., Lumpkin, P. W., & Carmichael, D. H. (1999). Treating anxiety disorders in children with group cognitive-behavioral therapy: A randomized controlled trial. *Journal of Consulting and Clinical Psychology, 67*, 995-1003.

Silverman, W. K., Kurtines, W. M., Ginsburg, G. S., Weems, C. F., Rabian, B., & Serafini, L. T. (1999). Contingency management, self-control, and education support in the treatment of childhood phobic disorders. *Journal of Consulting and Clinical Psychology, 67*, 675-687.

Silverman, W. K., & Serafini, L. T. (1998). Assessment of child behavior problems: Internalizing disorders. In A. S. Bellack & M. Hersen (Eds.), *Behavioral assessment: A practical handbook* (4th ed., pp. 342-360). Boston: Allyn and Bacon.

Simon, C. E., McNeil, J. S., Franklin, C., & Cooperman, A. (1991, June). The family and schizophrenia: Toward a psychoeducational approach. *Journal of Contemporary Human Services*, 323-333.

Simon, L. M. (1997). Do criminals specialize in crime types? *Applied and Preventive Psychology, 6*, 35-53.

Simon, L. M. (1998). Does criminal offender treatment work? *Applied and Preventive Psychology, 7*, 137-159.

Simons, A. D., Gordon, J. S., Monroe, S. M., & Thase, M. E. (1995). Toward an integration of psychologic, social, and biologic factors in depression: Effects on outcome and course of cognitive therapy. *Journal of Consulting and Clinical Psychology, 63*, 369-377.

Simpson, D. D., Joe, G. W., Rowan-Szal, G. A., & Greener, J. M. (1997). Drug abuse treatment process components that reduce retention. *Journal of Substance Abuse Treatment, 14*, 565-572.

Simpson, E. B., Pistorello, J., Begin, A., Costello, E., Levinson, J., Mulberry, S., et al. (1998). Use of dialectical behavior therapy in a partial hospital program for women with borderline personality disorder. *Psychiatric Services, 49*, 669-673.

Sisson, R., & Azrin, N. (1986). Family-member involvement to initiate and promote treatment of problem drinkers. *Journal of Behaviour Therapy and Experimental Psychiatry, 17,* 15–21.

Skinner, H.A. (1982).The Drug Abuse Screening Test. *Addictive Behaviors, 7,* 363–371.

Slater, J. M., Guthrie, B. J., & Boyd, C. J. (2001). A feminist theoretical approach to understanding health of adolescent females. *Journal of Adolescent Health, 28,* 443–449.

Slep, A. M. S., & Heyman, R. E. (2001). Where do we go from here? Moving toward an integrated approach to family violence. *Aggression and Violent Behavior, 6,* 353–356.

Sloan, R. B., Staples, F. R., Cristol, A. H., Yorkston, N. J., & Whipple, K. (1975). *Psychotherapy vs. behavior therapy.* Cambridge: Harvard University Press.

Smith, B. D., & Marsh, J. C. (2002). Client-service matching in substance abuse treatment for women with children. *Journal of Substance Abuse Treatment, 22,* 161–168.

Smith, D. E., Marcus, M. D., & Eldredge, K. L. (1994). Binge eating syndromes: A review of assessment and treatment with an emphasis on clinical application. *Behavior Therapy, 25,* 635–658.

Smith, G. R., Fischer, E. P., Nordquist, C. R., Mosley, C. L., & Ledbetter, N. S. (1997). Implementing outcomes management systems in mental health settings. *Psychiatric Services, 48,* 364–368.

Smith, M. L., Glass, G. V., & Miller, T. I. (1980). *The benefits of psychotherapy.* Baltimore: Johns Hopkins University Press.

Smith, P., Perrin, S., & Yule, W. (1998). In P. Graham (Ed.), *Cognitive-behaviour therapy for children and families* (pp. 127–142). New York: Cambridge University Press.

Smith, S. L., Sherrill, K. A., & Colenda, C. C. (1995). Assessing and treating anxiety in elderly persons. *Psychiatric Services, 46,* 36–42.

Smith, T. E., Bellack, A. S., & Liberman, R. P. (1996). Social skills training for schizophrenia: Review and future directions. *Clinical Psychology Review, 16,* 599–617.

Smokowski, P. R., & Wodarski, J. S. (1996). The effectiveness of child welfare services for poor, neglected children: A review of the empirical evidence. *Research on Social Work Practice, 6,* 504–523.

Smyth, N. J. (1996, December). Motivating persons with dual disorders: A stage approach. *Families in Society: The Journal of Contemporary Human Services,* 605–614.

Snyder, D. K., & Wills, R. M. (1989). Behavioral versus insight-oriented marital therapy: Effects on individual and interspousal functioning. *Journal of Consulting and Clinical Psychology, 57,* 39–46.

Snyder, D. K., Wills, R. M., & Grady-Fletcher, A. (1991). Long-term effectiveness of behavioral vs. insight-oriented marital therapy. *Journal of Consulting and Clinical Psychology, 59,* 146–149.

Sobell, L. C., Cunningham, J. A., & Sobell, M. B. (1996). Recovery from alcohol problems with and without treatment: Prevalence in two population surveys. *American Journal of Public Health, 86,* 966–972.

Sobell, L. C., Toneatto, T., & Sobell, M. B. (1994). Behavioral assessment and treatment planning for alcohol, tobacco, and other drug problems: Current status with an emphasis on clinical applications. *Behavioral Therapy, 25,* 533–580.

Solomon, P. (1992). The efficacy of case management services for severely mentally disabled clients. *Community Mental Health Journal, 28,* 163-180.

Solomon, S. D., & Davidson, J. R. T. (1997). Trauma: Prevalence, impairment, service use and cost. *Journal of Clinical Psychiatry, 58*(Suppl. 9), 5-11.

Sowers-Hoag, K. M. (1997). Case management with the elderly. In F. Safford & G. Krell (Eds.), *Gerontology for health professionals: A practice guide* (2nd ed., pp. 74-92). Washington, DC: NASW Press.

Spangler, D., Simons, A., Monroe, S., & Thase, M. (1996). Gender differences in cognitive diathesis-stress domain match: Implications for differential pathways to depression. *Journal of Abnormal Psychology, 105,* 653-657.

Spangler, D., Simons, A., Monroe, S., & Thase, M. (1997). Response to cognitive-behavioral therapy in depression: Effects of pretreatment cognitive dysfunction and life stress. *Journal of Consulting and Clinical Psychology, 65,* 568-575.

Spanier, G. B. (1976). Measuring dyadic adjustment: New scales for assessing the quality of marriage and similar dyads. *Journal of Marriage and Family Therapy, 38,* 15-28.

Spence, S. H. (1997). Structure of anxiety symptoms among children: A confirmatory factor-analytic study. *Journal of Abnormal Psychology, 106,* 280-297.

Spencer, T. J., Biederman, J., Wilens, T. E., & Faraone, S. V. (2002). Overview and neurobiology of attention-deficit/hyperactivity disorder. *Journal of Clinical Psychiatry, 63,* 3-9.

Sprock, J., & Yoder, C. (1997). Women and depression: An update on the report of the APA task force. *Sex Roles, 36,* 269-303.

Srebnik, D., Hendryx, M., Stevenson, J., Caverly, S., Dyck, D. G., & Cauce, A. M. (1997). Development of outcome indicators for monitoring the quality of public mental health care. *Psychiatric Services, 48,* 903-909.

Sroufe, L. A. (1997). Psychopathology as an outcome of development. *Development and Psychopathology, 9,* 251-268.

Stake, R. E. (1995). *The art of case study research.* Thousand Oaks, CA: Sage.

Staley, D., & El-Guebaly, N. (1990). Psychometric properties of the Drug Abuse Screening Test in a psychiatric patient population. *Addictive Behaviors, 15,* 257-264.

Stanley, M. A., Beck, J. G., Novy, D. M., Averill, P. M., Swann, A. C., Diefenbach, G. J., et al. (2003). Cognitive-behavioral treatment of late-life generalized anxiety disorder. *Journal of Consulting and Clinical Psychology, 71,* 309-319.

Stanley, M. A., & Turner, S. M. (1995). Current status of pharmacological and behavioral treatment of obsessive-compulsive disorder. *Behavior Therapy, 26,* 163-186.

Stanton, M. D., & Shadish, W. R. (1997). Outcome, attrition, and family-couples treatment for drug abuse: A meta-analysis and review of the controlled, comparative studies. *Psychological Bulletin, 122,* 170-191.

Stanton, M. D., Todd, T. C., et al. (1982). *The family therapy of drug abuse and addiction.* New York: Guilford Press.

Stark, K. D., Reynolds, W. M., & Kaslow, N. (1987). A comparison of the relative efficacy of self-control therapy and a behavioral problem-solving therapy for depression in children. *Journal of Abnormal Child Psychology, 15,* 91-113.

Stark, K. D., Rouse, L. W., & Kurowski, C. (1994). Psychological treatment approaches for depression in children. In W. M. Reynolds & H. F. Johnston (Eds.), *Handbook of depression in children and adolescents* (pp. 275-307). New York: Plenum Press.

Stark, K. D., Vaughn, C., Doxey, M., & Luss, L. (1999). Depressive disorders. In R. T. Ammerman, M. Hersen, & C. G. Last (Eds.), *Handbook of prescriptive treatments for children and adolescents* (2nd ed., pp. 114-140). Boston: Allyn and Bacon.

Staton, M., Leukefeld, C., Logan, T. K., Zimmerman, R., Lynam, D., Milich, R., et al. (1999). Risky sex behavior and substance use among young adults. *Health and Social Work, 24*, 147-153.

Steele, C. M, & Josephs, R. A. (1990). Alcohol myopia: Its prized and dangerous effects. *American Psychologist, 45*, 921-933.

Stein, L. I., & Test, M. A, (1980). Alternatives to mental hospital treatment: Part 1. Conceptual model, treatment program, and clinical evaluation. *Archives of General Psychiatry, 37*, 392-397.

Stein, R. I., Saelens, B. E., Dounchis, J. Z., Lewczyk, C. M., Swenson, A. K., & Wilfley, D. E. (2001). Treatment of eating disorders in women. *The Counseling Psychologist, 29*, 695-732.

Steinberg, A. M., Brymer, M. J., Decker, K. B., & Pynoos, R. S. (2004). The University of California at Los Angeles Post-traumatic Stress Disorder Reaction Index. *Current Psychiatry Reports, 6*, 96-100.

Steinglass, P., Bennett, L. A., Wolin, S. J., & Reiss, D. (1987). *The alcoholic family*. New York: Basic Books.

Steketee, G. S. (1993). *Treatment of obsessive compulsive disorder*. New York: Guilford Press.

Steketee, G. S. (1997). Disability and family burden in obsessive-compulsive disorder. *Canadian Journal of Psychiatry, 42*, 919-928.

Steketee, G. S., Chambless, D. L., & Tran, G. Q. (2001). Effects of Axis I and II comorbidity on behavior therapy outcome for obsessive-compulsive disorder with agoraphobia. *Comprehensive Psychiatry, 42*, 76-86.

Steketee, G. S., & Shapiro, L. J. (1995). Predicting behavioral treatment outcome for agoraphobia and obsessive compulsive disorder. *Clinical Psychology Review, 15*, 317-346.

Stern, A. (1938). Psychoanalytic investigation and therapy in the borderline group of neuroses. *Psychoanalytic Quarterly, 7*, 467-489.

Stern, M. I., Herron, W. G., Primavera, L. H., & Kakuma, T. (1997). Interpersonal perceptions of depressed and borderline patients. *Journal of Clinical Psychology, 53*, 41-49.

Stevens, J. R. (1992). Abnormal reinnervation as a basis for schizophrenia: A hypothesis. *Archives of General Psychiatry, 49*, 238-243.

Stewart, S. H. (1996). Alcohol abuse in individuals exposed to trauma: A critical review. *Psychological Bulletin, 120*, 83-112.

Stice, E., Fisher, M., & Martinez, E. (2004). Eating Disorder Diagnostic Scale: Additional evidence of reliability and validity. *Psychological Assessment, 16*, 60-71.

Stice, E., Telch, C. F., & Rizvi, S. L. (2000). Development and validation of the Eating Disorder Diagnostic Scale: A brief self-report measure of anorexia, bulimia, and binge eating disorder. *Psychological Assessment, 12*, 123-131.

Stiles, P. G., & McGarrahan, J. F. (1998). The Geriatric Depression Scale: A comprehensive review. *Journal of Clinical Geropsychology, 4*, 89-110.

Stith, S. M., Rosen, K. H., & McCollum, E. E. (2003). Effectiveness of couples treatment for spouse abuse. *Journal of Marital and Family Therapy, 29*, 407-426.

Stock, S. L., Werry, J. S., & McClellan, J. M. (2001). Pharmacological treatment of pae-diatric anxiety. In W. K. Silverman & P. D. A. Treffers (Eds.), *Anxiety disorders in children and adolescents: Research, assessment and intervention* (pp. 335-367). New York: Cambridge University Press.

Stoffelmayer, B. E., Mavis, B. E., & Kasim, R. M. (1994). The longitudinal stability of the Addiction Severity Index. *Journal of Substance Abuse Treatment, 11*, 373-378.

Strean, H. S. (1986). Psychoanalytic theory. In F. J. Turner (Ed.), *Social work treat-ment: Interlocking theoretical approaches* (3rd ed., pp. 19-45). New York: Free Press.

Streeter, C. L., & Franklin, C. (1992). Defining and measuring social support: Guide-lines for social work practitioners. *Research on Social Work Practice, 2*, 81-99.

Striegel-Moore, R. H. (1993). Etiology of binge eating: A developmental perspective. In C. G. Fairburn & G. T. Wilson (Eds.), *Binge eating: Nature, assessment and treat-ment* (pp. 144-172). New York: Guilford Press.

Striegel-Moore, R. H., & Cachelin, F. M. (2001). Etiology of eating disorders in women. *The Counseling Psychologist, 29*, 635-661.

Stuart, R. B. (1969). Operant-interpersonal treatment of marital discord. *Journal of Consulting and Clinical Psychology, 33*, 675-682.

Stuart, R. B. (1980). *Helping couples change*. New York: Guilford Press.

Stueve, A., Dohrenwend, B. P., & Skodol, A. E. (1998). Relationships between stressful life events and episodes of major depression and nonaffective psychotic disor-ders: Selected results from a New York risk factor study. In B. P. Dohrenwend (Ed.), *Adversity, stress and psychopathology* (pp. 341-357). New York: Oxford Univer-sity Press.

Sue, S., Zane, N., & Young, K. (1994). Research on psychotherapy with culturally diverse populations. In A. E. Bergin & S. L. Garfield (Eds.), *Handbook of psy-chotherapy and behavior change* (pp. 783-820). New York: Wiley.

Sullivan, P. F., Neale, M. C., & Kendler, K. S. (2000). Genetic epidemiology of major depression: Review and meta-analysis. *American Journal of Psychiatry, 157*, 1552-1562.

Sullivan, W. P., Hartmann, D. J., Dillon, D., & Wolk, J. L. (1994, February). Implementing case management in alcohol and drug treatment. *Families in Society: The Jour-nal of Contemporary Human Services*, 67-73.

Sunday, S. R., & Halmi, K. A. (2000). Comparison of the Yale-Brown-Cornell Eating Dis-orders Scale in recovered eating disorder patients, restrained dieters, and non-dieting controls. *International Journal of Eating Disorders, 28*, 455-459.

Sundel, M., & Sundel, S. S. (1998). Pharmacological treatment of panic disorder. *Research on Social Work Practice, 8*, 426-451.

Swanson, J. M. (1992). *School-based assessments and interventions for ADD stu-dents*. Irvine, CA: K. C. Publishing.

Swanson, J. M., Schuck, S., Mann, M., Carlson, C., Hartman, K., Sergeant, J., et al. (2002). *Categorical and dimensional definitions and evaluation of symptoms of ADHD: The SNAP and the SWAN ratings scales*. Retrieved from http://www .ADHD.net.

Swartz, M. S., Burns, B. J., Hiday, V. A., George, L. K., Swanson, J., & Wagner, H. R. (1995). New directions in research on involuntary outpatient commitment. *Psychiatric Services, 46*, 381-385.

Swartz, M. S., Swanson, J. W., Hiday, V. A., Borum, R., Wagner, H. R., & Burns, B. J. (1998). Violence and severe mental illness: The effects of substance abuse and nonadherence to medication. *American Journal of Psychiatry, 155*, 226-231.

Swenson, C. C., & Hanson, R. F. (1998). Sexual abuse of children: Assessment, research and treatment. In J. R. Lutzker (Ed.), *Handbook of child abuse research and treatment* (pp. 475-499). New York: Plenum Press.

Swenson, C. R., Sanderson, C., Dulit, R. A., & Linehan, M. M. (2001). The application of dialectical behavior therapy for patients with borderline personality disorder on inpatient units. *Psychiatric Quarterly, 72*, 307-324.

Szapocznik, J., Kurtines, W. M., Foote, F. H., Perez-Vidal, A., & Hervis, O. (1983). Conjoint versus one-person family therapy: Some evidence for the effectiveness of conducting family therapy through one person. *Journal of Consulting and Clinical Psychology, 51*, 889-899.

Szapocznik, J., Kurtines, W. M., Foote, F. H., Perez-Vidal, A., & Hervis, O. (1986). Conjoint versus one-person family therapy: Further evidence for the effectiveness of conducting family therapy through one person with drug-abusing adolescents. *Journal of Consulting and Clinical Psychology, 54*, 395-397.

Tarrier, N., & Barrowclough, C. (1995). Family interventions in schizophrenia and their long-term outcomes. *International Journal of Mental Health, 24*, 39-53.

Tarrier, N., Sommerfield, C., Pilgrim, H., & Faragher, B. (2000). Factors associated with outcome of cognitive-behavioural treatment of chronic post-traumatic stress disorder. *Behaviour Research and Therapy, 38*, 191-202.

Tarter, R., Vanyokov, M., Giancola, P., Dawes, M., Blackson, T., Miezzich, A., et al. (1999). Etiology of early age onset substance use disorder: A maturational perspective. *Development and Psychopathology, 11*, 657-683.

Task Force on Promotion and Dissemination of Psychological Procedures. (1995). Training in and dissemination of empirically-validated psychological treatments: Report and recommendations. *Clinical Psychologist, 48*, 3-23.

Taylor, E. H. (1987). The biological basis of schizophrenia. *Social Work, 32*, 155-121.

Taylor, S. (1995). Assessment of obsessions and compulsions: Reliability, validity and sensitivity to treatment effects. *Clinical Psychology Review, 15*, 261-296.

Taylor, S., Thordarson, D., Maxfield, L., Fedoroff, I. C., Lovell, K., & Ogrodniczuk, J. (2003). Comparative efficacy, speed, and adverse effects of three PTSD treatments: Exposure therapy, EMDR, and relaxation training. *Journal of Consulting and Clinical Psychology, 71*, 330-338.

Teague, G. B., Bond, G. R., & Drake, R. E. (1998). Program fidelity in assertive community treatment: Development and use of a measure. *American Journal of Orthopsychiatry, 68*, 216-232.

Teasdale, J. D. (1995). Clinically relevant theory: Integrating clinical insight with cognitive science. In P. M. Salkovskis (Ed.), *Frontiers of cognitive therapy* (pp. 26-47). New York: Guilford Press.

Tehrani, J. A., Brennan, P. A., Hodgins, S., & Mednick, S. A. (1998). Mental illness and criminal violence. *Social Psychiatry and Psychiatric Epidemiology, 33*, s81-s85.

Tengstrom, A., Grann, M., Langstrom, N., & Kullgren, G. (2000). Psychopathy (PCL-R) as a predictor of violent recidivism among criminal offenders with schizophrenia. *Law and Human Behavior, 24*, 45-58.

Teri, L. (1996). Depression in Alzheimer's disease. In M. Hersen & V. B. Van Hasselt (Eds.), *Psychological treatment of older adults: An introductory text* (pp. 209-222). New York: Plenum Press.

Terling, T. (1999). The efficacy of family reunification practice: Reentry rates and correlates of reentry for abused and neglected children reunited with their families. *Child Abuse and Neglect, 23*, 1359-1370.

Test, M. A., Burke, S., & Wallach, L. S. (1990). Gender differences of young adults with schizophrenic disorders in community care. *Schizophrenia Bulletin, 16*, 331-344.

Thase, M. E., Friedman, E. S., Fasiczka, A. L., Berman, S. R., Frank, E., Nofzinger, E. A., et al. (2000). Treatment of men with major depression: A comparison of seqential cohorts treated with either cognitive-behavioral therapy or newer generation anti-depressants. *Journal of Clinical Psychiatry, 61*, 466-472.

Thelen, M. H., Farmer, J., Wonderlich, S., & Smith, M. (1991). A revision of the Bulimia-Test: The BULIT-R. *Psychological Assessment: A Journal of Consulting and Clinical Psychology, 3*, 119-124.

Thibaut, J. W., & Kelly, H. H. (1959). *The social psychology of groups*. New York: Wiley.

Thomas, C., & Corcoran, J. (2001). Empirically-based marital and family interventions for alcohol abuse: A review. *Research on Social Work Practice, 11*, 549-575.

Thomas, E. J., & Ager, R. D. (1993). Unilateral family therapy with spouses of uncooperative alcohol abusers. In T. J. O'Farrell (Ed.), *Treating alcohol problems: Marital and family interventions* (pp. 3-33). New York: Guilford Press.

Thomas, E. J., & Santa, C. A. (1982). Unilateral family therapy for alcohol abuse: A working conception. *American Journal of Family Therapy, 10*, 49-58.

Thompson, L. W. (1996). Cognitive-behavioral therapy and treatment for late-life depression. *Journal of Clinical Psychiatry, 57*, 29-37.

Thorpe, G. L., & Olson, S. L. (1997). *Behavior therapy* (2nd ed.). Boston: Allyn and Bacon.

Thyer, B. A. (2001). Evidence-based approaches to community practice. In H. E. Briggs & K. Corcoran (Eds.), *Social work practice: Treating common client problems* (pp. 54-65). Chicago: Lyceum Books.

Thyer, B. A. (2004). Science and evidence-based social work practice. In H. E. Briggs & T. L. Rzepnicki (Eds.), *Using evidence in social work practice: Behavioral perspectives* (pp. 74-89). Chicago: Lyceum Books.

Tourse, R. W. C., & Sullick, J. (1999). The collaborative alliance: Supporting vulnerable children in school. In R. W. C. Tourse & J. F. Mooney (Eds.), *Collaborative practice: School and human service partnerships* (pp. 59-78). Westport, CT: Praeger.

Tran, T. V. (1993). Psychological traumas and depression in a sample of Vietnamese people in the United States. *Health and Social Work, 18*, 184-194.

Tran, T. V. (1997). Exploring the equivalence of factor structure in a measure of depression between black and white women: Measurement issues in comparative research. *Research on Social Work Practice, 7*, 500-517.

Treadwell, K. R. H., Flannery-Schroeder, E. C., & Kendall, P. C. (1995). Ethnicity and gender in relation to adaptive functioning, diagnostic status, and treatment outcome in children from an anxiety clinic. *Journal of Anxiety Disorders, 9*, 373-384.

Trimble, J. E. (1990). Ethnic specification, validation prospects, and the future of drug use research. *International Journal of the Addictions, 25*, 149-170.

Truax, C. B., & Carkhuff, R. R. (1967). *Toward effective counseling and psychotherapy*. Chicago: Aldine.

Trull, T. J., Sher, K. J., Minks-Brown, C., Durbin, J., & Burr, R. (2000). Borderline personality disorder and substance use disorders: A review and integration. *Clinical Psychology Review, 20*, 235-253.

Tryer, P. (1995). Are personality disorders well classified in *DSM-IV*? In J. Livesley (Ed.), *The DSM-IV personality disorders* (pp. 29–42). New York: Guilford Press.

Tubman, J. G., Windle, M., & Windle, R. C. (1996). Cumulative sexual intercourse patterns among middle adolescents: Problem behavior precursors and concurrent health risk behaviors. *Journal of Adolescent Health, 18,* 182–191.

Tuinstra, J., Groothoff, J. W., Van Den Jeuvel, W. J., & Post, D. (1998). Socio-economic differences in health risk behavior in adolescence: Do they exist? *Social Science and Medicine, 47,* 67–74.

Tuliatos, J., Perlmutter, B., & Holden, G. (Eds.). (2001). *Handbook of family measurement techniques: Vol. 2.* Thousand Oaks, CA: Sage.

Turkat, I. (1992). Behavioral intervention with personality disorders. In S. M. Turner, K. S. Calhoun, & H. E. Adams (Eds.), *Handbook of clinical behavior therapy* (2nd ed., pp. 117–134). New York: Wiley.

Turner, W. M., & Tsuang, M. T. (1990). Impact of substance abuse on the course and outcome of schizophrenia. *Schizophrenia Bulletin, 16,* 87–95.

Tutty, L. M. (1996). Post-shelter services: The efficacy of follow-up programs for abused women. *Research on Social Work Practice, 6,* 425–441.

Tversky, A., & Kahneman, D. (1974). Judgment under uncertainty: Heuristics and biases. *Science, 183,* 1124–1131.

Tyson, E. H., & Glisson, C. (2005). A cross-ethnic validity study of the Shortform Assessment for Children (SAC). *Research on Social Work Practice, 15,* 97–109.

Tyson, K. B. (1992). A new approach to relevant scientific research for practicioners: The heuristic paradigm, *Social Work,* 541–556.

Uba, L. (1994). *Asian Americans: Personality, patterns, identity and mental health.* New York: Guilford Press.

Uehara, E. S. (1994). Race, gender, and housing inequality: An exploration of the correlates of low-quality housing among clients diagnosed with severe and persistent mental illness. *Journal of Health and Social Behavior, 35,* 309–321.

Uehara, K., Morelli, P., & Abe-Kim, J. (2001). Somatic complaint and social suffering among survivors of the Cambodian killing fields. *Journal of Human Behavior in the Social Environment, 3,* 243–262.

Umbricht, D., & Kane, J. M. (1995). Risperidone: Efficacy and safety. *Schizophrenia Bulletin, 21,* 593–606.

U.S. Department of Health and Human Services. (1996a). *Child maltreatment 1994: Reports from the states to the National Center on Child Abuse and Neglect.* Washington, DC: U.S. Government Printing Office.

U.S. Department of Health and Human Services. (1996b). *Third national incidence study of child abuse and neglect: Final report (NIS-3).* Washington, DC: U.S. Government Printing Office.

U.S. Department of Health and Human Services. (1997). *Ninth special report to Congress on alcohol and health.* Washington, DC: U.S. Government Printing Office.

U.S. Department of Health and Human Services. (1998). *National household survey on drug abuse: Population estimates, 1997.* Washington, DC: U.S. Government Printing Office.

U.S. Department of Health and Human Services. (1999a). *Epidemiologic trends in drug abuse: Vol. 1. Proceedings of the Community Epidemiology Work Group.* Washington, DC: U.S. Government Printing Office.

U.S. Department of Health and Human Services. (1999b). *Epidemiologic trends in drug abuse: Vol. 2. Proceedings of the International Epidemiology Work Group on Drug Abuse.* Washington, DC: U.S. Government Printing Office.

U.S. Department of Health and Human Services. (1999c). *National survey results on drug use from the Monitoring the Future Study (1975-1998).* Washington, DC: U.S. Government Printing Office.

U.S. Department of Health and Human Services. (2000). *10th special report to Congress on alcohol and health.* Washington, DC: U.S. Government Printing Office.

U.S. Department of Health and Human Services. (2003). *Assessing alcohol problems: A guide for clinicians and researchers* (2nd ed.). Bethesda, MD: National Institute for Alcohol Abuse and Alcoholism.

U.S. Department of Justice. (2000). *Extent, nature, and consequences of intimate partner violence: Findings from the National Violence against Women Survey.* Washington, DC: Author.

U.S. Department of Justice. (2001). *National Institute of Justice Research in brief: Documenting domestic violence: How health care providers can help victims.* Washington, DC: Author.

Utsey, S. O., & Ponterotto, J. G. (1996). Development and validation of the Index of Race Relations (IRRS). *Journal of Counseling Psychology, 43,* 490-501.

Vaillant, G. (1983). *The natural history of alcoholism.* Cambridge: Harvard University Press.

Vaillant, G., & Hiller-Sturmhofel, S. (1996). The natural history of alcoholism. *Alcohol Health and Research World, 20,* 152-161.

Valois, R. F., Oeltmann, J. E., Waller, J., & Hussey, J. R. (1999). Relationship between number of sexual intercourse partners and selected health risk behaviors among public high school adolescents. *Journal of Adolescent Health, 25,* 328-335.

Van Balkom, A. J., De Haan, E., Van Oppen, P., Spinhoven, P., Hoogduin, A. L., & Van Dyck, R. (1998). Cognitive and behavioral therapies alone versus in combination with fluvoxamine in the treatment of obsessive compulsive disorder. *Journal of Nervous and Mental Disease, 186,* 492-499.

Van den Bree, M. B. M., Svikis, D. S., & Pickens, R. W. (2000). Antisocial personality and drug use disorders: Are they genetically related? In D. H. Fishbein (Ed.), *The science, treatment, and prevention of antisocial behaviors: Application to the criminal justice system* (pp. 1-19). Kingston, NJ: Civic Research Institute.

Van der Kolk, B. A., Weisaeth, L., & Van der Hart, O. (1996). History of trauma in psychiatry. In B. A. Van der Kolk, A. C. McFarlane, & L. Weisaeth (Eds.), *Traumatic stress: The effects of overwhelming experience on mind, body and society* (pp. 47-73). New York: Guilford Press.

Van der Krol, R. J., Oosterbaan, H., Weller, S. D., & Koning, A. E. (1998). Attention deficit hyperactivity disorder. In P. Graham (Ed.), *Cognitive-behaviour therapy for children and families* (pp. 32-44). New York: Cambridge University Press.

Van Etten, M., & Taylor, S. (1998). Comparative efficacy of treatments for posttraumatic stress disorder: A meta-analysis. *Clinical Psychology and Psychotherapy, 5,* 126-144.

Van Hook, M. (1999). Women's help-seeking patterns for depression. *Social Work in Health Care, 29,* 15-34.

Vasquez, M. J. T. (1994). Latinas. In L. Comas-Diaz & B. Greene (Eds.), *Women of color: Integrating ethnic and gender identities in psychotherapy* (pp. 114-138). New York: Guilford Press.

Vaughn, M. G., & Howard, M. O. (2004). Adolescent substance abuse treatment: A synthesis of controlled evaluations. *Research on Social Work Practice, 14,* 325-335.

Vaughn, M. J., & Matyastik Baier, M. E. (1999). Reliability and validity of the Relationship Assessment Scale. *American Journal of Family Therapy, 27,* 137-147.

Veeder, N. W. (2002). Care management as management. *Care Management Journal, 3,* 68-76.

Veltman, M. V. M., & Browne, K. D. (2002). The assessment of drawings from children who have been maltreated: A systematic review. *Child Abuse Review, 11,* 19-37.

Verheul, R., van den Bosch, L., Koeter, M., Ridder, M., Stijnen, T., & van den Brink, W. (2003). Dialectical behavior therapy for women with borderline personality disorder. *British Journal of Psychiatry, 182,* 135-140.

Verhulst, F. C. (2001). Community and epidemiological aspects of anxiety disorders in children. In W. K. Silverman & P. D. A. Treffers (Eds.), *Anxiety disorders in children and adolescents: Research, assessment and intervention* (pp. 273-292). New York: Cambridge University Press.

Vitelli, R. (1997). Comparison of early and late start models of delinquency in adult offenders. *International Journal of Offender Therapy and Comparative Criminology, 4,* 351-357.

Vito, G. F., & Tewksbury, R. A. (1998). The impact of treatment: The Jefferson County (Kentucky) drug court program. *Federal Probation, 62,* 46-51.

Vitousek, K. B. (2002). Cognitive-behavioral therapy for anorexia nervosa. In C. G. Fairburn & K. D. Brownell (Eds.), *Eating disorders and obesity: A comprehensive handbook* (2nd ed., pp. 308-313). New York: Guilford Press.

Vohs, K. D., Heatherton, T. F., & Herrin, M. (2001). Disordered eating and the transition to college: A prospective study. *International Journal of Eating Disorders, 29,* 280-288.

Vreven, D. L., Gudanowski, D. M., King, L. A., & King, D. W. (1995). The civilian version of the Mississippi PTSD scale: A psychometric evaluation. *Journal of Traumatic Stress, 8,* 91-109.

Wachtel, P. L. (1977). *Psychoanalysis and behavior therapy: Toward an integration.* New York: Basic Books.

Wachtel, P. L. (1987). *Action and insight.* New York: Guilford Press.

Wakefield, J. C. (1996). Does social work need the eco-systems perspective? *Social Service Review, 70,* 1-32.

Wakefield, J. C. (1997). When is development disordered? Developmental psychopathology and the harmful dysfunction analysis of mental disorder. *Development and Psychopathology, 9,* 269-290.

Wakefield, J. C., & Kirk S. A. (1995). Unscientific thinking about scientific practice: Evaluating the scientist-practitioner model. *Social Work Research, 20,* 83-95.

Walborn, F. S. (1996). *Process variables.* Pacific Grove, CA: Brooks/Cole.

Waldron, H. B. (1997). Adolescent substance abuse and family therapy outcome: A review of randomized trials. In T. H. Ollendick & R. J. Prinz (Eds.), *Advances in clinical child psychology: Vol. 19* (pp. 199-234). New York: Plenum Press.

Waldron, H. B., Brody, J. L., & Slesnick, N. (2001). Integrative behavioral and family therapy for adolescent substance abuse. In P. M. Monti, S. M.Colby, & T.A. O'Leary (Eds.), *Adolescents, alcohol and substance abuse: Reaching teens through brief interventions* (pp. 216-243). New York: Guilford Press.

Wall, A., Hinson, R. E., & McKee, S.A. (1998).Alcohol outcome expectancies, attitudes towards drinking, and the theory of planned behavior. *Journal of Studies on Alcohol, 59*, 409-419.

Walsh, T. C. (1997).Alcoholic offenders: A gender comparison. *Alcoholism Treatment Quarterly, 15*, 29-41.

Walters, S. T., Bennett, M. E., & Noto, J. V. (2000). Drinking on campus: What do we know about reducing alcohol use among college students? *Journal of Substance Abuse Treatment, 19*, 223-228.

Walton, E. (1997). Enhancing investigative decisions in child welfare: An exploratory use of intensive family preservation services. *Child Welfare, 76*, 447-461.

Walton, E. (2001). Combining abuse and neglect investigations with intensive family preservation services: An innovative approach to protecting children. *Research on Social Work Practice, 11*, 627-644.

Ware, J. E., Kosinski, M., & Keller, S. D. (1996). A 12-item short form health survey: Construction of scales and preliminary tests of reliability and validity. *Medical Care, 34*, 220-233.

Watson, J. C., Gordon, L. B., Stermac, L., Kalogerokos, R., & Steckley, P. (2003). Comparing the effectiveness of process-experiential with cognitive-behavioral psychotherapy in the treatment of depression. *Journal of Consulting and Clinical Psychology, 71*, 773-781.

Watson-Perczel, M., Lutzker, J. R., Greene, B. F., & McGimpsey, B. J. (1988). Assessment and modification of home cleanliness among families adjudicated for child neglect. *Behavior Modification, 12*, 57-81.

Weaver, T. L., & Clum, G. A. (1993). Early family environments and traumatic experiences associated with borderline personality disorder. *Journal of Consulting and Clinical Psychology, 61*, 1068-1075.

Webster-Stratton, C. (1997, March–April). From parent training to community building. *Families in Society: The Journal of Contemporary Human Services*, 156-171.

Webster-Stratton, C., & Hancock, L. (1998). Training for parents of young children with conduct problems: Content, methods and therapeutic processes. In J. M. Briesmeister & C. E. Schaefer (Eds.), *Handbook of parent training: Parents as co-therapists for children's behavior problems* (2nd ed., pp. 98-152). New York: Wiley.

Webster-Stratton, C., & Herbert, M. (1994). *Troubled families—problem children: Working with parents: A collaborative process.* New York: Wiley.

Webster-Stratton, C., Hollinsworth, T., & Kolpacoff, M. (1989). The long-term effectiveness and clinical significance of three cost-effective training programs for families with conduct-problem children. *Journal of Consulting and Clinical Psychology, 57*, 550-553.

Webster-Stratton, C., Kolpacoff, M., & Hollinsworth, T. (1988). Self-administered videotape therapy for families with conduct-problem children: Comparison with two cost-effective treatments and a control group. *Journal of Consulting and Clinical Psychology, 56*, 558-566.

Wechsler, H., Davenport, A., Dowdall, G., Moeykens, B., & Costillow, S. (1994). Health and behavioral consequences of binge drinking in college. *Journal of the American Medical Association, 272*, 1672-1677.

Wechsler, H., Dowdal, G., Davenport, A., & Rimm, E. (1995). A gender-specific measure of binge drinking among college students. *American Journal of Public Health, 85*, 982-985.

Wechsler, H., Lee, J. E., Kuo, M., Seibring, M., Nelson, T. F., & Lee, H. (2002). Trends in college binge drinking during a period of increased prevention efforts: Findings from four Harvard School of Public Health College Alcohol Study Surveys, 1993-2001. *Journal of American College Health, 50*, 203-217.

Wechsler, H., & McFadden, M. (1979). Drinking among college students in New England: Extent, social correlates, and consequences of alcohol use. *Journal of Studies on Alcohol, 40*, 969-996.

Weinberg, N., Rohdert, E., Colliver, J., & Glantz, M. (1998). Adolescent substance abuse: A review of the last 10 years. *Journal of the American Academy of Child and Adolescent Psychiatry, 37*, 252-261.

Weiner, E., & Wiener, J. (1997). University students with psychiatric illness: Factors involved in the decision to withdraw from their studies. *Psychiatric Rehabilitation Journal, 20*, 88-91.

Weinstein, D., Staffelbach, D., & Biaggio, M. (2000). Attention-deficit hyperactivity disorder and posttraumatic stress disorder: Differential diagnosis in childhood sexual abuse. *Clinical Psychology Review, 20*, 359-378.

Weisner, C., Matzger, H., & Kaskutas, L. (2003). How important is treatment? One-year outcomes of treated and untreated alcohol-dependent individuals. *Addiction, 98*, 901-911.

Weisner, C., & Schmidt, L. (1993). Alcohol and drug problems among diverse health and social service populations, *American Journal of Public Health, 83*, 824-829.

Weiss, B., Catron, T., Harris, V., & Phung, T. (1999). The effectiveness of traditional child psychotherapy. *Journal of Consulting and Clinical Psychology, 67*, 82-94.

Weiss, J. (1995). Empirical studies of the psychoanalytic process. In T. Shapiro & R. N. Emde (Eds.), *Research in psychoanalysis: Process, development, outcome* (pp. 7-30). Madison, CT: International Universities Press.

Weiss, R. L., & Heyman, R. E. (1997). A clinical-research overview of couples interactions. In W. K. Halford & H. J. Markham (Eds.), *Clinical handbook of marriage and couples intervention* (pp. 13-42). New York: Wiley.

Weissman, M. M., Markowitz, J. C., & Klerman, G. L. (2000). *Comprehensive guide to interpersonal psychotherapy.* New York: Basic Books.

Weisz, A. N., & Black, B. M. (2001). Evaluating a sexual assault and dating violence prevention program for urban youths. *Social Work Research, 25*, 89-102.

Weisz, J. R., Donenberg, G. R., Han, S. S., & Weiss, B. (1995). Bridging the gap between lab and clinic in child and adolescent psychotherapy. *Journal of Consulting and Clinical Psychology, 63*, 688-701.

Weisz, J. R., & Hawley, K. M. (1998). Finding, evaluating, refining, and applying empirically supported treatments for children and adolescent. *Journal of Child Clinical Psychology, 27*, 206-216.

Weisz, J. R., Weiss, B., Alicke, M. D., & Klotz, M. L. (1987). Effectiveness of psychotherapy with children and adolescents: A meta-analysis for clinicians. *Journal of Consulting and Clinical Psychology, 55*, 542-549.

Wekerle, C., & Wolfe, D. A. (1993). Prevention of child physical abuse and neglect: Promising new directions. *Clinical Psychology Review, 13*, 501-540.

Welch, G., Thompson, L., & Hall, A. (1993). The BULIT-R: Its reliability and clinical validity as a screening tool of *DSM-III-R* bulimia nervosa in a female tertiary education population. *International Journal of Eating Disorders, 14*, 95-105.

Wells, K., & Biegel, D. E. (1992). Intensive family preservation services research: Current status and future agenda. *Social Work Research and Abstracts, 28*, 21-27.

Wells, K. B., Astrachan, B. M., Tischler, G. L., & Unutzer, J. (1995). Issues and approaches in evaluating managed mental health care. *The Milbank Quarterly, 73*, 57-75.

Wells, K. C., Pelham, W. E., Kotkin, R. A., Hoza, B., Abikoff, H. B., Abramowitz, A., et al. (2000). Psychosocial treatment strategies in the MTA study: Rationale, methods, and critical issues in design and implementation. *Journal of Abnormal Child Psychology, 28*, 483-505.

Werch, C. E., Pappas, D. M., & Castellon-Vogel, E. A. (1996). Drug use prevention efforts at colleges and universities in the United States. *Substance Use and Misuse, 31*, 65-80.

Westenberg, P. M., Siebelink, B. M., & Treffers, P. D. A. (2001). Psychosocial developmental theory in relation to anxiety and its disorders. In W. K. Silverman & P. D. A. Treffers (Eds.), *Anxiety disorders in children and adolescents: Research, assessment and intervention* (pp. 72-89). New York: Cambridge University Press.

Wexler, D. B. (1991). Inducing therapeutic compliance through the criminal law. In D. B. Wexler & B. J. Winick (Eds.), *Essays in therapeutic jurisprudence* (pp. 187-218). Durham, NC: Carolina Academic Press.

Wexler, H. K. (1995). The success of therapeutic communities for substance abusers in American prisons. *Journal of Psychoactive Drugs, 27*, 57-66.

Whaley, A. L. (1998). Cross-cultural perspective on paranoia: A focus on the black American experience. *Psychiatric Quarterly, 69*, 325-343.

Wheaton, B. (1994). Sampling the stress universe. In W. R. Avison & I. H. Gotlib (Eds.), *Stress and mental health: Contemporary issues and prospects for the future* (pp. 77-114). New York: Plenum Press.

White, H. R., & Lebouvie, E. W. (1989). Towards the assessment of adolescent problem drinking. *Journal of Studies on Alcohol, 50*, 30-37.

White, J. D. (1999). Personality, temperament and ADHD: A review of the literature. *Personality and Individual Differences, 27*, 589-598.

Whiteman, M., Fanshel, D., & Grundy, J. F. (1987). Cognitive-behavioral interventions aimed at anger of parents at risk of child abuse. *Social Work, 32*, 469-474.

Widiger, T. A., & Corbitt, E. M. (1995). Antisocial personality disorder. In J. Livesley (Ed.), *The DSM-IV personality disorders* (pp. 103-126). New York: Guilford Press.

Widom, C. S. (1989). Does violence beget violence? A critical examination of the literature. *Psychological Bulletin, 106*, 3-28.

Widom, C. S. (1998). Childhood victimization: Early adversity and subsequent psychopathology. In B. P. Dohrenwend (Ed.), *Adversity and psychopathology* (pp. 81-95). New York: Oxford University Press.

Widom, C. S. (1999). Posttraumatic stress disorder in abused and neglected children grown up. *American Journal of Psychiatry, 156*, 1223-1229.

Widom, C. S., & Toch, H. (2000). The contribution of psychology to criminal justice education. In D. H. Fishbein (Ed.), *The science, treatment, and prevention of anti-*

social behaviors: Application to the criminal justice system (pp. 3-19). Kingston, NJ: Civic Research Institute.

Wilk, D. (1994). Women and alcoholism: How a male-as-norm bias affects research, assessment and treatment. *Health and Social Work, 19,* 29-35.

Williams, J. H., Stiffman, A. R., & O'Neal, J. L. (1998). Violence among urban African American youths: An analysis of environmental and behavioral risk factors. *Social Work Research, 22,* 3-13.

Williams, K. E., Chambless, D. L., & Steketee, G. (1998). Behavioral treatment of obsessive-compulsive disorder in African Americans: Clinical issues. *Journal of Behavior Therapy and Experimental Psychiatry, 29,* 163-170.

Wills, T., Sandy, J., & Yaeger, A. (2000). Temperament and adolescent substance use: An epigenetic approach to risk and protection. *Journal of Personality, 68,* 1127-1151.

Wilsnack, S. C., Wilsnack, R. W., & Hiller-Sturmhofel, S. (1994). How women drink: Epidemiology of women's drinking and problem drinking. *Alcohol Health and Research World, 18,* 173-184.

Wilson, G. T. (1993a). Assessment of binge eating. In C. G. Fairburn & G. T. Wilson (Eds.), *Binge eating: Nature, assessment and treatment* (pp. 227-249). New York: Guilford Press.

Wilson, G. T. (1993b). Binge eating and addictive disorders. In C. G. Fairburn & G. T. Wilson (Eds.), *Binge eating: Nature, assessment and treatment* (pp. 97-122). New York: Guilford Press.

Wilson, G. T. (1995). Behavior therapy. In R. J. Corsini & D. Wedding (Eds.), *Current psychotherapies* (5th ed., pp. 197-228). Itasca, IL: Peacock.

Wilson, G. T. (1996). Empirically-validated treatments: Realities and resistance. *Clinical Psychology: Science and Practice, 3,* 241-244.

Wilson, G. T., & Fairburn, C. G. (1993). Cognitive treatments for eating disorders. *Journal of Consulting and Clinical Psychology, 61,* 261-269.

Wilson, G. T., & Fairburn, C. G. (1998). Treatments of eating disorders. In P. E. Nathan & J. M. Gorman (Eds.), *A guide to treatments that work* (pp. 501-530). New York: Oxford University Press.

Wilson, G. T., & Vitousek, K. M. (1999). Self-monitoring in the assessment of eating disorders. *Psychological Assessment, 11,* 480-489.

Wilson, S. J., Lipsey, M. W., & Soydan, H. (2003). Are mainstream programs for juvenile delinquency less effective with minority youth than majority youth? A meta-analysis of outcomes research. *Research on Social Work Practice, 13,* 3-26.

Windle, M. (1996). Effect of parental drinking on adolescents. *Alcohol Health and Research World, 20,* 181-184.

Winefield, H. R., & Harvey, E. J. (1994). Needs of family caregivers in chronic schizophrenia. *Schizophrenia Bulletin, 20,* 557-566.

Winzelberg, A. J., Eldredge, K. L., Eppstein, D., Wilfley, D., Dasmahapatra, R., Dev, P., et al. (2000). Effectiveness of an Internet-based program for reducing risk factors for eating disorders. *Journal of Consulting and Clinical Psychology, 68,* 346-350.

Winzelberg, A. J., Taylor, C. B., Sharpe, T., Eldredge, K. L., Dev, P., & Constantinou, P. S. (1998). Evaluation of a computer-mediated eating disorder intervention program. *International Journal of Eating Disorders, 24,* 339-349.

Woerner, M. G., Mannuzza, S., & Kane, J. M. (1988). Anchoring the BPRS: An aid to improved reliability. *Psychopharmacology Bullentin, 24,* 112-117.

Wolfe, D.A., Edwards, B., Manion, I., & Koverola, C. (1988). Early intervention for parents at risk of child abuse and neglect: A preliminary investigation. *Journal of Consulting and Clinical Psychology, 56,* 40-47.

Wolfe, D.A., & McEachran, A. (1997). Child physical abuse and neglect. In E. J. Mash & L. G. Terdal (Eds.), *Assessment of childhood disorders* (3rd ed., pp. 523-568). New York: Guilford Press.

Wolfe, D.A., & Sandler, J. (1981). Training abusive parents in effective child management. *Behavior Modification, 5,* 320-335.

Wolfe, D.A., & St. Pierre, J. (1989). Child abuse and neglect. In T. H. Ollendick & M. Hersen (Eds.), *Handbook of childhood psychopathology* (2nd ed., pp. 377-398). New York: Plenum Press.

Wolfe, D.A., & Wekerle, C. (1993). Treatment strategies for child physical abuse and neglect: A critical progress report. *Clinical Psychology Review, 13,* 473-500.

Wolfe, J., & Kimerling, R. (1997). Gender issues in the assessment of posttraumatic stress disorder. In J. P. Wilson & T. M. Keane (Eds.), *Assessing psychological trauma and PTSD* (pp. 192-238). New York: Guilford Press.

Wolfe, R., Morrow, J., & Fredrickson, B. L. (1996). Mood disorders in older adults. In L. L. Carstensen, B. A. Edelstein, & L. Dornbrand (Eds.), *The practical handbook of clinical gerontology* (pp. 274-303). Thousand Oaks, CA: Sage.

Wolfe, V. V., & Birt, J. (1997). Child sexual abuse. In E. J. Mash & L. G. Terdal (Eds.), *Assessment of childhood disorders* (3rd ed., pp. 569-623). New York: Guilford Press.

Wolfe, V. V., & Gentile, C. (1991). *Children's Impact of Traumatic Events Scale-Revised (CITES-R)*. London, ON: Department of Psychology, London Health Sciences Centre.

Wolfe, V.V., Gentile, C., & Bourdeau, P. (1987). *History of victimization form.* Unpublished assessment instrument. London Health Sciences Centre, London, ON.

Wolfe, V.V., Gentile, C., & Wolfe, D.A. (1989). The impact of sexual abuse in children: A PTSD formulation. *Behavior Therapy, 20,* 215-228.

Wolfe, V.V., & Wolfe, D.A. (1988). The sexually abused child. In E. J. Mash & L. G. Terdal (Eds.), *Behavioral assessment of childhood disorders* (2nd ed., pp. 670-714). New York: Guilford Press.

Wolford, G. L., Rosenberg, S. D., Drake, R. E., Mueser, K. T., Oxman, T. E., Hoffman, D., et al. (1999). Evaluation of methods for detecting substance use disorder in persons with severe mental illness. *Psychology of Addictive Behaviors, 13,* 313-326.

Wolpe, J. (1958). *Psychotherapy by reciprocal inhibition.* Stanford, CA: Stanford University Press.

Wolpe, J. (1973). *The practice of behavior therapy.* Elmsford, NY: Pergamon Press.

Wong, S. (1999). Treatment of antosocial behavior in adolescent inpatients: Behavioral changes and client satisfaction. *Research on Social Work Practice, 9,* 25-44.

Wood, A., Harrington, R., & Moore, A. (1996). Controlled trial of a brief cognitive-behavioural intervention in adolescent patients with depressive disorders. *Journal of Child Psychology and Psychiatry and Allied Disciplines, 37,* 737-746.

Wood, K. (1978). Casework effectiveness: A new look at the research evidence. *Social Work, 23,* 437-457.

Woods, M. E., & Hollis, F. (1990). Classifications of casework treatment. In *Casework: A psychosocial therapy* (pp. 85-101). New York: McGraw-Hill.

Wright, K. N. (1993). Alcohol use by prisoners. *Alcohol Health and Research World, 17*, 157-161.

Xiaoming, L., Stanton, B., & Feigelman, S. (2000a). Impact of perceived parental monitoring on adolescent risk behavior over 4 years. *Journal of Adolescent Health, 27*, 49-56.

Xiaoming, L., Stanton, B., & Feigelman, S. (2000b). Perceived parental monitoring and health risk behaviors among urban low-income African-American children and adolescents. *Journal of Adolescent Health, 27*, 43-48.

Yates, B. T. (1996). *Analyzing costs, procedures, processes, and outcomes in human services* (Applied Social Science Research Methods Series, 42). Thousand Oaks, CA: Sage.

Yesavage, J. A., Brink, T .L., Rose, T. L., Lum, O., Huang, V., Adey, M., et al. (1983). Development and validation of a geriatric depression screening scale: A preliminary report. *Journal of Psychiatric Research, 17*, 37-49.

Yu, J., & Shacket, R. W. (2001). Alcohol use in high school: Predicting students' use and alcohol problems in four-year colleges. *American Journal on Drug and Alcohol Abuse, 27*, 775-793.

Yule, W., Perrin, S., & Smith, P. (2001). Traumatic events and post-traumatic stress disorder. In W. K. Silverman & P. D. A. Treffers (Eds.), *Anxiety disorders in children and adolescents: Research, assessment and intervention* (pp. 212-234). New York: Cambridge University Press.

Zabinski, M. F., Pung, M. A., Wilfley, D. E., Eppstein, D. L., Winzelberg, A. J., Celio, A., et al. (2001). Reducing risk factors for eating disorders: Targeting at-risk women with a computerized psychoeducational program. *International Journal of Eating Disorders, 29*, 401-408.

Zanarini, M. C., Frankenburg, F. R., Reich, B., Marino, M. F., Haynes, M. C., & Gunderson, J. G. (1999). Violence in the lives of adult borderline patients. *Journal of Nervous and Mental Disease, 187*, 65-71.

Zigler, E. F. (1989). Addressing the nation's child care crisis: The school of the twenty-first century. *American Journal of Orthopsychiatry, 59*, 484-491.

Zinbarg, R. E., Barlow, D. H., Brown, T. A., & Hertz, R. M. (1992). Cognitive-behavioral approaches to the nature and treatment of anxiety disorders. *Annual Review of Psychology, 43*, 235-267.

Zlotnick, C., Robertson, M. J., & Wright, M. (1999). The impact of childhood foster care and other out-of-home placement on homeless women and their children. *Child Abuse and Neglect, 23*, 1057-1068.

Zucker, R. A., & Fitzgerald, H. E. (1991). Early developmental factors and risk for alcohol problems. *Alcohol Health and Research World, 15*, 18-24.

Zucker, R. A., & Gomberg, E. S. L. (1986). Etiology of alcoholism reconsidered: The case for a biopsychosocial process. *American Psychologist, 41*, 783-793.

INDEX

David:
Is 3535
correct?